# VISION AND THE BRAIN

## Understanding Cerebral Visual Impairment in Children

**Amanda Hall Lueck and Gordon N. Dutton, Editors**

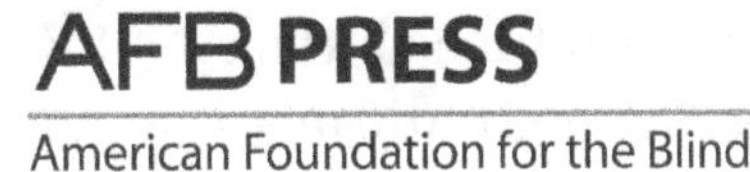
American Foundation for the Blind

Printed in the United States of America

Library of Congress Cataloging-in-Publication Data

Vision and the brain : understanding cerebral visual impairment in children / Amanda Hall Lueck and Gordon N. Dutton, editors.
pages cm
Includes bibliographical references and index.
ISBN 978-0-89128-639-4 (pbk. : alk. paper) — ISBN 978-0-89128-640-0 (online subscription) — ISBN 978-0-89128-642-4 (epub) — ISBN 978-0-89128-643-1 (mobi) 1. Vision disorders in children. 2. Pediatric neuroophthalmology. I. Lueck, Amanda Hall, 1949– II. Dutton, Gordon.
RE48.2.C5V495 2015
618.92'0977—dc23

2015001623

Every effort has been made to provide accurate and current information regarding websites that are mentioned in this book. However, because website addresses and the information posted on them are constantly changing, the accuracy of this information cannot be guaranteed.

The American Foundation for the Blind removes barriers, creates solutions, and expands possibilities so people with vision loss can achieve their full potential.

It is the policy of the American Foundation for the Blind to use in the first printing of its books acid-free paper that meets the ANSI Z39.48 Standard. The infinity symbol that appears above indicates that the paper in this printing meets that standard.

# CONTENTS

## PART III Assessment of Children with CVI



## PART IV Intervention for Children with CVI

# PREFACE

Cerebral visual impairment (CVI) has become the most common cause of visual impairment in children in our respective practices, but we were not always aware of this phenomenon. It started for Gordon in the early 1990s with a trickle of teenagers, accompanied by distraught parents, whose visual difficulties due to perceptual and cognitive visual impairment had been dismissed up to that point because the results of standard measures of vision had been in the normal range. Meanwhile, in the education community for children with visual impairments, Amanda began to see more and more children who had milder than usual visual disorders that couldn't be explained by visual acuity and visual field loss alone and that often did not fit the standard definition of visual impairment for entitlement to service in educational settings.

As we sought out more such cases, it became apparent that large proportions of children with cerebral palsy, hydrocephalus, and other conditions affecting the brain had visual disabilities that had been masked by and ascribed to their overall disorders. As more information came to light, and as more of these children were referred for services, it became clear that there was much to be understood, reevaluated, and disseminated in order to serve these children with CVI appropriately. Now, however, altered visual function is recognized as a discrete contributory element to the behavioral picture shown by affected children, but for both of us, many questions remain unanswered.

We have both been privileged to meet families, caregivers, and teachers of children with CVI from all over the world who have struggled to find accessible information about the subject, and to identify services that match the needs of the children under their care. These experiences highlighted for us the need for a basic textbook to explain CVI in a way that families and educational and medical professionals could understand and use to enhance these children's prospects. This is the aim of this book. We realize that this text is far from perfect and cannot encompass all the latest information, as the field is changing rapidly with new findings emerging all the time. Our hope is that this book will spur others to apply, refine, and redefine the current knowledge base, available best practices, and service delivery systems to best meet the needs of children who have CVI and their families.

# ACKNOWLEDGMENTS

We are indebted to all the gifted authors from the various disciplines who have contributed to this book. Input from their wide-ranging perspectives has created a richness and depth to the material presented. We would also like to thank all the children, families, and professionals who have been our teachers as we have sought to understand, learn about, and develop methods of addressing the multifaceted subject of cerebral visual impairment (CVI).

In addition, we thank Natalie Hilzen from AFB Press for her great persistence in the quest for a book about CVI and for her help in shaping its content, and we also thank George Abbott for his continued support of the project. Ellen Bilofsky and Alina Vayntrub, whose skill and care helped us to develop the book further, and guided the book from copyedits to production.

Finally we would like to thank our families for their continued support and patience throughout the conception, design, and writing of this book.

*—A.H.L. and G.N.D.*

# ABOUT THE CONTRIBUTORS

## EDITORS

**Amanda Hall Lueck, Ph.D.,** is a Professor in the Department of Special Education and Communicative Disorders and Coordinator of the Program in Visual Impairments at San Francisco State University, California, with more than 40 years of experience in the field of visual impairment, particularly the effects of early brain injury on vision in children and its educational consequences. She is the co-author of *Developmental Guidelines for Infants with Visual Impairments: A Guidebook for Early Intervention*, editor of *Functional Vision: A Practitioner's Guide to Evaluation and Intervention,* co-editor of *Proceedings of the Summit on Cerebral/Cortical Visual Impairment: Educational, Family, and Medical Perspectives,* and co-author of *Visual Impairment: An Overview.* In addition, she has authored or co-authored numerous chapters, journal articles, and conference presentations on cognitive development, education and rehabilitation of people with low vision, and promotion of vision skills and behaviors in children with visual impairments. Dr. Lueck has served as a consultant to various national and international organizations and was a Fulbright Professor in Nepal.

**Gordon N. Dutton, M.D., FRCOphth, FRCS,** is a Pediatric Ophthalmologist who has worked for over 20 years at the Royal Hospital for Sick Children in Glasgow, Scotland. He is currently Emeritus Professor of Visual Science at Glasgow Caledonian University, and an Honorary Senior Research Fellow at the University of Glasgow. He is the co-author of *Cerebral Visual Impairment in Children: Visuoperceptive and Visuocognitive Disorders,* co-editor of *Visual Impairment in Children Due to Damage to the Brain,* and chapter contributor to *Cerebral Palsy: Science and Clinical Practice.* In addition, he has authored or co-authored over 200 journal articles and taught an online course for the Association for Education and Rehabilitation of the Blind and Visually Impaired. Dr. Dutton is widely known for his expertise on visual dysfunction due to brain damage in children, has been invited to speak at conferences all over the world, and has served as a committee member and consultant for organizations throughout the United Kingdom and North America, including as a Visiting Professor at Boston Children's Hospital.

## CHAPTER AUTHORS

**Lizbeth A. Barclay, M.A.,** is recently retired from her position as Coordinator of the Assessment Program at the California School for the Blind in Fremont. A teacher of students with visual impairments and an orientation and mobility specialist for 25 years, Ms. Barclay is the editor of *Learning to Listen/Listening to Learn: Teaching Listening Skills to Students with Visual Impairments* and has authored or co-authored many chapters, journal articles, and conference presentations on the education of students with visual impairments.

**James Carreon, M.A.,** is a former Assistive Technology Specialist at the California School for the Blind in Fremont. He was a contributor to *Itinerant Teaching: Tricks of the Trade for Teachers of Students with Visual Impairments* and has authored a number of technology guides for the California School for the Blind.

**Zaira Cattaneo, Ph.D.,** is Research Scientist in Neuropsychology in the Department of Psychology of the University of Milano-Bicocca in Milan, Italy. She is co-author of *Blind Vision: The Neuroscience of Visual Impairment* and has authored or co-authored numerous journal articles and conference presentations on the study of cognitive brain functioning in individuals with visual impairments. Dr. Cattaneo is the 2015 recipient of the European Society of Cognitive Psychology Paul Bertelson Award for making a significant contribution to European Cognitive Psychology.

**Sylvie Chokron, Ph.D.,** is Senior Researcher, head of the Vision and Cognition Unit, and head of the Perception, Action, and Cognitive Development Team of the Fondation Ophtalmologique Adolphe de Rothschild–CNRS in Paris, France. She has contributed chapters to several books and has authored or co-authored many journal articles and conference presentations on the assessment and management of neuropsychological and visual behaviors in babies, children, and adults.

**Debbie Cockburn, MSc, DipCOT,** is an occupational therapist at the Glasgow Caledonian University Royal Hospital for Sick Children in Glasgow, Scotland. She is a chapter contributor to *Visual Impairment in Children Due to Damage to the Brain.*

**Elisa Fazzi, M.D., Ph.D.,** is Chief of the Unit of Child Neuropsychiatry and Early Neurorehabilitation at the Civil Hospital in Brescia, Italy, and Professor and Director of the Specialization School in Child Neuropsychiatry, Department of Clinical and Experimental Sciences at the University of Brescia in Italy. She is the author or co-author of over 130 papers on child development, neuropsychiatry, and neurodevelopmental problems in the first years of life. Dr. Fazzi is member of the board of the Société Europeénne de Neurologie Pédiatrique.

**Marion Felder, M.Ed., Ph.D.,** is Professor of Inclusion and Rehabilitation in the Department of Social Sciences at the Koblenz University of Applied Sciences in Germany.

**Elizabeth Hartmann, Ph.D.,** a certified teacher of students with visual impairments and students with severe or intensive special needs, is Assistant Professor in the Department of Education at Lasell College in Newton, Massachusetts. She is co-author of *Developmental Guidelines for Infants with Visual Impairments: A Guidebook for Early Intervention.* Her practice and research interests include universal design for learning, teachers' collaborative practice, and the development of symbolic understanding in learners with deafblindness and multiple disabilities.

**Anne Henriksen, M.A.,** is a teacher of visually impaired students and a low vision therapist at the State Center for Visually Impaired, Schleswig, Germany, and a university lecturer with specialization in low vision at the University of Hamburg in Germany.

**Lea Hyvärinen, M.D., Ph.D., FAAP,** is Honorary Professor in Rehabilitation Sciences at the Technical University of Dortmund in Germany, and was Senior Lecturer in Developmental Neuropsychology at the University of Helsinki, Finland. She is co-author of *WHAT and HOW Does This Child See?* and has authored or co-authored over

200 articles and conference presentations on early intervention, pediatric services, and vision screening programs. Dr. Hyvärinen has developed more than 40 tests for clinical assessment and screening of vision. She served as an adviser for the World Health Organization on early intervention, management of low vision, and standards for characterization of vision loss and visual functioning.

**Namita Jacob, Ph.D.,** is Education Specialist, Asia/Pacific Region, Perkins International, and Program Director, Chetana Charitable Trust, Chennai, India. She is the co-author of *WHAT and HOW Does This Child See?* and *Helping Children Who Are Blind: Family and Community Support for Children with Vision Problems.* She has written and edited numerous resources for families and professionals working in the areas of deafblindness, complex sensory impairment, special education, and early intervention. Dr. Jacob works as a consultant with national and international organizations in the areas of sensory impairment, multiple disabilities, and early childhood development.

**John Kingston, M.A.,** a certified orientation and mobility specialist, is Orientation and Mobility Supervisor at the Western Blind Rehabilitation Center of the U.S. Department of Veterans Affairs Palo Alto Health Care System in Palo Alto, California. He has published articles and presented on neurological vision loss and rehabilitation.

**Barry S. Kran, O.D., FAAO,** is Faculty Chair and Professor of Optometry at the New England College of Optometry in Boston, Massachusetts, and Optometric Director of the New England Eye Low Vision Clinic at Perkins in Watertown, Massachusetts. He is the former chair of the Low Vision Division of the Association for Education and Rehabilitation of the Blind and Visually Impaired (AER). His research and service interests include identifying barriers to eye care for individuals with visual and other disabilities and pursuing improved ways of treating individuals with cerebral visual impairment. Dr. Kran has contributed chapters, journal articles, and presentations on vision care and individuals with multiple disabilities. He was the recipient of the 2007 Thomas Caulfield Award of the Northeast AER for excellence in assisting persons with visual impairments.

**Angela Martyn, M.S.,** is a teacher of students with visual impairments and an orientation and mobility specialist, and is Coordinator of the Assessment Program at the California School for the Blind in Fremont.

**D. Luisa Mayer, M.Ed., Ph.D.,** is Associate Professor of Vision Science and Individuals with Disabilities at the New England College of Optometry in Boston and is a member of the clinical staff of the New England Eye Low Vision Clinic at the Perkins School for the Blind in Watertown, Massachusetts. She is also Clinical Assistant Professor of Ophthalmology at the Harvard Medical School and is Affiliate Clinical Associate in Ophthalmology at Children's Hospital in Boston, Massachusetts. She has published many articles on vision testing with pediatric patients.

**Amanda McKerracher, Ph.D.,** is a school psychologist and adjunct professor in British Columbia, Canada. She has published and presented widely on reading and mathematics achievement among students with visual impairments.

**Lotfi B. Merabet, MPH, O.D., Ph.D.,** is Associate Professor of Ophthalmology in the Department of Ophthalmology and Director of the Laboratory for Visual Neuroplasticity of the Massachusetts Eye and Ear Infirmary at the Harvard Medical School in Boston. His work focuses on understanding neuroplasticity as it relates to vision loss of ocular and cerebral causes.

**Anna Molinaro, M.D., Ph.D.,** is a clinician in the Departmental Unit of Child Neuropsychiatry and Early Rehabilitation, Civil Hospital, University of Brescia, Brescia, and the Department of Reproductive and Developmental Science, University of Trieste, Trieste, Italy. She has collaborated on Phase IV clinical trials and has co-authored numerous articles and presented internationally on genetic and clinical findings in cases of epilepsy, as well as psychosocial symptoms in young patients.

**John L. Morse, Ed.D.,** is a clinical psychologist and certified school psychologist in private practice in New Hampshire. He is a former president of the New Hampshire Society of Psychologists; former board member of the New Hampshire Psychological Association and recipient of its Lifetime Achievement Award; and president of the New Hampshire Association of School Psychologists and recipient of its Lifetime Achievement Award. He is also the recipient of the Thomas Carroll Award of the Northeast Chapter and the Lifetime Achievement Award from the Association for Education and Rehabilitation of the Blind and Visually Impaired and the School Psychologist of the Year Award from the National Association of School Psychologists. Dr. Morse has authored many journal articles on the psychological aspects of assessing and treating individuals who are blind or have low vision.

**Mary T. Morse, M.Ed., Ph.D.,** is a special education consultant and certified teacher of students with visual impairments, as well as of students with emotional and behavioral, learning, and intellectual/developmental disabilities in private practice in the United States and other countries. She is the recipient of the 2000 Outstanding Practice Award from the Association for Education and Rehabilitation of the Blind and Visually Impaired (AER), Division for Individuals with Deafblindness/Multiple Disabilities; the 2010 Lifetime Achievement Award from the New Hampshire Excellence in Education Awards; the 2002 Special Friend of Children Award from the National Association of School Psychologists; and the 2014 Robert Lambert Lifetime Achievement Award from AER. She is a chapter contributor and author of many journal articles on cortical visual impairment, multiple disabilities, and associated neurological issues.

**Carlene Creamer O'Brien** is an orientation and mobility specialist and a former team member of the Assessment Program at the California School for the Blind in Fremont. She has presented several workshops for parents and professionals on orientation and mobility and skills of daily living. She has raised four successful adult children, two with low vision.

**Terese Pawletko, Ph.D.,** is a certified school psychologist in private practice in New England, performing specialty evaluations, and consulting on children with autism spectrum disorders and individuals with visual impairments nationally and internationally. Dr. Pawletko is the author or co-author of several book chapters and journal articles and numerous conference presentations and workshops on autism in children who are blind or visually impaired.

**Kathryn J. Saunders, Ph.D., FCOptom,** is Professor and Head of Optometry and Vision Science at the School of Biomedical Sciences, University of Ulster, Coleraine, Northern Ireland. She is a fellow and elected councilmember of the UK College of Optometrists. Dr. Saunders has published over 50 peer-reviewed scientific papers and authored several book chapters. Her research interests center around vision and visual development in both typically developing children and those with developmental disabilities.

**Marieke Steendam, B.S.**, is an occupational therapist at Koninklijke Visio (Royal Dutch Visio) in the Netherlands. She is the author of *Cortical Visual Impairment in Children: A Handbook for Parents and Professionals* and *Weet Jij Wat Ik Zie?* [*Do You Know What I See?*]. She has presented papers at various conferences on the topics of cerebral visual impairment and occupational therapy.

**Adam Wilton, M.A.**, is a Ph.D. candidate in Special Education at the University of British Columbia, Vancouver, Canada. He is a teacher of students with visual impairments and a certified orientation and mobility specialist and has authored articles and presentations on the use of print and tactile graphics and early intervention, among other topics.

**Darick Wright, M.A.**, is Coordinator of the New England Eye Low Vision Clinic at the Perkins School for the Blind in Watertown, Massachusetts; Adjunct Assistant Professor of Vision Rehabilitation at the New England College of Optometry; and an adjunct faculty member the University of Massachusetts, Boston. Prior to that, was a full-time faculty member at the University of Arkansas at Little Rock. He has served in a variety of regional and international leadership positions and has taught and lectured nationally and internationally on topics related to visual impairment.

**Sander Zuidhoek, Ph.D.**, is a children's neuropsychologist and Chairman of the Expertise Group on Cerebral Visual Impairment in Children at Koninklijke Visio (Royal Dutch Visio), the Netherlands. He is a coauthor of many journal articles on visual and spatial imagery and haptic perception.

## OTHER CONTRIBUTORS

**Ian L. Bailey, O.D., FBCO, FAAO,** is Professor of Optometry and Vision Science at the University of California, Berkeley. He is widely known for his research on functional visual abilities and clinical measures of visual function. Dr. Bailey co-authored *Visual Impairment: An Overview,* as well as many journal articles on topics related to optometry and ophthalmology. Among his many international awards, he received the 2014 Meritorious Award for Lifetime Contributions to the Field of Low Vision from the Low Vision Rehabilitation Division of the Association for Education and Rehabilitation of the Blind and Visually Impaired.

**Hubertine Burgers** is an occupational therapist and specialist in assistive technology at Koninklijke Visio (Royal Dutch Visio) in the Netherlands.

**Deborah Chen, Ph.D.**, is Professor in the Department of Special Education at California State University, Northridge, where she coordinates and teaches in the Early Childhood Special Education Program. She is the editor of *Essential Elements in Early Intervention: Visual Impairment and Multiple Disabilities*, and co-author of *Developmental Guidelines for Infants with Visual Impairments, Adapting Early Childhood Curricula for Children with Special Needs,* and *Tactile Strategies for Children Who Have Visual Impairments and Multiple Disabilities*, as well as the creator of several videos on young children with multiple disabilities.

**Frances Dibble, M.A.**, is a retired teacher of students with visual impairments, with more than three decades of experience. She worked for the California School for the Blind, Fremont, as its Coordinator of State Assessment Services and for the Oakland Unified School District as Administrator for Programs for Special Needs Students.

**Gregory L. Goodrich, Ph.D.**, recently retired as Supervisory Research Psychologist and Optometric Research Fellowship Coordinator, Psychology Service and Western Blind Rehabilitation Center, U.S. Department of Veterans Affairs Palo Alto Health Care System, Palo Alto, California. He is coauthor of *Low Vision—The Reference,* contributed chapters to several books, and is author of over 150 journal articles on low vision rehabilitation and its history. Dr. Goodrich has also served as President of the Association for Education and Rehabilitation of the Blind and Visually Impaired and received a Lifetime Achievement Award from its Low Vision Division, and was a founding member, treasurer, and board member of the International Society for Low Vision Research and Rehabilitation.

**Bernadette Jackel, B.S.**, is a parent of a child with cerebral visual impairment. She has co-authored a number of articles on parents of children with CVI.

**Iain Livingstone, MBChB, FRCOphth,** is an Ophthalmology Specialist Registrar at the National Health Service, Greater Glasgow and Clyde, in Glasgow, Scotland, and a Clinical Research Fellow at the National Health Service Glasgow Centre for Ophthalmic Research.

**Fiona Lovett** is a parent of a child with cerebral visual impairment.

**Yue-Ting Siu, M.A.**, is a doctoral candidate at the Joint Doctoral Program for Special Education at the University of California at Berkeley and San Francisco State University. She is a lecturer in the Department of Special Education and Communicative Disorders, San Francisco State University, and a teacher of students with visual impairments in Bay Area public schools. She has contributed articles and presentations on the use of technology with students who are visually impaired.

# INTRODUCTION

Over 40 percent of the brain is involved in processing and supporting vision (Nakayama, 2012), so it is not surprising that damage to the brain commonly impairs vision in a wide range of ways. Damage to the brain that impairs vision is often called *cerebral visual impairment* (CVI) and can be related to a number of conditions.

Premature birth places infants at risk of brain injury. The number of children who are born prematurely is increasing worldwide, with a variety of contributing factors in both high-income and low-income countries. Of the 15 million children born prematurely in 2010 (more than 1 in 10 babies), about 14 million survived, and many had disabilities (March of Dimes Foundation et al., 2012). One of these disabilities may result from damage to the visual brain—the various segments of the brain that help create and sustain vision (Donahue, 2007)—which can lead to profound visual impairment in the most severely affected children or to more subtle visual perceptual problems that may or may not be detected by school age (Dutton, 2013; Macintyre-Béon et al., 2013). With the survival of increasing numbers of premature children, and smaller and smaller infants, the population of prematurely born children with CVI is rising.

Successful resuscitation at the time of birth is one factor that has led to the increased survival of children who have experienced poor oxygen supply and blood flow to the brain. Infection of the brain (in the form of meningitis or encephalitis), retained water in the water spaces or ventricles in the brain (or hydrocephalus), and head injury are further causes that are being managed more effectively, leading to the survival of yet more children with brain injury, with some developing CVI.

In contrast, immunization for rubella (German measles) has decreased the frequency of congenital retinal damage and damage to the lens of the eye, causing cataract. Congenital cataract resulting from other causes is now successfully treated, as is congenital glaucoma. As a result, these once leading causes of poor vision are now rare.

The combination of increasing survival rates of brain-injured children and greater success in managing eye disorders causing low vision and blindness has led CVI to become the most frequent cause of visual impairment in children in high-income countries, including Canada (Matsuba & Jan, 2006), Denmark (Nielsen, Skov, & Jensen, 2007), Greenland (Rosenberg, 1994), Ireland (Flanagan, Jackson, & Hill, 2003), Sweden (Blohmé & Tornqvist, 1997), the United Kingdom (Alagaratnam, Sharma, Lim, & Fleck, 2002; Bunce & Wormald, 2008; Mitry, Bunce, Wormald, & Bowman, 2013; Rogers, 1996), and the United States (Hatton, Schwietz, Boyer, & Rychwalski, 2007), among others. In addition, CVI has been increasingly associated with cerebral palsy and a variety of other conditions, which in turn has contributed to more cases being identified and registered (Bamashmus, Matlhaga, & Dutton, 2004). While precise prevalence figures are not available due to lack of identification of the full range of children who have the condition, the number of children with CVI is in all likelihood significantly higher than current reports indicate.

There is increasing awareness of the complexity of the subject of CVI. The individual pattern of visual dysfunction in CVI is arguably unique to each child. It is important to recognize CVI in children with profound visual impairment, but it can also cause difficulties in those with milder manifestations that can impinge considerably on their ability to perform school tasks such as reading and math, as well as compromise independent orientation and mobility (O&M), social interaction, and daily living skills.

## Purpose

Knowledge of the role the brain plays in vision is increasing rapidly. There is considerable literature concerning the ways in which vision is processed by the normal brain and about recent discoveries relating to neuroplasticity of brain functions. This information indicates that processing of visual data takes place throughout the brain (Jan et al., 2013). Nevertheless, in both adults and children, localized (or focal) damage to the brain leads to specific patterns of disordered visual function and behavior (Dutton, 2003). The approaches described in this book apply practical models of thinking aimed at helping practitioners understand these patterns. This knowledge can be used to optimize the environment, the materials, and the approaches taken to enhance the ultimate outcome for affected children.

This book presents a snapshot in time of current research and thought and recommended practices for children whose vision is compromised by brain damage. The material has been organized into an integrated text to present current knowledge that may evolve into a coherent system for practitioners. The overarching purpose of the book is to provide sufficient information for readers to recognize, understand, and assess the behavioral manifestations of damage to the visual brain in order to develop effective interventions based on identification of the spectrum of individual needs.

Information about a wide range of children with damage to the visual brain is presented in this work, and it is hoped that professionals find this approach instructive and useful. The book does not dwell on intricate details of brain functions, a very complex topic, but attempts to present basic information about the visual brain and to relate common patterns of visual behavior to specific patterns of damage to the brain. Technical terminology has been minimized and definitions have been provided to enable readers to gain an understanding of a complicated phenomenon. References are provided throughout the book for those interested in pursuing topics in further detail. Although the subject is challenging, it is to be hoped that the challenge of understanding the nature of CVI will be met so that professionals can make informed and appropriate decisions about assessment and intervention methods for the children with whom they work.

The detailed foundational information presented in the following pages is designed to serve as a resource for courses and educational programs concerned with this now common visual condition in children. As professional understanding of CVI increases, it will be incumbent upon medical and educational systems internationally to explore ways to best provide services to the full spectrum of affected children. This collaboration may lead to additional, mandatory training for specialists, reconsideration of guidelines and regulations for entitlement to services related to visual impairment, and reconfiguration of educational environments to accommodate, as part of universal design, the learning needs of this population.

## Organization and Use of this Book

*Vision and the Brain* reflects the complex nature of CVI in children, which requires assessment and intervention methods drawn from a variety of related disciplines. Since CVI is a condition that has affected children around the globe, this book draws on the expertise of contributors who present what is happening in the field internationally. Chapter contributions come from writers with backgrounds in education, occupational therapy, neuropsychology, ophthalmology, optometry, orientation and mobility, pediatrics, psychology, and vision science. Illustrative cases and stories of children and their families are found throughout the book, including a section with stories about individual cases "in their own words."

Divided into four main parts, the book presents information in a stepwise fashion with the intention of creating a systematic body of knowledge for professionals. Chapters build upon one another and are designed to help those working with children with CVI ascertain the nature and degree of visual impairment in each child, so that they can "see" and appreciate the world through the child's eyes and put measures in place to ensure that every child is served appropriately.

Part 1, "Vision and the Brain: An Introduction," provides a discussion of the history of thought about CVI, a review of terminology, basic information about the brain's role in vision, and a discussion of brain plasticity. In addition, the possible developmental effects of CVI in children, the role of attention and executive functions, and considerations in behavioral diagnoses are addressed.

Part 2, "Related Visual Issues," examines eye movement disorders and ocular issues associated with refractive errors and impaired focusing that can contribute to visual impairment in children with CVI.

Part 3, "Assessment of Children with CVI," begins with an overview of assessment needs for children with CVI, followed by several chapters on the assessment of visual functions and functional vision, including a review of history-taking methods to assess functional vision, assessments of visual processing, and observational assessment for young children with multiple disabilities who have CVI. Additional chapters examine assessments tied to interventions in the core and expanded core curricular areas of literacy, math, independent living skills, O&M, and assistive technology.

Part 4 focuses on "Intervention for Children with CVI." An overview of the principles of intervention methods is followed by a chapter that addresses combined assessment and intervention for very young children with profound cerebral visual impairment, as these issues are so closely interconnected for this population. Following this are chapters that address interventions for children who have CVI and multiple disabilities; compensatory strategies; supports for children and families; and insights from adult neuro-vision rehabilitation with rehabilitative considerations for children.

It is important that, in this nascent field, the worldwide effort to address the needs of children with CVI is recognized and embraced. Although different methods of service delivery and statutory regulations exist even within individual countries, readers are asked to consider and to adapt the techniques presented here to conform to the needs of their own unique service delivery models and, at this early juncture, to consider ways to incorporate material deemed relevant to advance existing methods and systems to better serve children with CVI.

Many potential readers of this book are teachers and caregivers. While some of the material is technical, the background information provided is essential to place current thinking about CVI in perspective. *Vision and the Brain* provides practical suggestions throughout, but a precise, step-by-step guidebook that addresses the complex needs of the wide array of children with CVI is not possible within a single text. Rather, this work has been written as a basic text with the goal of creating a climate of constructive and positive inquiry among practitioners around the world in order to promote deeper questioning and healthy debate.

## Concluding Remarks

Research related to children with cerebral visual impairment is in its infancy. As a result, a number of recommendations throughout the text are based on evidence from current practice. This book may therefore be viewed as a stepping-stone, pointing the way toward the development and provision of services for children with damage to the visual brain. It is hoped that future studies will lead to further refinement of the information presented here.

As with all areas of inquiry, terms and methods change as bodies of evidence emerge and theoretical paradigms are modified and improved. As the complexity of new knowledge grows, the need to maintain memorable and effective models of thinking that all can apply remains essential. Readers are encouraged to continue to add to their knowledge base, using and amending the framework provided in this book for ongoing investigation, refinement, and revision. Research and practice must advance hand in hand, and it is hoped that the material in this book will be one contribution to this essential and cumulative process.

## References


Alagaratnam, J., Sharma, T. K., Lim, C. S., & Fleck, B. W. (2002). A survey of visual impairment in children attending the Royal Blind School, Edinburgh using the WHO childhood visual impairment database. *Eye, 16*(5), 557–561.

Bamashmus, M. A., Matlhaga, B., & Dutton, G. N. (2004). Causes of blindness and visual impairment in the West of Scotland. *Eye, 18*(3), 257–261.

Blohmé, J., & Tornqvist, K. (1997). Visual impairment in Swedish children. III. Diagnoses. *Acta Ophthalmologica Scandinavica, 75*(6), 681–687.

Bunce, C., & Wormald, R. (2008). Causes of blind certifications in England and Wales: April 1999–March 2000. *Eye, 22*(7), 905–911.

Donahue, K. V. (2007). Cortical visual impairment: Etiology, associated findings, and prognosis in a tertiary care setting. *Journal of the American Association of Pediatric Ophthalmology and Strabismus, 11*(3), 235–239.

Dutton, G. N. (2003). The Edridge Green Lecture. Cognitive vision, its disorders and differential diagnosis in adults and children: Knowing where and what things are. *Eye, 17,* 289–304.

Dutton, G. N. (2013). The spectrum of cerebral visual impairment as a sequel to premature birth: An overview. *Documenta Ophthalmologica, 127*(1), 69–78.

Flanagan, N. M., Jackson, A. J., & Hill, A. E. (2003). Visual impairment in childhood: Insights from a community-based survey. *Child Care Health and Development, 29*(6), 493–499.

Hatton, D. D., Schwietz, E., Boyer, B., & Rychwalski, P. (2007). Babies count: The national registry for children with visual impairments, birth to 3 years. *Journal of the American Association of Pediatric Ophthalmology and Strabismus, 11*(4), 351–355.

Jan, J. E., Heaven, R. K. B., Matsuba, C., Langley, M. B., Roman–Lantzy, C., & Anthony, T. L. (2013). Windows into the visual brain: New discoveries about the visual system, its functions, and implications for practitioners. *Journal of Visual Impairment & Blindness, 107*(4), 251–261. Retrieved July 3, 2013, from http://www.afb.org/afbpress/pubjvib.asp?DocID=jvib070402

Macintyre-Béon, C., Young, D., Dutton, G. N., Mitchell, K., Simpson, J., Loffler, G., & Hamilton, R. (2013). Cerebral visual dysfunction in prematurely–born children in mainstream school. *Documenta Ophthalmologica, 127*(2), 89–102.

March of Dimes Foundation, Partnership for Maternal, Newborn & Child Health, Save the Children & World Health Organization. (2012). *Born too soon: The global action report on preterm birth.* Geneva: WHO.

Matsuba, C. A., & Jan, J. E. (2006). Long-term outcome of children with cortical visual impairment. *Developmental Medicine & Child Neurology, 48*(6), 508–512.

Mitry, D., Bunce, C., Wormald, R., & Bowman, R. (2013). Childhood visual impairment in England: A rising trend. *Archives of Diseases in Childhood, 98*(5), 378–380.

Nakayama, K. (2012). Retrieved July 5, 2013, from http://visionlab.harvard.edu/members/ken/nakayama.html

Nielsen, L. S., Skov, L., & Jensen, H. (2007). Visual dysfunctions and ocular disorders in children with developmental delay. I. Prevalence, diagnoses and aetiology of visual impairment. *Acta Ophthalmologica Scandinavica, 85*(2), 149–156.

Rogers, M. (1996). Vision impairment in Liverpool: Prevalence and morbidity. *Archives of Diseases of Childhood, 74*(4), 299–303.

Rosenberg, T. (1994). Congenital and hereditary visual impairment in Greenland. *Arctic Medical Research, 53*(2), 91–96.

# PART I

## Vision and the Brain

### *An Introduction*

# 1

# Impairment of Vision Due to Damage to the Brain

*Gordon N. Dutton and Amanda Hall Lueck*

This book concerns cerebral visual impairment (CVI) and the many ways in which this complex and multifaceted condition can affect how children see and behave. The ultimate aim is to provide teachers of students with visual impairments and other professionals working with and caring for children who have CVI with the information necessary to understand the resulting impairment of vision, allowing them to put carefully selected measures in place to address these students' needs and ensure that they receive appropriate services. As the focus in these pages will be CVI, which is neurologically based, readers who require basic information about educational assessment and intervention for ocular visual impairments are encouraged to review such texts as Corn & Erin, 2010 or Lueck, 2004a.

At the outset, it may be helpful to address some of the confusion surrounding CVI, and to present a functional definition of this complex phenomenon. Although vision as a sense has typically been associated with the eyes, they comprise only a part of the system that supports and sustains the sense of vision. The term *cerebral visual impairment* was introduced in the 1990s to describe deficits of vision and visual perception in children (Ortibus, De Cock, & Lagae, 2011) that result from damage to the brain. In this book the term is applied as an inclusive concept relating to children with visual disorders or visual perception issues of any type or severity resulting from damage to the visual pathways and centers of the brain.

As explained in the introduction, many areas of the brain are involved in sustaining the sense of sight. As a result, the term "visual brain" has recently emerged as part of discussions surrounding CVI. The *visual brain* is a conceptual term referring to the totality of brain elements serving or supporting vision. The visual brain serves to map, search, give attention to, as well as recognize and interpret visual input. It also provides mapping information to the motor planning centers of the brain. When areas of the visual brain are damaged in children, the ability to learn and perform tasks of daily life is affected and must be addressed in educational programs. The current understanding that visual functions are dealt with throughout the brain by means of a highly complex array of interconnected networks (Jan et al., 2013) has given rise to a number

### SIDEBAR 1.1

## Key Terms and Definitions

| | |
|---|---|
| Blindness | Absence of vision. *Total blindness* is complete absence of vision, and is rare. |
| Cerebral visual impairment (CVI) | Visual impairment due to damage or disorder of the visual pathways and visual centers in the brain, including the pathways serving visual perception, cognition, and visual guidance of movement. |
| Functional vision | The ways in which a person uses available visual skills and abilities in typical tasks of daily life. |
| Habilitation | Services that enable a person to learn, keep, or improve skills and functional abilities that have never developed or have not developed in a typical manner. |
| Higher visual functions | The combination of visual perception, visual cognition, guidance of movement, and the capacity to choose to give visual attention. |
| Legal blindness | A central visual acuity of 20/200 or less in the better eye with the best possible correction, or a visual field of 20 degrees or less, used in the United States to determine eligibility for certain services. |
| Low vision | Vision impairment that is severe enough to impede a person's ability to learn or perform usual tasks of daily life but still allows some functionally useful visual discrimination. It covers a range from mild to severe visual impairment, but excludes total blindness. |
| Perception | The ability to see, hear, or become aware of something through the senses. |
| Rehabilitation | Training to improve skills or behaviors that have been lost or decreased due to disease or injury. |
| Vision loss | Acquired damage to a previously intact visual system. |
| Visual brain | The totality of brain elements serving or supporting vision that serves to map, search, give attention to, recognize, and interpret visual input. Also provides mapping information to motor planning centers of the brain. |
| Visual cognition | The capacity to process what is seen, to think about its significance, and to manipulate and use both incoming image data and remembered imagery in the context of creative thought. |
| Visual dysfunction | Disorder of visual perception, visual guidance of movement, and/or visual attention. |
| Visual functions | Measurable components of vision, including visual acuity, contrast sensitivity, color perception, visual fields, and the perception of movement. |
| Visual guidance of movement | Mapping of incoming visual information in the mind that is employed to guide movement of the limbs and body. |
| Visual impairment | Damage to the visual system that impedes the ability to learn or perform usual tasks of daily life, given a child's level of maturity and cultural environment. The term includes both low vision blindness. |
| Visual perception | Ability to interpret the immediate environment by processing incoming information from visible light that is sent from the eyes to the brain. |
| Visual system | Network that produces sight, including both the eyes and the brain. |

of terms being used to describe CVI and related issues. This terminology has been open to interpretation among the research and medical communities (Colenbrander, 2010, Fazzi et al., 2009; Jan et al., 2013; Ortibus et al., 2011). For this reason, it is necessary to explain some basic terms as they are applied in this book. (See Sidebar 1.1 for a summary of key terms used in this chapter.)

## Principal Terminology

### Visual Impairment

Before a discussion of *cerebral* visual impairment can begin, it is important to discuss how the term visual impairment is used in this book since definitions for, and interpretations of, this term vary. The term *visual impairment* is applied here as an overarching descriptor for all aspects of impaired vision.

It is important to note that a social, as opposed to clinical, model of disability has come into widespread use internationally as a way to emphasize a person's capabilities and to determine methods of support so that individuals can participate more fully in situations that arise in everyday life (National Research Council, 2002; World Health Organization, 2007). For this reason, a functional definition of visual impairment for children is used throughout this book, with a focus on the use of vision in learning and in the performance of critical and meaningful tasks. For children, a functional definition of visual impairment would be "damage to the visual system that impedes the ability to learn or perform usual tasks of daily life, given a child's level of maturity and cultural environment" (adapted from Lueck, 2004b, p. 3). The visual system, in this definition, includes both the eyes and the brain, and damage can affect one or both of these areas.

In the United States, according to the Individuals with Disabilities Education Act (IDEA, 2004, P. L. 108–446), the current federal definition of visual impairment for entitlement to special education services is:

> Visual impairment, including blindness, means an impairment in vision that, even with correction, adversely affects a child's educational performance. The term includes both partial sight and blindness.
> (Sec. 300.8)

### Visual Functions and Functional Vision

*Visual functions* (such as visual acuity, visual field, and contrast sensitivity) refer to and describe how the eye and visual system function, with measures taken at the eye or organ level (Colenbrander, 2002). They refer to measurements of the limits of vision. These threshold measures of vision (for example, the smallest element that can be perceived at a given distance or the least amount of contrast that can be detected) are measured quantitatively, are usually measured for each eye separately, and evaluate a single variable at a time (Colenbrander, 2002). For example, the measurement of visual acuity is used for the diagnosis and management of ophthalmological disorders. (See Chapter 12 for additional discussion.) Tests of visual functions are usually performed in a static, controlled environment.

In contrast, *functional vision* describes how an individual functions using vision and involves evaluation of that person's visual skills and abilities as applied to the performance of usual tasks of daily life, such as reading (for example, the optimum print size needed for a person to read a particular style of running text most efficiently). Functional vision is often described qualitatively, although quantitative measures are available for some tasks, such as reading. It is measured binocularly (both eyes viewing) to replicate "real world" performance, and examines supra-threshold (above threshold) performance so that a person's comfort level for an activity is identified and taken into account. For example, a person may be able to see the footnotes in a textbook, but for sustained reading, a larger (supra-threshold) print size is required. An evaluation of functional vision involves categories that are less precise than measures of visual function, and is often affected by multiple variables at one time. Functional vision evaluations are usually performed in dynamic environments (Colenbrander, 2002) that are intended to represent the daily activities and surroundings of the person being assessed. (See Chapter 12 for a detailed discussion of functional vision assessment.)

There will be occasional references throughout this book to a child's "visual functioning." This term is used in the everyday sense of how well a child is managing with his or her vision and is not a technical term.

## Entitlement to Services: Legal Blindness

*Total blindness* is complete absence of vision and is rare. The term *legal blindness,* however, is a broader term that includes individuals who have some vision. It is used in some countries, including the United States, to qualify individuals for specialized medical, educational, and social services. (For a history of how the definition of legal blindness for entitlement of services has changed over time in the United States, see Sidebar 1.2.) In the United States, legal blindness is commonly defined as a visual acuity of 20/200 (6/60) or less in the better eye with best correction, or a visual field of less than 10 degrees from the fixation point or with a visual field whose greatest diameter is less than 20 degrees (National Research Council, 2002, p. 36). There is currently no federal definition in the United States for *low vision* (see Sidebar 1.1) or for *partial sight* (a term that is rarely used today but still appears in IDEA) for entitlement to services, although some local, regional, or state agencies use the definition of a visual acuity of 20/70 or less in the better eye with best correction for partial sight.

There are children whose visual capabilities fall within the functional definition of visual impairment as used in this book, but who, in some countries or regions, do not meet the statutory definition of legal blindness or low vision for entitlement to services related to their disability. Thus, practitioners may confront situations in which a child is visually impaired, but is not considered eligible for special educational services related to vision.

## Visual Perception, Visual Attention, and Related Terms

Perception can be thought of as the ability to see, hear, or become aware of something through the senses. *Visual perception* is thus the act of detecting and recognizing what is seen. *Visual cognition* is considered an extension of visual perception and involves the capacity to process what is seen, to think about its significance, and to manipulate and use both incoming image data and remembered imagery in the context of creative thought. Thus, the way in which something

SIDEBAR 1.2

## The Evolution of the Definition of Legal Blindness

*Gregory L. Goodrich*

In 1935, one of the most far-reaching events in education and rehabilitation of individuals in the United States who are visually impaired took place: The enactment of the Aid to the Blind Act within the 1935 Social Security Administration Act by the U.S. Congress (Social Security Administration, 1935). This event was intended to be meaningful, though it may not have been intended to be far-reaching in its import, but in fact it was both.

The Aid to the Blind provision was a response to both the unemployment created by the Great Depression, and the congressional view that individuals who were blind were at a substantial financial disadvantage as a result of their visual condition. Congress recognized that blindness was not limited to total absence of vision and included in the definition those who had vision substantially less than normal both in its consideration of aid and benefits and in its efforts to define eligibility criteria for this aid. Thus, in 1934, it asked the American Medical Association to develop a quantifiable definition of blindness to be used for eligibility determinations ("Report of the Committee," 1934). The empirical definition arrived at by a panel appointed by the American Medical Association was a definition of what was termed "legal blindness," which was identified as a best-corrected visual acuity of 20/200, or a visual field subtending no more than 20 degrees at its greatest extent.

This moment in history is of interest for at least two reasons. First, it may reflect the intent of Congress at a particular juncture in time, and second, the implications of the definition that emerged, which considers only visual acuity and visual field independently of one another rather than reflect the complex nature of vision as we understand it today, are still being felt today. The intent of Congress in 1935 was not necessarily to create a definition to be used by educational institutions, states, private organizations, or even federal agencies other than the Social Security Administration, but the widespread use of the definition did in fact ensue. The adoption of the definition by other organizations may result from the fact that it was founded on easy and inexpensive measures of vision. It is possible that it may also have been adopted because some organizations believed that individuals included in the definition warranted inclusion and that those excluded warranted exclusion.

Since 1935 there has been vigorous debate about whether or not the inclusive and exclusive nature of the definition is valid. As early as the 1950s, both Father Thomas Carroll (1956) and Dr. Richard Hoover (1958) criticized the definition. This debate has continued over the past 80 years as more has been learned concerning the complexity of the human visual system, as well as its deficiencies and resulting disabilities when it is disordered. The debate calls into question the validity of the definition of legal blindness, signifying that the definition is arbitrary and not founded on a meaningful understanding of the outcomes of the numerous conditions that cause visual impairment.

For most of its existence, the U.S. Department of Veterans Affairs (VA, previously known as the Veterans Administration) used this definition of legal blindness as a key criterion for veterans' eligibility for blind rehabilitation services. These services did not only include services for totally blind individuals, but also extended to those who had a visual impairment that met the criteria of the original definition of legal blindness. Traditional practice changed in 2008 as increasing numbers of troops returned from combat in Afghanistan and Iraq with hemianopia and other severe visual impairments that often did not meet the criteria defining legal blindness. That is, these individuals

*(continued on next page)*

**SIDEBAR 1.2** *(continued from previous page)*

maintained better than 20/200 visual acuity (with some having acuities of 20/15) and/or had visual fields that exceeded 20 degrees, but they nevertheless had difficulty reading, traveling safely and independently, and/or performing many activities of daily living as a result of their visual impairment and other factors related to their injury. This reality presented a dilemma for the VA as an agency charged with providing care for those injured during their military service, because the definition of legal blindness used to determine eligibility for services excluded this group of veterans who had significant visual impairments.

The situation was resolved in 2008 when the VA amended its eligibility requirements to include the concept of "excess disability." This term refers to vision loss that has a substantial impact on the individual's functional independence that is out of proportion to the degree of impairment as measured by visual acuity or visual field (Department of Veterans Affairs, 2008). More recently, the U.S. National Eye Institute (NEI, n.d.) has also updated its definition of visual impairment to indicate that it "can be defined as any chronic visual deficit that impairs everyday functioning and is not correctable by ordinary eyeglasses or contact lenses."

The VA's experience is not unique. Other attempts have been made to differentiate vision as defined by clinical measurements such as those used to delineate legal blindness from functional vision, which addresses the abilities and impairments individuals may have (International Society for Low Vision Research and Rehabilitation, 1999). Other organizations have used a model similar to that used by the VA to clarify the provision of services to visually impaired persons. In the United Kingdom, for example, the legal definition of severe sight impairment (blindness) is when "a person is so blind that they cannot do any work for which eyesight is essential" (National Health Service, 2013). These are not unique attempts to overcome the limitations imposed by definition (see, for example, Social Security Administration, 2014; U.S. Equal Employment Opportunity Commission, n.d.).

The definition of legal blindness established in 1935 conflicts with our current understanding of the complexity of vision and society's intent to provide needed rehabilitation where appropriate. The challenge to society today is to not be limited by a definition that was never intended to do what it has been asked to do.

Human vision is not limited solely by either visual acuity or visual field or a combination of both, as the changes to the definitions used by both the VA and NEI emphasize. As our understanding of vision and vision rehabilitation grows, a useful definition of "legal blindness" may never be developed. However, terminology should not be a limiting factor in addressing the needs of individuals with visual impairments, regardless of their specific causes or manifestations. Rather, professional practice should be limited only by our ever-increasing understanding of disorders of human vision and our capacity to provide rehabilitation.

is seen, known, and understood is called visual perception. The mental action or process of acquiring knowledge and understanding through vision is referred to as visual cognition. The phrase visual guidance of movement refers to the mapping of incoming visual information in the mind that is utilized to guide movement of the limbs and body. The conscious visual process of choosing to pay visual attention—that is, focusing on specific elements in the visual scene—is known as an *executive function.* The term *higher visual functions* is used to encompass the combination of visual perception, visual cognition, visual guidance of movement, and the capacity to choose to give visual attention. (Visual attention is discussed further in Chapter 2.)

## Visual Dysfunction

The term *visual dysfunction* is applied in this book to disorders of visual perception, visual guidance of movement, and visual attention. Many children with such disorders also have measurable impairments of primary (or "lower") visual functions, such as visual acuity, color vision, contrast sensitivity, and visual field (Colenbrander, 2010) that can be either ocular or neurological in origin. Whether children who only have visual dysfunctions are entitled to services related to visual impairment remains under review in the medical, rehabilitation, and education communities. In the United States, some of these children receive special education services related to visual impairment, while others do not. As described in Sidebar 1.2, war veterans in the United States with visual perceptual disorders alone are currently receiving comprehensive services related to their vision. Functional definitions of impairment that are based on skills, abilities, and quality of life speak to the inclusion of children with visual dysfunctions for services related to vision, while definitions based on visual functions alone lead to their exclusion. At this juncture there is no easy resolution to this dilemma. As the debate about services for these children evolves, current classification systems will either be accepted as they are, or will be amended to embrace more functional standards related to visual impairment. In the meantime, the challenge for practitioners is how to classify and approach intervention for children with visual perceptual dysfunctions so they are not disadvantaged because they do not meet criteria for entitlement to services, are incorrectly labeled, or are not provided with appropriate resources.

## Congenital and Acquired Cerebral Visual Impairment

The most common causes of cerebral visual impairment typically occur while the child is in the womb or is being born. They are therefore *congenital.* Less frequently, a child who has developed normal vision for his or her age may later develop a condition or be subject to injury or trauma that damages parts of the brain that serve vision. Such cases are considered *acquired* cerebral visual impairment or vision loss.

## Vision Loss

Although the terms *visual impairment* and *vision loss* (or loss of vision) are commonly used interchangeably in the literature, a distinction is made in this book. While the term *visual impairment* applies to all children whose vision is deficient, the term *vision loss* is applied only in cases with acquired damage to a previously intact visual system. This distinction is made because prior vision allows a child to attain a range of knowledge and skills that may still be present once some vision has been lost and may be used to assist in rehabilitation.

## Cerebral Visual Impairment: Definition and Implications

This section describes the meaning and the history of the term *cerebral visual impairment.* For a brief historical overview of how the understanding of the condition described by that term came about, see Sidebar 1.3.

*Cerebral visual impairment,* or CVI, as applied in this book, refers to disordered vision or visual perception of any type or severity as a result of damage or disorder to the visual pathways or centers of the brain. The eyes act like a pair of movie cameras to

**SIDEBAR 1.3**

## Historical Background: A Brief Overview

The process by which vision is created and sustained primarily takes place in the brain. Acquired damage in adulthood to the individual parts of the brain that serve vision is relatively rare, but more than a century of careful observation of how different brain injuries affect vision has helped to establish a picture of how the brain "sees." (Grusser & Landis, 1991, provide a comprehensive review of how this knowledge came about.)

### The Brain's Role in the Vision System

Current knowledge of the role of the brain in the vision process originated in the early 1900s, mainly from careful observational studies of soldiers with shrapnel injuries to the brain, and noting how these injuries affected their vision. Publications from both Japan and the United Kingdom provided similar results showing that damage to the brain's occipital lobes led to a variety of patterns of visual loss depending on where the damage was (Grusser & Landis, 1991; Holmes, 1918a). Visual field assessment, the careful mapping of the soldiers' remaining areas of vision, revealed a correspondence between areas of field loss and the sites of the brain damage sustained, and showed that the pattern of loss of the field of vision was very similar, or identical, in both eyes (homonymous). In addition, the area of loss of vision is upside down and horizontally reversed with respect to where the brain damage is (see Chapter 2 and Figure 2.4). These observations led to the notion that the picture or image of an object formed in the eyes is carried to the occipital lobes of the brain, where the picture is "seen." This basic conceptual model still holds sway, despite considerable evidence that there is much more to the story (Milner & Goodale, 2006).

In a less well recognized account, Holmes, in 1918(b), described six soldiers with similar visual symptoms and signs as a result of shrapnel damage to the top of the brain, just in front of the occipital lobes (the posterior parietal area; see Figure 2.1). Despite intact clarity of vision (visual acuity) in five of the six cases and intact ability to see in three dimensions (stereopsis) with good recognition of individual detail, these soldiers had very similar patterns of profound visual difficulties, but were not completely aware of them. The damage to the brain had caused loss of vision in the lower visual field of both eyes. In addition, when shown a picture, these subjects were able to see only one or two parts of it at a time; the other parts were missing. The soldiers were unable to move around freely without bumping into everything. They could not negotiate steps or stairs, and when they reached out for what they were looking at, their reach was inaccurate. Holmes gave the following description: The patients "collided with obstacles chiefly because they did not recognize how near they were to them, and ran into walls and screens for the same reason" (Holmes, 1918b, p. 508).

In 1909, Rudolph Balint published a detailed account of an elderly patient who had very similar visual difficulties due to damage to the same areas of the brain (Rizzo & Vecera, 2002). Despite being able to recognize what he was looking at, the patient could not see more than one or two things at once. As with the soldiers, he too could not reach accurately, nor use vision alone as a means of guiding the movement of his upper and lower limbs. Another observation that Balint made was that although his patient could, when asked, move his eyes quickly, he could not easily look from one item to another. The significance of Balint's paper was recognized a few years later when additional cases had shown that damage to the posterior parietal area on both sides gave rise to:

- the ability to see only one or two things at once (later given the term *simultanagnosia)*
- considerable disability using vision to guide movement of the arms, the legs, and the body, referred to as *optic ataxia*

*(continued on next page)*

- the inability to move the eyes to look at different parts of the surrounding scene (despite a normal eye movement control system in the brain)

This group of visual difficulties, when severe, is now known as *Balint's syndrome* (also discussed in Chapters 2 and 3), and is commonly accompanied by lack of vision in the lower visual field because the incoming pathways serving the lower visual field pass through the lower part of the posterior parietal lobes, where they, too, are damaged. Since then, there have been a number of published reports of adults and children with the same set of visual difficulties associated with damage to the same area of the brain. (This topic is well reviewed by Rizzo & Vecera [2002]. Readers should note that data from a recent epidemiological study [Williams et al., 2011] suggest that this type of CVI, now often referred to as *dorsal stream dysfunction* and explained in Chapter 2, is not uncommon.)

Further observations were reported related to the casualties of World War I. Riddoch (1917) noticed that his patients with shrapnel injuries of the visual brain leading to focal areas of loss of their visual field, were sometimes aware of the perception of movement in the field of vision that had lost vision. The brain processes the perception of the static image and the perception of the moving image in different areas, and it has been found that the motion perception centers can be spared (Weiskrantz, 2009). As first described by Zihl and colleagues in 1983 (Zeki, 1991), these centers can also be selectively damaged, leading to an inability to see moving targets despite the remaining ability to see static objects fairly clearly.

When it comes to the conscious recognition of what we see, there have been many descriptions over the last century of loss of the ability to recognize specific people or objects, often associated with disorientation and impaired route finding, despite retained clarity of vision and the ability to move around freely. This range of difficulties arises from focal damage to the temporal lobes of the brain (Grusser & Landis, 1991)—the bottom of the brain at the back on both sides.

### A Unifying Hypothesis

Many years elapsed before a unifying hypothesis describing how visual imagery is processed in the mind gained influence. In the 1980s, the neuroscientists David Milner and Melvyn Goodale created a synthesis of the abundance of diverse information available (Goodale & Milner, 2013; Milner & Goodale, 2006). They had studied in detail a subject, DF, who took a shower in a room with a malfunctioning gas boiler that had given off carbon monoxide. This exposure damaged the part of the brain serving visual recognition, yet she could still perceive movement, and with sufficient confidence, could accurately grasp moving objects that she could not identify. She could walk around obstacles she could not properly see, without bumping into them and without understanding how she did it. She had essentially the reverse of Balint's syndrome. These observations demonstrated that the posterior parietal lobes, which for DF remained intact, serve the ability to use vision to plan and guide our movements through three-dimensional space, and that this process ostensibly takes place unconsciously. In other words, an automatic system seemingly exists in our brain that prevents us from bumping into things without our necessarily knowing how we do it.

These accounts show how damage to the visual brain in one location but not another can result in paradoxical visual behaviors. On the one hand, how can the person with posterior parietal brain damage see clearly and identify things, but only one or two things at a time, as well as bump into everything and reach inaccurately? On the other hand, how can the person who has damage to the temporal lobes be able to move freely through the visual world without really being able to see it? Milner and Goodale have advanced a model of thinking that the visual brain can be

*(continued on next page)*

**SIDEBAR 1.3** *(continued from previous page)*

divided into a number of functional components (Goodale & Milner, 2013; Milner & Goodale, 2006), and this topic is discussed in further detail in Chapters 2 and 3.

The model developed by Goodale and Milner, while a simplified description of how the brain "sees," is used in this book as the basis for understanding patterns of behavioral manifestations of CVI in children and has proven to be highly useful to practitioners. Vision scientists, neuropsychologists, neuro-ophthalmologists, electrophysiologists, neuroimaging specialists, and many others are now all contributing to a current explosion of new literature on the complex role the brain plays in sustaining vision. This model of thinking, formed on what goes wrong with vision when there is damage to the brain, is well-founded on historical precedents and is applied in leading pediatric neuro-ophthalmic texts (for example, Brodsky, 2010).

capture flowing images of the surrounding environment. The visual information the eyes capture is carried along the optic nerves emerging from the back of the eyes to a pair of relay stations in the brain called the lateral geniculate bodies (see Chapter 2 and Figure 2.2 for more information). The information is relayed from there (either directly or indirectly) along bundles of nerve fibers, called visual pathways, to different locations in the brain, where a range of different visual processes are served. These include:

- The analysis of incoming visual information in terms of clarity, contrast, and color, as well as the overall area seen (the visual fields).
- The analysis and interpretation of the moving elements of the visual scene.
- The maintenance of a continuous process of forming a map of the visual scene within the brain that is constantly being updated. This visual map is built up automatically and subconsciously as the head and eyes move to look around the scene. The map contains each element of the surroundings. The picture of the visual scene is captured, held for a short time, and then replaced by new incoming image data. The brain uses this dynamic, constantly changing, subconsciously held visual map to
  - make accurate body and limb movements
  - search the scene
  - give visual attention, and
  - move the eyes at will to look at an item of choice
- The process of recognition of what is being looked at, whether it is a face, a facial expression, a shape, an object, or the surrounding environment, to enable orientation and navigation.

As used in this book, the term *cerebral visual impairment* is employed as an inclusive term to describe disorders of the visual pathways or centers of the brain that compromise visual processes in any combination and in any severity.

In addition, the process of vision is also supported by a range of other brain systems. For example:

- An automatic subconscious visual system (served by the thalamus and upper midbrain) that spots and initiates protective avoidance of hazards.
- Eye movement control systems.

- The balance system in the inner ear and brain (the labyrinthine system) that keeps the eyes, and the picture that is seen, steady.
- The system (in the cerebellum) that coordinates body movements and helps to synchronize them with the moving visual image.

Disorder of these systems can sometimes interfere with vision and can also contribute to the manifestations of cerebral visual impairment, particularly in children with extensive damage to the brain.

A more technical definition of cerebral visual impairment that uses terminology explained in more detail in Chapter 2, combines descriptions given by Boot et al. (2010), Fazzi et al. (2009), and Ortibus et al. (2011):

> Cerebral visual impairment is a term that describes deficiency in the functions of vision, due to damage or malfunction of visual pathways and visual centers in the brain (specifically those behind the lateral geniculate bodies), including the optic radiations, the occipital cortex and the visual associative areas, which may be accentuated by associated disorders of the control of eye movements.

It should also be noted that the term cerebral visual impairment has historically been applied in a variety of ways, as has the term *cortical visual impairment.* At times these terms have been used interchangeably to refer to visual impairment resulting from damage or malfunction of the brain (see, for example, Dennison & Lueck, 2006). However, terminology is a changing and unresolved issue associated with visual disorders due to brain anomalies, and to date, "terminology has yet to be definitively established by the international medical community" (Lueck & Goodrich, 2011).

In the past, the term cortical visual impairment often referred to visual impairment related to the cortical area of the brain and/or the optic radiations. While some in the medical community have suggested that the terms cortical and cerebral have similar meanings (Good, 2009), others have indicated the need for a term that could be applied to injuries that are anatomically outside the cortical region of the brain. This led to a movement to adopt a term that encompassed more than the cortical region, and the term cerebral visual impairment was introduced (Ortibus et al., 2011). Differing views on the definition of cerebral visual impairment have persisted in the United States and Europe (see, for example, Jan, 2011; Lueck & Goodrich, 2011; & Colenbrander, 2011). However, in light of dramatically expanding understanding of the role of the brain and the widespread neuronal networks that participate in supporting vision, the use of terminology continues to evolve (Jan et al., 2013). Currently, in the United States, the term cortical visual impairment continues to be in common use and is often also abbreviated as CVI (Ortibus et al., 2011). In this book, CVI refers to the term cerebral visual impairment.

## Types of Children with Cerebral Visual Impairment

From a practical perspective of working with children who have cerebral visual impairment, they can be considered to fall into three groups:

- Children with profound visual impairment due to CVI, many of whom have additional disabilities

- Children with CVI who have functionally useful vision and cognitive challenges
- Children with CVI who have functionally useful vision and who work at or near the expected academic level for their age group

The first group, children with profound visual impairment due to CVI, encompasses those for whom nonvisual approaches to learning need to be applied to substitute for their lack of vision, as well as many children who have rudimentary but identifiable elements of visual functions that may respond to interventions. Infants and very young children in this category may develop more functionally useful vision over time, particularly those whose primary brain damage is located in the visual cortex (Hoyt, 2003). Often children in this group have multiple disabilities; however, vision alone may be affected, particularly when the condition is acquired at later ages.

The second group, children with CVI who have functionally useful vision and cognitive challenges, typically includes children who have widespread damage to the brain that affects vision, intellect, and often mobility. Children with cerebral palsy, for example, may have this type of widespread brain damage.

The third group, children with CVI who have functionally useful vision and who work at or near the expected academic level for their age, may be the least severely affected by CVI, but some may have additional minor disorders of intellectual function and mobility. Others may have good central visual functions (such as acuity and contrast sensitivity) but their principal visual difficulties relate to disorders of visual perception, which may also affect how vision is used to guide movement of the limbs and body.

It should be noted that these three broad categories are not mutually exclusive and may overlap. For example, a child who has developed poor visual acuities due to an episode of low oxygen and low blood delivery to the parts of the brain that serve vision (the occipital lobes) can retain the ability to move around and be intellectually unaffected. These categories are considered in more detail when assessment is discussed in Chapter 10.

## Other Terms

A distinction will often be made in this book between the concepts of *rehabilitation* and *habilitation*. Rehabilitation takes advantage of capabilities gained prior to acquired damage to the brain; habilitation progressively assists in the development of skills that have been affected by congenital damage to the brain or damage occurring shortly after birth.

## Diagnostic Terminology and Its Interpretation

Diagnostic terms ideally refer to a known underlying cause; however, they are conceptually less precise when the cause is not known (Walton, Beeson, & Scott, 1986). For example, "meningococcal meningitis" describes the cause—the meningococcus bacterium—and the affected structure—the meninges (the lining around the brain). On the other hand, the diagnosis "autistic spectrum disorder" is less precise because its diagnosis is typically based primarily on patterns of behavior, in many cases without a known cause.

Similarly, the diagnostic term cerebral visual impairment may be based on a known primary diagnosis such as meningococcal meningitis. In this case a known germ has caused damage to the visual pathways, leading to CVI. However, another child may show typical behavioral features of CVI, despite normal brain imaging in the visual areas (Ortibus et al., 2011). Such children still warrant a diagnosis of CVI because they show features typical of CVI (see Chapter 3), even though the diagnosis is less precise since the underlying cause has not been determined. Although it is not always a simple undertaking, children with CVI need to be identified, their visual difficulties characterized, and their needs met.

## The Importance of Identifying CVI in Children

Damage to the brain of a child before birth may result in impaired movement of the limbs, or cerebral palsy, which is obvious to the observer. In contrast, impaired vision as a result of CVI is not so evident, unless the child has very poor vision or lacks vision completely. Even marked visual impairment may go undetected because the resulting behavior displayed by the individual is not recognized or is misinterpreted (see Chapter 7). Such misinterpretation can be problematic for a child with CVI, whose inaccurate visual guidance of movement, for example, may be misinterpreted as clumsiness; whose problems finding objects due to impaired visual search may be considered willful; whose inability to look at people's faces while listening may be ascribed to bad behavior; and whose problems recognizing people may be attributed to poor social integration. Meanwhile, the child may be doing his or her best, yet is criticized at every turn. The outcome can be disheartening for a child, leading to low self-esteem and a sense of being misunderstood. In the authors' experience, the act of recognizing and accurately characterizing the range of visual disorders, and adopting approaches to overcome the resulting difficulties, can be life changing. The child is no longer criticized, but is understood and helped.

Young children with any type of visual impairment, whether as a result of abnormal optics, damage to the eyes, or injury to the visual pathways or visual centers of the brain, may not even be aware that their vision is limited. If they have always seen the world a certain way, they have no way of comparing how they see with how others see. They are, in a sense, asymptomatic, because a symptom is a disease manifestation of which the patient complains, and this requires awareness (Walton et al., 1986). Thus, they cannot inform others about what they are unable to see. If their visual limitations are not recognized, children affected in this way may be taught using materials they cannot adequately see, which puts them at risk of falling behind their peers.

Up-to-date knowledge of the limits of what each child is able to easily see in daily life—their functional vision—in both optimal and less than optimal circumstances (such as when tired, in busy and noisy environments, or in poor lighting conditions), is needed to ensure that this information is conveyed accurately and appropriately to those who interact with the child at home, at school, and at leisure, in order to provide appropriate interventions to promote the use of vision and alternative strategies for learning. Nevertheless, the assessment of functional vision is not carried out in standard ophthalmic practice, except in dedicated low vision clinics. Assessment, documentation, and communication of functional vision need to be carried out by members of a collaborative medical and educational team. This includes teachers who can collect educational assessment data related to functional vision over time in the child's school, home, and community settings.

Participation of the child's family in this process is essential. Often family members are the best source of information about their child's behaviors. Family members of children who have CVI may be able to identify behaviors in their children that require attention, even though they may not understand that limitations in functional vision are their cause.

By observing a child's daily activities and participating in the collaborative assessment of vision themselves, teachers and family members can better understand how a child functions visually and attempt to see the world "through the child's eyes." Such insight helps these caregivers ensure that all information is routinely presented in formats that are readily accessible to the child. It also ensures that any difficulties experienced by the child are readily identified and acted upon through instructional approaches that meet the specific needs of each child, thereby reducing the expectations of a visual performance that is unattainable. To teach using material that cannot be fully seen by a visually impaired child is not only a waste of resources, but is disabling for children who may be blamed for not paying attention to something, which to them is not visible. For children with CVI, what cannot be seen usually goes beyond issues related to visual acuity and visual field and involves aspects of visual attention and perception, as well as the use of vision to guide movement. These additional visual limitations must be understood and carefully addressed by the medical-educational team.

## Services for Children with CVI

Educational services for children with cerebral visual impairment in the United States have been implemented since the late 1980s, largely in response to the groundbreaking work of Dr. James Jan and his associates in Vancouver, Canada (see Good, Jan, Burden, Skoczenski, & Candy, 2001; Jan & Groenveld, 1993; Jan, Groenveld, Sykanda, & Hoyt, 1987). Since then, approaches aimed at integrating medicine with education have been progressively developing (Dutton & Bax, 2010; Hyvärinen & Jacob, 2011; Hyvärinen, Walthes, Freitag, & Petz, 2012). Interventions have tended to focus primarily on children with significant visual acuity impairment, and most, if not all, of these children have had additional disabilities (Baker-Nobles & Rutherford, 1995; Groenveld, Jan, & Leader, 1990; Morse, 1990). Intervention programs worldwide continue to address the needs of this specific population of children and provide guidance for educators in the areas of assessment and instruction (Roman-Lantzy, 2007; Steendam, 2008).

However, the growing body of evidence detailing the wide range of additional behavioral manifestations of damage to the visual brain that can occur with or without decreased visual acuity (Jacobson et al., 1996; Dutton et al., 1996; Dutton, 2003; Dutton, 2008; Hoyt, 2003; Fazzi et al., 2009; Ortibus et al., 2011), coupled with increased awareness and concern for the population of children in schools who tend to have less severe visual acuity impairment but additional visual difficulties, has created a call for further information on best practices (Hyvärinen & Jacob, 2011; Lueck, 2006) and increased services for this large population of children who have CVI.

Concerns have been raised by some educators and educational administrators regarding who should provide educational services for children with CVI when they do not fit within the parameters of a country's or region's usual definitions for entitlement based on visual impairment. Finding ways to obtain such services can be problematic for the many children with CVI who "fall between the cracks" of existing service regulations. In addition, some professionals may not be aware of the complex array of possible behaviors that may manifest themselves as a result of CVI and therefore may not be equipped to identify children with this condition.

As mentioned in Sidebar 1.2, definitions of visual impairment based on measurement of visual acuity and visual field are slowly being replaced by functional definitions. These new classification systems move away from medical models that attempt to identify the extent of damage to organs, and instead focus on the behavioral effects of a condition within critical daily tasks that may affect the child's ability to participate optimally in society (Colenbrander, 2010). Over time, it is hoped, these newer methods used to characterize visual impairments will fully enter the mainstream and have an effect on entitlement criteria for governmental service programs for all children with CVI. Until this occurs, however, ways need to be found to serve these children through collaborative and cooperative efforts. Teachers of students with visual impairments, occupational therapists, orientation and mobility specialists, speech-language therapists, psychologists, medical specialists, caregivers, and other professionals need to work together to develop appropriate instructional programs and parenting strategies that address the multidimensional needs of children with CVI and their families within the framework of existing systems. In addition, advocacy efforts to modify existing service delivery systems are essential so that processes can be adjusted to support the growth, development, and learning of all children with CVI.

It is difficult when a new population of children with disability develops and is identified, as this places strains on existing service systems and stretches the limits of current professional expertise. This has happened before in the field of educating students with visual impairments as well as in other fields. One example took place with the move away from segregated schools for children who were blind to integrated local school programs, resulting from the increased number of children with visual impairment caused by retrolental fibroplasia (now called retinopathy of prematurity) in the 1940s and 1950s. Another significant change occurred when the number of children with visual impairments and multiple disabilities increased greatly as a consequence of the rubella epidemic in the 1960s. An additional instance was the profound shift in educational philosophy in the 1960s, when so-called sight conservation classes were discontinued and children with low vision were encouraged to use their vision. In all of these cases, professionals were required to expand their repertoire of skills and new service delivery methods were introduced (Hatlen, 2000). Similar changes are needed to promote the education of children who have CVI, guided by increased educational research in this area, expansion of training of personnel in professional preparation programs, improved design of accessible instructional environments, and advocacy that focuses on improved school services and service definitions.

## Conclusion

Although cerebral visual impairment is now the most common cause of visual impairment among children in the developed world (as documented in the introduction to this book), the understanding of how to characterize the disorder to make best use of vision and effectively teach children with CVI is in its infancy. Obtaining an in-depth knowledge and understanding of how each affected child sees the surrounding world and applying this knowledge to ensure that all children receive the services they need is now the primary focus of professionals working with children with CVI. The chapters that follow focus on important aspects of CVI and on related issues such as assessment and intervention in an effort to support professionals as they strive to gain and apply this understanding.

## References


Baker-Nobles, L., & Rutherford, A. (1995). Understanding cortical visual impairment in children. *American Journal of Occupational Therapy, 49*, 899–903.

Boot, F. H., Pel, J. J., Van der Steen, J., & Evenhuis, H. M. (2010). Cerebral visual impairment: Which perceptive visual dysfunctions can be expected in children with brain damage? A systematic review. *Research in Developmental Disability, 31*, 1149–1159.

Brodsky, M. C. (2010). *Pediatric neuro-ophthalmology* (2nd ed.). New York: Springer.

Carroll, T. J. (1956, August). Address to the Blinded Veterans Association, Milwaukee, WI. Accessed October 1, 2013 from http://carroll.org/about-the-carroll-center/our-founder/father-carrolls-transcripts/

Colenbrander, A. (2002, August). *Visual standards: Aspects and ranges of vision loss with emphasis on population surveys.* Report presented at the 29th International Congress of Ophthalmology, International Council of Ophthalmology, Sydney, Australia.

Colenbrander, A. (2010). Towards the development of a classification of vision related functioning—A potential framework. In G. N. Dutton & M. Bax (Eds.). *Visual impairment in children due to damage to the brain.* London: Mac Keith Press.

Colenbrander, A. (2011). Further response to the Letter to the Editor from James E. Jan [Letter to the editor]. *Journal of Visual Impairment & Blindness, 105*(2), 71–72.

Corn, A. L., & Erin, J. N. (Eds.). (2010). *Foundations of low vision: Clinical and functional perspectives* (2nd ed.). New York: AFB Press.

Dennison, E., & Lueck, A. H. (Eds.). (2006). *Proceedings of the summit on cerebral/cortical visual impairment: Educational, family, and medical perspectives, April 30, 2005.* New York: AFB Press.

Department of Veterans Affairs. (2008). *Blind rehabilitation outpatient specialist program procedures.* Washington, DC: Author. Accessed October 1, 2013 from http://www.va.gov/vhapublications/ViewPublication.asp?pub_ID=1763

Dutton, G. N., Ballantyne, J., Boyd, G., Bradnam, M., Day, R., McCulloch, D., . . . Saunders, K. (1996). Cortical visual dysfunction in children: A clinical study. *Eye, 10*, 302–309.

Dutton, G. N. (2003). Cognitive vision, its disorders and differential diagnosis in adults and children: Knowing where and what things are. *Eye, 17*(3), 289–304.

Dutton, G. N. (2008). Dorsal stream dysfunction and dorsal stream dysfunction plus: A potential classification for perceptual visual impairment in the context of cerebral visual impairment? *Developmental Medicine & Child Neurology, 10*, 1–2.

Dutton, G. N., & Bax, M. (Eds.). (2010). *Visual impairment in children due to damage to the brain.* London: Mac Keith Press.

Fazzi, E., Bova, S., Giovenzana, A., Signorini, S., Uggetti, C., & Bianchi, P. (2009). Cognitive visual dysfunctions in preterm children with periventricular leukomalacia. *Developmental Medicine & Child Neurology, 51*, 974–981.

Good, W. V. (2009). Cortical visual impairment: New directions. *Optometry and Visual Science, 86*, 663–665.

Good, W. V., Jan, J. E., Burden, S. K., Skoczenski, A., & Candy, R. (2001). Recent advances in cortical visual impairment. *Developmental Medicine & Child Neurology, 43*, 56–60.

Goodale, M. A., & Milner, A. D. (2013). *Sight unseen: An exploration of conscious and subconscious vision* (2nd ed.). New York: Oxford University Press.

Groenveld, M., Jan, J. E., & Leader, P. (1990). Observations on the habilitation of children with cortical visual impairment. *Journal of Visual Impairment & Blindness, 84,* 11–15.

Grusser, O.-J., & Landis, T. (1991). Visual agnosias and other disturbances of visual perception and cognition. In J. R. Cronly-Dillon (Ed.), *Vision and visual dysfunction: Vol. 12.* London: Macmillan Press.

Hatlen, P. (2000). Historical perspectives. In M. C. Holbrook & A. J. Koenig (Eds.), *Foundations of education: Volume I. History and theory of teaching children and youths with visual impairments* (2nd ed., pp. 1–54). New York: AFB Press.

Holmes, G. (1918a). Disturbances of vision caused by cerebral lesions. *British Journal of Ophthalmology, 2*, 353–384.

Holmes, G. (1918b). Disturbances of visual orientation. *British Journal of Ophthalmology, 2*, 449–468, 506–516.

Hoover, R. E. (1958). An American definition of blindness. *Optician, 136*(3514), 94–96.

Hoyt, C. S. (2003). Visual function in the brain-damaged child. *Eye, 17,* 371–386.

Hyvärinen, L., & Jacob, N. (2011). *WHAT and HOW does this child see?* Helsinki, Finland: VISTEST Ltd.

Hyvärinen, L., Walthes, R., Freitag, C., & Petz, V. (2012). Profile of visual functioning as a bridge between education and medicine in the assessment of impaired vision. *Strabismus, 20*, 63–68.

International Society for Low Vision Research and Rehabilitation. (1999). *Guide for the evaluation of visual impairment.* Presentation at Vision '99: International Conference on Low Vision, New York, NY. Accessed October 1, 2013 from http://www.ski.org/Colenbrander/Images/Visual_Impairmnt_Guide.pdf

Jacobson, L., Ek, U., Fernell, E., Flodmark, O., & Broberger, U. (1996). Visual impairment in preterm children with periventricular leukomalacia—Visual, cognitive and neuropaediatric characteristics related to cerebral imaging. *Developmental Medicine & Child Neurology, 38*(8), 724–735.

Jan, J. E. (2011). Cortical visual impairment is not the same as cerebral visual impairment [Letter to the editor]. *Journal of Visual Impairment & Blindness, 105*(2), 68–70.

Jan, J. E., & Groenveld, M. (1993). Visual behaviors and adaptations associated with cortical visual and ocular impairment in children. *Journal of Visual Impairment & Blindness, 87,* 101–105.

Jan, J. E., Groenveld, M., Sykanda, A. M., & Hoyt, C. S. (1987). Behavioural characteristics of children with permanent cortical visual impairment. *Developmental Medicine & Child Neurology, 29,* 571–576.

Jan, J. E., Heaven, R. K. B., Matsuba, C., Langley, M. B., Roman-Lantzy, C., & Anthony, T. L. (2013). Windows into the visual brain: New discoveries about the visual system, its functions, and implications for practitioners. *Journal of Visual Impairment & Blindness, 107*(4), 251–261.

Lueck, A. H. (Ed.). (2004a). *Functional vision: A practitioner's guide to evaluation and intervention.* New York: AFB Press.

Lueck, A. H. (2004b). Comprehensive low vision care. In A. H. Lueck (Ed.), *Functional vision: A practitioner's guide to evaluation and intervention* (p. 3). New York: AFB Press.

Lueck, A. H. (2006). Issues in intervention for children with visual impairment or visual dysfunction due to brain injury. In E. Dennison & A. H. Lueck (Eds.), *Proceedings of the summit on cerebral/cortical visual impairment: Educational, family, and medical perspectives, April 30, 2005* (pp. 121–130). New York: AFB Press.

Lueck, A. H., & Goodrich, G. L. (2011). Response to the letter to the editor from James E. Jan [Letter to the editor]. *Journal of Visual Impairment & Blindness, 105*(2), 70–71.

Milner, D., & Goodale, M. (2006). *The visual brain in action* (2nd ed.). New York: Oxford University Press.

Morse, M. T. (1990). Cortical visual impairment in young children with multiple disabilities.

*Journal of Visual Impairment & Blindness, 84*(5), 200–203.

National Eye Institute. (n.d.). Low vision and blindness rehabilitation. In *National plan for eye and vision research.* Bethesda, MD: Author. Accessed October 1, 2013 from http://www.nei.nih.gov/strategicplanning/np_low.asp

National Health Service. (2013, October). Visual Impairment [Online resource]. Accessed October 1, 2013 from http://www.nhs.uk/Conditions/Visual-impairment/Pages/Introduction.aspx

National Research Council. (2002). *Visual impairments: Determining eligibility for social security benefits.* Washington, DC: The National Academies Press.

Ortibus, E. L., De Cock, P. P., & Lagae, L. G. (2011). Visual perception in preterm children: What are we currently measuring? *Pediatric Neurology, 45,* 1–10.

Report of the Committee on the Definition of Blindness. (1934). *Journal of the American Medical Association, 103*(19), 1445–1446.

Riddoch, G. (1917). Dissociation of visual perception due to occipital injuries, with especial reference to the appreciation of movement. *Brain, 40,* 15.

Rizzo, M., & Vecera, S. P. (2002). Psychoanatomical substrates of Bálint's syndrome. *Journal of Neurology, Neurosurgery & Psychiatry, 72,* 162–178.

Roman-Lantzy, C. A. (2007). *Cortical visual impairment: An approach to assessment and intervention.* New York: AFB Press.

Social Security Administration. (1935). *The Social security act of 1935.* Woodlawn, MD: Author. Accessed October 1, 2013 from http://www.ssa.gov/history/35act.html

Social Security Administration. (2014). *If you are blind or have low vision–How we can help* [Publication No. 05-10052]. Woodlawn, MD: Author. Accessed October 1, 2013 from http://www.ssa.gov/pubs/EN-05-10052.pdf

Steendam, M. (2008). *Weet jij wat ik zie? Cerebrale visuele stoornissen bij kinderen, een handleiding voor professionals* [Do you know what I see? Cerebral visual impairment in children, a handbook for professionals]. Huizen, The Netherlands: Royal Dutch Visio.

U.S. Equal Employment Opportunity Commission. (n.d.). *Questions and answers about blindness and vision impairments in the workplace and the Americans with Disabilities Act (ADA).* Washington, DC: Author. Accessed October 1, 2013 from http://www.eeoc.gov/facts/blindness.html

Walton, J., Beeson, P. B., & Scott, R. B. (1986). *The Oxford companion to medicine.* New York: Oxford University Press.

Weiskrantz, L. (2009). *Blindsight: A case study spanning 35 years and new developments.* New York: Oxford University Press.

Williams, C., Northstone, K., Sabates, R., Feinstein, L., Emond, A., & Dutton, G. N. (2011). Visual perceptual difficulties and underachievement at school in a large community-based sample of children. *PLoS ONE, 6*(3), e14772.

World Health Organization. (2007). *International classification of functioning, disability and health: Children and youth version (ICF-CY).* Geneva, Switzerland: WHO Press.

Zeki, S. (1991). Cerebral akinetopsia (visual motion blindness): A review. *Brain, 114*(2), 811–824.

# 2

# The Brain and Vision

*Gordon N. Dutton*

The complexity of how the brain sees is enormous. Visual information provided by the eyes is processed in myriad interconnected processing elements throughout the brain, in which data provided by vision and the other senses are handled in an integrated way (Jan et al., 2013). For this reason, a simplified but workable model that explains what happens to vision when different parts of the brain are damaged is needed to guide a practical approach to thinking about assessment and intervention. This chapter, therefore, discusses the relationship between various parts of the brain and the roles they play in bringing about and sustaining vision. (Interested readers can find more detailed information in texts dedicated to this topic listed under "For Further Reading" at the end of this chapter.) Knowing how the visual system works and what can go wrong with it enables those working with children with cerebral visual impairment (CVI) to envision their difficulties and optimally plan their day-to-day management.

## The Parts of the Brain

At a very basic level (see Figure 2.1), the brain can be viewed as comprising the following parts:

- ***The occipital lobes,*** at the back of the brain, process information about visual images received by, and then transferred from, the eyes. They work in harmony with the posterior part of the parietal lobes, and with the temporal lobes (located under the temples), to generate vision.
- ***The frontal lobes,*** at the front of the brain, and particularly the prefrontal cortex on both sides, think, plan, and control behavior.
- ***The parietal lobes,*** in the middle of the brain, feel and move the body. They also process language—usually in the left side (or hemisphere) of the brain. As explained later in this chapter, the posterior portions support visual search and attention and serve visual guidance of movement.
- ***The temporal lobes,*** under the temples, analyze the input from the senses. They process language and speech production—according recognition and meaning—and provide the memory banks that underpin knowledge and image recognition.
- ***The cerebellum*** serves as a timekeeper, ensuring that emotion controlled by the frontal lobes, movement of the body processed by the parietal lobes, and vision processed by the occipital lobes are

FIGURE 2.1
**The Principal Regions of the Brain**

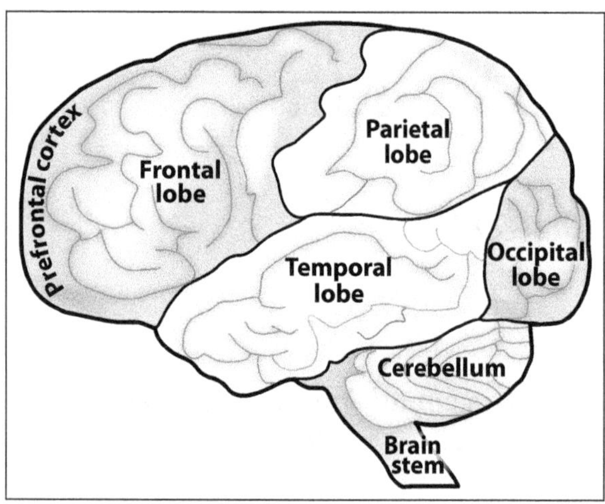


This illustration shows the left hemisphere of the brain.

synchronized and coordinated (Kaeser & Borruat, 2010; Kossorotoff et al., 2010).

- ***The brain stem,*** and above this, the midbrain (not shown), carry the nerves running in both directions between the brain and the spinal cord, to supply the body with nerves that bring about movement, sensation, and knowledge of position. The midbrain and brain stem also receive and process input from the nerves in the head (the cranial nerves) that serve hearing, eye movement, sensation of the head, and movement of the face and tongue. They also contribute to the maintenance of balance, control of heart and breathing rates, and auditory and visual alertness to hazards.

## The Brain's Role in Vision: How the Brain 'Sees'

Vision is automatic, and we take it for granted. We can look at a group of people and instantly recognize one of them, and, without thinking about it, *not* recognize everybody else. How does this happen? When we look at an apple, pick it up, and eat it, the tasks we perform are very complex, but we don't even think about them. How does the visual system help us accomplish these amazing feats?

The eye (see Figure 2.2) first creates a visual image that is conveyed to the brain. Sidebar 2.1 provides an overview of the structures of the eye and how the eye creates an image that is perceived by the brain. Not only does the photographic image of the people or the apple that is made inside the eye have to be converted into electrical signals, the information in these signals has to be carried to the brain and processed in a way that lets us "know" that what we are viewing is out in front of us. The picture of the visual scene, which the brain creates, gives us the overwhelming and compelling feeling that it is laid out in a three-dimensional array in front of us, yet the entire time, the picture that we see is actually being produced inside our brains.

Being able to recognize someone in a group and not recognize everyone else essentially means that we have a picture "library" in the brain that we can use to instantly compare with incoming image data. The matching face is recognized, but all the other incoming face pictures are instantly known to be "not known." We must therefore have a meaningful stored image library of everything that we may see, readily available and accessible, so that everything we look at is not only recognized, but its nature and character are implicitly understood. This library needs to be linked to predictive knowledge of the features of the particular image and available for forward planning

SIDEBAR 2.1

## How the Eye Creates an Image

Figure 2.2 depicts an eye that has been sliced through horizontally, as if viewed from above, to show the structures involved in receiving an image in the form of light, and converting it to electrical signals that are transmitted to the brain.

The *conjunctiva* is the transparent protective membrane that covers the white of the eye and the inside of the eyelids. It fuses with the surface of the *cornea*, the clear structure at the front of the eye like the glass on a watch, which transmits and focuses light as it enters the eye.

Light passes through the circular hole in the center of the colored *iris*, the *pupil*, and is focused by the *lens* onto the receptive lining inside the back of the eye, the *retina*.

The iris has muscle within it that makes the pupil constrict in light conditions and dilate in dark conditions.

The iris is continuous with the ciliary body that encircles and supports the transparent lens. Muscle inside the ciliary body contracts or elongates to change the shape of the lens. To view a visual target nearby, the ciliary muscles contract, and the supporting ligaments of the lens, or *zonules*, relax, making the lens more convex to bring the object into focus. When the ciliary muscles relax to bring distant targets into focus, this process, called *accommodation*, is reversed.

A clear liquid, called *aqueous fluid*, fills the space between the cornea and the lens. The fluid is made by the ciliary body. It flows through the posterior chamber and pupil and escapes into the bloodstream by permeating into the *canal of Schlemm*.

The eye is moved by six muscles that are attached to it. The *medial* (inner) *rectus* muscle turns the eye in and the *lateral* (outer) *rectus* muscle turns the eye out.

The retina receives the focused image of the eye's visual target. This image is converted by myriad elements—analogous to pixels—called *rods* (that see in the dark) and *cones* (that see in the light), into electrical signals that are transferred to over a million ganglion cells for onward transfer along the optic nerve to the brain.

The *fovea* is the part of the retina that provides more detailed perception to the central part of the image being seen. The *choroid* that underlies the retina is filled with blood vessels that supply nourishment and cool the retina. The tough *sclera* merges seamlessly with the cornea; together these two structures make up the protective outer coating of the eye.

FIGURE 2.2

### The Principal Structures of the Eye

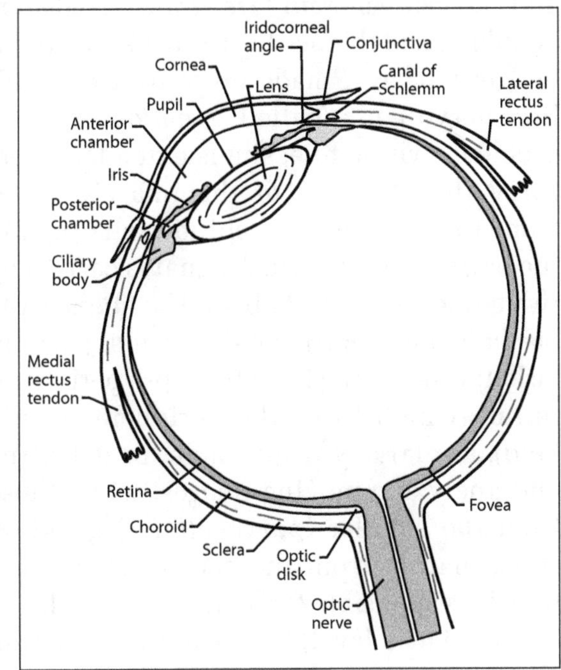

of our actions: "Ah! There are some apples in that basket. They'll be cold, smooth, firm, and round to the touch. I know what they will smell and taste like. I'll pick up the top one and eat it."

Conceptually, we are endowing the apple with the characteristics that its image conveys to our minds. The knowledge that the apple *is* an apple, and the knowledge of where it is with respect to our body, are processed in such a way that we can see the apple for what it is, choose it, reach out for it, and eat it. This complex set of visual recognition skills and visual guidance of movement skills is so ubiquitous throughout the animal kingdom that it tends to be taken for granted.

We are able to move freely and confidently without bumping into anything, when in fact we are in a sense, moving through the image generated inside our minds, making the tacit, automatic, and subconscious assumption that the image coincides with external reality. Even though everything we see is out in front of us, the "picture" of what we are seeing is inside our heads, and it is this mind picture that we know, attend to, see, learn from, recognize, react to, and move through.

Children who are born with disorders of the brain's visual system, and those who acquire such a disorder at an early age, have their own form of vision that is less effective than those with typical vision. The apple may not be seen or it may not be recognized; it may not be found, or it may not be accurately reached for. Only by understanding how normal vision works can one start to understand how vision that is impaired, in any of its manifestations, may affect the day-to-day living of an affected child.

## Conversion of Images into Electrical Signals

If you look closely at a picture on a television screen, you will see that it is made up of thousands of triplets of dots, which are very closely spaced. The dots, or pixels, are red, green, and blue. For seeing in daylight conditions, the retina functions in a similar way. Millions of color-registering cells called *cones* (which are interspersed among many more *rod* cells for seeing in dark conditions in shades of gray) are arrayed in a single layer in the outer part of the retina.

During daylight, the image entering the eye is registered by three types of cone cells that separately detect and determine the amount of incoming red, green, or blue light, which is then converted into electrical impulses. The electrical signals that the rods and cones generate are transferred—via double-ended (bipolar) nerve cells—to an inner retinal layer made up of over one million nerve cells (called *ganglion cells*) in each eye, whose fine, single extended fibers carry the elements of the image's signal along the optic nerves behind each eye, into the brain. This electrical signal is carried by two enmeshed sets of fibers. The fibers of the big (*magnocellular*) ganglion cells, particularly those coming from the more peripheral retina (which "see" the peripheral visual field), are largely responsible for detecting and analyzing moving images, while those from the smaller (*parvocellular*) ganglion cells, mainly from the central retina, are largely responsible for analyzing detail.

At a basic level, the visual information about an apple that is seen is principally relayed to the parts of the brain responsible for recognition by nerve fibers connecting to the parvocellular ganglion cells. Information about the location of the apple and its moment-to-moment position with respect to a moving hand about to grasp it is primarily relayed to the parts of the brain responsible for using vision to guide movement by fibers connecting to the magnocellular ganglion cells. The detail and identity of the apple (required to recognize it), and its location and size (required to bring about visual guidance of movement), are processed in two separate but interconnected parts of the brain.

FIGURE 2.3
**Visual Pathways from the Eyes to the Visual Cortex**

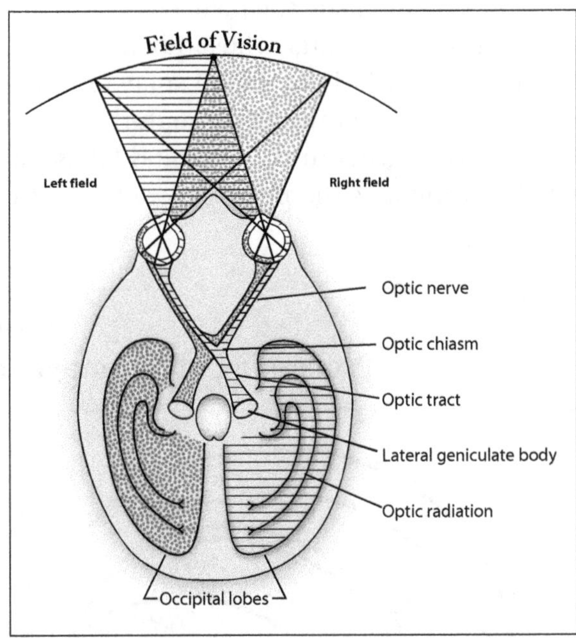


The shading in the diagram is used to illustrate how an image coming from different areas of the field of vision is transmitted to the eyes, through the optic nerves (which cross at the optic chiasm), and eventually reaches the visual cortex in the occipital lobes. The image on the right of the visual field is served by the left occipital lobe, and the field of vision on the left is served by the right occipital lobe.

## Transfer of Image Data to the Visual Cortex

### The Visual Pathways from the Eyes to the Occipital Lobes

The eye functions in a way similar to a digital camera, and the optic nerves and visual pathways (bundles of nerves) are analogous to the connections that run between the digital camera and a digital recorder. The electrical signals carried by the two main types of ganglion cells are conveyed to the brain. They are layered like transparent threads of silk over the back of the eye as they travel to, and coalesce in, the optic nerve head. From there they exit the eye through a circular channel into the optic nerve itself (see Figure 2.2). The constantly changing pictures that are formed by each eye are slightly different, and the information carried to the brain is joined together to generate a sensation of seeing in three dimensions, or *stereopsis*. (Stereopsis is deficient or absent in about 3 percent of the population, and commonly caused by misalignment of the eyes due to strabismus.)

Figure 2.3 illustrates the visual pathways from the eyes to the visual cortex located in the occipital lobes at the back of the brain. As the two optic nerves enter the skull they combine together in a cross (called the *optic chiasm*) where the nerve fibers intermingle in such a way that the picture "seen" on the right side by both eyes is sent to the left side of the brain, and the picture "seen" on the left side by both eyes is sent to the right side of the brain.

The two bundles of retinal ganglion cell nerve fibers that emerge out of the back of the optic chiasm, one on each side, are called the *optic tracts*. The optic tracts terminate in little knee-shaped structures deep inside the brain called the *lateral geniculate* (from the Latin: resembling a knee) bodies. Here, the magnocellular and parvocellular fibers relay their information, in separate layers, to the next set of nerve cells whose fibers emerge as the optic radiations. These splay out and pass in curved pathways through the brain before terminating in the occipital lobes, in what is known as the *primary visual cortex* (or V1), where fundamental image processing takes place.

The processing of an image in the primary visual cortex is illustrated in Figure 2.4, which shows a person looking straight at the center of a clock face. The clock face is divided into four quadrants, each indicated by a different pattern, so that the location in the brain of that portion of the image

FIGURE 2.4
**Processing of an Image in the Primary Visual Cortex**

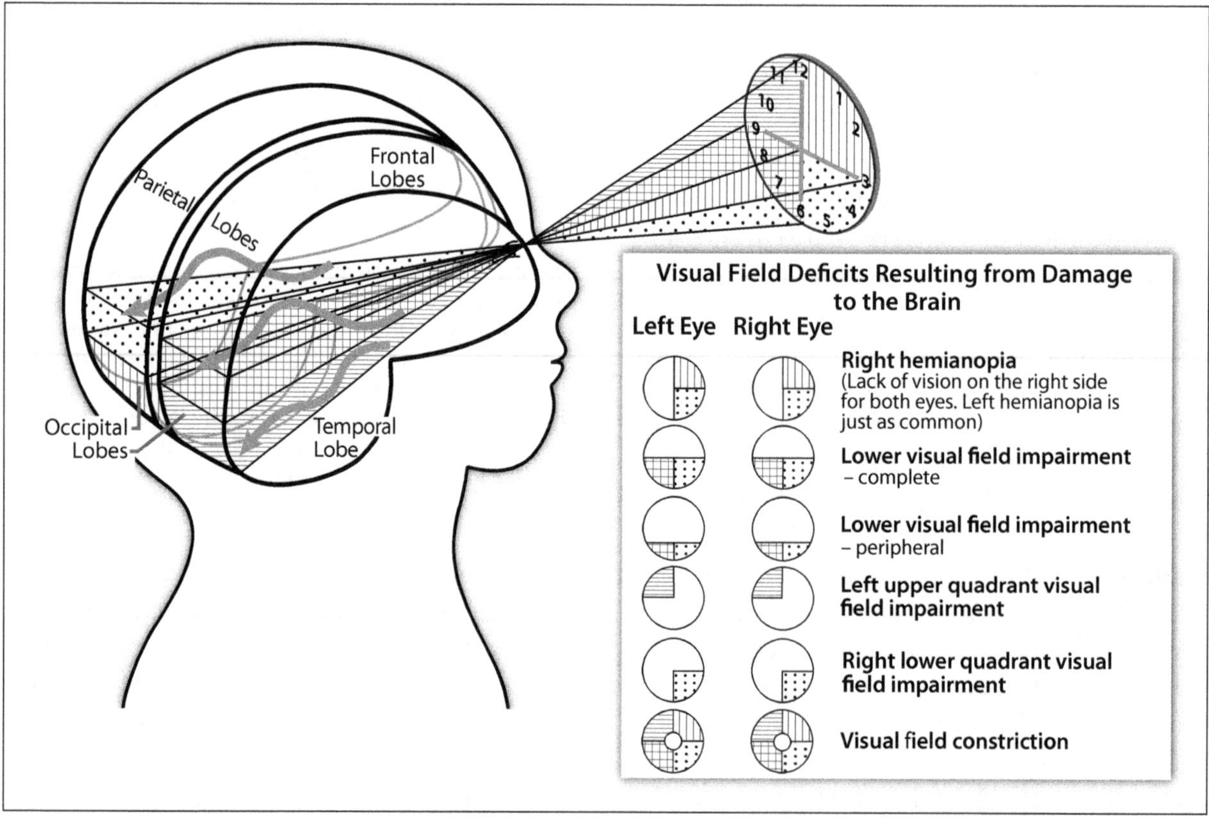


The shading of the four quadrants of the clock face in this diagram corresponds to the shading of the location of the image in the brain, when the individual stares directly at the center of the clock face. The upper flowing arrows denote the upper optic radiation pathways running over the top of the lateral ventricles in the parietal lobes. The lower sinuous arrows denote the lower optic radiation pathways that curve around the lateral ventricles, into the temporal lobes, before reaching the occipital lobes. Typical patterns of visual field deficits and approximate locations of the causative damage in the brain are indicated in the box within the figure. The shading indicating missing vision in these diagrams of the visual field of each eye corresponds to the location in the brain where the damage causing the visual field loss is located.

can be traced. For both eyes, the image is optically formed both horizontally and vertically inverted on the retina. The image data are conveyed to and processed in this same orientation in the occipital lobes. So, for example, the area on the clock between the numbers 12 and 3, in the upper right-hand quadrant of the clock, is conveyed to and processed in the lower portion of the left occipital lobe.

The wavy arrows in Figure 2.4 represent the pathways taken by nerve fibers in the optic radiations, where, if they are damaged, the patterns of visual field impairment shown in the diagram occur. The upper visual optic radiations arch up and over the top of the *lateral ventricles* (the water spaces in the brain), through the posterior parietal lobes. The lower visual pathways loop around the "horns" of the lateral ventricles through the temporal lobes.

## Patterns of Visual Field Impairment Due to Damage in the Optic Tract and Optic Radiations

The box in Figure 2.4 illustrates some common patterns of visual field impairment due to damage to the brain. The circles represent the visual field of each eye; the shading matches the locations of the damage within the brain, as well as the portion of the visual image (in this case, the clock face) that the individual would be unable to see.

If there is damage to an optic tract, it causes a blind spot in the field of vision on the side opposite to the damage. Similarly, if there is a discrete area of damage in one optic radiation, it will also cause a small blind area (which is either very similar or identical for each eye) in the corresponding visual field. By plotting the size and location of the blind area or areas within the field of vision in each eye, one can work out where the damage in the brain is likely to be. For example, damage to the left optic tract or optic radiation causes right-sided lack of vision called *hemianopia*, which is very similar (or *homonymous*) in both eyes. The result is *homonymous hemianopia*, a term and condition frequently encountered by those working with children with visual impairments as a result of damage to the brain.

Similarly, if there is damage to the optic radiations at the top of the brain at the back on both sides, where the nerve fibers of the optic radiations curve into the posterior parietal lobes, then it is important to check for lower visual field impairment in both eyes. Reversing the concept, if a child has impairment of the lower visual field of both eyes, then the most likely cause is damage to the upper *periventricular* fibers (or white matter) in the posterior parietal lobes. When bilateral lower visual field impairment is marked, the damage can be seen on MRI imaging. However, in the author's experience, when damage affects the peripheral portions of the lower visual field only, MRI imaging may appear normal, making an analysis of the visual field a useful way of knowing, by inference, that there is damage in this area of the brain, and plotting it, even though the damage is not necessarily evident on MRI scanning.

Damage to the visual pathways in the brain can be more localized and less extensive so that only a quarter of the visual field is affected. As shown in Figure 2.4, a child who cannot see the numbers 1 and 2 while looking at the center of a clock likely has damage at the back of the brain in the temporal lobe, on the left at the bottom, because the lower optic radiation fibers curve into this area. The child who cannot see the numbers 4 and 5 probably has damage at the back of the brain in the posterior parietal lobe, on the left at the top. Similar inferences can be made for inability to see the numbers 10 and 11 (damage to the right temporal lobe), and 7 and 8 (damage to the right posterior parietal lobe). (When the eyes look around the clock face, the numbers flit in and out of view as the eyes move and the visual field deficit moves with them; it is only when the center of the clock face is viewed that this description and analysis apply.)

## Analysis of the Image Data by the Occipital Lobes and Motion Perception Centers

The visual cortex in the occipital lobes receives the electrical signals from the optic radiations and sorts the information out into its component parts. The elements of the visual scene are analyzed by tens of millions of cells that are responsible for seeing detail (the lower limit at maximum contrast comprising the individual's visual acuity), discriminating shades of gray from one another (contrast sensitivity), color perception, three-dimensional perception (*stereopsis*), the area which can be seen (the visual fields), and the orientation and dimensions of the elements of the image. As already mentioned, the left occipital lobe "sees" the right side of the visual scene and the right occipital lobe "sees" the left side of the visual scene. Moreover, the lower visual cortex in the occipital lobes "sees" the upper part of the scene and the upper visual cortex "sees" the lower part of the scene.

Children with damage to the occipital lobes, shown as boxes at the back of the brain in Figure 2.4, can therefore also have a range of different visual field defects corresponding to the damage in the same manner already described for damage to the optic tracts and radiations. Thus, damage to the right occipital lobe causes loss of vision on the left side (for both eyes), and damage to the upper part of both occipital lobes (or the upper incoming pathways to the occipital lobes) results in the lower visual field being impaired, so that an affected child is unable to see the ground when looking straight ahead and may tend to trip over things.

The middle temporal lobes are the motion perception centers, and are shown in Figure 2.5 (the boxes labeled "motion" in the diagram). They are found on each side of the brain just in front of the occipital lobes. They not only register and perceive movement within the visual scene, they also contribute crucial information to inform visual guidance of movement. As one moves, the surroundings are seen to "move" in an equal and opposite direction.

Both the parvocellular visual pathways, mainly serving the perception of image, and the magnocellular visual pathways, mainly serving the perception of movement, are conducted to the occipital lobes, but there is evidence that some of the magnocellular fibers go directly to the middle temporal lobes, and are thought to contribute to visual guidance of movement of the body as an automatic, subconscious visual function. This relationship becomes very significant in the rare adults and children whose occipital lobes are damaged by lack of a blood supply, but whose middle temporal lobe territories and their functions have been spared, leading to the paradox of the persisting ability to move accurately through a scene that is ostensibly invisible to the individual (as noted in Chapter 1 and discussed in Chapter 3) (Goodale et al., 2008).

FIGURE 2.5

**Principal Locations and Pathways in the Brain for Image Processing**

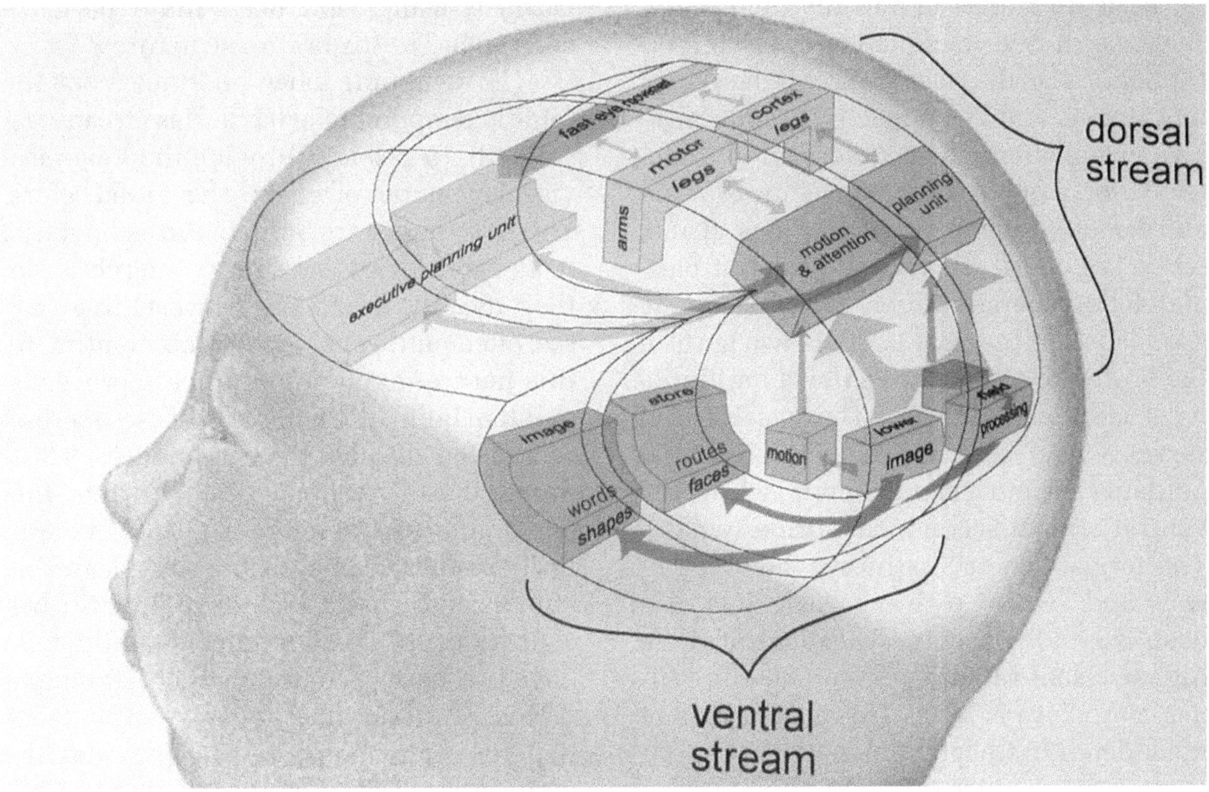

This stylized diagram illustrates the locations in the brain where image processing takes place and the principal interconnecting pathways, including the dorsal stream and the ventral stream.

*Source:* Reproduced with permission from Nature Publishing Group from Dutton, G. N. (2003). Cognitive vision, its disorders and differential diagnosis in adults and children: Knowing where and what things are. *Eye, 17*(3), 289–304.

## Ventral and Dorsal Stream Pathways

It takes about one-tenth of a second for information that is received about the visual scene to reach the occipital lobes. During the next tenth of a second, the visual information is conveyed to be analyzed in two separate ways by two main areas—the temporal lobes and the posterior parietal lobes. As shown in Figure 2.5, the visual pathway between the occipital lobes and the temporal lobes is called the *ventral stream;* it supports the process of visual recognition and is therefore sometimes called the "what" pathway. The visual pathway between the occipital lobes and the posterior parietal lobes is called the *dorsal stream* (sometimes called the "where" pathway). The posterior parietal lobes subconsciously capture, and briefly hold on to, the moment-to-moment visual information about all the visible items in the surrounding scene needed to bring about visual guidance of movement, visual search, and the facility to switch attention from one element of the scene to another.

In-depth studies of how the "higher" visual system (the combination of visual perception, visual cognition, guidance of movement, and the capacity to choose to give visual attention, as described in Chapter 1) works indicate that the ventral stream and temporal lobes serve conscious vision, while the dorsal stream and posterior parietal lobes operate largely subconsciously (Goodale & Milner, 2013). These two parts of the brain are closely linked by a multiplicity of additional pathways. The dorsal stream serves visual search (where?) and visual guidance of movement (how?), while the ventral stream serves recognition (what?). The terms "where" pathway, "how" pathway, and "what" pathway have thus also been used to conceptually represent these higher visual functions (Goodale and Milner, 1992; Vecera, 2002). This is described in more detail in Chapter 6.

## Visual Recognition and Orientation: The Temporal Lobes and Ventral Stream Pathways

When you walk down a busy street and recognize someone, your brain has accomplished a fantastic computing task for you. First, you probably know where you are going. Then, for every person you do not recognize, you have compared the facial appearance of that person with your personal store of hundreds, if not thousands, of faces. When it does not match, you walk past that person. When you meet the person you recognize, you have a matching comparison, which allows you to greet your friend. You can also communicate freely by recognizing the language conveyed by the facial expressions that your friend is using. How does this experience correspond to the brain's structures?

The temporal lobes (distinct from the middle temporal lobe territories already described), in essence, provide the long-term visual memories of what we have seen before. These memories are built up throughout life. If one carefully observes very young children, they usually try to touch everything they see, often putting objects in their mouths. As this natural exploration process proceeds, children build up their image libraries, cross-referenced through the other senses. (Children whose cerebral palsy restricts this exploration are therefore likely to have similarly restricted image libraries.) Scanning studies of the brain (Schiltz, Dricot, Goebel, & Rossion, 2010) and studies of adults who have had damage to the right or left temporal lobe (Dutton, 2003) have shown evidence that the right temporal lobe provides the main image library of all the faces one has remembered and recognizes, while the left temporal lobe provides the main library of the shapes and objects one expects to recognize in everyday life, like a pen in the foreground or a tree in the distance (see the two areas labeled "image store," one for "words and shapes," the other for "routes and faces" in Figure 2.5).

Brain scans of infants shown pictures of faces display increased activity in the right temporal lobe, with extra activity in the left temporal lobe when their mother's faces are shown (Nakato et al., 2011). This remarkable phenomenon begins to shed light on how we learn to recognize what we are looking at. In a sense, the temporal lobes resemble a computer search engine. Image data that come in are sent to the search engine to identify whether what is being looked at is known. If it is, recognition takes place. If it is not, the person being viewed is seen to be a stranger, and the new incoming image data are stored for future recognition, but are slowly lost with time if the stranger is not seen again.

People who have had damage to the right temporal lobe can lose the ability to recognize faces, and also tend to lose their ability to find their way around and can become profoundly lost. The progressive brain disorder of Alzheimer's disease and other forms of dementia lead to gradual onset impairment in recognition of people, often accompanied by a tendency to get lost, as a result of the right temporal lobe being affected. Inability to recognize people (which can be complete or incomplete) is called *prosopagnosia* and the tendency to get lost is called *topographic agnosia* (as discussed further in Chapter 3). If the left temporal lobe is damaged, the ability to recognize shapes and objects can be diminished or lost, and this is known as *shape and object agnosia*. However, these general assertions are not absolutely specific, and a range of patterns of visual disability can be seen when the temporal lobes of the brain are damaged (Milner & Goodale, 2006).

Children who have had damage to the ventral stream functional pathways, or the temporal lobes, or both—most commonly on both sides—can experience difficulty in distinguishing objects and different types of animals, as well as recognizing people's faces. They may also be unable to recognize language conveyed by facial expressions. Similarly, route finding can be very difficult, both on a large scale when out and about, and on a small scale in the home, where, for example, it can be particularly difficult to know in which drawer items are kept.

## Visual Guidance of Movement, Visual Search, and Attention: The Posterior Parietal Lobes and Dorsal Stream Pathways

The back of the brain at the top (or *posterior parietal cortex)* is responsible for handling a lot of information at the same time. It works in a way analogous to the RAM in a computer: it allows us to hold open lots of functions simultaneously. If you look at a complicated visual scene such as a class of school children, while looking at one child in the middle, you are able to pick out another child and immediately change your gaze and attention to that second child. In order to do this, you have to maintain an awareness of the whole class. This is an enormously complex computing task. To make matters more complicated, you may have had to make this choice while all the children were trying to attract your attention and create a lot of background noise. While your frontal lobes are making the choices, the posterior parietal lobes of your brain are providing them with the unconscious framework for you to do this. They temporarily store the three-dimensional image data from moment-to-moment, in such a way that you can move freely without bumping into anything (Milner & Goodale, 2006).

If there is damage to the dorsal stream pathways on both sides, the posterior parietal lobes, or both, the ability to handle a lot of information at one time is decreased. A child with such damage probably sees the world in a way similar to a baby. Babies, in their first few months of life, tend to concentrate on one thing at a time. That is why books for babies present large single images, because it is known that infants respond to one or two pictures, but not more. Likewise, when babies listen to music, they are less aware of other things happening around them.

The motor cortex of the brain is responsible for bringing about movement of the body. In an adult who has had a stroke and who cannot move the right side of the body, it is commonly the left motor cortex or its pathways that have been damaged. The top of the motor cortex is responsible for moving the foot, and the side of the motor cortex is responsible for moving the hand (see Figure 2.5).

The task of picking up an apple involves both the visual system and the motor cortex. The apple has to be recognized, and this information is provided by the temporal lobes. The size, orientation, and location of the apple are plotted in the moment-to-moment, unconscious, three-dimensional virtual map provided by the posterior parietal lobes. The decision to pick up the apple is made in the frontal lobes, and this information is used by the motor cortex, which brings about the act of picking up the apple. To do this, the hand is shaped so that the fingers are separated far enough apart to encompass the apple. Once the hand has reached the right position, the fingers grasp the apple and pick it up. Throughout this task, the visual system and the movement system are working in perfect harmony. The picture of the apple was formed in the occipital lobes, and recognized in the temporal lobes. It was mapped by the parietal lobes. The choice to pick it up was made by the frontal lobes, the action was brought about by the motor cortex, while the whole performance was integrated by the ventral stream (consciously), the dorsal stream (subconsciously), and many other brain pathways.

When we cross a road and step up onto a curb, a similar instruction has to be given to the feet. Children with damage to the dorsal stream may have difficulty reaching accurately for objects or moving their feet to a correct location in visual space. This can mean that they have difficulty interpreting whether a line or pattern on the floor is a step or not (needing to first probe the floor junction with their foot to provide additional information through touch) and difficulty working out how far the foot has to be lifted up in order to navigate over a curb. It is possible that dorsal stream fibers responsible for moving the feet through visual space are damaged, while the dorsal stream fibers responsible for moving the hands are not, in which case reaching is accurate but movement of the legs is not. Associated impairment of the lower visual field, resulting from damage to the incoming visual pathways of the occipital lobe, which are likely to be close to the dorsal stream pathways, may compound the problem and make it difficult to determine the relative contribution of each element (Dutton et al., 2004). (These statements by the author are currently observational in nature and await further research.)

The dorsal stream works automatically and unconsciously. When it is damaged, the resulting outcomes of impairment in visual search (due to lack of ability to simultaneously process multiple elements of the visual scene) and impaired visual guidance of movement (known as optic ataxia) do not usually give rise to complaint (because one cannot easily be aware of loss of a subconscious function). The result is a difficulty finding things, associated with clumsiness, which is noticeable by others. However, these problems are often not interpreted as visual difficulties, despite being profoundly disabling. In children with cerebral palsy and impaired dorsal stream function, impaired subconscious visual guidance of movement commonly compounds the motor impairment; the term for this is *visual-motor dysfunction.*

The front part of the brain (the frontal lobes) has many functions. One of these is to bring about movement of the head and eyes to look at a new target location. When the dorsal stream is damaged, the ability to accurately move the head and eyes to this new location is decreased, and such movements can either be inaccurate or may not be possible at all. This means that it can be difficult to follow and track moving objects because the dorsal stream pathway, which "tells" the head and eyes where to look next, via the frontal lobes, is not functioning properly. This is known as *apraxia of gaze.*

In light of this information, reading difficulties experienced by individuals with damage to the dorsal stream can be understood (Vidyasagar & Pammer, 2010). Not only can printed information on the same page not all be seen and appreciated at the same time, but it may be difficult to move the head and eyes accurately to a new location in order to access the information. (An effective educational approach in such cases would include presenting small numbers of words at the same time, enlarging them, increasing their spacing in both directions, or when especially difficult, showing them one after another, for example, on a computer screen. The amount of information that can be handled at one time varies considerably, and has to be determined for each child.)

In essence, the parietal lobe houses three automatic, subconscious functional systems: one that informs the prefrontal cortex of the location of an item, so that attention can be given and choices can be made; one that provides an internalized three-dimensional map of the surroundings to visually guide movement brought about by the premotor and motor areas of the brain; and one that facilitates navigation interlinked with the memory systems of the hippocampi (a seahorse-shaped structure within each temporal lobe), which contribute to spatial awareness and memory (Kravits, Saleem, Baker, & Mishkin, 2011).

The dorsal stream and ventral stream pathways work together in harmony, because when something is seen and recognized using our temporal lobes, we are able to elect (with the frontal lobes) to reach out and pick it up, using the dorsal stream system. However, when brain damage takes place, specific elements of these tasks are deficient, and it can be difficult to understand why an affected child is seen to be able to do one thing but not another.

## Conscious and Subconscious Vision

The conscious visual system allows us to see and understand the world around us. Incoming visual information is processed, analyzed, understood, and acted upon. At birth, the visual brain is rather like an empty library with different sections reserved for different sets of books. As a young child grows and develops, the visual system is being programmed. New experiences are progressively stored, and the visual system is being built up.

How often have we heard the expression, "Look where you're going!"? The fact is, we do not look where we are going. Like all other sighted animals, we move through the visual world without giving it a thought, by using our subconscious visual systems. Most people, when they first learn how to drive a car, find steering difficult until they look into the distance, at which point it becomes much easier. Although we check the view ahead to choose where we are going, we use our peripheral vision in a subconscious way to drive a car, move through a crowd, or walk over uneven ground.

We often need to take evasive action. Whether one is ducking one's head to avoid hitting a kitchen cupboard door or dodging an oncoming child, it is our subconscious safety system that is coming into play.

Progressive improvement in driving skill shows that certain aspects of our subconscious visual system can be trained, whereas the remarkable automatic systems that we and other animals have for self-protection are based on reflexes that develop spontaneously. From a practical point of view there are two subconscious visual systems that guide movement: the high-level system facilitated by the dorsal stream that allows us to move effortlessly through the visual world while talking or thinking about something else; and an additional protective reflex system, which makes us brake suddenly when a child runs out in front of the car. This second system calls forth our adrenaline and makes us feel drained afterward because of the amount of effort involved in such subconsciously generated evasive action. Only after the event do we recognize what our visual system and reflex evasive action have done for us.

## The Reflex Visual Centers: The Primitive Visual Brain

A child with profound damage to the visual brain might appear to have no vision but may respond to a moving target, particularly if it is in the peripheral field of vision. Another child with profound visual impairment due to brain damage may be able to move around without bumping into things. This kind of vision, which appears to be a low-level form of *blindsight* (Boyle, Jones, Hamilton, Spowart, & Dutton, 2005), sometimes also referred to as "travel vision" (Jan, Wong, Groenveld, Flodmark, & Hoyt, 1986), can be thought of as the ability to respond to visual stimuli that one cannot consciously see.

The primitive visual brain is supported by the upper midbrain and part of the thalamus, deep within the brain. These parts of the brain are responsible for protecting us from danger. We are not truly aware of this visual system until after it has worked, because it functions subconsciously. If you dodge a moving ball or have a near miss while driving, it is your primitive visual brain that helps protect you. It detects a peripheral movement and automatically initiates movement of your body before you are even aware of what you are doing (Tamietto et al., 2010).

There is an even more remarkable visual reflex that the primitive visual brain is thought to serve: the ability to respond to a facial expression, despite having little or no detectable vision as a result of damage to the visual pathways in the brain. This condition has been observed in a number of adults and has been called *affective blindsight* (deGelder, Vroomen, Pourtois, & Weiskrantz, 1999).

In children who have profound brain damage that has caused very poor vision, peripheral motion detection can be present and appears to function at a subconscious level. Many such children who are mobile may be able to walk around objects in their path despite appearing to have little, if any, detectable vision. Some children who cannot move their four limbs may detect a moving spoon if it is at their side and open their mouths more readily than if the spoon comes from straight ahead. This reaction may be caused by the primitive visual system. In some such cases, the system may be affected by fatigue, because it may appear to work initially, then doesn't work, but will work again after resting (Boyle et al., 2005).

## Visual Attention

*Visual attention*, or the ability to focus on specific elements in the visual scene, is needed to register what we see (Das, Bennett, & Dutton, 2007) and is related to visual processing. (In Chapter 6, visual attention is considered from the perspective of how the frontal area of the brain serves the capacity to choose what to give attention to.) The amount we can see at any moment is limited by the amount that can be processed by the brain at one time, and how quickly it can be processed. While awake and alert, we constantly see what is around us, but we can only look at and react to part of the scene at once. We miss things that move too quickly to be seen, do not stand out, or are not being given attention, especially if our attention is focused elsewhere (Boynton, 2005).

Attention is both subconscious and conscious. Background, subconscious visual attention prevents us from bumping into things, by simultaneously dealing with the salient items of the moving visual scene through parallel processing of the relevant information. Elements that are sufficiently different, due to their movement, bright color, or contrast, are drawn to our conscious attention because they "pop out." In contrast, the conscious visual attention that we use to recognize faces and words, for example, is slower, because it functions sequentially (processing information in a series), focusing on one thing after another.

A large part of the brain is devoted to the process of visual attention. The brain stem, at the top of the spinal cord, and the thalamus help deal with the subconscious computing process required to move around freely using visual guidance. The act of making a choice, paying conscious attention, and moving toward and picking something up, is initiated in the frontal lobes. This process is integrated with conscious analysis of imagery carried out by the occipital lobes and ventral stream structures. (These processes give an identity to the salient items that were unconsciously seen and processed by the parietal lobes.)

The act of looking at a scene and choosing an item from within it involves a lot of brain activity. The ability to find and identify someone in a crowd requires that person's image to be retrieved from the memory store in the temporal lobe area of the brain, in order to compare it with the faces in the crowd, until the face being sought is found and identified. During this process, distractions are actively relegated into the background (Nobre, 2001). This process also involves considerable "computing power."

Visual attention develops progressively as a child grows up. The newborn infant is only able to attend to one thing at a time, but learns to split attention between his or her parents a few weeks later. This ability develops progressively. Visual attention competes with sound, smell, discomfort, pain, and the child's thoughts and imagination. Teachers, in general, are aware of the advantages of minimizing these distractors (Lueck & Heinze, 2004).

Damage in any area of the brain related to visual attention—whether subtle or severe—can interfere with subconscious or conscious visual attention, depending on which parts of the attention and visual brain systems have been damaged. Impairment of subconscious attention may lead to colliding with obstacles, tripping and being clumsy, and an inability to find people or objects in patterned or cluttered scenes. Impairment of conscious attention leads to an apparent lack of focus and concentration, with errors being made in relation to recognition. The outcome of both types of difficulty, as far as an observer is concerned, is that an affected child does not appear to see as well as other children, particularly when tired. When CVI interferes significantly with attention, the affected child who is listening may not appear to be able to see until the distracting sound is eliminated. As a result, many children with CVI show improvement in visual performance and behavior when visual and other distractions are kept to a minimum; therefore, distractions from pattern, clutter, and sound need to be kept to a minimum.

## The Mirror Neuron System

Children learn by copying the behavior they see in others. This imitation is a complex process. There is considerable evidence that there is a network of visual processing in the human brain, called the *mirror neuron system*, which helps in understanding the actions of others. This system also underpins the ability to learn by observing the actions of others and copying them appropriately and in context (Cattaneo & Rizzolatti, 2009). As yet, little is known about the development of this system in children and how it is impaired by disorders of vision, but it may be affected in children who have difficulties with visual input or processing.

Professionals involved in the education and habilitation of children with early-onset CVI, therefore, need to recognize that limitations in the capacity of the mirror neuron system to facilitate imitation may impair the ability to learn. Children can only learn by copying the actions of others if their intent and purpose are accessible to them.

## Conclusion

The process of vision is complex. The eyes function like a pair of cameras that are constantly kept in focus by changing the shape of the lens, or accommodation. The information about the image that they create is fed as a constant data stream along the optic nerves to the brain. The optic chiasm rearranges the visual information so that the left side of the brain "sees" the right visual scene and vice versa. The visual information is processed at a fundamental level in the occipital lobes of the brain. Two principal systems serve the higher visual functions. The posterior parietal lobes (via the dorsal stream system) underpin visual search and attention and bring about visual guidance of movement. They function unconsciously. The temporal lobes (via the ventral stream system) provide image recognition, a conscious function. These two systems are closely interconnected. Finally, the upper midbrain affords the ability to rapidly, unconsciously, and reflexively avoid hazards. Visual attention is controlled by the frontal lobe of the brain, making use of this network.

These complex visual systems are seamlessly interconnected, but when they are damaged, the ways in which they work can become apparent. Chapter 3 provides a more detailed account of how disorders of the brain in children affect their vision.

## For Further Reading

Duckman, R. H. (2006). *Visual development, diagnosis, and treatment of the pediatric patient.* Philadelphia: Lippincott Williams & Wilkins.

Goldberg, S., & Trattler, W. (2012). *Ophthalmology made ridiculously simple* (5th ed.). Miami, FL: Medmaster Books.

Goodale, M., & Milner, D. (2013). *Sight unseen: An exploration of conscious and unconscious vision* (2nd ed.). New York: Oxford University Press (This book provides a basic account of the dorsal and ventral stream systems and how they function.)

Ledford, J. K. (2008). *The little eye book: A pupil's guide to understanding ophthalmology* (2nd ed.). Thorofare, NJ: Slack Incorporated.

## References

Boyle, N. J., Jones, D. H., Hamilton, R., Spowart, K. M., & Dutton, G. N. (2005). Blindsight in children: Does it exist and can it be used to help the child? Observations on a case series. *Developmental Medicine & Child Neurology, 47,* 699–702.

Boynton, G. M. (2005). Attention and visual perception. *Current Opinion in Neurobiology, 15,* 465–469.

Cattaneo, L., & Rizzolatti, G. (2009). The mirror neuron system. *Archives of Neurology, 66*(5), 557–560.

Das, M., Bennett, D. M., & Dutton, G. N. (2007). Visual attention as an important visual function: An outline of manifestations, diagnosis and management of impaired visual attention. *British Journal of Ophthalmology, 91,* 1556–1560.

deGelder, B., Vroomen, J., Pourtois, G., & Weiskrantz, L. (1999). Non-conscious recognition of affect in the absence of striate cortex. *NeuroReport, 10*(18), 3759–3763.

Dutton, G. N. (2003). Cognitive vision, its disorders and differential diagnosis in adults and children: Knowing where and what things are. *Eye, 17*(3), 289–304.

Dutton, G. N., Saaed, A., Fahad, B., Fraser, R., McDaid, G., McDade, J., . . . Spowart, K. (2004). Association of binocular lower visual field impairment, impaired simultaneous perception, disordered visually guided motion and inaccurate saccades in children with cerebral visual dysfunction—A retrospective observational study. *Eye, 18,* 27–34.

Goodale, M. A., & Milner, A. D. (1992). Separate visual pathways for perception and action. *Trends in Neurosciences, 15*(1), 20–25.

Goodale, M. A., & Milner, A. D. (2013). *Sight unseen: An exploration of conscious and unconscious vision* (2nd ed.). New York: Oxford University Press.

Goodale, M. A., Wolf, M. E., Whitwell, R. L., Brown, L. E., Cant, J. S., Chapman C. S., . . . Dutton, G. N. (2008). Perception and action: How dissociated are they? Preserved motion processing and visuomotor control in a patient with large bilateral lesions of occipitotemporal cortex. *Journal of Vision, 8*(6), 371.

Jan, J. E., Heaven, R. K. B., Matsuba, C., Langley, M. B., Roman-Lantzy, C., & Anthony, T. L. (2013). Windows into the visual brain: New discoveries about the visual system, its functions, and implications for practitioners. *Journal of Visual Impairment & Blindness, 107*(4), 251–261.

Jan, J. E., Wong, P. K., Groenveld, M., Flodmark, O., & Hoyt, C. S. (1986). Travel vision: "Collicular visual system"? *Pediatric Neurology, 2,* 359–362.

Kaeser, P. F., & Borruat, F. X. (2010). Altered vision during motion: An unusual symptom of cerebellar dysfunction, quantifiable by a simple clinical test. *Acta Ophthalmologica, 88,* 791–796.

Kossorotoff, M., Gonin-Flambois, C., Gitiaux, C., Quijano, S., Boddaert, N., Bahi-Buisson, N., . . . Desguerre, I. (2010). A cognitive and affective pattern in posterior fossa strokes in children: A case series. *Developmental Medicine & Child Neurology, 52,* 626–631.

Kravits, D. J., Saleem, K. S., Baker, C. I., & Mishkin, M. (2011). A new neural framework for visuospatial processing. *Neuroscience, 12,* 217–230.

Lueck, A. H., & Heinze, T. (2004). Interventions for young children with visual impairments and students with visual and multiple disabilities. In A. H. Lueck (Ed.), *Functional vision: A practitioner's guide to evaluation and intervention* (pp. 277–351). New York: AFB Press.

Milner, A. D., & Goodale, M. A. (2006). *The visual brain in action* (2nd ed.). New York: Oxford University Press.

Nakato, E., Otsuka, Y., Kanazawa, S., Yamaguchi, M. K., Honda, Y., & Kakigi, R. (2011). I know this face: Neural activity during mother's face perception in 7- to 8-month-old infants as investigated by near-infrared spectroscopy. *Early Human Development, 87,* 1–7.

Nobre, A. C. (2001). The attentive homunculus: Now you see it, now you don't. *Neuroscience & Biobehavioral Reviews, 25,* 477–496.

Schiltz, C., Dricot, L., Goebel, R., & Rossion, B. (2010). Holistic perception of individual faces in the right middle fusiform gyrus as evidenced by the composite face illusion. *Journal of Vision, 26*(10), 25.1–16.

Tamietto, M., Cauda, F., Corazzini, L. L., Savazzi, S., Marzi, C. A., Goebel, R., et al. (2010). Collicular vision guides nonconscious behavior. *Journal of Cognitive Neuroscience, 22,* 888–902.

Vecera, S. P. (2002). Dissociating "what" and "how" in visual form agnosia: A computational investigation. *Neuropsychologia, 40*(2), 187–204.

Vidyasagar, T. R., & Pammer, K. (2010). Dyslexia: A deficit in visuo-spatial attention, not in phonological processing. *Trends in Cognitive Science, 14,* 57–63.

# 3

# Disorders of the Brain and How They Can Affect Vision

*Gordon N. Dutton*

In the same way that successful medical treatment needs accurate diagnosis and knowledge of the underlying disorder, successful education and habilitation of children with cerebral visual impairment (CVI) hinges on an appreciation of how and why they see the way they do. Recognizing and understanding the capabilities of children affected by CVI is essential to ensure that interventions and educational endeavors are rendered visible and accessible, so as to be efficient and successful.

Disorders of the eye and optic nerve impair vision in a limited range of predictable ways, but when vision is affected by damage to the brain, the range of possible outcomes is wider, and the resulting nature of each affected child's vision and visual behavior is arguably unique. This means that educational approaches need to be "made to measure" for each child (Dutton, 2003; Dutton & Bax, 2010; McKillop et al., 2006).

The ways in which vision can be disturbed as a result of damage to the brain are complex (Fazzi et al., 2007; Jan et al., 2013). The approach described in this book applies the model explained in Chapters 1 and 2 that is derived from the long history of how damage to the brain affects vision (see Sidebar 1.3). This model (reviewed in detail by Brodsky, 2010) has been found to provide a practical means of characterizing and working with children with CVI. This chapter describes the common ways that vision can be affected by damage to the brain so as to provide a structure for developing customized approaches for children with functional vision. The features of profound visual impairment resulting from CVI are presented in relation to habilitative approaches explained in Part 4 of this book. A more in-depth neuropsychological approach to CVI is described by Zihl and Dutton (2015).

The features described in Tables 3.2–3.9 throughout this chapter have been compiled from experience attained first-hand from many hundreds of children with CVI seen over a period of more than 20 years. Recognition of a child's condition, along with useful strategies to help, can be life changing for both children and their families. To find out that the condition is not progressive, and that the child is neither clumsy nor stupid, but that there is a specific explanation for the child's behaviors, leads to positive changes in the behavior of parents, caregivers, and teachers.

Practitioners should be especially alert to the potential visual origin of the behaviors described in these tables in order to aid identification of the underlying disorders, and identification of children who have CVI, when organic evidence from brain imaging is not currently available.

## Location, Timing, and Causes of CVI

### Location of Brain Damage

This chapter considers, in turn, the effects of both bilateral and unilateral damage to the occipital lobes and their incoming visual pathways, the dorsal stream pathways and posterior parietal lobes, and the ventral stream pathways and temporal lobes (see Figures 2.1 and 2.5 in Chapter 2). As explained in Chapter 2, the occipital, temporal, and parietal lobes are discrete but integrated structures. By contrast, the ventral and dorsal streams represent functional concepts of pathways that connect those structures, not specific discrete pathways that can easily be imaged by an MRI of the brain. The ventral stream may be rendered dysfunctional by damage in the region of the occipital and temporal lobes, and likewise the dorsal stream may be rendered dysfunctional by damage in the region of the occipital and parietal lobes. In the experience of the author and others, ventral and dorsal stream pathways can, in some cases, be dysfunctional even though no evidence of anatomical damage to the visual areas of the brain has been obtained from commonly used imaging techniques (Ortibus et al., 2009).

Each of these areas of the brain can be damaged, alone or in combination, leading to fairly predictable disorders of vision, behavioral adaptations, and behavioral reactions. Appendix 3A at the end of this chapter presents a more detailed comparison between damage to the brain as seen on an MRI and possible resulting visual dysfunction.

In addition to the location of the brain damage, the way that a child is affected by CVI also depends on the timing and cause of the damage.

### Timing of the Damage

As discussed in Chapter 1, the timing of damage to the brain—whether it occurs before birth, during a child's early development, or after development is essentially complete—can affect the visual outcome.

#### *Acquired Damage to the Visual Brain of an Adult or Developed Child*

Damage to the brain of an adult or a child whose vision is already developed leads to predictable patterns of loss of visual function. Unaffected functions are preserved and prior knowledge and abilities learned through vision are retained. The effects of acquired brain damage on vision are discussed in more detail later in this chapter.

#### *Damage to the Visual Brain during Early Development*

Patterns of visual disability and behavior resembling those of acquired damage result from damage to the visual brain during early development. However, lack of prior vision to aid learning and the ways in which the child adapts developmentally to the visual deficits lead to a wider range of patterns of visual dysfunction and adaptive behaviors.

#### *Damage while in the Womb*

Damage to the visual brain of the fetus affects its growth and development. In general, very early damage tends to be the most severe, and the outcome may include combined intellectual disability, cerebral palsy, and visual impairment. However, the remarkable capacity of the developing brain to grow and change means that visual outcome is unpredictable, with remarkably good outcomes in some children.

### Causes of Cerebral Visual Impairment

Table 3.1 describes the principal causes of damage to the visual brain. Readers can refer to these descriptions while reading about the effects of brain damage in different locations in the following sections. These conditions may affect much of the brain, or they may be focal, affecting only a discrete part of the visual system. All the conditions listed can occur very early in life, while a number can also develop in later childhood. (Appendix 3B at the end of this chapter details specific effects on visual functioning from some of these conditions.)

## Types of Cerebral Visual Impairment

CVI can be considered in the context of which parts of the brain are dysfunctional and which are not:

- the visual pathways and occipital lobes
- the middle temporal lobes (for perception of movement)
- the ventral stream and temporal lobes (for recognition and orientation)
- the dorsal stream and parietal lobes (for search and visual guidance of movement)

### Damage to the Visual Pathways and Occipital Lobes

As described in Chapter 2, the occipital lobes and their incoming neural pathways serve visual acuity, color perception, contrast perception, and the visual fields. Both brain hemispheres support central vision. The right side serves the left visual field for both eyes, and the left side serves the right visual field for both eyes (see Figures 2.3 and 2.4). This means that the principal outcome of damage to an occipital lobe or its incoming pathway on one side is loss of the field of vision on the opposite side (similarly and symmetrically for both eyes, as shown in Figure 2.4), but the central visual functions of acuity, color perception, and contrast perception are usually unaffected. Damage to both sides (most often due to poor oxygen levels or poor blood supply during early development, or very low blood sugar in the newborn period) impairs visual acuity and contrast sensitivity and affects the visual fields on both sides. Typical visual behaviors seen in children with poor central vision with low visual acuities are shown in Table 3.2. When there is involvement of the *thalamus* (a structure situated between the cerebral cortex and the midbrain involved in relaying and processing sensory and motor signals to the cerebral cortex), the visual impairment tends to be more profound (Ricci et al., 2006).

#### *Early-Onset Damage to One Occipital Lobe*

In most cases, damage to one occipital lobe in early childhood probably relates to impaired blood supply from one posterior cerebral artery. It causes lack of vision in the visual field on the opposite side for both eyes. It can, however, spare the parts of the brain—the middle temporal lobes—that serve perception of movement. Formal visual field testing with static targets shows lack of vision on the side opposite the side of the damage, yet perception of movement,

**TABLE 3.1**

## Causes of Damage to the Visual Brain*

| *Cause* | *Comment* |
|---|---|
| Anatomical disorders of the visual brain | For example, *occipital encephalocele* (protrusion of brain tissue through the skull in the occipital region). |
| Brain malformations | A wide range of abnormalities of brain structure can impair vision. |
| Blocked shunts in hydrocephalus* | If the plastic tube used to treat hydrocephalus gets blocked, vision can be severely affected. |
| Chromosomal and other genetic disorders | Disorders of both brain structure and function can impair vision. |
| Closed head injury* | Bleeding, blunt injury, and high pressure in the head all contribute to a range of patterns of visual impairment. |
| Focal damage to specific brain locations | Disorders of visual function depend on the brain structures damaged. |
| Hemorrhage* | A broken blood vessel leaks blood into a part of the brain. |
| Tumors* | A wide range of tumors can cause damage in specific locations. |
| Cortical dysplasia | A part of the cortex of the brain does not develop properly. Vision can be affected if the visual brain is involved. |
| Hydrocephalus* | Water (cerebrospinal fluid) is unable to escape normally from the spaces where it is made. The water spaces expand under pressure, causing damage to white matter. |
| Hypoxic ischemic encephalopathy at term | A blocked blood vessel in the brain, or poor blood and oxygen delivery to the brain, causes damage in a single location or in many locations in the brain. |
| Infantile spasms, and epilepsy* | The electrical discharge in the brain resulting from seizures can impair vision. This may be the first sign of the disorder. |
| Injury to the periventricular white matter | Damage to the white matter nerve fibers (or *cabling*) surrounding the water spaces, or ventricles in the brain, has many patterns, and is mainly due to poor oxygen or blood supply during early development. Vision is commonly impaired. Premature birth and *spastic diplegia* (a form of cerebral palsy) are common, but not universal, associations. |
| Metabolic disorders* | A wide range of rare disorders of how brain cells function can impair visual functioning. Some of these conditions can be progressive in nature. |
| Meningitis and encephalitis* | Viruses, bacteria, and the parasite toxoplasma can all cause damage. |
| Neonatal hypoglycemia (low blood sugar) | Low blood sugar shortly after birth causes damage. |

*All causes listed can occur early in life. Asterisks denote conditions in which damage to the visual system can also develop in later childhood.

which is reflexive, automatic, and largely subconscious, may be intact. Therefore, the lack of vision on the opposite side may not be debilitating since the surrounding world appears to move as the person moves. There have been cases of skilled drivers attending a vision test and discovering they have a hemianopia, yet their good movement perception on the "blind" side prevented them from being aware of any visual difficulty.

The possible range in the severity of the visual impairment that may result from

TABLE 3.2

### Visual Behaviors and Adaptations Exhibited by Children with CVI with Low Corrected Visual Acuities for Distance, Near Vision, or Both, as Well as Adaptive Strategies that May Be Used by the Children and Their Families

| *Typical Age (years) of Behavior* | *Difficulty* | *Behavior or Adaptation* | *Reason* |
|---|---|---|---|
| 0–adult | Inability to see facial expressions or recognize people, unless nearby | Children may be incorrectly considered to have, and may be being managed as having impaired social interaction. Families may have learned to interact within the "facial expression recognition distance." | Low visual acuities lead faces to appear blank and meaningless at a critical distance. |
| 0–adult | Inability to see at near | Material tends to be enlarged, without recognizing why the child cannot see at near. Some children discover that their grandparents' eyeglasses for presbyopia markedly improve near vision. | Impaired focusing (accommodation), causing low near visual acuity, is seen in over 55 percent of children with cerebral palsy and in most children receiving hyoscine patches. |
| 1–adult | Inability to see pictures and text | Children may move closer to pictures, text, and television in order to gain the magnification obtained by being near the object. | Low visual acuity precludes access to subthreshold detail. |
| 2–adult | Inability to see to navigate | Children may be accompanied by a sighted person to assist them to make their way, | Low vision precludes identification of obstacles, hazards, and landmarks. |
| 5–adult | Inability to see in the distance | Children learn to move closer to things to determine what they are, or ask questions of family members about what is in the distance. Some families and children may have found alternative ways of enlarging distant objects, such as viewing them through the camera of a mobile phone. | Visual acuity for near vision is better in children with nystagmus. Images are enlarged and crowding is diminished. |

*Source*: Adapted with permission from Dutton, G. N., Bowman, R., & Fazzi, E. (2014). Visual function. In B. Dan, M. Mayston, N. Paneth, & L. Rosenbloom (Eds.), *Cerebral palsy: Science and clinical practice*. London: Mac Keith Press.

damage to one or both occipital lobes is considerable, as illustrated in Figure 3.1. Disabilities can occur in a wide variety of combinations and degrees of severity.

### *Later-Onset Damage to One Occipital Lobe during Childhood*

Damage to one occipital lobe acquired later in childhood is more disabling than in early development and is more likely to interfere with mobility when crossing streets and accessing information, including reading. In two such cases, the author has seen children aged 7 and 8 with acquired hemianopia who spontaneously adapted to their resulting reading difficulty by rotating the text clockwise through 90 degrees, reading vertically upward (for right hemianopia) or vertically downward (for left hemianopia), as this meant that the blind area did not intrude into the text that was about to be read (see Figure 3.2). Instead, as the eye moved down the page, the blind area progressively covered over the text that had just been read.

### *Early-Onset Damage to Both Occipital Lobes*

Severe damage to the optic radiations and occipital lobes on both sides—before or around the time of birth causes profound

FIGURE 3.1

**Range of Visual Disabilities in Children Resulting from Damage to the Occipital Lobes**

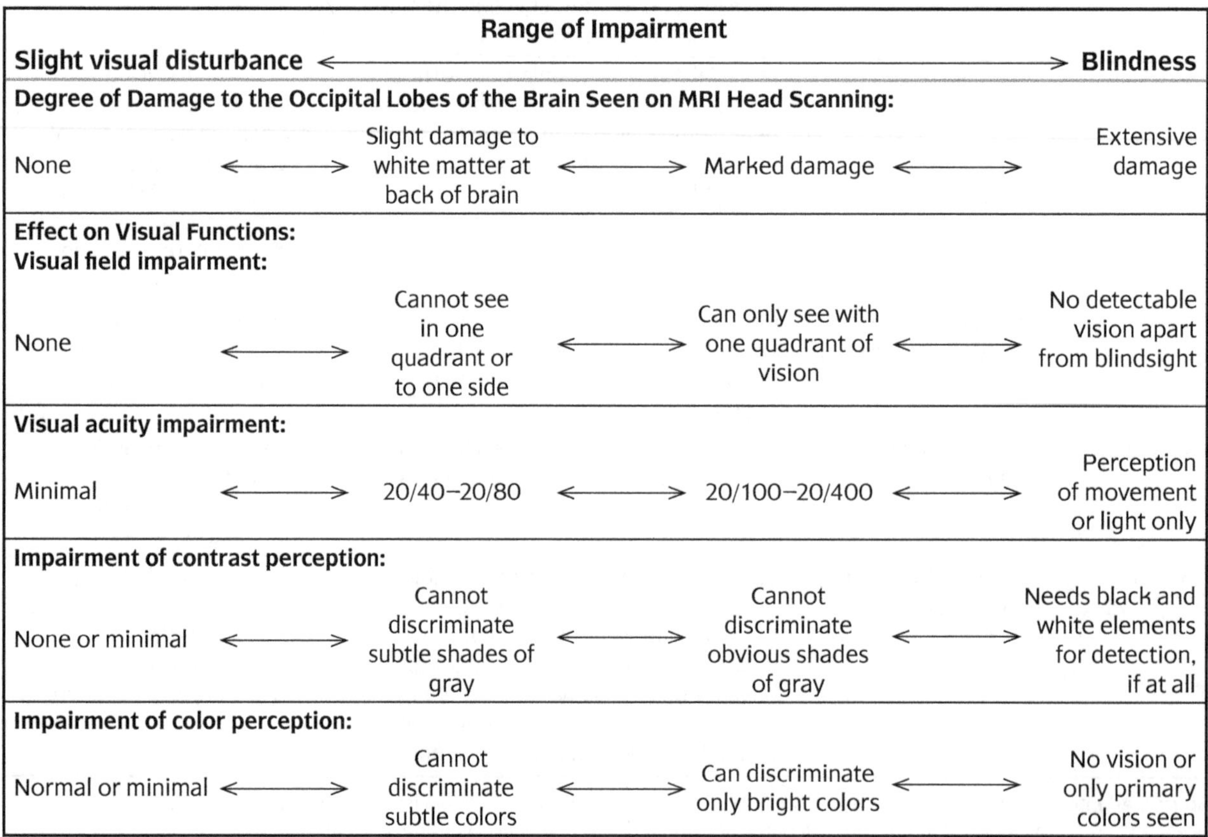

| Range of Impairment | | | |
|---|---|---|---|
| **Slight visual disturbance** ⟵ | | | ⟶ **Blindness** |
| **Degree of Damage to the Occipital Lobes of the Brain Seen on MRI Head Scanning:** | | | |
| None ⟷ | Slight damage to white matter at back of brain ⟷ | Marked damage ⟷ | Extensive damage |
| **Effect on Visual Functions:**<br>**Visual field impairment:** | | | |
| None ⟷ | Cannot see in one quadrant or to one side ⟷ | Can only see with one quadrant of vision ⟷ | No detectable vision apart from blindsight |
| **Visual acuity impairment:** | | | |
| Minimal ⟷ | 20/40–20/80 ⟷ | 20/100–20/400 ⟷ | Perception of movement or light only |
| **Impairment of contrast perception:** | | | |
| None or minimal ⟷ | Cannot discriminate subtle shades of gray ⟷ | Cannot discriminate obvious shades of gray ⟷ | Needs black and white elements for detection, if at all |
| **Impairment of color perception:** | | | |
| Normal or minimal ⟷ | Cannot discriminate subtle colors ⟷ | Can discriminate only bright colors ⟷ | No vision or only primary colors seen |

FIGURE 3.2

## How Vertical Reading Can Compensate for Acquired Loss of Vision on One Side (Hemianopia) in Childhood

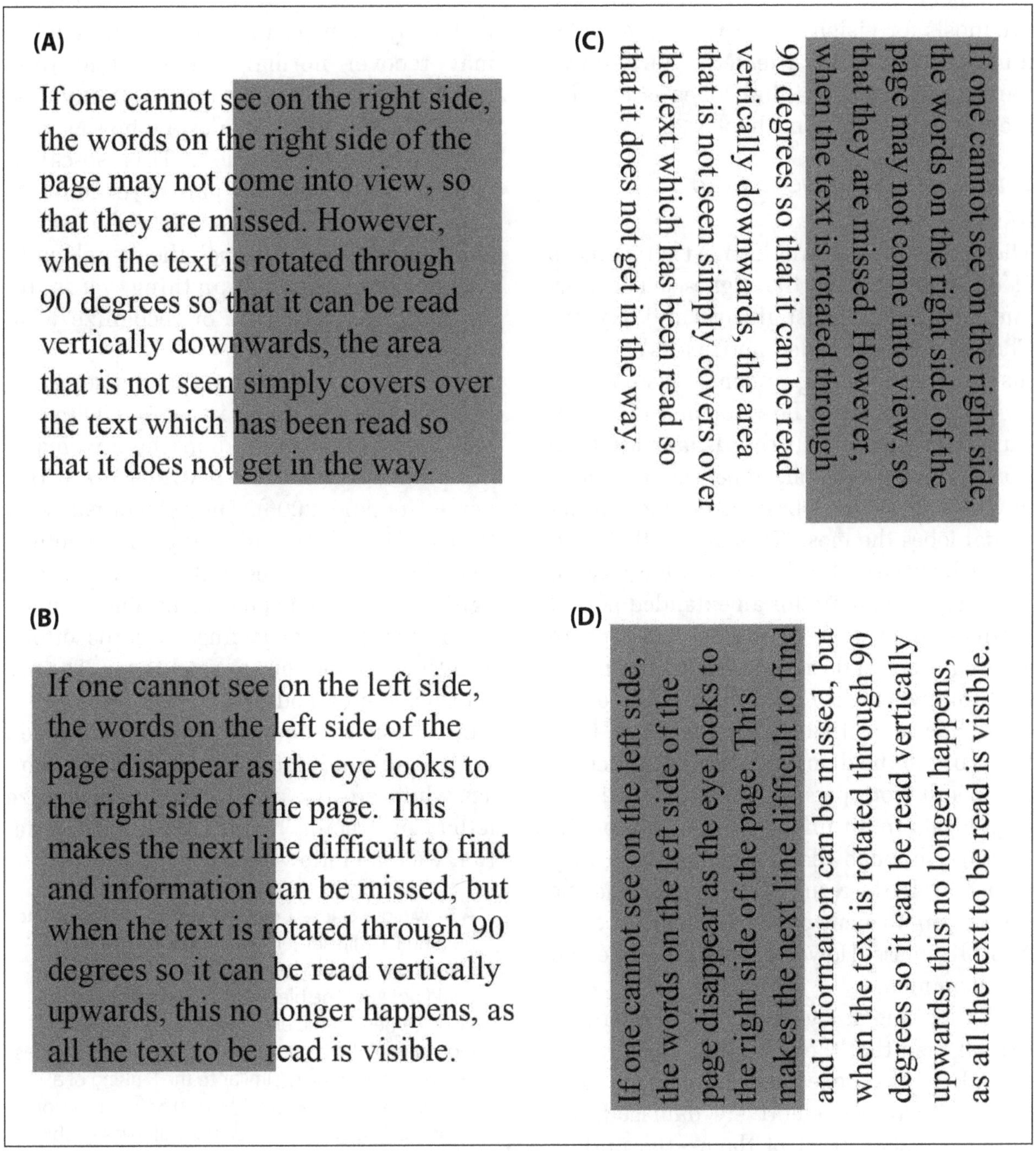

**(A)**

If one cannot see on the right side, the words on the right side of the page may not come into view, so that they are missed. However, when the text is rotated through 90 degrees so that it can be read vertically downwards, the area that is not seen simply covers over the text which has been read so that it does not get in the way.

**(B)**

If one cannot see on the left side, the words on the left side of the page disappear as the eye looks to the right side of the page. This makes the next line difficult to find and information can be missed, but when the text is rotated through 90 degrees so it can be read vertically upwards, this no longer happens, as all the text to be read is visible.

**(C)**

If one cannot see on the right side, the words on the right side of the page may not come into view, so that they are missed. However, when the text is rotated through 90 degrees so that it can be read vertically downwards, the area that is not seen simply covers over the text which has been read so that it does not get in the way.

**(D)**

If one cannot see on the left side, the words on the left side of the page disappear as the eye looks to the right side of the page. This makes the next line difficult to find and information can be missed, but when the text is rotated through 90 degrees so it can be read vertically upwards, this no longer happens, as all the text to be read is visible.

When a child has hemianopia, the blind area—represented by the shaded area in each image—blocks part of the text on one side (A and B). However, when the text is rotated clockwise 90 degrees (C and D), the entire line can be read vertically and the blind area progressively covers the portion of the text that has already been read. This is explained by the text embedded in the figures.

visual impairment—is often accompanied by cerebral palsy and intellectual dysfunction when other parts of the brain serving movement and intellect are affected. The prognosis for vision is best when the thalamus has not been affected. (Early-onset damage to both occipital lobes is considered in more detail in Chapter 20.)

### *Later-Onset Damage to Both Occipital Lobes*

The occipital lobes are the most active parts of the brain, having the highest blood flow and needing the most glucose and oxygen. Those who have fainted notice loss of vision just before becoming unconscious because the impaired blood flow to the brain that caused the faint affects the visual brain first. Consequently, a prolonged period of reduced oxygen supply to the brain can affect the occipital lobes the most. This means that children who have suffered from very low oxygen delivery to the brain for an extended period of time—for example, as the result of a severe asthma attack or decreased blood pressure—find that when they recover, they have lost vision because their occipital lobes bore the brunt of the damage. A similar outcome can result from persistently low blood glucose levels in an infant (infantile hypoglycemia). Although the rest of the brain may recover well, the result of the damage may be severe impairment of vision or even cerebral blindness. However, this kind of event is uncommon.

By looking at Figure 2.5 in Chapter 2, it can be seen that the occipital lobes, represented by the boxes labeled "image processing," can be selectively damaged, but the area just in front of them—the middle temporal lobes of the brain, represented by the boxes labeled "motion," and responsible for perception of movement—may survive. The middle temporal lobes are connected to the dorsal stream pathways that serve accurate visual guidance of movement. This can lead to the paradox that children affected by damage to both occipital lobes may recover normal intellect and limb movement, and in some cases retain visual guidance of movement, despite having very limited conscious vision. This so-called "high-level blindsight" can be difficult to understand because the affected child is able to move freely through the visual world without bumping into anything, yet is unable to consciously see or recognize what they are looking at.

As noted in Chapter 1, this phenomenon was described in detail in a case where carbon monoxide toxicity damaged a woman's occipital lobes (Goodale & Milner, 2013; Milner & Goodale, 2006). The subject was able to accurately trace with a finger large letters that she could not see, but was able to recognize them. Later she became able to imagine the movement of her finger over the letters, and this enabled her to read them. The author has seen an adult (Culham, Witt, Valyear, Dutton, & Goodale, 2008) and children with acquired bilateral occipital lobe damage who were also able to learn to recognize letters by tracing them. One child's situation was the following:

> **A 5-YEAR-OLD GIRL FELL OUT OF A WINDOW AND FRACTURED** her skull. Brain surgery was needed to stop the bleeding inside her head. When she woke up she could not see. The bleeding led to downward displacement of the brain which, in turn, led to blockage of the blood vessels to the occipital lobes as a result of kinking (similar to the kinking of a garden hose). As the child recovered, some vision returned, but one year later, the child was unable to recognize what she was looking at. Despite her poor perceptual vision, this child was able to move freely around her visual world, of which she had limited conscious awareness.

When asked to pick up a small coin from a plain play mat, she was able to do so easily if this was the only item; but when she had to choose the coin from among other items, she could not do so without touching each item in turn. Remarkably, however, she was able to move her finger over lines drawn with a felt-tip pen, depicting circles, triangles, and rectangles and name them correctly, using the knowledge that she had before the accident. Her rehabilitation took advantage of this prior knowledge and nine months later she was able to recognize most of the letters of the alphabet—printed on cards the size of playing cards—by imagining the movement of her fingers over them, as well as the braille equivalents that she had been taught.

Testing the visual acuity of this girl was challenging, as she was unable to name any shape or letter, but when asked to trace the lines of the visual acuity targets, she could do so to a visual acuity level estimate equivalent to 20/60.

The apparent paradox in this girl's visual behavior results from the fact that the principal damage was to her occipital lobes and ventral stream pathways, but her dorsal stream pathways were functioning well. Thus, she had good recovery of movement perception functions, with the result that she could move freely through the environment, which she could see consciously only in a limited fashion. She could not recognize objects in the environment unless she used her other senses such as touch, haptic analysis, and her knowledge of the movement of her limbs (*kinesthesia*), which provided alternative routes to interpreting her surrounding world.

## Damage to the Middle Temporal Lobes: Impaired Movement Perception

As one might expect from the fact that the middle temporal lobes are the motion perception centers of the brain (see Chapter 2), damage to the middle temporal lobes or the white matter (nerve fiber) pathways that support them impairs perception of movement. This occurs only rarely in children as an isolated phenomenon. The condition was first described in the early 1980s (Zihl, Von Cramon, & Mai, 1983) in an adult who had other visual disorders resulting from adjacent brain damage. She was able to see things only when they were not moving: the condition was given the term *akinetopsia*.

There are few reports of akinetopsia occurring in children (Ahmed & Dutton, 1996). More frequently, the impairment of perception of movement is relative and not absolute (Dutton et al., 2004; Morrone et al., 2008; Saidkasimova, Bennett, Butler, & Dutton, 2007); the term given to this disorder is *dyskinetopsia*.

This author has followed a number of children with CVI who had difficulty seeing moving targets as a result of damage to the periventricular white matter (Guzzetta et al., 2009). When these children were younger, they walked out in front of traffic they did not appear to see. (It should be noted that when children commit such acts as walking out in front of moving traffic, it may be related to impaired perception of movement, but it can also be due to lack of appreciation of risk, and possibly to difficulty knowing how large targets should appear at different distances, leading to difficulty estimating how close a moving car is.)

As a young teenager, one boy with CVI explained why he always chose to play soccer as a goalkeeper. He said "I can only see a ball when it is moving slowly, of course, but when it is moving toward or away from me, I can see it all the time." He was asked, "What does a ball look like when it is kicked?" The answer was, "It disappears, of course, for the first few feet, then it reappears once it has slowed down." The words "of course,"

TABLE 3.3

## Visual Behaviors and Adaptations Exhibited by Children with CVI with Impaired Perception of Movement, as Well as Adaptive Strategies that May Be Used by the Children and Their Families

| *Typical Age (years) of Behavior* | *Difficulty* | *Behavior or Adaptation* | *Reason* |
|---|---|---|---|
| 0–adult | Fast-moving stimuli, such as small animals, cause distress | Affected children are startled and upset by fast-moving small animals. | Small, fast animals seem to appear out of nowhere as a result of impaired visual perception of movement or slow visual attentional processing. |
| 0–adult | Movement makes things seem to disappear | The child is unable to move quickly. | Impaired visual perception of movement. |
| 1–adult | Language conveyed by facial expression is occasionally missed | The child is thought to have difficulties with social engagement, when in fact, fast-moving elements of facial expression are not visible and go unidentified. | Fast facial expressions are not seen, but slow facial expressions and expressions in photographs are seen and understood. |
| 3–adult | Fast movement on video is not seen | The child chooses to watch TV shows and films that have limited movement and avoids fast-moving films. | Impaired visual perception of movement. |
| 5–adult | Fast-moving stimuli while walking are not seen | Child only sees slow traffic. | Impaired visual perception of movement. |

*Source*: Adapted with permission from Dutton, G. N., Bowman, R., & Fazzi, E. (2014). Visual function. In B. Dan, M. Mayston, N. Paneth, & L. Rosenbloom (Eds.), *Cerebral palsy: Science and clinical practice*. London: Mac Keith Press.

reflect his interpretation of his own visual experiences as being normal. Since then, the same question has been asked of many young people with CVI and similar descriptions have been forthcoming on a number of occasions. This phenomenon can also be observed when the blades of a propeller are watched as they start moving; for most people, the blades seem to disappear as the rate of rotation increases. For individuals with dyskinetopsia, the propeller blades disappear when the rotation is significantly slower. Table 3.3 highlights some of the behaviors and adaptations shown by children with impaired visual perception of movement.

### *Clinical Observation of Disordered Perception of Movement*

Formal standardized clinical tests for disordered perception of movement have yet to be designed. In clinical practice, the author uses the simple expedient of moving a hand horizontally to and fro across the subject's line of sight, raising one, two, three, or four fingers while the hand is moving quickly. The hand is then gradually slowed down. The child is initially asked to count the number of fingers shown when the hand is static, to check that he or she can do so. The child is then asked to do the same on the moving hand. Children who say that balls disappear after being kicked are uniformly able to count the fingers only when the hand is moving very slowly. This is only a crude test, and more objective tests are needed.

### *Assessment of the Ability to See Fast-Moving Facial Expressions*

Another important practical test that is worth administering to children suspected of having impaired perception of movement is to sit in front of the child and to ask him or her to tell you what facial expression is being presented (happy, sad, or angry), while offering the expressions at different speeds and for different durations. Expressions that are adopted only briefly are not seen, while the more prolonged ones are. (The social and educational implications of an inability to pick up on the nuances of rapid changes in facial expression may need to be addressed.)

Aside from damage to the middle temporal lobes, other possible causes for a child not seeing fast-moving targets include:

- overall slow mental processing
- difficulty with visual search
- limited ability to give attention to more than one thing at a time
- difficulty shifting attention from one thing to another

However, a child whose inability to see fast-moving events results from one of these other causes is usually able to count fingers on a fast-moving hand when concentrating on the task.

### *Perception and Recognition of Biological Motion*

Perception and recognition of biological motion—that is, the typical movement of a living creature such as a person—is a discrete function of the visual brain that is probably served by the temporal lobes working in harmony with the cerebellum. It can be investigated by means of moving dots on a computer screen that are configured to represent key locations on a moving body. An individual with typical perception of biological motion can distinguish the nature of the movement represented by the dots, such as whether they depict a walking or running person, by simple observation. The Pepi Test (Hyvärinen & Jacob, 2011) is designed to examine biological motion in children (see Chapter 13). Children born prematurely who have CVI as a result of periventricular white matter damage, and who have limited abilities to interact socially, have been shown to perform poorly on such tests of biological movement (Pavlova, 2012).

### *Damage to the Temporal Lobes and Disorders of Ventral Stream Function*

The ventral stream and the visual functions it serves are described in Chapter 2. As noted there, the ventral stream serves the process of visual recognition and is sometimes called the "what" pathway. Disordered ventral stream function alone is rare, but it needs to be considered in all children with evidence of CVI. It rarely occurs in isolation because it is commonly associated with impaired visual acuities, visual field disorders, and varying patterns of dorsal stream dysfunction (described in the next section). These associations can make it difficult to determine whether it is poor visual acuity that prevents recognition of an image or object, or whether impaired recognition is an additional impairment. The distinction can be verified by making the salient elements of any images being shown more visible (for example, making them larger, bolder, and of higher contrast) to minimize the effects of poor visual acuity.

When there has been early-onset damage in ventral stream functions, the principal difficulty is one of overall recognition and orientation. The child may have difficulty recognizing people's faces, both in real life and from photographs. Animals may be recognized only from the way they move or the sounds they make. Lack of ability to recognize faces (*prosopagnosia*) can occur in isolation, or it may accompany other difficulties with recognition. It is often associated with difficulty recognizing the language of facial expression. Affected children may choose not to look at people and are not aware of the meaning of a disciplining look.

Problems with recognition of faces and facial expressions can go unidentified, and may come to light only when other clues to recognizing someone, like the voice, are not available. This might occur, for example, when a child fails to recognize a family member looking through a double-glazed window. Children who are more profoundly affected may also have difficulty recognizing shapes. For example, the shape of the family car does not help the child identify it; instead the child relies on color to do so.

Profoundly impaired orientation, although rare, can be a major obstacle for those who are affected. Not only are severely affected children unable to find their way around places they are familiar with, they may also not be able to find their way to their school desk and can have a hard time remembering where their possessions are kept, even if these locations are shown to them over and over again.

A common finding in affected children is that they can have trouble judging the length and orientation of lines. Profound difficulty in learning shapes, numbers, and letters by means of vision may be evident. Tactile recognition is better for some, but not all.

In the author's experience, the group of children most commonly affected by difficulties with recognition and orientation are those with hydrocephalus that has been severe enough to require the insertion of a plastic tube (a shunt) to drain the water out of enlarged water spaces in the brain (the ventricles) and into the abdominal cavity. Over 50 percent of children with shunted hydrocephalus have a range of patterns of perceptual visual dysfunction, which at present are best determined by taking a carefully structured history from parents (Andersson et al., 2006; Houliston, Taguri, Dutton, Hajivassiliou, & Young, 1999). However, children who also have spina bifida are at a lower risk (Andersson et al., 2006).

Acquired focal damage to the temporal lobes is rare in children, but can give rise to prosopagnosia. Removal of part of the right temporal lobe to treat epilepsy can cause prosopagnosia (Glosser, Salvucci, & Chiaravalloti, 2003) that can be temporary (Mesad, Laff, & Devinsky, 2003).

Children who have impaired recognition of objects frequently have great difficulty creating visual memories and tend to rely on their alternative strengths, particularly language. They may pose the apparent paradox of not being able to remember their way around their grandparent's garden, nor the appearance of their grandparents, despite having visited many times. Yet they may be able to remember word for word what their grandfather said a number of months earlier.

Geometry, technical drawing, and artwork all rely on an ability to create a mental representation of the requisite imagery, and the ability to perceive, remember, and imagine three-dimensional geometric shapes and rotate them in one's mind. Children with evidence of ventral stream dysfunction who have problems with visual recognition are also likely to have difficulty with these abilities. Creating alternative tactile representations of geometric shapes to explore and remember can help children with this type of visual disorder conceptualize such forms through tactile rather than visual approaches. Table 3.4 describes some of the typical behaviors and adaptations shown by children with ventral stream dysfunction.

Although more research evidence is needed, it has been reported many times to this author that among prematurely born children whose blindness in infancy resulted from bilateral damage to the retina (retinopathy of prematurity), those who also developed hydrocephalus because of bleeding inside the water spaces in the brain (intraventricular hemorrhage) had greater difficulty than other students who are visually impaired in finding their way around. When they grew older, navigation remained difficult for them. It is likely that damage to the temporal lobe areas resulting from loss of white matter due to hydrocephalus led to problems with forming a mental map, thus leading to disorientation (*topographic agnosia*). These reports suggest that it is not primarily vision that is responsible for mapping our past, present, and future locations in our surroundings, but that it is the functions of memory and prediction that are deficient in topographic agnosia.

The degree of severity of ventral stream dysfunction can vary considerably, as illustrated in Figure 3.3. Moreover, because poor visual acuity also affects the ability to recognize objects, ventral stream dysfunction is evident only when the child's central visual functions are sufficient to recognize the object they are looking at.

## Damage to the Parietal Lobes and Disorders of Dorsal Stream Function: Visual Guidance of Movement, Visual Search, and Attention

The dorsal stream and its functions are described in Chapter 2 and involve visual guidance of movement (the component accomplished automatically without conscious thought); visual search, the facility to elect to move the eyes to other targets; and through connection with the frontal lobes, attention. (The dorsal stream is sometimes called the "where" pathway.) Impairment of dorsal stream function can affect children in a number of ways related to these abilities.

### *Impairment of Dorsal Stream Function Affecting Both Sides of the Brain*

Bilateral damage to the posterior parietal lobes or the white matter supplying this area disrupts dorsal stream functions (Fazzi et al., 2009; Jacobson & Dutton, 2000; Macintyre-Béon et al., 2010). Dorsal stream dysfunction as a result of damage to the periventricular white matter is commonly associated with impairment of the lower visual field, cerebral palsy (particularly *spastic*

TABLE 3.4

## Visual Behaviors and Adaptations Exhibited by Children with CVI with Ventral Stream Dysfunction, as Well as Adaptive Strategies that May Be Used by the Children and Their Families[a]

| *Typical Age (years) of Behavior* | *Difficulty* | *Behavior or Adaptation* | *Reason* |
|---|---|---|---|
| 2–adult | Impaired orientation within the surrounding environment (topographic agnosia) | Children become easily lost, even in places that are familiar to them. In cases of severely impaired orientation, children, families, and teachers may have developed strategies such as the use of color-coded lines on the floor in the classroom or color coding of doors in the home. | Temporal lobe damage can lead to severe impairment of the ability to recognize and navigate. The disorientation of ventral stream dysfunction is more severe than that as a result of the clutter-induced disorientation of dorsal stream dysfunction. |
| 2–adult | Difficulty or inability recognizing people's faces (prosopagnosia), as well as difficulty recognizing the language of facial expressions | Affected children and adults may not look at people's faces when communicating. Children may go up to strangers thinking that they are a person they know. A young child may turn her parent's head to look straight at her to make the face easier to recognize. Alternative identifiers, such as color of clothing or voice recognition, may be substituted to such a degree that the difficulty may go unrecognized for many years. Family members may go out together wearing clear identifiers, such as brightly colored clothing. | Prosopagnosia accompanies temporal lobe damage to a structure called the fusiform gyrus. Lack of ability to see the language conveyed by facial expression is a common accompaniment. |
| 2–adult | Difficulty or inability to recognize animals | Four-legged animals may be indistinguishable from one another, particularly when they are moving. Families may take the child to a farm where they can interact with the animals at close range. | This problem occasionally accompanies prosopagnosia. |
| 2–adult | Difficulty recognizing objects (object agnosia) | The child may pick up one object after another before retrieving the chosen one by means of touch. | Tactile recognition is being used instead of visual object recognition. |
| 5–adult | Difficulty identifying family car in parking lot | Color tends to be used instead of shape, so that it is easy to miss the car. Some families use a distinct identifier such as a recognizable picture pasted on the car's bumper. | Object agnosia results in alternative and less robust recognition strategies. |

[a]Isolated severe ventral stream dysfunction with good visual acuity is rare. Affected children are able to move around with their dorsal stream dysfunction intact and appear sighted, yet are unable to easily recognize what they are looking at. Ventral stream dysfunction is more commonly identified as an accompaniment to dorsal stream dysfunction.

*Source*: Adapted with permission from Dutton, G. N., Bowman, R., & Fazzi, E. (2014). Visual function. In B. Dan, M. Mayston, N. Paneth, & L. Rosenbloom (Eds.), *Cerebral palsy: Science and clinical practice*. London: Mac Keith Press.

FIGURE 3.3
## Range of Visual Disabilities in Children Resulting from Ventral Stream Dysfunction

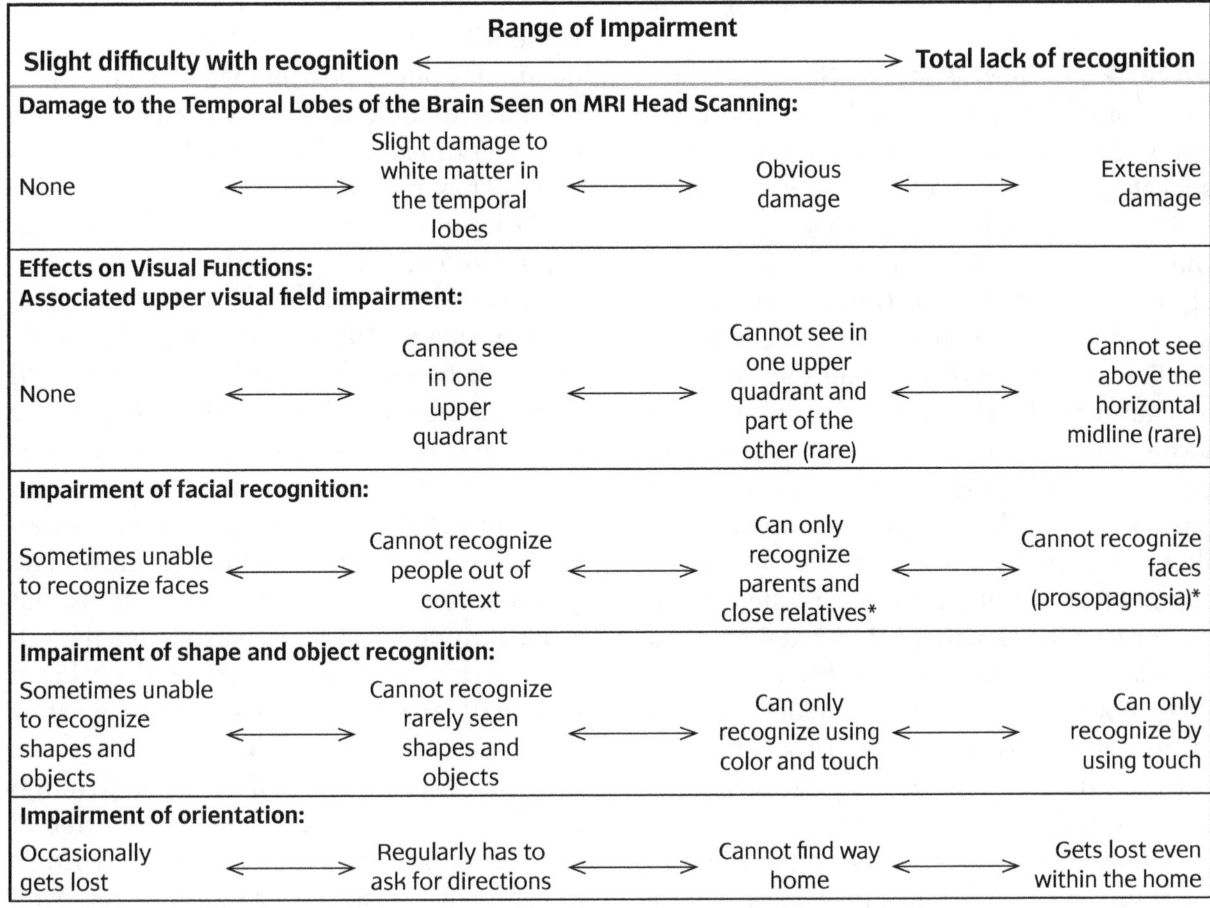

| Range of Impairment: Slight difficulty with recognition ⟷ Total lack of recognition | | | | | | |
|---|---|---|---|---|---|---|
| **Damage to the Temporal Lobes of the Brain Seen on MRI Head Scanning:** | | | | | | |
| None | ⟷ | Slight damage to white matter in the temporal lobes | ⟷ | Obvious damage | ⟷ | Extensive damage |
| **Effects on Visual Functions:** | | | | | | |
| **Associated upper visual field impairment:** | | | | | | |
| None | ⟷ | Cannot see in one upper quadrant | ⟷ | Cannot see in one upper quadrant and part of the other (rare) | ⟷ | Cannot see above the horizontal midline (rare) |
| **Impairment of facial recognition:** | | | | | | |
| Sometimes unable to recognize faces | ⟷ | Cannot recognize people out of context | ⟷ | Can only recognize parents and close relatives* | ⟷ | Cannot recognize faces (prosopagnosia)* |
| **Impairment of shape and object recognition:** | | | | | | |
| Sometimes unable to recognize shapes and objects | ⟷ | Cannot recognize rarely seen shapes and objects | ⟷ | Can only recognize using color and touch | ⟷ | Can only recognize by using touch |
| **Impairment of orientation:** | | | | | | |
| Occasionally gets lost | ⟷ | Regularly has to ask for directions | ⟷ | Cannot find way home | ⟷ | Gets lost even within the home |

*Inability to recognize facial expressions commonly accompanies impaired face recognition.

*diplegia*, which results in weakness and stiffness of the lower limbs), or both (Pagliano et al., 2007). Other causes of damage to dorsal stream function include a history of hypoxia after respiratory arrest (Drummond & Dutton, 2007) and focal brain infection secondary to heart valve infection (Gillen & Dutton, 2003).

When there is damage to the dorsal stream, there are fewer brain cells and nerve fibers in this region of the brain. Thus, the brain's data-processing capacity is reduced, and fewer elements are available to build up and maintain an unconscious virtual map of the surroundings. Movement of the body through visual space is therefore less accurate since visual guidance is impaired (see Chapter 2), a condition called *optic ataxia*. In children with associated impaired movement, the term applied is *visual-motor impairment*. Fewer objects in the surrounding environment can be handled subconsciously and simultaneously. The individual with optic ataxia tends to bump into objects that are not perceived or not found through visual search because, effectively, they are not available to the frontal areas of the brain that would otherwise elect to give them attention.

### Balint's syndrome in children

The frontal lobes support the ability to actively search for an item of interest, give it visual attention, and rapidly move the eyes to it. This ability requires clear image data across the whole visual field—provided by the occipital lobes—as well as the construction of an internalized virtual map of elements in the field of vision created from source material gathered by the dorsal stream and posterior parietal lobes. As a result, when there is severe damage to the bilateral posterior parietal lobes, the affected person can neither move freely through the visual environment (optic ataxia) nor see more than one or two items within the visual scene at once (*simultanagnosia*). In addition, the ability to move the eyes from one target to another is limited (*apraxia of gaze*). This condition is called *Balint's syndrome* (Rizzo & Vecera, 2002), introduced in Chapter 1.

This author has seen large numbers of such children with similar but less severe visual difficulties as in Balint's syndrome, often associated with impairment in the peripheral lower visual field (Dutton et al., 2004), and occasionally, impaired perception of movement. This less severe condition is known as *dorsal stream dysfunction* (Brodsky, 2010).

### Lower visual field impairment and impaired visual guidance of movement

Children affected by disorders of the dorsal stream usually, but not always, have impairment of the lower visual field in both eyes ranging in extent from affecting the entire lower visual field below the horizontal midline to affecting only the lowermost visual field. This may not be detected by standard formal visual field testing because this testing method does not extend far enough peripherally, or because testing in sufficient detail may not be possible. Affected children may not be able to see movement of their own feet unless the feet are extended far forward. They may walk over toys or obstacles as if they are not there (particularly children 4 years old or younger in the author's experience). Even when they are looking down to compensate for their lower visual field deficit, or in cases where no lower visual field defect can be identified, such children may probe the ground ahead with their foot, particularly flat boundaries between different areas of the floor that they have not previously seen. This appears to be because they do not know whether there is a step present or not, which suggests impaired visual guidance of foot movement. Affected children may walk around patterns on the carpet as if they are obstacles. If furniture such as a coffee table is moved, children tend to bump into it. Such children have been reported to become angry and insist that the furniture never be moved again, or that it be removed altogether. (The fact that furniture kept in the same place is not bumped into as often suggests that the affected child is using learned information to compensate for the degraded mental map provided by the dorsal stream.) Another feature occasionally seen in the young child with bilateral posterior parietal damage is reaching for patterns on a plate as if they are three-dimensional. In this author's experience, behaviors of this type have been observed in some young affected children (aged 1–3) as a temporary phase in their development.

Many of these behaviors frequently observed in children with dorsal stream dysfunction closely resemble those first described in soldiers with posterior parietal lobe injuries (Holmes, 1918; see Sidebar 1.2). These observations suggest that lower visual field impairment and impaired visual guidance of movement (optic ataxia) of the lower limbs may coexist. However, objective validation of these observations has yet to be carried out.

Detailed visual field examination of older children with *periventricular leukomalacia* (damage to the white matter adjacent to the lateral ventricles in the brain) has shown that the lower visual field can be inefficient, providing the ability to see moving targets, but not to see detail. This may be because earlier damage to the developing visual brain left fewer nerve fibers to "pixelate" the lower visual field (Jacobson, Flodmark, & Martin, 2006).

***Adaptive strategies for lower visual field impairment and presumed lower limb optic ataxia.*** The extent of lower visual field impairment and impairment of visual guidance of movement of both the upper and lower limbs varies considerably among affected children, as do the character and nature of the adaptive strategies that children discover and use. Affected children whose CVI has gone unrecognized, as is frequently the case among children with normal or near-normal visual acuities, can often be identified on the basis of these patterns of behavior and adaptive strategies. It is therefore crucial for professionals who work with these children to understand and recognize these behavioral manifestations of CVI. Interviews and careful observation can reveal these patterns (as described in Part 3 of this book). Parents also commonly develop adaptive methods to care for and teach their affected child.

Many children with dorsal stream dysfunction also have stiffness and weakness of the lower limbs, resulting from spastic diplegia, but they are taught to walk upright, and their walking frames have been designed to help them do so. Yet these children commonly insist on bending forward and looking down. The likely explanation is that they may have an undetected lower visual field defect (with or without other visual difficulties), and are compensating by looking down to see the ground ahead of them so as to avoid tripping, as noted earlier. They may also probe the ground ahead with their foot at previously unencountered floor boundaries. A small proportion of affected children are described by their parents as tending to run quickly from place to place. This could perhaps be an adaptive strategy of aiming to get to the more distant visible ground ahead, while it remains in visual memory.

Young adults with lower visual field impairment have described their sense of "walking on clouds," and bumping into low obstacles. Others have described an inability to find shoes on the floor, and their strategy of storing their shoes on a higher shoe rack. Table 3.5 describes some of the typical behaviors and adaptations shown by children with lower visual field impairment and presumed lower limb optic ataxia.

#### Impaired Visual Guidance of Movement of the Upper Limbs

Impaired visual guidance of movement of the upper limbs also occurs with dorsal stream dysfunction, but is observed and described less frequently. The typical trait is that as the child's hand is extended to reach an item, the gap between the fingers as the hand approaches the object is much wider than normal, or the whole hand may be extended flat and brought down upon the object to gather it up. An alternative strategy

TABLE 3.5

## Visual Behaviors and Adaptations Exhibited by Children with CVI with Lower Visual Field Impairment or Presumed Impaired Visual Guidance of the Lower Limbs Due to Dorsal Stream Dysfunction, as Well as Adaptive Strategies that May Be Used by the Children and Their Families

| *Typical Age (years) of Behavior* | *Difficulty* | *Behavior or Adaptation* | *Reason* |
|---|---|---|---|
| 0–3 | Difficulty learning to walk | May choose to lie on older sibling's skateboard, pushing along with hands, to get around. | Being closer to the ground allows the child to use the intact upper visual field to see the ground ahead. |
| 0–adult | Wheelchair users cannot find items on their tray | Parents have found that the tray on the wheelchair needs to be elevated or moved further away to become visible for children with lower visual field impairment. | Items need to be made visible by being placed in area of intact vision, higher up in the visual field. |
| 1–8 | Difficulty walking without tripping or bumping into things | The child wants to take a push-along wheeled toy wherever possible. | The push toy provides a tactile guide to the height of the ground ahead, and affords a mobile protective boundary. |
| 1–10 | Inability to see ground immediately ahead | The child, apparently paradoxically, tends to run from place to place. | Running may enable the child to get to the more distant ground, which can be seen, before it is lost from memory. |
| 1–adult | Difficulty crossing floor boundaries or walking over patterned floor surfaces, such as tiles or carpeting | Uses a foot to probe the height of ground ahead when there are floor boundaries or large patterns, especially in new places. (Parents have often already adapted by installing a plain boundary-free floor surface in the house.) | Those affected look down and use central vision to inspect floor boundaries and patterns, but still probe with the foot, suggesting impaired visual guidance of movement of the feet. (The ability to see with three-dimensional perception, or stereopsis, is often intact.) |
| 1–adult | Issues with jumping off a wall or a bench | The child either refuses to jump or jumps but is prepared to fall. Some parents may teach a "commando roll," a movement to absorb the energy and minimize the impact of the fall. | The child cannot see the ground to land on. |

*(continued on next page)*

**TABLE 3.5** *(continued from previous page)*

| *Typical Age (years) of Behavior* | *Difficulty* | *Behavior or Adaptation* | *Reason* |
|---|---|---|---|
| 2–8 | Issues with going down slides | The child may refuse to go down the slide in a sitting position, but rather may insist on going down headfirst. | In the seated posture, the child cannot see the slide below, but in the lying posture, it can be seen using the upper visual field. |
| 2–10 | Misses the bottom of the TV screen | The child may choose to lie on his or her back on the ground, a sofa, or chair, and to watch TV upside down. Or the child may choose to watch TV from lower down than usual. | Child prefers to use upper visual field to watch TV, despite the picture being upside down. |
| 2–adult | Issues with walking downstairs | Initially the child goes down step-by-step on his or her backside. Later the child may grip a bannister with both hands while going down sideways. When older, the child may have learned to use the heel to slide down each stair riser as a way of judging height. | Cannot see the stairs going down and has difficulty estimating their height. |
| 3–adult | Difficulty walking down slopes or over uneven ground | The child holds onto clothing or belt of an accompanying person, while pulling down and walking slightly behind. They prefer not to hold a hand, unless it is consistently extended and held backwards. Older children may simply touch the elbow of an accompanying person. The mobile child may independently discover and use a normal stick, walking stick, or hiking pole on country walks. | These strategies provide a tactile guide for the height of the ground ahead, with advance notice. (The "loose" hand of an accompanying person gives no such guidance unless it is extended and the elbow fixed to give a consistent tactile height guide.) |
| 4–8 | Difficulty seeing buttons | It is difficult to do up buttons, but the task may be much easier in front of a full-length mirror. | Buttons cannot be seen even when looking down if the visual field impairment involves the whole lower visual field; however, they can still be seen in a mirror. |
| 4–adult | Difficulty negotiating escalators | Avoids escalators and instead uses elevators. | Stepping onto a moving surface is very difficult. |
| 4–adult | Difficulty jumping or diving into a swimming pool | The child is frightened of jumping or diving into a swimming pool. | Cannot see or judge the height of the water, or may collide with another swimmer. |
| 4–adult | Issues with putting on shoes | Lifts foot high onto step, or lies on back lifting the foot to put their shoes on. | Cannot see feet well enough in lower visual field. |

*(continued on next page)*

**TABLE 3.5** *(continued from previous page)*

| *Typical Age (years) of Behavior* | *Difficulty* | *Behavior or Adaptation* | *Reason* |
|---|---|---|---|
| 4–adult | Avoiding and having difficulty with negotiating low obstacles | Coffee tables are bumped into, especially if they have been moved. The child becomes angry if this happens. Families have often removed these obstacles, or have ensured that they are in a fixed location. The family should also inform the child when furniture has to be moved. | Position of items in lower visual field is difficult to see and estimate. |
| 5–adult | Inability to estimate the height of the bottom of a bath | Families have learned to use a colored bath mat and may also install a handrail. Often the child prefers to use a shower with a handrail to cope with the step. | Lack of clearly visible contours renders the height of the bottom of the bath difficult to estimate. |
| 5–adult | Difficulty reaching for items | May automatically use a wide finger gap or an outstretched hand when reaching for an item in the impaired lower visual field. Or the child may reach beyond the item to gather it up. | Variable combination of lower visual field impairment with dorsal stream dysfunction means that hand movement is clumsy, and the child compensates automatically. |
| 5–adult | Difficulty putting items down | Items are often misplaced. A child may have already learned to use the little finger as a tactile guide to locate and estimate heights of surfaces. | Visual guidance of movement needs to be supplemented by touch when putting items down, especially when tired. |
| 5–adult | Misses the lower part of a page | The child prefers text to be held up high, or placed on a book or music stand. May have learned that text placed further away on a desk allows the lower part of page to be read more easily. | Although one reads with the center of the visual field, the lower visual field guides the gaze as it moves down the page. |
| 8–adult | Difficulty finding shoes on floor | The child learns to put shoes in a specific location on the floor or on a higher surface to make them easier to find. | Shoes and other possessions are often lost when on the floor. |
| 8–adult | Cannot see hand extended for a handshake | The child avoids handshakes. | The proffered hand in the lower visual field may not be seen, and this can cause embarrassment. |
| 8–adult | Cannot see friends when looking down into a crowd | Families recognize this problem, and thus wave and call out to their child so they can identify them. | Search is affected in lower visual field impairment. |

*Source*: Adapted with permission from Dutton, G. N., Bowman, R., & Fazzi, E. (2014). Visual function. In B. Dan, M. Mayston, N. Paneth, & L. Rosenbloom (Eds.), *Cerebral palsy: Science and clinical practice*. London: Mac Keith Press.

that such children use, is to reach the hand beyond the object and sweep it toward themselves as a means of getting hold of and grasping it.

There is a need to develop objective approaches beyond the author's clinical observations, to classify disorders of visual guidance of hand movement in children, akin to such recent developments in adults (Borchers, Müller, Synofzik, & Himmelbach, 2013). Table 3.6 describes some of the typical behaviors and adaptations shown by children with lower visual field impairment and presumed upper limb optic ataxia.

### Problems with Visual and Auditory Search and Attention

A large proportion of children with lower visual field impairment, often with impaired visual guidance of the lower (and less often, the upper) limbs, also have difficulties with visual search and giving attention to more than one or two things at once. This combination is often seen with early-onset bilateral posterior parietal damage leading to dorsal stream dysfunction, with or without cerebral palsy (Jacobson & Dutton, 2000). It can also be seen in able-bodied children affected by bilateral dorsal stream dysfunction in mainstream schools (Dutton et al., 2004). Additionally, there is epidemiological evidence that less severe variants of the condition are not uncommon, but tend to go unrecognized (Williams et al., 2011). These features become more prominent when the child is tired. Thus, teachers may not see the features at school, but parents are likely to be more aware of clumsiness and poor visual search when the child comes home.

TABLE 3.6

## Visual Behaviors and Adaptations Exhibited by Children with CVI and Impaired Visual Guidance of the Upper Limbs Due to Dorsal Stream Dysfunction, as Well as Adaptive Strategies that May Be Used by the Children[a]

| *Typical Age (years) of Behavior* | *Difficulty* | *Behavior or Adaptation* | *Reason* |
|---|---|---|---|
| 3–adult | Inaccuracy of reach | The child is not able to accurately match the movement of a hand in the air (Milner & Goodale, 2006) to its spatial location. The gap between finger and thumb is wide, a whole hand is extended to grasp a target object, or the object is gathered up. Some, with good control of movement, learn to extend the pinkie finger as a tactile guide to the location of the target surface to avoid accidents or the misplacement of an object. Larger objects may also be used to facilitate grasp. | The posterior parietal cortices are damaged, leading to optic ataxia, commonly accompanied by simultanagnosia. (This may be combined with, or diagnosed as dyspraxia or as being motor in origin.) |

[a]Motor difficulties may mask aspects of impairment of visual guidance of movement, but for those with little or no motor difficulties, impaired visual guidance of movement (optic ataxia) may be evident as the principal issue.

*Source*: Adapted with permission from Dutton, G. N., Bowman, R., & Fazzi, E. (2014). Visual function. In B. Dan, M. Mayston, N. Paneth, & L. Rosenbloom (Eds.), *Cerebral palsy: Science and clinical practice*. London: Mac Keith Press.

An individual's subconscious mental map of the surroundings also includes auditory information (Isenburg, Vaden, Saberi, Muftuler, & Hickok, 2012). This author has seen many children with visual dorsal stream dysfunction who are unable to localize the source of a voice or other sounds, particularly in background conversation or noise, suggesting that visual mapping and auditory mapping are linked. Table 3.7 describes some of the typical behaviors and adaptations shown by children with difficulties giving attention to more than one issue at once and impaired visual search related to dorsal stream dysfunction.

TABLE 3.7

**Visual Behaviors and Adaptations Exhibited by Children with CVI and Difficulties Giving Attention to More Than One Issue at Once Associated with Impaired Visual Search Related to Dorsal Stream Dysfunction**

| *Typical Age (years) of Behavior* | *Difficulty* | *Behavior or Adaptation* | *Reason* |
|---|---|---|---|
| 1–8 | Difficulty finding toys | Difficulty finding toys is compensated for by emptying toy box and spreading toys out; lining toys up; asking a parent or caregiver to find the toy; choosing a random toy instead; or not bothering with toys at all. Parents have found that a few well-placed toys overcome this difficulty. | The three-dimensional disarray of the contents of a toy box is difficult to cope with. |
| 1–12 | Cannot see all the information on a TV screen | The child chooses to watch material with slow presentation, such as a weatherman. The child also gets very close to the TV, shifting their head and eyes to the elements which attract their attention the most. | The combination of fast-moving images and multiple details compel a child to get very close to the TV to view everything, even if their visual acuities are normal or near normal. |
| 1–adult | Difficulty seeing and listening at the same time | Appears not to see when listening, in severe cases. | Profound difficulty dividing attention between sight and sound. |
| 1–adult | Does not watch cartoons and films with a lot of visual and auditory information | The child either does not watch TV, or chooses to watch the person who reads the news or explains the weather, or programs with similarly limited visual information. Films made before the invention of the zoom lens, since they contain no zooming or panning, are preferred. | Simultanagnostic visual dysfunction, often with other visual processing difficulties, means that complex imagery cannot be fully seen and appreciated. |
| 2–adult | Will not look at a face and listen at the same time | Looks away from people when listening to them. | Difficulty giving attention to a face and the spoken word at the same time. |

*(continued on next page)*

**TABLE 3.7** *(continued from previous page)*

| *Typical Age (years) of Behavior* | *Difficulty* | *Behavior or Adaptation* | *Reason* |
|---|---|---|---|
| 2–adult | Finding a relative or friend among a group of people | Parents learn to meet in a specific location, to wave, to call, and to wear distinct clothing when picking up a child from school, or going out as a family. They know this is normal for their child. Older children use a friend or sibling as a guide, or stay at the side of the playground and know that it is normal not to be able to identify friends. Good friends work out the problem and adapt by accepting and helping the child. | Impaired ability to identify a person in a group as a result of impaired visual search is a typical feature of dorsal stream dysfunction. |
| 2–adult | Easily gets lost in crowded places | The child tends to avoid crowded places, which can be distressing. Older children and adults know it is normal to frequently ask for directions. Families have found that walkie-talkies or mobile phones are essential for older children, who can contact them if they get lost. (Inability to locate where sounds are coming from means that calling out to the child may not help.) | Crowded places with a lot of people and noise cause confusion. |
| 2–adult | Easily gets lost in busy towns and shops | A young child can wander off and get lost. Children often are not allowed to go out with friends. Visits are only made to known locations with limited distractions. Families have learned to visit places ahead of time to learn the "lay of the land." | Town centers and shops can present too much visual input to analyze. |
| 4–adult | Items pointed out in the distance cannot be seen | Some families physically rotate the child toward the target and get them to look along a pointing arm. Digital cameras with zoom capabilities have already been found to be a way of circumventing the problem. | In general, the further away one is, the more there is to see. |
| 4–adult | Impaired reading of crowded text | Some children learn to occlude surrounding text by using their fingers, a ruler, or a self-made typoscope (a plastic screen with a slot cut out through which to read text). | Simultanagnostic dysfunction can focally affect access to the written word, which can be overcome by minimizing crowding with a typoscope or a well-spaced text layout. |
| 4–adult | Impaired ability to access numbers from the printed page | The problem relates to an inability to access columns or rows of numbers accurately, unless they are both presented and written on squared paper, which makes the numbers easier to distinguish. | Visual crowding can lead to numbers in columns and rows becoming jumbled. |

*(continued on next page)*

**TABLE 3.7** *(continued from previous page)*

| *Typical Age (years) of Behavior* | *Difficulty* | *Behavior or Adaptation* | *Reason* |
|---|---|---|---|
| 4–adult | Inability to identify and find items of clothing from a pile | Clothes get spread out to find a chosen item. Parents have also found that using a small number of clothing items placed in specific locations, or hung up and arranged in groups, helps deal with the problem. | A partially covered item of clothing can be difficult to identify. |
| 5–18 | Problems finding items on school workstation | The school workstation and tray easily becomes messy and disorganized. Learned strategies, such as a template for where to put things, help to deal with this difficulty. | Overlapping objects may not be identified and found. |
| 5–18 | Problems changing clothes at school | Items of clothes can get mixed up. Some children learn that a strategy of hanging up clothes sequentially as they come off can be reversed successfully in order to get dressed again. | Overlapping clothing renders individual items difficult to find. |
| 7–adult | Great difficulty copying | Takes a very long time to copy information and does so imperfectly. | The dual task of visual search of both source and target documents, and visually remembering the information, is impaired. |

*Source*: Adapted with permission from Dutton, G. N., Bowman, R., & Fazzi, E. (2014). Visual function. In B. Dan, M. Mayston, N. Paneth, & L. Rosenbloom (Eds.), *Cerebral palsy: Science and clinical practice*. London: Mac Keith Press.

#### Discomfort and Anxiety Related to Dorsal Stream Dysfunction

Lack of ability to simultaneously handle (or parallel process) visual and auditory information related to posterior parietal damage leading to dorsal stream dysfunction can, perhaps not surprisingly, lead to discomfort and distress. Typical behaviors of affected children and adaptive strategies that families may have already found to be effective are outlined in Table 3.8.

#### The Spectrum of Expression of Bilateral Dorsal Stream Dysfunction

As described previously, the severity of the difficulties from bilateral dorsal stream dysfunction ranges from mild dysfunction to profound difficulties (Balint's syndrome) (see Figure 3.4).

In cases in which dysfunction is severe, there is extensive and obvious damage to the posterior parietal brain (Gillen et al., 2003; Drummond et al., 2007). In cases in which it is moderate, the damage is less severe (Saidkasimova, Bennett, Butler, & Dutton, 2007). In cases in which dysfunction is mild—although it is evident when given detailed consideration—imaging of the brain may show only subtle abnormalities (Saidkasimova, Bennett, Butler, & Dutton, 2007). The cluster of visual behaviors typical of dorsal stream dysfunction is common. In

TABLE 3.8

## Behavioral Features of Discomfort and Anxiety Commonly Seen in Children Who Show Evidence of Dorsal Stream Dysfunction and Adaptive Strategies that Families Have Commonly Identified

| *Typical Age (years) of Behavior* | *Difficulty* | *Behavior or Adaptation* | *Reason* |
|---|---|---|---|
| 1–7 | Having temper tantrums in busy places and situations | The distress caused by busy places can cause temper tantrums, which are difficult to manage. Families have learned to avoid these situations with the child. | The noise, combined with the inability to escape, becomes overwhelming. |
| 3–12 | Experiencing distress on car journeys | More profoundly impaired children can be distressed by the sensory input from car journeys. Parents have found that window shields or dark glasses diminish the visual stimulation, while playing music through headphones causes sufficient distraction. | Engine noise and the moving scene can be distressing. |
| 3–adult | Inability to go to family events and parties | Many families adapt by going to an event early, while it is still quiet, and allowing the party to build up, taking the child away if they become distressed. | Gradual build-up of crowding is less distressing. |
| 3–adult | Shopping in supermarkets causes distress | Families learn to take their child to the store early or late, when shops are quiet, or avoid taking the child altogether. Younger children like to sit in the shopping cart. Older children may like to push a small shopping cart to feel safer (but this can be difficult to manage). Children who get lost can be difficult to find and cannot identify where a calling voice is coming from. Older children can be given mobile phones to compensate for this. | The visual and auditory noise, accompanied by inability to know whether shopping trolleys will collide into one another, can be very distressing. |

*Source*: Adapted with permission from Dutton, G. N., Bowman, R., & Fazzi, E. (2014). Visual function. In B. Dan, M. Mayston, N. Paneth, & L. Rosenbloom (Eds.), *Cerebral palsy: Science and clinical practice*. London: Mac Keith Press.

one epidemiological study of 4,512 children aged 13 years, behavioral features identified as typical of such visual perceptual dysfunction were associated with underachievement in reading and mathematics (Williams et al., 2011).

Exploration of the surroundings with the head and eyes is commonly impaired in children with more severe dorsal stream dysfunction. This may be the reason why objectively measured visually attracted and guided eye movement is prolonged in children with CVI (Pel et al., 2011), and why children with spastic diplegia make fewer searching fast eye movements (*saccades*) than normal (Fedrizzi et al., 1998).

FIGURE 3.4

## Range of Visual Disabilities in Children Resulting from Bilateral Dorsal Stream Dysfunction

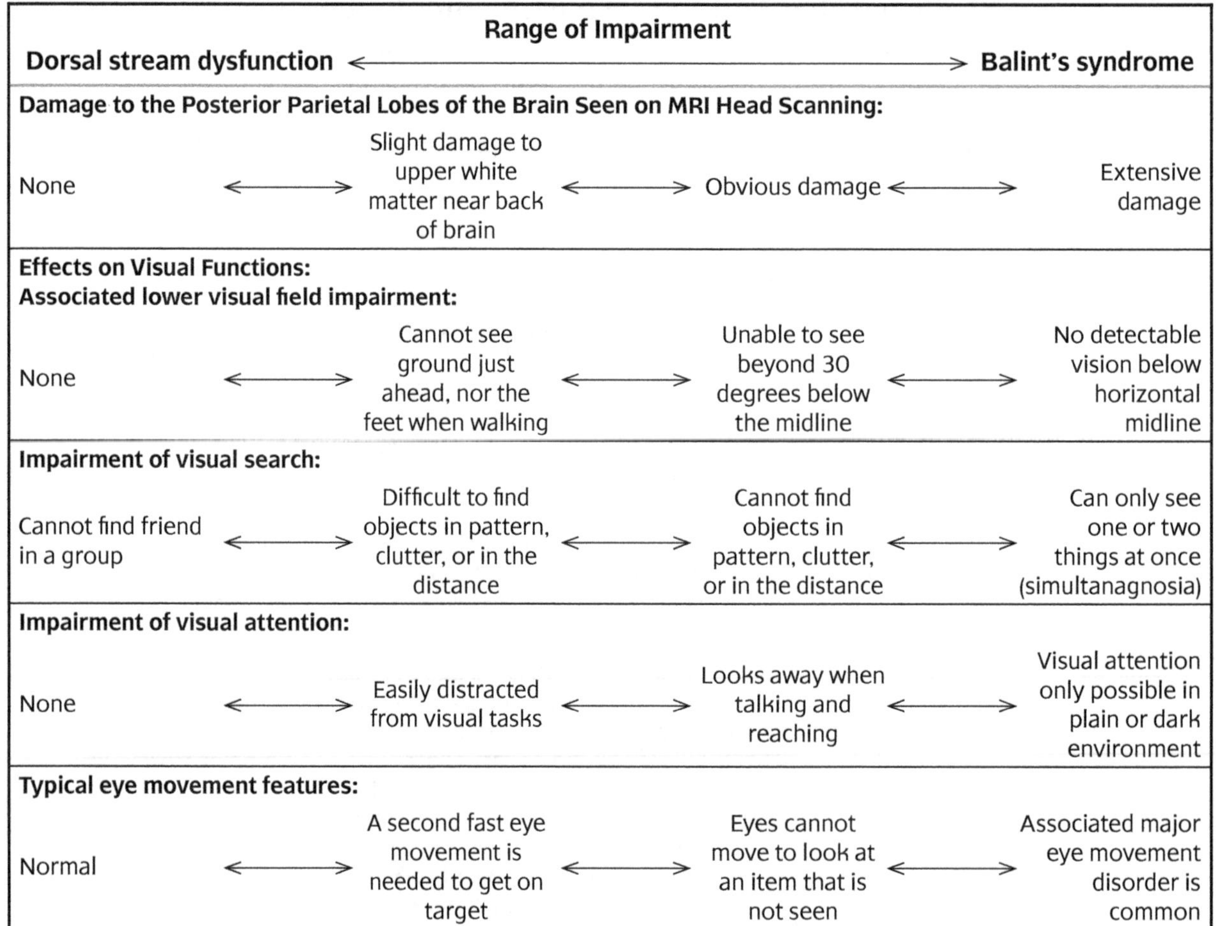

| Range of Impairment<br>Dorsal stream dysfunction ⟷ Balint's syndrome | | | |
|---|---|---|---|
| **Damage to the Posterior Parietal Lobes of the Brain Seen on MRI Head Scanning:** | | | |
| None | Slight damage to upper white matter near back of brain | Obvious damage | Extensive damage |
| **Effects on Visual Functions:**<br>**Associated lower visual field impairment:** | | | |
| None | Cannot see ground just ahead, nor the feet when walking | Unable to see beyond 30 degrees below the midline | No detectable vision below horizontal midline |
| **Impairment of visual search:** | | | |
| Cannot find friend in a group | Difficult to find objects in pattern, clutter, or in the distance | Cannot find objects in pattern, clutter, or in the distance | Can only see one or two things at once (simultanagnosia) |
| **Impairment of visual attention:** | | | |
| None | Easily distracted from visual tasks | Looks away when talking and reaching | Visual attention only possible in plain or dark environment |
| **Typical eye movement features:** | | | |
| Normal | A second fast eye movement is needed to get on target | Eyes cannot move to look at an item that is not seen | Associated major eye movement disorder is common |

### THE POSSIBILITY OF BILATERAL DORSAL STREAM DYSFUNCTION IN CHILDREN WITH QUADRAPLEGIC CEREBRAL PALSY

Features of Balint's syndrome can be observed or inferred in children with evidence of generalized brain dysfunction. Children with spastic quadriplegic cerebral palsy commonly have profound visual impairment to the extent that it is difficult to assess their vision beyond an estimate of visual acuity obtained through preferential looking methods (see Chapter 12 for details about assessment methods). Yet many of these children become much more attentive when in a sensory room—a controlled environment—with a single stimulus, or when playing together with a caregiver while in a low tent or under a cover that eliminates surrounding visual and auditory distractions (see Chapters 20 and 21). All of a sudden the child seems to "wake up" and becomes more attentive and easier to communicate with.

A hypothesis to explain this behavior is that the child may have previously unrecognized additional profound Balint's syndrome, resulting in the child's being able to find and give attention to only one or two things at a time. This will always remain a hypothesis, however, because the presumed syndrome is masked by the child's overall condition. Nevertheless, it is important to consider an approach that assumes that the child can pay attention to only one or two things at a time, minimize background auditory and visual stimulation, and then evaluate the results for each child.

Some children with these more profound visual difficulties may not reach out at all. A potentially important hypothesis is that they may have very limited visual guidance of movement as a result of unrecognized (and effectively undiagnosable) Balint's syndrome, and that they do not know, by means of vision, where their limbs are. In the author's experience, such children may respond to forms of "tactile bridging" by reaching along the top of a parent's moving and outstretched hand. This allows them to start exploring their surroundings safely, without risking the unpleasant surprise of having their hand collide with what they are reaching for—an experience that may contribute to future tactile defensiveness.

### *Unilateral Dorsal Stream Dysfunction: Visual Neglect and Inattention on One Side*

Adults who have had damage to the posterior parietal area on one side, most commonly due to stroke, can develop *visual neglect*—lack of attention to visual space on one side leading to that side being neglected—affecting the opposite side of the body (Ting et al., 2011). Children and young adults can also experience this condition, but it is rare.

In common parlance, the word *neglect* implies a conscious act of failing to pay attention, but in medical use, the term has no implication of consciousness. On the contrary, a person with visual neglect usually has no knowledge of his or her visual disability, nor is the person aware of having no knowledge, despite being taught otherwise. The affected person is unaware of the disability and cannot tell the doctor about it. Since this can only be communicated by caregivers, visual neglect can often remain undiagnosed.

Visual neglect is even more complicated because of the way we comprehend the world around us. We have a set of concepts about the external space around us that includes: (1) our location within that space, (2) our knowledge of the presence of our own bodies, and (3) our knowledge of the interaction of our bodies with the environment. Depending on the location, nature, and extent of damage to the brain, neglect can affect any of these three concepts of external space, in any combination or degree.

Neglect of the left side of the body due to right-sided damage to the brain tends to be more severe than mirror image damage to the other side, because the right side of the brain also gives some visual attention to the right side of visual space. In contrast, damage to the left side of the posterior parietal lobe tends to cause more minor features of neglect on the right side.

#### VISUAL INATTENTION VS. IMPAIRED VISUAL FIELDS

The occipital lobes support vision in such a way that when there is damage on one side, vision on the opposite side is lost or impaired. This affects the visual field of both eyes equally. When the head or eyes are turned to the left, the area lacking vision moves with the eyes and head.

In contrast, the posterior parietal area of the brain provides awareness of the surrounding environment by creating a virtual construct, or map, of the external environment, to enable accurate visual guidance of movement of the limbs and body (see Chapter 2). This requires the virtual image to integrate accurately with the location of the body from moment to moment, rather than with the location of the head. Therefore, damage to the posterior parietal lobe on one side creates a lack of awareness of visual space on the other side of the body, along with lack of attention to that space (despite evidence of intact vision on that side if the occipital lobes are functioning). This lack of awareness and attention relates to the position of the body and is independent of the position of the head and eyes (Ting et al., 2011).

Lack of vision on one side resulting from damage to the occipital lobes (*hemaniopia*)

FIGURE 3.5

**The Role of Head Position and Body Position in Giving Awareness to the Left in a Child with Left Hemianopia and Left Inattention**

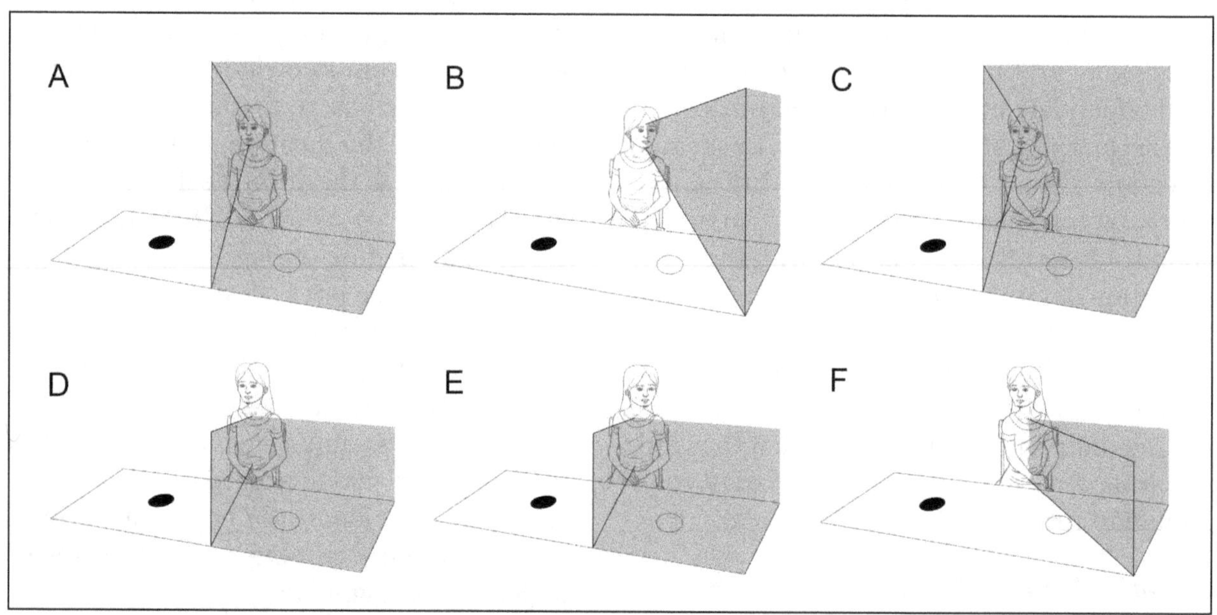


Left hemianopia: The visual fields move with the head and eyes.

**A.** When the child is sitting and looking straight ahead, the white disc is not seen.
**B.** Turning the head to the left reveals the white disc.
**C.** Turning the body to the left without turning the head does not reveal the white disc.

Left inattention: Visual attention to external space relates to, and moves with the body.

**D.** When the body is facing straight ahead, the child does not identify the white disc.
**E.** The head is turned to the left, but the disc is not revealed.
**F.** The body is turned to the left, but the head is still looking straight ahead. This affords attention to the white disc, despite the head not being turned, because the disc has entered "attended space."

*Source*: Reprinted from Zihl, J., & Dutton, G. N. (2015). *Cerebral visual impairment in children: Visuoperceptive and visuocognitive disorders.* Vienna: Springer-Verlag Wien.

moves with the head and eyes, but lack of awareness and knowledge of the position of objects in surrounding space as a result of damage to the posterior parietal lobes does not. Therefore, for objects to be seen, recognized, and reacted to, the body has to rotate.

For example, if an affected child is seated at a desk to attempt a task involving perception of objects, the desk—or the objects on the desk, the visual targets—have to be displaced to the better-functioning side of the body, or the body has to be rotated, as illustrated in Figure 3.5. This diagram contrasts the role of head position and body position in attending to the left in a child with left hemianopia, as compared with a child with left inattention. In hemianopia, turning the head suffices to shift the blind area and reveal an object that has previously been invisible (Figure 3.5A–C). In visual neglect, as already noted, the body must shift (Figure 3.5D–F). When both the visual field and attention to the left are limited, turning the head and body together best helps to reveal the white disc. A mirror image diagram would apply for lack of vision and attention to the right. However, attention to the right is less frequently impaired to the same degree, because the intact right posterior parietal area is able to give a degree of attention to the right in addition to giving attention to the left.

The following case study shows an example of a young girl with left visual neglect who developed ways of coping on her own:

**Emily was 18 months old when abnormal blood** vessels (an arteriovenous abnormality) inside the right parietal lobe ruptured, bled, and caused damage. When seen at the age of 6, she had partially recovered from the resulting impaired movement in her left leg. Although her left leg remained weak and stiff, she was still able to walk. Her left hand and arm, however, had limited movement, and she tended to ignore them.

Emily was able to turn to look at a target that was moved from behind her into her visual field on both sides, a reflex action. However, when she was seated on a chair directly facing a table and asked to pick up a counter placed on one or the other side, she only picked up the counter on the right side. Despite moving her head and eyes to search the whole table, she could not find the counter on her left (see Figure 3.5E). At this point, she rotated her chair into the usual position that she adopts to eat at a table. She turned it 30 degrees counterclockwise so that it was facing toward the left side of the table. This time, she consistently picked up the counters on both sides with no difficulty, even when looking straight ahead (Figure 3.5F).

Her parents explained that Emily had been turning her body in this way to eat at a table for more than two years. She had discovered for herself that by doing this, she would not leave food on the left side of her plate.

When Emily walked down the school corridor, she turned the upper part of her body in the same way. This most likely allowed her to attend to both sides of the corridor so that she could find her classroom. However, her left leg had a tendency to collide with her right leg, perhaps as a result of the chosen body position.

By combining a slight turn in her chair with displacement of her schoolwork to her right, Emily's accuracy and rate of schoolwork increased considerably.

Thus, Emily's visual field—the area she was capable of seeing—differed from her field of visual attention—the area to which she was able to pay attention. Her visual fields were elicited by attracting attention, which requires only a reflexive response, whereas her field of visual attention was elicited by getting her to consciously search on both sides. (It was only visual search to her left that was impaired.) The visual field test required a reactive attentional reflex, but assessment of her field of visual attention required proactive search. (See Chapter 12 for a discussion of assessment of visual neglect.)

#### Strategies to Manage Visual Neglect

The individuals most commonly affected by visual neglect are those with hemiplegic cerebral palsy. The main blood vessels supplying the central part of the brain are the middle cerebral arteries. Blockage of these blood vessels causes brain damage leading to lack of movement on the opposite side of the body. In addition, the resulting damage to the brain can also affect the posterior parietal area. This, in turn, can lead to features of visual neglect that become apparent as the child develops. However, because damage to the brain occurs very early on, there is also potential for healing and growth, for recovery of brain tissue, as well as improvement of function owing to neuroplasticity—the brain's ability to reorganize itself by forming new neural interconnections throughout life. This means that the patterns of lack of awareness and lack of attention affecting the same side as the limb weaknesss are variable and unique for each person. It also means that standardized tests that measure lack of performance ability in specified tasks may not reveal the true nature of the problem (see Appendix 13A for an example of a screening test that has been standardized for children with CVI). The professional needs to apply a deductive approach with considerable imagination to elicit the problems. Careful history taking and keen observation (see Chapters 11 and 14) are needed to understand the deficits of the individual child as they experience the world around them, if one is to intervene constructively with habilitational strategies that are matched to the child's individual needs, as illustrated in the following example:

**Amy is 8 years old. She was born with weakness of** her right side as a result of a vascular accident affecting the left side of her brain around the time of birth. Her case came to the author's attention because her drawings were always very clear on the left, but had a poorer quality on the right. For example, the right eye may be missing when she draws a face, and the right limbs of a person tend to be distorted. She draws with her left hand and shows evidence of good dexterity for the left side of the picture, but not for the right. Moving the paper so that it is placed off-center to her left significantly improves the overall quality of her drawings. Turning the paper upside down to finish her picture allows her to view the right side of the drawing within her left field of view, so that she automatically refines her picture.

Amy has, for a long time, insisted on sitting at a table with her table setting placed off-center to her left. She also eats with her plate fully within her left field of view, with the right margin of her plate placed at the center of her body, presumably as a subconscious adaptation. Her parents indicate that, prior to doing this, she would often miss the food on the right side of the plate.

The recommendation that Amy sits near the front of class with the teacher to her left has been followed by significant improvement in her behavior, discipline, and performance. Common among other children whose right side of the body has been affected, Amy has a subtle disorder of language that also needs to be evaluated, understood, and managed, because the language centers of the brain are located primarily on the left side, where the damage took place. Behaviors commonly seen in children with hemianopia or hemianopic lack of attention, or both, are outlined in Table 3.9.

## Combined Occipital, Dorsal, and Ventral Stream Dysfunction

An open-minded approach is essential when evaluating a child with evidence of CVI. If there is evidence of one impaired function, one must always check to see whether any other functions are impaired as well. Combined impairment of the occipital lobe and dorsal and ventral stream functions is ob-

**TABLE 3.9**

## Behaviors Commonly Seen in Children with Hemianopic Visual Field Defects and/or Hemianopic Lack of Visual Attention[a]

| *Typical Age (years) of Behavior* | *Difficulty* | *Behavior or Adaptation* | *Reason* |
|---|---|---|---|
| 2–adult | Toys and material in books are not seen on affected side | Toys and books are displaced off center to the "good" side by children. | Lack of attention on the weakest side is common and easy to identify. As in adults, right posterior parietal lesions tend to cause greater inattention (on the left) than left lesions. |
| 3–adult | Food on one side of a plate is missed | Children or family members rotate the plate to bring food into view. Children lacking attention on one side may discover that food can be moved off center to the sighted side. The child may consistently sit at table with the better functioning side turned slightly toward the table. | Food on affected side becomes accessible when adaptations are made. |
| 3–adult | Books, toys, and place settings are incompletely seen on one side | Children may discover for themselves that body rotation is compensatory. For example, they may sit at a table with chair rotated to one or other side, to turn the midline of the body so that the intact area of attention encompasses the material of interest. (Affected children who are mobile sometimes also turn their body to one side when walking, perhaps for the same reason.) | Inattention is related to the body and, unlike hemianopia, tends not to be compensated for by head and eye turns. |
| 5–16 | Learning is impaired when the teacher is positioned at the affected side | The child with impaired visual attention on one side is placed with the teacher on the attended side. | Inattention is related to the body and, unlike hemianopia, tends not to be compensated for by head and eye turn. |
| 5–18 | People are not seen on the affected side | Teachers, friends, and family may have learned to communicate when positioned on the side with best visual function. | People may not be seen and may not be attended to when on affected side. |
| 5–adult | Traffic is missed on affected side | Mobile children may turn the body to look to the affected side because unilateral lack of attention, which may be isolated or may accompany hemianopia, relates to and moves with the body rather than the head and eyes. | Inattention relates to the body schema and is not compensated for by head and eye turns. The body needs to turn to compensate. This also deals with hemianopia, as the head turns with the body. |

[a]Many children with hemianopia have good compensation, and difficulties resulting from early-onset hemianopia can diminish with time.

*Source*: Adapted with permission from Dutton, G. N., Bowman, R., & Fazzi, E. (2014). Visual function. In B. Dan, M. Mayston, N. Paneth, & L. Rosenbloom (Eds.), *Cerebral palsy: Science and clinical practice*. London: Mac Keith Press.

served more frequently than individual disturbances of function. In essence, any of the visual disorders described in this chapter can occur in any combination or degree (see Figures 3.1, 3.3, and 3.4). This means that detection of any one visual disability resulting from damage to the brain should automatically trigger a search for additional disabilities, initially by means of structured history taking, followed by corroboration with observation of the child's behaviors, and if available, appropriate investigation.

Dorsal stream dysfunction may occur in isolation, or may be accompanied by evidence of ventral stream dysfunction, whereas isolated ventral stream dysfunction as a result of CVI is rare. This has led to the suggestion that the terms "dorsal stream dysfunction" and "dorsal stream dysfunction plus" be used to help convey conceptual awareness of the patterns of visual perceptual dysfunction commonly seen in children (Dutton, 2009).

## Acquired Brain Injury Causing Visual Impairment in Later Childhood

Although brain injury of very early onset—before or right after birth—is the most common cause of CVI, acquired damage to the visual brain later in childhood, although rare, is important to understand and manage as well. The deficits that result tend to differ from those of early-onset brain injury for the following reasons:

- The child has already learned a range of skills when vision was intact.
- The child has a prior memory of skills and a conceptual framework for these learned skills.
- Language and concepts have been learned in a visual context.
- Knowledge and memories related to vision have been gained.

These aspects of prior knowledge, the potential for recovery of vision (initially over weeks, but later, over many years), and the fact that residual vision can be employed to great advantage by learning adaptations (such as using visual search to compensate for lack of visual field), make it possible to apply previously acquired skills and knowledge in the rehabilitation of these children. The more common acquired brain disorders that can interfere with vision are outlined below, along with the issues that render the potential outcomes somewhat different from early-onset CVI.

### *Epilepsy*

Epilepsy, manifesting as a seizure, can affect the whole body. However, it can also affect distinct parts of the brain, giving rise to continuing dysfunction of the affected area. If the part of the brain that moves one hand is affected, then twitching of the hand may occur, although this is rare. Similarly, if the occipital lobes are affected, then vision can be impaired intermittently at varying times and to varying degrees. Any aspect of vision may be affected. The electrical activity in the brain can also cause hallucinations, causing the child to see colors and patterns that are not there.

If vision deteriorates or fluctuates markedly in a child with CVI, epilepsy affecting the visual brain needs to be considered as a possible cause, so that appropriate drug treatment can be provided. If vision fluctuates, a strategy of brief assessment of vision is needed at the start of each school day to match the educational material to the visual abilities at that moment in time. Those who have controlled epilepsy but develop a seizure out of the blue can occasionally experience visual impairment afterward that, in some cases, can persist for days.

### Acquired Occipital Brain Injury Due to Lack of Oxygen Delivery

As described earlier, the occipital lobes have the greatest metabolic need because they are always active while the individual is awake. This means they are particularly susceptible to damage from lack of a blood supply as a result of cardiac arrest, or low oxygen levels resulting from very severe respiratory disease.

Occipital damage varies in degree and impairs basic visual functions. Ventral stream recognition functions can be affected, with preservation of dorsal stream functions, facilitating movement despite poor conscious vision. This can lead to the false impression that conscious vision is better than it appears from observable behavior.

### Spontaneous Bleeding Inside the Brain

Congenitally abnormal blood vessels inside the brain can rupture. Taking into consideration the area involved and the extent of the resulting damage, vision can be affected in a wide variety of ways, depending on the specific functions that are lost or disordered.

### Nonaccidental Head Injury

Children who survive a severe non-accidental head injury can sustain a variety of severe impairments as a result, including damage to the retina, the optic nerve of one or both eyes, or damage to both structures.

The injury can also affect any part of the brain with predictable consequences. Damage to the occipital lobes diminishes visual fields and can affect visual acuities. Damage to the parietal lobes tends to cause dorsal stream dysfunction with impaired visual guidance of movement, leading to the mobile child bumping into walls and not recognizing whether there is a step present or not. This is associated with significant problems with visual search and giving visual attention. Temporal lobe damage affects orientation and recognition, while frontal damage can impair intellect, learning, and emotion.

### Accidental Head Injury

Depending on the location and extent of the injury, any part of the visual brain can be damaged in any combination.

### Viral Encephalitis

Brain infection by a virus (*viral encephalitis*) tends to cause visual difficulties that are unique to each child. This author has seen a child who, during recovery, had lost the ability to recognize certain individual letters (called *literal alexia*), but whose ability to read other letters remained intact. Similarly, the child may be able to recognize some people but not others. Taking an in-depth history from the family together with detailed observation will help to untangle and to characterize what may appear to be a confusing set of visual dysfunctions. Regular evaluation, possibly even on a weekly basis at the beginning of recovery, may be needed. Recovery tends to continue over a period of years, particularly with good teaching that recognizes and rehabilitates the consequences of the specific visual difficulties. It is important to have and convey an optimistic outlook.

### Acute-Onset Congenital Disorders of Brain Function

There are a number of rare congenital conditions that can cause stroke-like events later in life. For example, there are several inheritable disorders of the mitochondria—the microscopic parts of a cell that function as its powerhouse—and in some of those variants, the brain can be suddenly and focally affected (as in MELAS syndrome). The affected child grows up normally, but then, out of the blue, sudden onset brain damage resembling a stroke takes place, giving rise to a range of possible brain dysfunctions. The visual effects depend on the structures damaged and the extent of the damage. Visual rehabilitation comprises part of the overall management.

### *Chronic Progressive Congenital Disorders of Brain Function*

There are a number of rare, chronic, progressive brain disorders of childhood in which ongoing deterioration of brain function takes place. Vision is frequently affected. It is important that an approach be taken that informs families and schools of current visual functional levels, to ensure that toys or gifts or materials being shown or used for education are rendered visible, audible where appropriate, and if possible, intelligible. A positive and supportive approach should be taken that enhances the experience of these children by making sure the materials are accessible and by matching them to each child's declining functions.

## Recognizing CVI in Children

This section focuses on the identification of children who have visual difficulties as a result of CVI that may be missed but that have functional consequences. These functional difficulties may be masked by other conditions in children who have profound disabilities. In the child without other disabilities, these difficulties may be attributed to a behavioral disorder, or they may simply go undetected by parents, especially when there is no sibling for comparison.

The key to identifying children affected by CVI is to be aware of the clues that lead one to suspect that a child has the condition, as well as the cluster of associated features to look for in order to validate the initial hypothesis that CVI may be present. The table in Appendix 3B is divided into "Indications" and associated clusters of "Visual Features to Look For." It is by no means a comprehensive list, and each practitioner in a position to identify affected children may well develop his or her own sets of clues and clusters to add to this list.

Appendix 3A outlines how findings reported on an MRI scan can also act as indicators for the practitioner by providing a list of specific visual behaviors characteristic of CVI to watch out for. Although MRI scans do not accurately predict visual outcomes and behaviors (Boot et al., 2010), the associations indicated on the list occur commonly enough to be considered.

Finally, typical behaviors and adaptations that the author has observed, along with their significance, have been described in Tables 3.2–3.9 as a means of helping practitioners identify children with CVI through the range of patterns that they and their families frequently exhibit when CVI has gone unidentified, particularly when evidence from brain imaging is not available. Professionals working with children who have this condition may wish to implement some of these strategies and suggest them to families.

Once CVI is suspected, full assessment is required to identify and characterize the disorder, its cause, and effective strategies for its management. (See the chapters in Part 3 for in-depth discussions of assessment.)

## Indicators for Identifying CVI in a Child Who Has Become Aware of a Visual Difficulty

Young children with CVI are not aware that they are different. As they grow older, however, these children can become aware that their vision is different from that of other people or, when questioned, they may be surprised to discover that what they consider to be their "normal" vision is not in fact typical. Upon learning this, the visual difficulty becomes apparent to the children, and thus symptomatic. (Symptoms are defined by the individual's subjective awareness of the evidence of a change or condition, so that a disorder that an individual is not aware of is asymptomatic. Once an individual is aware of the condition, it becomes symptomatic.)

In this author's experience, the most common set of symptoms of this type relate to perceptual visual dysfunction and are characterized by difficulties with the following aspects of vision:

- Finding things among pattern and clutter, or in the distance
- Seeing something, or someone, that has been pointed out
- Seeing numbers in columns and rows, when there are no additional reference lines
- Perception of moving objects (they can disappear when moving quickly, and reappear when they slow down)
- Finding their way around without bumping into things
- Recognizing people and objects

There is considerable variability from one child to the next because all these features may not be present in the same child. If an older child becomes aware of one of these difficulties, it should act as a signal that it may be worthwhile to investigate other possible features of perceptual visual impairment, since some features may be asymptomatic and therefore go unreported because the child is not aware of them.

## CVI Masked by Severe Disability

The way in which a severely disabled child with profound CVI sees can only be inferred from observing the characteristics of visual dysfunction in less severely disabled children, or from the features reported on head scans. The information provided in this chapter can be used to identify similar visual difficulties. For example, a child with profound CVI who focuses his attention on a single stimulus in a sensory room most likely also has severe dorsal stream dysfunction (Balint's syndrome). Adopting intervention strategies that take into account all possible difficulties can be immensely beneficial for the child.

When one comes across certain features that are indicative of potential CVI, it is always worth seeking further evidence of possible additional features. By having an open mind, and employing the range of approaches described in this book, many readers are likely to suspect hitherto unidentified CVI, both in children with known neurological disorders and those with no other difficulties, so that appropriate action can be taken. In the author's experience, parents are delighted when an explanation is offered for what were previously inexplicable and inconsistent behaviors. The affected children and young adults are even more delighted, not least because the criticism they were used to experiencing evaporates, replaced instead by concern and understanding.

FIGURE 3.6

## Tree of Vision: The Principal Functions of the Visual System and How They Are Connected

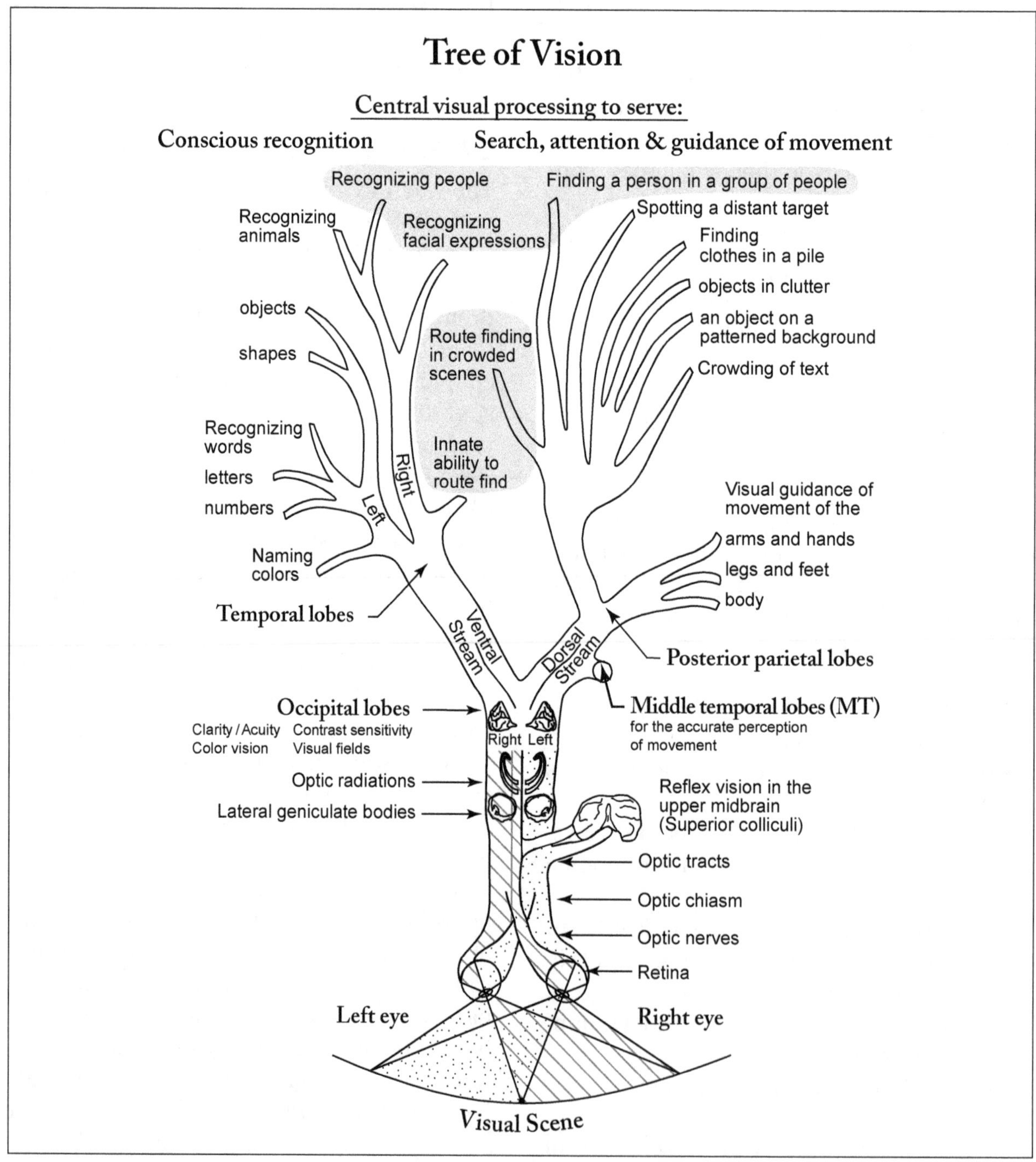


Damage at any location in the tree leads to impairment of the functions above that level.

*Source*: Reproduced with permission from Dutton, G. N., Bowman, R., & Fazzi, E. (2014). Visual function. In B. Dan, M. Mayston, N. Paneth, & L. Rosenbloom (Eds.), *Cerebral palsy: Science and clinical practice*. London: Mac Keith Press.

## Conclusion

Visual impairment as a result of damage to the visual brain is complex, but an overview of the system that the author likes to keep in mind may be helpful to readers. Figure 3.6 provides a summary in the form of a functional visual map for the visual system, showing the types of functions and tasks that are handled in each area.

The diagram is in the form of a tree. The eyes—the roots of the tree—receive the image. The image data are transferred along the visual pathways of the trunk to the occipital lobes, with some data being transferred to the upper midbrain to serve reflex vision. Data are transferred from the occipital lobes along the dorsal and ventral streams, represented as the two main tree branches. Any of the visual functions illustrated at the ends of the branches can be impaired to a variable degree. The tree-branching pattern symbolizes the clusters of visual difficulties that are commonly observed. Any significant damage lower down on the tree in turn impairs everything further up the tree.

The author keeps this map in mind when taking a history from, or examining, a child with CVI. It provides a conceptually helpful way of ensuring that no key information is overlooked.

## References

Ahmed, M., & Dutton, G. N. (1996). Cognitive visual dysfunction in a child with cerebral damage. *Developmental Medicine & Child Neurology, 38*, 736–739.

Andersson, S., Persson, E. K., Aring, E., Lindquist, B., Dutton, G. N., & Hellstrom, A. (2006). Vision in children with hydrocephalus. *Developmental Medicine & Child Neurology, 48,* 836–841.

Boot, F. H., Pel, J. J., van der Steen, J., & Evenhuis, H. M. (2010). Cerebral visual impairment: Which perceptive visual dysfunctions can be expected in children with brain damage? A systematic review. *Research in Developmental Disabilities, 31*, 1149–1159.

Borchers, S., Müller, L., Synofzik, M., & Himmelbach, M. (2013). Guidelines and quality measures for the diagnosis of optic ataxia. *Frontiers of Human Neuroscience, 7*, 324.

Brodsky, M. C. (2010). *Pediatric neuro-ophthalmology* (2nd ed.). New York: Springer.

Culham, J. C., Witt, J. K., Valyear, K. F., Dutton, G. N., & Goodale, M. A. (2008). fMRI and behavioral testing reveal preserved motion processing and visuomotor control in a patient with extensive occipitotemporal lesions. *Journal of Vision, 8*(6), 372.

Drummond, S. R., & Dutton, G. N. (2007). Simultanagnosia following perinatal hypoxia: A possible pediatric variant of Balint syndrome. *Journal of American Association for Pediatric Ophthalmology and Strabismus, 11*, 497–498.

Dutton, G. N. (2003). The Edridge Green Lecture. Cognitive vision, its disorders and differential diagnosis in adults and children: Knowing where and what things are. *Eye, 17,* 289–304.

Dutton, G. N. (2009). "Dorsal stream dysfunction" and "dorsal stream dysfunction plus": A potential classification for perceptual visual impairment in the context of cerebral visual impairment? *Developmental Medicine & Child Neurology, 51*(3), 170–172.

Dutton, G. N., & Bax, M. (2010). *Visual impairment in children due to damage to the brain.* London: Mac Keith Press.

Dutton, G. N., Bowman, R., & Fazzi, E. (2014). Visual function. In B. Dan, M. Mayston, N. Paneth, & L. Rosenbloom (Eds.), *Cerebral palsy: Science and clinical practice.* London: Mac Keith Press.

Dutton, G. N., Saaed, A., Fahad, B., Fraser, R., McDaid, G., McDade, J., . . . Spowart, K. (2004). The association of binocular lower visual field impairment, impaired simultaneous perception, disordered visually guided motion and inaccurate saccades in children with cerebral visual dysfunction—A retrospective observational study. *Eye, 18*, 27–34.

Fazzi, E., Bova, S., Giovenzana, A., Signorini, S., Uggetti, C., & Bianchi, P. (2007). Spectrum of visual disorders in children with cerebral visual impairment. *Journal of Child Neurology, 22*, 294–301.

Fazzi, E., Bova, S., Giovenzana, A., Signorini, S., Uggetti, C., & Bianchi, P. (2009). Cognitive visual dysfunctions in preterm children with periventricular leukomalacia. *Developmental Medicine & Child Neurology, 51*, 974–981.

Fedrizzi, E., Anderloni, A., Bono, R., Bova, S., Farinotti, M., Inverno, M., et al. (1998). Eye-movement disorders and visual-perceptual impairment in diplegic children born preterm: A clinical evaluation. *Developmental Medicine &Child Neurology, 40*(10), 682–688.

Gillen, J. A., & Dutton, G. N. (2003). Balint's syndrome in a 10-year-old male [Case report]. *Developmental Medicine & Child Neurology, 45*, 349–352.

Glosser, G., Salvucci, A. E., & Chiaravalloti, N. D. (2003). Naming and recognizing famous faces in temporal lobe epilepsy. *Neurology, 61*, 81–86.

Goodale, M., & Milner, A. D. (2013). *Sight unseen: An exploration of conscious and subconscious vision* (2nd ed.). New York: Oxford University Press.

Guzzetta, A., Tinelli, F., Del Viva, M. M., Bancale, A., Arrighi, R., Pascale, R., et al. (2009). Motion perception in preterm children: Role of prematurity and brain damage. *Neuroreport, 20*, 1339–1343.

Holmes, G. (1918). Disturbances of visual orientation. *British Journal of Ophthalmology, 2*, 449–468, 506–516.

Houliston, M. J., Taguri, A. H., Dutton, G. N., Hajivassiliou, C., & Young, D. G. (1999). Evidence of cognitive visual problems in children with hydrocephalus: A structured clinical history-taking strategy. *Developmental Medicine & Child Neurology, 41*, 298–306.

Hyvärinen, L., & Jacob, N. (2011). *WHAT and HOW does this child see?* Helsinki, Finland: VISTEST Ltd.

Isenberg, A. L., Vaden, K. I. Jr., Saberi, K., Muftuler, L. T., & Hickok, G. (2012) Functionally distinct regions for spatial processing and sensory motor integration in the planum temporale. *Human Brain Mapping, 33*, 2453–2463.

Jacobson, L., Flodmark, O., & Martin, L. (2006). Visual field defects in prematurely born patients with white matter damage of immaturity: A multiple-case study. *Acta Ophthalmologica Scandinavica, 84*, 357–362.

Jacobson, L. K., & Dutton, G. N. (2000). Periventricular leukomalacia: An important cause of visual and ocular motility dysfunction in children. *Survey of Ophthalmology, 45*, 1–13.

Jan, J. E., Heaven, R. K. B., Matsuba, C., Langley, M. B., Roman-Lantzy, C., & Anthony, T. L. (2013). Windows into the visual brain: New discoveries about the visual system, its functions, and implications for practitioners. *Journal of Visual Impairment & Blindness, 107*(4), 251–261.

Macintyre-Béon, C., Hussein, I., Hay, I., Cockburn, D., Calvert, J., Dutton, G. N., et al. (2010). Dorsal stream dysfunction in children. A review and an approach to diagnosis and management. *Current Pediatric Reviews, 6*, 166–182.

McKillop, E., Bennett, D., McDaid, G., Holland, B., Smith, G., Spowart, K., et al. (2006). Problems experienced by children with cognitive visual dysfunction due to cerebral visual impairment—And the approaches which parents have adopted to deal with these problems. *British Journal of Visual Impairment, 24*, 121–127.

Mesad, S., Laff, R., & Devinsky, O. (2003). Transient postoperative prosopagnosia. *Epilepsy Behavior, 4*, 567–570.

Milner, A. D., & Goodale, M. (2006). *The visual brain in action* (2nd ed.). New York: Oxford University Press.

Morrone, M. C., Guzzetta, A., Tinelli, F., Tosetti, M., Del Viva, M., Montanaro, D., . . . Cioni, G. (2008). Inversion of perceived direction of motion caused by spatial undersampling in two children with periventricular leukomalacia. *Journal of Cognitive Neuroscience, 20*, 1094–1106.

Ortibus, E., Lagae, L., Casteels, I., Demaerel, P., & Stiers, P. (2009). Assessment of cerebral visual impairment with the L94 visual perceptual battery: Clinical value and correlation with MRI findings. *Developmental Medicine & Child Neurology, 51*, 209–217.

Pagliano, E., Fedrizzi, E., Erbetta, A., Bulgheroni, S., Solari, A., Bono, R., . . . Riva, D. (2007). Cognitive profiles and visuoperceptual abilities in preterm and term spastic diplegic children with periventricular leukomalacia. *Journal of Child Neurology, 22*(3), 282–288.

Pavlova, M. A. (2012). Biological motion processing as a hallmark of social cognition. *Cerebral Cortex, 22*(5), 981–995.

Pel, J., Does, L. V., Boot, F., Faber, T. D., Steen-Kant, S. V., Willemsen, S., et al. (2011). Effects of visual processing and congenital nystagmus on visually guided ocular motor behaviour. *Developmental Medicine & Child Neuroogy, 53,* 344–349.

Ricci, D., Anker, S., Cowan, F., Pane, M., Gallini, F., Luciano, R., . . . Mercuri, E. (2006). Thalamic atrophy in infants with PVL and cerebral visual impairment. *Early Human Development, 82,* 591–595.

Rizzo, M., & Vecera, S. P. (2002). Psychoanatomical substrates of Bálint's syndrome. *Journal of Neurology, Neurosurgery & Psychiatry, 72,* 162–178.

Saidkasimova, S., Bennett, D. M., Butler, S., & Dutton, G. N. (2007). Cognitive visual impairment with good visual acuity in children with posterior periventricular white matter injury: A series of 7 cases. *Journal of the American Association for Pediatric Ophthalmology and Strabismus, 11,* 426–430.

Ting, D. S., Pollock, A., Dutton, G. N., Doubal, F. N., Ting, D. S., Thompson, M., et al. (2011). Visual neglect following stroke: Current concepts and future focus. *Survey of Ophthalmology, 56,* 114–134.

Williams, C., Northstone, K., Sabates, R., Feinstein, L., Emond, A., & Dutton, G. N. (2011). Visual perceptual difficulties and underachievement at school in a large community-based sample of children. *PLoS ONE, 6*(3), e14772.

Zihl, J., & Dutton, G. N. (2015). *Cerebral visual impairment in children: Visuoperceptive and visuocognitive disorders.* Vienna: Springer-Verlag Wien.

Zihl, J., Von Cramon, D., & Mai, N. (1983). Selective disturbance of movement vision after bilateral brain damage. *Brain, 106,* 313–340.

# APPENDIX 3A

# Visual Features of CVI to Consider Looking for in Relation to Damage in Specific Brain Locations Reported on a Brain MRI Scan

| *Area of Damage Seen on MRI Scan* | *Visual Features to Look For* |
|---|---|
| **Occipital Lobes** | |
| Left occipital lobe | • Lack of visual field on the right side for both eyes |
| Right occipital lobe | • Lack of visual field on the left side for both eyes |
| Both occipital lobes | • Impaired central visual functions of acuity, contrast, and color<br>• Lack of visual field on both sides (often manifesting as visual field constriction)<br>• Severe damage causes profound visual impairment |
| **Posterior Parietal Lobes** | |
| Left posterior parietal lobe | • Intermittent lack of attention on the right side<br>• A tendency to miss people and events on the right side<br>• A tendency to bump into people and objects on the right side, especially when upset or tired<br>• Reduced accuracy of visual guidance of movement of the right side of the body<br>• A tendency to be left-handed (because this becomes the dominant hand)<br>• Weakness of the right side of the body (as a result of damage further forward in the brain)<br>• Difficulties with spoken or written language (because the left parietal lobe serves language)<br>• When drawing, the right side of the picture can be distorted |
| Right posterior parietal lobe | • Significant lack of attention on the left side and intermittent lack of attention on the right side (Ting et al., 2011)<br>• People and events on the left side are frequently missed<br>• People and objects on the left side are frequently bumped in to<br>• A tendency to be right-handed<br>• Weakness of the left side of the body |
| Both posterior parietal lobes<br>*Severe damage affecting the cortex, white matter, or both* | • Inability to see more than one or two items in a visual scene at once (simultanagnosia), despite the requisite visual field<br>• Inability to use vision to guide movement, accurately despite sometimes having clear three-dimensional vision (stereopsis), in rare cases, resulting in colliding with walls and obstacles, bumping into people and objects, and not being aware of drop-offs<br>• Inability to give attention to more than one or two things at once<br>• Noise or conversation can make the child lose visual attention<br>• Inability to move the eyes from one target to another at will, despite ability to move the eyes<br>• Profound lack of ability to see moving targets is common<br>• Lack of lower visual field below the horizontal midline<br>• Impaired movement of all four limbs as a result of quadriplegic cerebral palsy is common |

*(continued on next page)*

| *Area of Damage Seen on MRI Scan* | *Visual Features to Look For* |
|---|---|
| *Limited damage to parietal white matter* | • Behavioral patterns of dorsal stream dysfunction<br>• Lack of ability to see moving targets is occasionally observed<br>• Lack of the peripheral lower visual field means that the feet cannot be seen while walking<br>• Impaired ability to move feet over floor boundaries, or walking around patterns despite looking at them, suggests optic ataxia of the lower limbs<br>• Reaching for patterns on plates as if they are three-dimensional is observed in some young children |
| **Temporal Lobes**<br>(The patterns described for damage to one side apply to acquired damage, but can be variable. Damage from birth tends to affect all forms of recognition.) | |
| Left temporal lobe | • Impaired object recognition (object agnosia); color recognition may be used to compensate<br>• Impaired shape recognition (shape agnosia)<br>• Difficulty learning the shapes of letters (alexia) |
| Right temporal lobe | • Impaired face recognition (prosopagnosia)<br>• Impaired ability to see meaning in facial expressions<br>• Difficulty being orientated (may be profound) and navigating known environments (topographic agnosia) |
| Both temporal lobes | • Combination of the impaired abilities described for the left and right temporal lobes (integrative agnosia)<br>• Difficulty knowing the length and orientation of lines, or size of objects<br>• Impaired visual memory (often with reliance on auditory memory and language ability) |

# APPENDIX 3B

# Common Clues to the Possibility of CVI and Its Potential Features

| *Possible Indications of the Presence of CVI* | *Visual Features to Look For* |
|---|---|
| **Medical Features** | |
| Premature birth (if damage is subtle, MRI may be normal) | • Low visual acuities with no optical or eye disorder<br>• Inability to find someone in a group, or objects in a pile<br>• Lower visual field impairment (very peripheral in mild cases)<br>• Inaccurate visual guidance of limb movement<br>• Difficulty reading crowded text |
| Hydrocephalus (can have periventricular white matter injury) | • Many have visual acuity or visual field impairment<br>• Over 50 percent have perceptual impairments that can affect both dorsal and ventral streams |
| History of seizure | • *West syndrome (infantile spasms or early-onset epilepsy):* low vision (low vision may lead to the diagnosis)<br>• *Grand mal seizures:* CVI symptoms and reduced vision lasting for hours or days after a seizure<br>• *Continuous epilepsy with variable vision* that can be controlled with anti-epileptic drugs<br>• *Occipital seizures:* unformed images that are not actually there (hallucinations), resulting from electrical activity in the visual brain |
| Low blood sugar or respiratory arrest in early weeks after birth (leads to damage to visual brain if sugar or oxygen does not reach the brain cells) | • Occipital or posterior parietal lobe damage, or both; severity of damage and outcome varies<br>• Low visual acuities with visual field reduction unexplained by eye or refractive disorders<br>• Features of dorsal stream dysfunction common<br>• Possible Balint's syndrome<br>• Ventral stream dysfunction can predominate in some cases |
| Meningitis (infection around lining of brain) or encephalitis (infection of brain) (can lead to multiple foci of damage with outcome ranging from mild to severe visual dysfunction) | • Photophobia<br>• Visual acuity impaired (worse when tired)<br>• Vision can fluctuate during recovery<br>• Visual field constriction<br>• Visual perceptual disorders (impaired color naming, inability to recognize shapes, letters, or words)<br>• Faces can look distorted or are not recognized<br>• Getting lost<br>(Note: Progressive recovery needs to be sought and the approach to the child modified accordingly) |
| Hyoscine patches to control salivation | • Large pupils, causing photophobia<br>• Poor or absent accommodation (ability to focus) causing reduced vision in the long farsighted (long sited), and minimal near vision |
| History of major head injury | • Any type of CVI can result |

*(continued on next page)*

| *Possible Indications of the Presence of CVI* | *Visual Features to Look For* |
|---|---|
| **Appearance** | |
| Microcephaly (small head), with flattening at the back, more so on one side | • Low visual acuities<br>• Lack of vision/visual field on side opposite to the greatest degree of flattening |
| Spastic diplegia | • Lower visual field impairment<br>• Impaired visual search<br>• Difficulty reading crowded text |
| Hemiplegic cerebral palsy *or* Consistent repeated bruising on one leg | • Lack of vision (often relatively asymptomatic) or impaired visual attention on the weak or bruised side |
| Spastic quadriplegia | • Any aspect of visual functioning can be impaired |
| Dyskinetic cerebral palsy | • Impaired focusing (accommodation) |
| Horizontal nystagmus (some children have undiagnosed periventricular white matter disease [PVWMD]) | • The same features as for premature birth need to be looked for (only a small proportion of cases affected) |
| **Visual Behaviors** | |
| Visual search difficulties (any of these features should trigger a search for the others) | • Inability to find a distant target being pointed out<br>• Inability to find a person in a group<br>• Inability to find a clothing item in a pile of clothes<br>• Inability to find a toy in a toy box<br>• Inability to read crowded text |
| Running out in front of traffic | • Low visual acuities<br>• Visual field impairment<br>• Impaired visual attention<br>• Impaired perception of movement<br>• Visual inattention |
| Not looking at someone who is talking to him or her | • Low visual acuity precluding interpretation of facial appearance and expressions<br>• Evidence of dorsal stream dysfunction with impaired splitting of attention between sight and sound<br>• Impaired perception of movement precluding fast-moving facial expressions from being seen<br>• Inability to recognize faces<br>• Inability to interpret the language of facial expression |
| Refusing to run down a hill | • Lower visual field impairment, often very peripheral, precluding the extended foot from being seen |
| Drawings poor on one side of the page | • Evidence of visual inattention on the side of the poor drawing |
| Reading difficulties, starting around age 8 (resulting from smaller print size and increased crowding) | • Lack of focusing (accommodation)<br>• Difficulties with visual crowding |

*(continued on next page)*

| *Possible Indications of the Presence of CVI* | *Visual Features to Look For* |
|---|---|
| **Reactive Behaviors** | |
| Not looking at what is being reached for | • Lack of central vision<br>• Features of ventral or dorsal stream dysfunction |
| Striking an adjacent restless child, while continuing to work | • Limited visual attention, leading to a need not to be distracted when completing a task |
| Displaying anger when furniture is moved | • Lower visual field impairment<br>• Features of dorsal stream dysfunction |
| Exhibiting fear in straight symmetrical corridors | • Lack of visual attention on one side can render symmetrical environments frightening, perhaps because one side becomes less evident |
| Exhibiting distress in crowded places | • Features of dorsal stream dysfunction |
| **Compensatory Behaviors** | |
| Sitting very close to the TV | • Low visual acuity<br>• Features of dorsal stream dysfunction |
| Watching the TV upside down, lying on back with head back | • Lower visual field impairment (using the intact upper field to watch the TV) |
| Feeling the ground ahead at floor boundaries | • Low vision<br>• Lower visual field impairment<br>• Other features of dorsal stream dysfunction |
| Organizing possessions in fixed locations | • Other features of dorsal stream dysfunction |

# 4

# The Potential Impact of Visual Impairment and CVI on Child Development

*Elisa Fazzi, Anna Molinaro, and Elizabeth Hartmann*

How does cerebral visual impairment (CVI) affect child development? There is no simple answer to this question. It is well known that vision contributes significantly to early cognitive, motor, and social development (Baird, Mayfield, & Baker, 1997; Chen, 1999; Jakobson, Frisk, & Downie, 2006; Rogers & Puchalski, 1984). For example, vision enables children to recognize their caregivers, to know whether they are present or absent, and motivates children to move toward them. In addition, vision is qualitatively different from other senses in that it is constantly active, or *tonic*, in contrast to other senses that function intermittently and are *phasic* in nature. Vision enables children to actively, and often without pause, take in a massive amount of information about events, objects, and people in their surroundings.

Despite our growing knowledge of the impact of vision on development in general, there is still much to learn about how visual functioning relates to specific etiologies, such as CVI. Understanding how CVI, in all its manifestations, affects development can be complex, as CVI and visual impairment in general co-occur with additional impairments (Hatton, Bailey, Burchinal, & Ferrell, 1997). What is known is that the visual functioning of children with CVI can be quite variable, and this fluctuating visual performance can affect development in a number of areas. Even if visual acuity values do not indicate poor vision, children with CVI may have complex visual difficulties that cannot be explained by visual acuity alone (Dutton et al., 1996). Nevertheless, children with CVI can develop free from any cognitive, motor, or social challenges, and where difficulties do emerge, they may be overcome and may ultimately be viewed simply as delays (Pring & Tadic, 2010).

The aim of this chapter is to explore the development of children with CVI. First, early identification of CVI will be discussed, as the early identification of visual impairment has implications for almost all areas of development. Then, specific issues regarding cognitive, motor, and social development will be addressed. Both seminal works and recent research will be reviewed and connected to the development of children with CVI. Lastly, the chapter will conclude with implications for practice, including suggestions for assessment and intervention.

## Early Identification of Cerebral Visual Impairment

The newborn infant has a measurable visual acuity and contrast sensitivity just hours after birth (Mercuri, Baranello, Romeo, Cesarini, & Ricci, 2007; Ricci et al., 2008), and uses vision to explore and learn about the surrounding environment. These visual capabilities become more efficient during the first weeks of life. Measurements of these capabilities as they develop can help to identify functionally significant CVI in those at risk, such as very preterm infants, in order to gauge plasticity and recovery from perinatal brain damage in early life, through measured changes over time (Atkinson & Braddick, 2007). Early signs of CVI that can be identified in the first months of life are reduced visual acuity, reduced visual field, and malfunctioning of basic visual functions (Good, Jan, Burden, Skoczenski, & Candy, 2001).

Early identification of CVI is critical because it can lead to the provision of intervention services while there is maximum potential to employ the processes of maturation, plasticity, and adaptation of the visual system (Spolidoro, Sale, Berardi, & Maffei, 2009). As neuroimaging techniques have been refined and used as a way to identify brain damage, a correlation between children's visual profiles and structural brain lesions has been identified. For example, damage that appears on neuroimaging helps to understand a child's visual abilities related to visual acuity and visual field (as explained in Chapter 3). However, it has been more difficult to demonstrate the correlation between higher visual functions and conventional MRIs. What is known is that cognitive visual impairments (see Chapter 3) depend on atypical processing of information in the network of associative areas of the brain served by the ventral and dorsal stream pathways (Fazzi et al., 2009), and are linked to well-known neurological impairments such as cerebral palsy, as a consequence of preterm brain damage or encephalopathy (Volpe, 1996). Therefore, conventional neuroimaging is useful in helping to identify the presence of problems that might indicate a child has CVI, but do not yet provide reliable information on a range of visual functions. More detailed information might be achieved through the use of new functional investigative tools such as fMRIs.

Two of the authors, Fazzi and Molinaro, recently assessed visual function in full-term and preterm newborns through an easily administered clinical instrument called NAVEG (Neonatal Assessment Visual European Grid), which provided a detailed analysis of visual functioning using a grid made up of three main sections—ocular, motor, and perceptual visual components (Rossi et al., 2013). They found it was possible to differentiate the visual functioning profiles of preterm infants, particularly those with brain lesions, from those that were full-term. The NAVEG showed good discrimination power between healthy preterm infants and those with pathology in relationship to neurological and neuroimaging data, proving it to be an effective assessment tool.

Evaluation of early behavioral markers of CVI, through interviews, observations, and direct assessments of the child (Pueyo et al.,

2014; Roman, 1996; Rossi et al., 2013), can be used to follow changes in specific behavioral characteristics evidenced in infants. Children whose CVI manifests early in life can have a range of visual characteristics, including light gazing, poor visual attention, color preference, low visual acuities, restricted visual field, difficulty discriminating or interpreting complex visual patterns, difficulty finding an object at a distance, better recognition of familiar objects than novel ones, attention to moving objects, and looking away when reaching. The CVI Range (Roman-Lantzy, 2007) is an assessment that addresses these visual characteristics of children with CVI and determines how each characteristic impacts visual functioning. Using information obtained through this systematic assessment of the child's visual and behavioral characteristics, educators and therapists can formulate specific intervention programs and environmental adaptations to overcome the child's difficulties.

Children with CVI can have a range of vision, from total blindness to normal or near-normal visual functions, and this variation in visual functioning is often related to variation in developmental outcomes. Many children with CVI identified at very young ages have additional disabilities (Fazzi, Signorini et al., 2012; Hatton et al., 1997; Roman-Lantzy, 2007) since their CVI is more likely to be detected as a result of screening related to their other neurological impairments. On the other hand, there are also many children with CVI who have visual perceptual disabilities that can affect performance even when their visual acuity, field, and contrast are close to typical levels. These children, who are usually identified later in life when they reach school age, may have near-normal visual functions. In all of these children with CVI, cerebral damage occurring during development probably leads to a reorganization of maturing visual processing functions as a result of cerebral plasticity (Guzzetta et al., 2010; Ortibus, De Cock, & Lagae, 2011), and children can exhibit some intact vision that often improves over time (Fazzi et al., 2007).

To understand the impact that CVI has on children's development, it is important to note that visual functioning changes as the central nervous system matures and as the child attains different developmental milestones. The assessment of visual dysfunctions cannot be narrowed to traditional components associated with ocular visual impairment, but has to be extended to include higher levels of integration of attentional, perceptual, and visual-spatial functions (Fazzi, Signorini et al., 2012; Atkinson & Braddick, 2011; see Chapter 1). In addition, the development of children with CVI can vary greatly and must be understood in a functional context, and specifically in relation to cognitive, motor, and social development. This is particularly true at school age, when visual skills come into play with learning and cognitive processes. These areas of development will be explored in the next section. Given that there is limited research on CVI and development, each section begins with a review of relevant research on the development of children with visual impairments, and then discusses implications for children with CVI.

## The Effects of Visual Impairment and CVI on Development

While generalizations cannot be applied to individual children, many studies have found that, overall, children with visual impairments, particularly those whose vision is severely affected, attain many developmental milestones at later ages than typically sighted peers (Ferrell, 1998; Hatton et al., 1997). Some of these children appear to follow different trajectories in various developmental domains since they experience their world in different ways from children with typical vision (Donnelly, Stewart, & Hollinger, 2005; Ferrell, 1998; Warren, 1994). In general, congenital or early-onset visual impairments may interfere with many aspects of development. These include organization of sleep-wake patterns, gross and fine motor functions, spatial concepts, cognitive abilities, attention and memory, communication skills, learning processes, behavior, bonding, social responsiveness, and communication (Burlingham, 1975; Fraiberg, 1977; Lueck, Chen, Kekelis, & Hartmann, 2008; Pérez-Pereira & Conti-Ramsden, 1999; Sonksen & Dale, 2002; Warren, 1994).

Fewer developmental differences have been noted in children who have low vision with no additional disabilities compared to those with very little available sight who have co-occurring conditions (Ferrell, 1998; Hatton et al., 1997). Given that many children identified early with CVI have additional disabilities, their patterns of development follow those of children with visual impairments with co-occurring conditions, which may result in different developmental trajectories and slower rates of skill attainment in various developmental domains (Hatton et al., 1997). Those children identified as having CVI later in life, and without co-occurring conditions, may have fewer of these differences in development.

It is also important to note that behaviors exhibited by some children with visual impairments can be hard for sighted adults to interpret because these behaviors may serve a different purpose than in typically sighted children (Bigelow, 2003). For example, infants with visual impairments may show that they are orienting to an object by becoming still, as if to quiet their body in order to gain more sensory information. Caregivers may incorrectly interpret this "quieting" of the body as disinterest, since, in contrast, children without visual impairments may begin to move toward the object and show more outward signs of interest. Therefore, it is important to understand that the development of children who are blind or visually impaired may differ from that of sighted children, and comparisons between the two groups may not be appropriate (Lueck et al., 2008), unless they help us to better understand and support development for all children.

## Cognitive and Motor Development

### *Object Permanence, Mental Images, and Mobility*

One of the most important cognitive developmental milestones for all children is *object permanence* (the concept that objects exist and continue to exist even when not seen). Children typically learn object permanence through vision, and this, in turn, leads to the attainment of other important cognitive and motor milestones, such as early notions of causality and the motivation to move to interact with objects. Children who are visually impaired or blind often do not have the same sensory and perceptual experiences with objects that make them as accessible and recognizable to sighted children. Without vision, which helps to organize and integrate incoming information from different senses, children with limited or no vision must draw upon and organize different perceptual data to arrive at cognitive achievements—such as object permanence—through alternative developmental routes (Bigelow, 1983, 1986, 1992).

Another key milestone in early cognitive and motor development that supports the development of object permanence is the formation of mental images, which is an important step in giving meaning to the world. Vision is helpful, but not essential, to understanding space, spatial relationships, and internal spatial representation (Pring & Tadic, 2010). As with object permanence, children who are blind or visually impaired gain this understanding through the use of alternative sensory channels such as hearing and touch (Brambring & Asbrock, 2010). For example, children who are visually impaired or blind learn to grasp an object that makes a sound by using a mental image derived from prior sensory experience, such as tactile experience.

It has long been known that the development of infants who are visually impaired or blind can be delayed, especially with regard to self-initiated mobility, posture, and locomotion (Fazzi et al., 2002; Fraiberg, 1977; Levtzion-Korach, Tennenbaum, Schnitzer, & Ornoy, 2000; Tröster & Brambring, 1992). When children become interested in sound-making toys and begin meaningful exploration and understanding of them, this indicates that the concept of object permanence is being acquired, and sound is leading to motor experience and exploration. At this stage, compensatory strategies are developing (Prechtl, 2001). Vision and motor skills typically evolve together, but children who are blind, whose hands remain at shoulder height for much of the time during the first months of life, and who do not show evidence of exploratory tactile function, may be at risk for delayed development of object permanence and mental image formation (Fraiberg, 1977).

Fraiberg (1977) hypothesized that lack of sight impairs the ability to build up a picture of the world, and without this, there is decreased incentive for developing voluntary skills. She suggested that the development of the visually impaired child can be divided into two stages. During the first 6 months of life, attainment of gross motor milestones is only slightly delayed. However, delay becomes more evident during the second 6 months of life, when normal development of movement is progressively learned through search and exploration. At this second stage, children who are visually impaired may start to show alternative routes to upright mobility with the development of crawling, standing, and walking skills, although walking may be delayed in some children with severe visual impairment. Some children may adopt solutions such as "bottom shuffling," or scooting along in a sitting position, which may be a more secure position for them (Strickling & Pogrund, 2002).

Research on the early development of cognitive and motor skills in children with CVI is limited. However, it has been shown in adolescents that periventricular leukomalacia (PVL) can give rise to impaired navigational skills, which are most affected in those who lack mobility due to their cerebral palsy, arguably through lack of practice and training (Pavlova, Sokolov, & Krägeloh-Mann, 2007). Other recent studies have reported children with difficulties in their ability to recognize objects as a result of impairment in their ventral or occipitotemporal streams (Fazzi et al., 2004; Stiers et al., 2001). These studies suggest that children with neurological impairments that co-occur with CVI may not be motivated to move toward objects they do not recognize (Ortibus et al., 2011).

### *Reach on Sound*

Other research has found that children who are blind or have low vision may have unique ways of reaching key cognitive and motor milestones. Fazzi et al. (2002) have found the "reach and touch on sound" milestone (the ability to reach out for and grasp an object that has been presented exclusively through the medium of sound) to be a critical developmental phase in children who are visually impaired or blind, and one that may provide insights on how development occurs when children are not easily able to use vision.

The task of reaching for an object that makes a sound requires the child with visual impairments to overcome a conceptual problem. How can an object be identified solely by means of the sound it makes? An internal representation of the object needs to have been built up in advance (Fraiberg, Siegel, & Gibson, 1966). In general, the sighted infant will stretch out his or her arms toward a visually perceived object by the age of 5–6 months. In contrast, the visually impaired infant will become aware of an object through sound by 7–8 months, his facial expression showing that he recognizes it. When a musical toy is placed near a child who touches it, and it is then removed for a moment, the child will open his hand and move it slightly in an attempt to get it back. By the age of 11 months, the sound-making object only needs to be shaken near the child for it to be located by hand (Bigelow, 1983, 1986, 1992; Fazzi, Signorini, & Lanners, 2010; Fraiberg, 1977; Fraiberg et al., 1966).

The development of "reach on sound" probably relates to a growing awareness of object permanence in the absence of sight, indicating progressive cognitive development (Bigelow, 1983, 1986, 1992). However, this process is commonly impaired in children with CVI, probably as a result of dorsal stream (occipitoparietal) dysfunction, limiting both attention and the capacity to form an internal mental representation of external space with sufficient detail (Dutton, personal communication, 2013).

Unlike the child with vision, the child with visual impairment or blindness has to be equipped with memory and an emerging concept of object permanence before being able to reach out a hand to grasp an object that makes sound. Opportunities to learn about their environment can be very limited for children with visual impairments, especially for those children who do not receive early intervention services. Many objects do not make sounds, or the sounds they do make may provide insufficient information to motivate children to reach for them or to understand their permanence. If an object brought into contact with the hands is released, it can seem to the child to disappear completely, which limits learning from experience. Furthermore, research has shown that ear-hand coordination is more complex than hand-eye coordination, and is established later (Clifton, Rochat, Litovsky, & Perris, 1991; Pérez-Pereira & Conti-Ramsden, 1999). Therefore, it is easy to understand how children who are blind or visually impaired may have difficulty finding adaptive solutions for learning about the environment, and how their skills may remain stagnant and focused upon their own bodies. (One suggestion to encourage exploratory activity and "reach on sound" is, once children acquire the ability to sit unsupported, to furnish the surrounding space with objects that will arouse curiosity, arranging them in a way that encourages exploratory activity by the hands.)

The development of the "reach on sound" function was studied in 37 children who were congenitally blind, comparing the children with normal mental development on the Reynell-Zinkin Scales, and without associated motor disabilities or focal signs at the neurological examination, to children who had disabilities associated with their visual impairment, such as cerebral palsy and developmental delay (Fazzi et al., 2011). The main type of visual damage in the first group of children was retinal disorders (75 percent, mostly Leber's congenital amaurosis), while CVI accounted for 94 percent of cases in the second group. The children were followed up every 3 months for 6 to 36 months, and assessed on their ability to reach for objects presented through sound and tactile cues. For children whose primary disability was visual impairment without associated neuromotor and/or cognitive disabilities, the study found that they

- reached for objects they had previously touched rather than those they had previously heard;
- had difficulty reaching for an object that made a sound when it is was concealed by a cover or when it was taken from their hands; and
- were motivated to retrieve objects if they could predict their location.

In contrast, the children who were visually impaired with associated neuromotor or cognitive disabilities, or both

- used their hands mainly for self-stimulation instead of reaching;
- rarely achieved, or achieved only with marked delay, the ability to reach an object presented through sound;
- made movements indicating excitement and oriented to sound; and
- found it difficult to separate themselves from environmental points of reference and contact (e.g., moving away from a piece of furniture or getting up from the floor).

The findings from this study support previous findings (Fazzi et al., 2002) that when a child's visual deficit is associated with other impairments, the capacity to explore surroundings is profoundly limited. The study (Fazzi et al., 2002) assessed early neuromotor development in 20 children between the ages of 4 and 30 months, and followed up for a period of 3 to 36 months those who were congenitally blind or severely visually impaired (9 were blind only, and 11 were blind and had multiple disabilities such as cerebral palsy or intellectual disability). Results confirmed Fraiberg's (1977) earlier findings showing that children who were blind reached all motor milestones, but with a delay. When compared with the motor development of sighted children, the children in the study who were visually impaired with no additional disabilities

- were slightly delayed in achieving head control and independent sitting;
- achieved the "reach on sound" task between 8 and 10 months of age (in sighted children, coordination of vision with reach takes place by the age of 5 months);
- were delayed in spatial orientation, standing upright, and walking independently;
- improved their motor development only when they were able to reach out for and grasp an object presented through sound; and
- walked independently only after gaining the ability to get their bearings guided by

sound (approximately half of the children never crawled).

The profile was very different in the children with visual impairments and multiple disabilities. These children

- did not walk independently by the age of 3 years (with the exception of two participants), owing to their multiple complex disabilities;
- did not reach toward a sound in the majority of instances;
- had marked delays in postural-motor abilities;
- had difficulties letting go of reference points in their environment, such as contact with the floor or the bed; and
- had the common behavior of "freezing" in response to interesting stimuli (Pring & Tadic, 2010).

From the studies just reviewed, it can be deduced that "reach on sound" is a breakthrough skill in children's development, and for children who are visually impaired or blind, this skill is at once a condition of, and a catalyst to, all their subsequent cognitive and motor achievements. The capacity to reach for an object presented by sound seems to serve as the organizer of motor experience and appears to be a hallmark that indicates the child's readiness to achieve locomotion.

As already noted, children with CVI and multiple disabilities may struggle with these early cognitive and motor skills and need extensive support. As described in Chapter 3, children with isolated damage to the posterior parietal lobes of the brain causing optic ataxia were commonly observed by one of the authors (Fazzi) to not only have impaired visual guidance of reach and body movement, but were also commonly unable to locate the source of sounds. A hypothesis can therefore be suggested that this mental process is also deficient in children with occipital pathology and cerebral palsy because of additional damage to the posterior parietal lobe, leading to an impaired internal representation or map of the outside world. In other words, children with CVI have specific impairments in the part of the brain that supports their understanding of space and how they move through it.

Children with profound CVI who have difficulty locating objects around them may be helped by having the early interventionist allow them to move their hands along tactile guides to locate playthings around them, starting with the forearm and hand of an attendant, and then moving on to custom-designed guides that lead the child's hand to safely explore interesting and informative objects. This allows the child to be rewarded by finding the toy or other object, and can help avert any tactile defensiveness that might arise from previous search attempts when a misreaching hand has been hurt by a collision.

### *Cognitive Visual Dysfunction in Children without Additional Disabilities*

CVI may not be recognized in children without additional disabilities until later in life, when visual tasks become more challenging and dysfunction in higher visual functions such as visual cognition (see Chapter 1) becomes more noticeable. The term *cognitive visual disorder* refers to problems in visual cognition or misinterpretation of the visual world with respect to where things are or what things are, and can be present even when visual acuity and visual field are normal or only mildly impaired (Dutton, 2003). Cognitive visual dysfunction is related to damage to the visual associative areas in the temporal and posterior parietal lobes and their incoming pathways, leading to impairment of more complex functions such as visual-spatial skills and visual recognition of objects.

Impairment of these higher visual functions in children with CVI can interfere with the timely acquisition of an array of skills and have an adverse impact on development. The challenges may first manifest during school age. At this age, preterm children with CVI may have difficulties establishing the correct grip for holding a pencil, reading when print size diminishes, using scissors, buttoning up buttons, tying shoelaces, and building with construction toys (Fazzi, Galli, & Micheletti, 2012). Research has found that these children complain about aching hands while writing, miss lines and margins, and make inappropriately sized and spaced letters. These disabilities are signs of visual problems related to the expansion and processing of visual information (Dutton, 2003). During the school years, the presence of behaviors such as visual latency (delay in processing visual information), poor visual attention, extremely shortened gaze, and a characteristic head turn when reaching for objects, could result in frequent misperceptions of these children as easily distracted, inattentive, or unmotivated, when, in reality, some of their behaviors result from CVI (Good et al., 1994; Jan & Groenveld, 1990; Smith & Kelley, 2007). The visual components of a task frequently become even more difficult when combined with the demands of listening, maintaining position in space, and simultaneously performing complex motor actions (Dutton et al., 1996). Moreover, visual performance tends to vary both during the day and from one day to another, because visual perception (see Chapter 1) is subject to fatigue (Dutton, 2011). For many of these children, professionals need to understand behaviors exhibited by the child, not only in terms of their functional vision, but also in relation to their ability to modulate states of arousal, determine which aspects of a task are important to attend to, and employ memory. Educators regularly recommend incorporating a wide range of adaptations, such as visual supports (such as modifications to the visual environment), compensatory use of additional senses, and adaptive positioning, based on the functional needs of each student (Shaman, 2009).

## Visual Impairment and Social Development

The intimate connection between early cognitive and motor development with social development cannot be overstated. During early development, reaching and locomotion may be delayed because children who are visually impaired or blind have difficulty understanding their position within the physical environment and their position in relation to objects. Therefore, they are at risk for becoming socially contracted (closed or focused) around their body sensations, which, in turn, limits the connection they have between themselves and the outside world (Fazzi et al., 2010).

### *Joint Attention*

One of the most important social developmental milestones that encourages children to make connections with the outside world is the ability to engage in *joint attention.* Joint attention is defined as an exchange that involves both the child's and the partner's awareness of the other's mutual focus of attention on a third object or event (Bigelow, 2003). Joint attention is attained when an object or event is shared by both the child and the partner through mutual gaze, gesture, or language. Toward the end of their first year, typically developing infants are able to direct others' attention to objects they find interesting (called referential communication). Infants develop sustained joint attention when they learn to perceive the intentions of others. This requires infants to understand how they can set a goal and then choose to cause an effect (Bigelow, 2003).

Visual impairment appears to have a profound effect on social-communicative development, particularly in the areas of joint attention and referential communication (Dale & Salt, 2008). In addition, the ability to engage in joint attention is the initial indicator that two forms of early self-knowledge are evolving: the *interpersonal self* and the *ecological self*. The interpersonal self relates to the perception of the self in relation to others, while the ecological self concerns the idea of the self in relation to the local physical environment. Visual impairment and blindness challenge the development of both these forms of self-knowledge, particularly limiting ecological self-knowledge (Neisser, 1991, 1993). Children who are visually impaired or blind may have difficulty perceiving what others are attending to as well as understanding the emotional reactions of others. In addition, they cannot readily perceive the physical layout of their environment, the objects in that environment, the spatial relations among the objects, or the spatial relation of self to the objects and their surrounding physical space (Bigelow, 2003). All of these challenges in perceiving objects, people, and space can create barriers to developing joint attention and delays in developing self-knowledge.

### Caregiver-Child Relationship

Vision also plays a crucial role in the caregiver-child relationship. After just a few weeks of life, infants begin to observe caregivers' faces and smile in response, pleasing caregivers and encouraging mutual attachment. For infants, the fact that they can see their caregivers helps with bonding, even when they are not physically in contact. It helps infants to develop an emotional attachment to caregivers and interact with them in meaningful ways, aiding the development of their relationship (Malekpour, 2007; Rogers & Puchalski, 1986; Spitz, 1946).

Through these early interactions, infants move from their chaotic and disorganized world of elementary and fragmentary sensations toward the interpersonal awareness that underpins the development of relationships. Trevarthen and Aitken (2001) stated that infants' behavioral systems bring about actions on the part of the caregiver that are aimed at promoting interaction in daily life. In this way, infants establish emotionally significant relationships with specific key individuals during their first 18 months of life. The development of permanent human bonds during this period becomes evident from the way infants choose to interact with preferred individuals through social smiling, discriminating between the caregiver and the stranger, as well as separation and reunion behaviors. All these behaviors, without exception, are brought about through the infants' use of vision.

### Research on Early Social Development and Visual Impairment

In a world where visual information is limited or not consistently understood, how do children learn to distinguish preferred individuals from other people? How do they develop a preference for certain individuals and communicate this preference? Voice seems to be the principal means of promoting the development of the ability to differentiate between familiar and unfamiliar people, as well as the development of emotional language in children with visual impairments or blindness (Loots & Devisé, 2003). Infants who are visually impaired or blind also respond to the way they are touched. During the first year of life, they use their hands preferentially to explore parents' faces and surrounding objects, presumably to build up tactile recognition memory.

The seminal work of Fraiberg (1977) also supports the importance of voice during early social development of children who are blind or visually impaired. Observing the sequential development of selective and preferential behaviors in a group of non-sighted children, Fraiberg (1977) found that a familiar voice is the primary activator of smiling. As early as 4 weeks of age, the children display a selective, but irregular, smile in response to the voices of their parents, and their mothers in particular, while the same smile is not evoked by unfamiliar voices. However, no circumstance that can regularly evoke a smile has been observed. From 2.5 to 6 months of age, children with visual impairment or blindness continue to smile selectively in response to a caregiver's voice; but smiling, evoked by voice, remains inconstant. From 6 to 11 months of age, the production of smiles of children with visual impairment or blindness still does not alter substantially compared with the previous phase.

Touch is an equally important sense in the social development of all children. Research has found that in the course of the first year of life, tactile language is crucial in the construction of object relations for learners with visual impairments (Preisler, 1991). *Tactile language* is defined as the sharing of intent and emotion through touch. During the first weeks of life, children who are blind or visually impaired connect with others in a very similar way to that of sighted children (with the exception that, for sighted children, tactile experience is just one of a range of possible ways of establishing contact). For the first few months, children who are blind or visually impaired are able to establish contact with caregivers when their caregivers' presence is established through touch and voice (Tröster & Brambring, 1992). By the fifth month of life, children with visual impairment or blindness become increasingly discriminatory and intentional in their use of touch. Between 5 and 8 months of age, children with visual impairment or blindness begin to use their hands to explore the faces of their parents and other familiar individuals, and only rarely will they explore the face of a stranger. Thus, this is a first form of recognition. Between 7 and 15 months of age, children with visual impairment or blindness, like sighted peers, reject strangers, refuse their embraces and care, cry in protest, and can be consoled only by their caregivers' voice or touch (Als, Tronick, & Brazelton, 1980; Preisler, 1991; Tröster & Brambring, 1992).

Children's negative reaction to strangers is regarded as a criterion for evaluating the positive bonds established with the caregiver and with other preferred individuals; the manifestation of separation anxiety may correspond to the emergence of a concept of the caregiver's permanence. Until the caregiver has been established as "an object," there cannot be any concept of loss or absence (Fraiberg, 1971; Howe, 2006; Rogers & Puchalski, 1988; Troster & Brambring, 1992). In the second year of life, children who are blind or visually impaired can present episodes of intense attachment to the caregiver when separated. Problems may arise if parents overprotect their visually impaired child and do not allow the child to achieve independence appropriate to his or her age. Overprotectiveness prevents the visually impaired child from discovering the world on his or her own. The potential consequences are difficulties in building up feelings of security and extended mechanisms of dependence. In contrast, being treated "like the other kids" can help the child's self-image and self-esteem.

Many children who are blind or visually impaired show healthy and substantially harmonious social development. Research has found that an intuitive caregiver (one who understands the power of touch and sound) can create a valid and gratifying emotional atmosphere and can foster harmonious social development for infants with visual impairment and blindness (Kekelis & Prinz, 1996; Kelly & Barnard, 2000; Loots, Devisé, & Sermijn, 2003; McCollum & Hemmeter, 1997; Perez-Pereira & Conti-Ramsden, 2001; Preisler, 1991). Caregivers' ability to develop effective modes of interaction, combined with the ability to adapt to the ways children understand their world, can compensate for the children's impairment in vision.

The way caregivers react to a child's visual impairment or blindness also plays a fundamental role in their social development. It is possible to observe reactions of denial, overprotection, or even profound depression in the caregiver, which prevent effective social and emotional interaction with the child (Tröster & Brambring, 1992). The risk is that the child with visual impairment and blindness, who needs to receive extra input to compensate for lack of vision, may receive less than a typical child does, and this can have profound effects on his or her emotional development. Nonetheless, many caregivers do prove able from the outset to interpret the needs and behaviors of their children and to adapt to them, keeping the interaction going (Campbell, 2003; Perez-Pereira & Conti-Ramsden, 2001). The caregivers' sensitivity to the needs of their children, and the capacity to predict their behavior, are essential elements for secure attachment. It has been noted that some parents of children who are blind or visually impaired may develop a relationship with their child where the child becomes overly dependent, which can hinder later achievement of personal autonomy in daily life (Tröster & Brambring, 1992). Early intervention programs address these issues by guiding caregivers to understand their children's reactions and respond in meaningful ways (Campbell, 2007; Ferrell, 2011).

Children with visual impairment and blindness are slow to internalize the caregiver as an object, and thus may demand that their recently acquired sense of security and protection be constantly reinforced by the caregiver's physical presence. In this situation, the normally healthy dependent relationship between the child and caregiver will last much longer than is usual, and attempts at separation could become difficult (Fazzi et al., 2010). The presence of such strong anxieties in these children can become an obstacle to their development and their building of optimal relationships. This risk is greater when visual deficit is associated with multiple disabilities.

### *Signs of Social Isolation and Impaired Social Development*

Given these findings, early developmental differences in children with visual impairments might reflect the influence of the visual deficit on early interactive experiences, rather than the coexistence of a primary impairment of social interaction and communication (Pring & Tadic, 2010). A greater understanding of what hinders and supports early social development may lead to the advancement of specific intervention strategies designed to encourage alternative channels of communication and promote environmental exploration (Fazzi et al., 2007). With this in mind, it is crucial that professionals who come into contact with children who are visually impaired or blind are able to recognize the signs that a child's social development may be at risk. The main signs are the presence, persistence, and entrenchment of a series of behaviors that impede joint attention and thus social development, and are expressions of considerable social isolation. These behaviors include:

- Lack of self-initiated motor experience
- Lack of attention to environmental stimuli
- Absence of smiling or difficulty eliciting smiling (absence of smiling may not be a major issue for the child, but it has the potential to impair bonding with caregivers due to their adverse reaction to this behavior)
- Poor adaptive use of the hands to explore and recognize objects
- Absent or poor "reach on sound" after the first 3 months of life
- Persistence of excessive and nonfunctional use of the mouth as the main interface with the environment (Fazzi et al., 2011; Fraiberg, 1977)
- Tendency to create an exclusive bond with certain caregivers

Although there is a great deal of variability in the personality profiles of children who are blind or visually impaired, it is possible to recognize certain traits in children who rely on senses other than vision to develop socially. For example, the behavioral traits more often associated with deafness, namely aggressive or angry reactions (Bailly, Dechoulydelenclave, & Lauwerier, 2003; Carvill, 2001), are not typical in children with visual impairment or blindness. Nevertheless, it has been reported that some children who are blind and visually impaired may exhibit with great frequency difficulty in social interaction with peers, a tendency toward isolation, imitative and echolalic speech, and increased stereotypical behaviors (Carvill, 2001; Fazzi et al., 2007; Fraiberg, 1977; Minter, Hobson, & Pring, 1991; Pring & Tadic, 2010; Rogers & Puchalski, 1986).

Rather than this being a psychopathological problem, the most likely explanation is that these behaviors reflect a specific way of acquiring social-cognitive abilities by those who are blind (Brambring & Asbrock, 2010). The child who is blind may require much more stimulation to reliably elicit a response, but these children are more isolated and receive less social stimulation in activities with sighted peers. This reduced social interaction may be observed in activities with high demand for orientation and mobility and manual skills, and which therefore are unsuitable for children who are blind (Bambring, 1998). Furthermore, sighted peers may not be able to anticipate the needs of their blind peers (Preisler, 1993). Stereotypical behaviors may have a functional value for children who are blind, by reducing stress or uncertainty (Tröster, Brambring, & Beelmann, 1994). Echolalia and excessive production of speech (with declarative rather than communicative intent) may possibly be explained by a different process of language acquisition in children who are blind. Echolalia can provide the blind child with a way to participate in a conversation before he has the requisite verbal skills to carry on a true dialog. It also provides a feeling of inclusion in the social aspect of conversation, which would normally be fulfilled by eye contact and body language (Brambring & Asbrock, 2010; Tadic, Pring, & Dale, 2008).

### *Development of Language*

Language production and use is a later, yet equally important, developmental milestone for social development, following the development of preverbal communication. Research on the development of language in children with visual impairment and blindness is not conclusive. For example, recent research (Tadic, Pring, & Dale, 2010) shows that there is variability in the language abilities of children with visual impairment and blindness, with general evidence of good structural language skills (e.g., syntax), but a weaker use of pragmatic language (language used in a social context), which is a key feature required for social communication. It has, however, been argued that unusual speech patterns in toddlers may serve a true purpose, and that they play an important function by providing an adaptive strategy to promote cognition and social interaction (Perez-Pereira & Conti-Ramsden, 1999).

### *Social Development and Children with CVI*

Recent research has emphasized that CVI can affect social development in both mildly and severely affected children (McDaid & Dutton, 2007), especially those with multiple disabilities. The capacity of children with CVI to see the external world both on a global and detailed scale may be limited by the characteristics of their visual functioning, such as diminished visual acuity, visual field, color vision, and contrast perception; visual fatigue, limited recognition of objects and faces; and impaired visual guidance of movement. The world may appear to them as inconsistent, confusing, and unfriendly. Understanding how aspects of CVI affect social development leads to suggestions for appropriate intervention strategies. (See Part 4 of this book for more detailed consideration of interventions.)

For example, as children with CVI may have variations in degree of visual impairment, visual field, fluctuation of visual performance, and visual crowding problems, it is important to identify elements that are reinforcing and interesting to the child, such as sound, familiar objects, rhythm, song, and movement. Children with CVI will need additional time to make sense of incoming visual information and to recognize patterns in what they see. Specific to this, the simultaneous use of touch and vision, of selective colors, of appropriate lighting, and simplification of the visual environment may help the child respond to and process external stimuli, as well as participate in a dynamic environment and construct meaningful experiences with people (Morgan, 2004).

Children with CVI may experience various types of visual agnosia (decreased ability to visually recognize or identify objects or people) (Good et al., 2001), including the inability to recognize familiar faces (prosopagnosia). Types and severity of prosopagnosia are variable, but an inability or disability in recognizing one's peers can affect early socialization experiences. If this is compounded by not being able to interpret facial expressions, children may feel even further isolated from their peers (Dutton, 2006). (It is important that prosopagnosia be properly diagnosed so that children are not inappropriately diagnosed as having autism; see Chapter 7.) When teaching a child with these challenges, one has to be aware that people are recognized by the tone of their voice and that the language component of facial expression may not be apparent. The voice, therefore, needs to convey all the language (Shaman, 2009; Swift, Davidson, & Weems, 2008).

Many children diagnosed with CVI at an early age also have severe multiple disabilities, in particular cerebral palsy and developmental delay or mental retardation. These additional conditions may restrict opportunities for the child to reach out and actively participate in his environment, as a result of decreased mobility or cognitive impairment. Children with CVI and multiple disabilities may have fewer experiences in using their other sensory systems to extract knowledge, and may have more difficulty confirming and associating their sensory experiences (Morse, 1992). For many of these children, movement itself may provide the most meaningful and pleasurable feedback about the world and may be central to learning and participation. Yet, these children may be passively moved by caregivers or school staff to make them reach or touch something, without the child being actively engaged in the social interaction. It is essential to include the child as an active participant in the play partnership.

Most young children with CVI like to learn from touch and may prefer play and interactions that involve direct touch. Moreover, it is important to consider the child's communication level and formal communication strategies, because children with multiple disabilities can express themselves in unconventional and sometimes unpredictable manners (such as knocking materials from a table as a signal of rejection or closing their eyes and bowing their head as an indication of fatigue) (Swift et al., 2008).

Children with CVI identified at early ages, who have profound visual difficulties, like all young children, need to have access to familiar and repetitive activities with a distinct beginning, middle, and end, but with a shortened duration, in order to increase the child's sense of readiness and enjoyment of the activity. However, whereas other young children may be adaptable to novelty, children with CVI and profound visual difficulties need routines or rituals for locating objects in space and to inform them when an activity begins and ends (Groenveld, Jan, & Leader, 1990). Examples include ritualized beginning and ending through a special clap sequence, song, or entry and exit from a specific location in the classroom (Shaman, 2009). Moreover, young children with CVI come to understand their visual world better when verbal and tactile cues are associated with language concepts (Hodgdon, 1997; Lane, 1996; Morse, 1992). It may be helpful to keep colors and background features of a specific activity consistent in order to correlate activities, people, and places in the room and present visual stimuli at the child's current level of visual skills (Roman-Lantzy, 2007).

## Implications for Practice

Visual impairment is a common outcome of preterm birth that may not only be a result of peripheral (retina or optic nerve) problems but also a widespread involvement of visual pathways at different levels of cerebral structures (Fazzi, Galli, & Micheletti, 2012). CVI is a neurological disorder that results in unique visual responses to people, educational materials, and the environment. Despite its label, the term cerebral visual impairment refers not to an eye condition but to a brain condition. CVI clinical profiles are widely heterogeneous, and every child can present a different spectrum of features that vary according to the different levels of involvement of the visual pathways (ocular, oculomotor, perceptual, and cognitive). Profiles can also vary as a result of environmental influences and neuroplasticity that can induce a reorganization of maturing visual functions.

Despite this heterogeneity and variability, three recommendations can be made to guide intervention that will facilitate the development of children with CVI. First, it is critical that early identification of CVI be a focus of pediatricians and other early interventionists. Second, intervention should be focused on the use of integrated sensory information. Lastly, intervention should be family focused.

## Importance of Early Identification and Intervention

The existence of many different causes and features makes CVI difficult to define and detect. This is especially true during the school-age years when a child shows normal or near-normal visual acuity and visual field but has difficulties with daily living and academic skills as a result of perceptual dysfunction. It is important for pediatricians to identify and recognize CVI as a common cause of visual impairment in children with a history of prematurity or of pre- or perinatal insults, because early detection and recognition of CVI is the first step toward the implementation of adapted habilitation programs. As recommended by the American Academy of Pediatrics, the American Academy of Ophthalmology, and the American Association for Pediatric Ophthalmology and Strabismus, an age-appropriate visual screening by primary care providers is indicated for all children before they are discharged from neonatology units, at 6 months of age, at 3–4 years of age, and annually during the school years, in order to identify those with, or at risk of developing, visual deficits. A full investigation of all the different aspects of visual function is thus mandatory in order to arrive at a precise definition of the clinical picture, and it is crucial that professionals who come into contact with these children are able to recognize the signs of developmental risk. Although the amount of vision present can be difficult to demonstrate in children who have multiple disabilities, it is fundamental to persevere in the endeavor because these signs have considerable value and important repercussions, not only on these children's diagnoses, but also on their habilitation. Indeed, by engaging in interventions to make children aware of the vision they have, professionals and parents can help them to further their own psychomotor development and relationship with the world.

It is crucial that the child with CVI be assisted in acquiring, through available senses, knowledge that cannot be acquired through sight. Recent studies have shown that growth in an "enriched" environment (i.e., an environment with modifications that make it more easily perceptible) may influence the development of the visual system in animal models (Cancedda et al., 2004; Sale et al., 2004; Scali, Baroncelli, Cenni, Sale, & Maffei, 2012). These enriched environments seem to have effects on the development and plasticity of the central nervous system, in particular on the visual pathways, by changing the start and end of the "critical or sensitive period" for the development of functions such as visual acuity (see Chapter 5). In addition, they play a key role in the activation of brain plasticity (Prusky, Silver, Tschetter, Alam, & Douglas, 2008), especially in the postnatal period when cortical circuits show the greatest sensitivity to sensory stimuli induced by experience (Hooks & Chen, 2007; Spolidoro, Sale, Berardi, & Maffei, 2009). These experimental data corroborate the importance of providing the child with CVI with environmental contexts that are meaningful and enriched, and which encourage the development of skills that can be used in their interaction with the world. Enriched environments for children with CVI often require the simplification of visual stimuli to encourage use of vision. For example, they may be plain, with limited decoration and regular removal of clutter, to increase children's ability to extract meaningful information that is presented clearly and accessibly.

### Integrated Sensory Approach

An integrated sensory approach meaningfully brings together the components of incoming sensory information by presenting them in such a way that the child can understand and respond. The approaches and instruments that are used bring together touch with sound and sight (the child responding to different levels of each at the same time). The aim is to ensure optimal coupling of incoming information in ways that promote attention, so that the information has meaning and promotes recognition and understanding of the incoming multisensory data. This approach aims to improve the child's ability to integrate information, enhance cognitive skills, and produce motor actions that progressively become more accurate, goal-oriented, and meaningful. (Integrated sensory approaches are covered in detail in Chapters 19, 20, 21, and 22.)

### Family-Centered Therapy

Family-centered therapy is crucial for effective therapeutic intervention with children with CVI, taking into account the need to involve all family members in the choice of priorities, the habilitation plan, and its implementation. It is crucial to recognize that each family is unique in order to be able to provide appropriate support, gain trust, and promote cooperation from each family member. Optimal development of the child takes place within the family and the community. Every family member needs to be supported and encouraged to participate, and should have the opportunity to decide their level of their involvement in the child's care. To be effective, interventions should take into account the child in their specific family and social context, with its own characteristics, difficulties, and strengths (see Chapter 23).

## Conclusion

Efforts to identify children with CVI in the early years most often lead to children with more severe visual impairments, many of whom also have additional disabilities. Developmental risk factors are compounded for children with CVI since they can have visual processing disorders in addition to limitations in lower visual functions such as visual acuity or visual field. This complex disorder can affect social, cognitive, communication, and motor development and requires knowledge of the range of potential intervention approaches described in later chapters.

## References

Als, H., Tronick, E., & Brazelton, B. (1980). Stages of early behavioral organization: The study of a sighted infant and a blind infant in interaction with their mother. In T. M. Field, S. Goldberg, D. Stern, & A. M. Sostek (Eds.), *High-risk infants and children: Adult and peer interaction* (pp. 181–204). New York: Academic Press.

Atkinson, J., & Braddick, O. (2007). Visual and visuocognitive development in children born very prematurely. *Progress in Brain Research, 164,* 123–149.

Atkinson, J., & Braddick, O. (2011). Linked brain development for vision, visual attention and visual cognition in typical development and in development disorders. In D. Riva, C. Njiokiktjien, & S. Bulgheroni (Eds.), *Brain lesion localization and developmental functions* (pp. 247–270). Montrouge, France: John Libbey Eurotext.

Bailly, D., Dechoulydelenclave, M. B., & Lauwerier, L. (2003). Hearing impairment and psychopathological disorders in children and adolescents. Review of the recent literature. *Encephale, 29*(4 Pt 1), 329–337.

Baird, S. M., Mayfield, P., & Baker, P. (1997). Mothers' interpretations of the behavior of their infants with visual and other impairments during interactions. *Journal of Visual Impairment & Blindness, 91*(5), 467–483.

Bigelow, A. E. (1983). The development of the use of sound in the search behavior of infants. *Journal of Developmental Psychology, 19*(3), 317–321.

Bigelow, A. E. (1986). The development of reaching in blind children. *British Journal of Developmental Psychology, 4,* 355–366.

Bigelow, A. E. (1992). Locomotion and search behavior in blind infants. *Infant Behavior and Development, 15,* 179–189.

Bigelow, A. E. (2003). The development of joint attention in blind infants. *Development and Psychopathology, 15,* 259–275.

Brambring, M. (1998). *Lessons with a child who is blind: Development and early intervention in the first years of life.* Okemos, MI: Blind Children's Fund.

Brambring, M., & Asbrock, D. J. (2010). Validity of false belief tasks in blind children. *Journal of Autism and Developmental Disorders, 40*(12), 1471–1484.

Burlingham, D. (1975). Special problems of blind infants. Blind baby profile. *The Psychoanalytic Study of the Child, 30,* 3–13.

Campbell, J. (2003). Maternal directives to young children who are blind. *Journal of Visual Impairment & Blindness, 97*(6), 353–363.

Campbell, J. (2007). Understanding the emotional needs of children who are blind [Research report]. *Journal of Visual Impairment & Blindness, 101*(6), 351–355.

Cancedda, L., Putignano, E., Sale, A., Viegi, A., Berardi, N., & Maffei, L. (2004). Acceleration of visual system development by environmental enrichment. *The Journal of Neuroscience, 24*(20), 4840–4848.

Carvill, S. (2001). Sensory impairments, intellectual disability and psychiatry. *Journal of Intellectual Disability Research, 45*(6), 467–483.

Chen, D. (1999). Interactions between infants and caregivers: The context for early intervention. In D. Chen (Ed.), *Essential elements in early intervention: Visual impairment and multiple disabilities* (pp. 22–54). New York: AFB Press.

Clifton, R. K., Rochat, P., Litovsky, R. Y., & Perris, E. E. (1991). Object representation guides infants' reaching in the dark. *Journal of Experimental Psychology, 17,* 323–329.

Dale, N., & Salt, A. (2008). Social identity, autism and visual impairment (VI) in the early years. *British Journal of Visual Impairment, 26*(2), 135–146.

Donnelly, U. M., Stewart, N. M., & Hollinger, M. (2005). Prevalence and outcomes of childhood visual disorders. *Ophthalmic Epidemiology, 12*(4), 243–250.

Dutton, G. N. (2003). Cognitive vision, its disorders and differential diagnosis in adults and children: Knowing where and what things are. *Eye, 17,* 289–304.

Dutton, G. N. (2006). Cerebral visual impairment: Working within and around the limitations of vision. In E. Dennison & A. H. Lueck (Eds.), *Proceedings of the summit on cerebral/cortical visual impairment: Educational, family, and medical perspectives, April 30, 2005.* New York: AFB Press.

Dutton, G. N. (2011). Structured history taking to characterize visual dysfunction and plan optimal habilitation for children with cerebral visual impairment. *Developmental Medicine & Child Neurolology, 53*(5), 390.

Dutton, G. N., Ballantyne, J., Boyd, G., Bradnam, M., Day, R., McCulloch, D., et al. (1996). Cortical visual dysfunction in children: A clinical study. *Eye, 10*, 302–309.

Fazzi, E., Bova, S. M., Giovenzana, A., Signorini, S., Uggetti, C., & Bianchi, P. (2009). Cognitive visual dysfunctions in preterm children with periventricular leukomalacia. *Developmental Medicine & Child Neurology, 51*, 974–981.

Fazzi, E., Bova, S. M., Uggetti, C., Signorini, S. G., Bianchi, P. E., Maraucci, I., . . . Lanzi, G. (2004). Visual-perceptual impairment in children with periventricular leucomalacia. *Brain & Development, 26*, 506–512.

Fazzi, E., Galli, J., & Micheletti, S. (2012). Visual impairment: A common sequel of preterm birth. *NeoReviews, 13*(9), 542–550.

Fazzi, E., Lanners, J., Ferrari-Ginervra, O., Achille, C., Luparia, A., Signorini, S., et al. (2002). Gross motor development and reach on sound as critical tools for the development of the blind child. *Brain & Development, 24*(5), 269–275.

Fazzi, E., Signorini, S. G., Bomba, M., Luparia, A., Lanners, J., & Balottin, U. (2011). Reach on sound: A key to object permanence in visually impaired children. *Early Human Development, 87*(4), 289–296.

Fazzi, E., Signorini, S. G., Bova, S. M., La Piana, R., Ondei, P., Bertone, C., . . . Bianchi, P. E. (2007). Spectrum of visual disorders in children with cerebral visual impairment. *Journal of Child Neurology, 22*, 294–301.

Fazzi, E., Signorini, S. G., & Lanners, J. (2010). The effect of impaired vision on development. In G. Dutton & M. Bax (Eds.), *Visual impairment in children due to damage to the brain* (pp. 162–173). London: Mac Keith Press.

Fazzi, E., Signorini, S. G., La Piana, R., Bertone, C., Misefari, W., Galli, J., . . . Bianchi, P. E. (2012). Neuro-ophthalmological disorders in cerebral palsy: Ophthalmological, oculomotor, and visual aspects. *Developmental Medicine & Child Neurology, 54*(8), 730–736.

Ferrell, K. A. (1998). *Project PRISM: A longitudinal study of developmental patterns of children who are visually impaired* [Executive summary]. Retrieved July 11, 2013, from www.unco.edu/ncssd/research/prism/execsumm.pd

Ferrell, K. A. (2011). *Reach out and teach: Helping your child who is visually impaired learn and grow* (2nd ed.). New York: AFB Press.

Fraiberg, S. (1971). Smiling and stranger reaction in blind infants. In J. Hellmuth (Ed.), *Exceptional infant: Vol. 2* (pp. 110–127). New York: Brunner/Mazel.

Fraiberg, S. (Ed.). (1977). *Insights from the blind: Comparative studies of blind and sighted infants.* New York: Basic Books.

Fraiberg, S., Siegel, B. L., & Gibson, R. (1966). The role of sound in the search behavior of a blind infant. *Psychoanalytic Study of the Child, 21*, 327–357.

Good, W. V., Jan, J. E., Burden, S. K., Skoczenski, A., & Candy, R. (2001). Recent advances in cortical visual impairment. *Developmental Medicine & Child Neurology, 43*(1), 56–60.

Good, W. V., Jan, J. E., de Sa, L., Barkovich, A. J., Groenveld, M., & Hoyt, C. S. (1994). Cortical visual impairment in children. *Survey of Ophthalmology, 38*, 351–364.

Groenveld, M., Jan, J. E., & Leader, P. (1990). Observations on the habilitation of children with cortical visual impairment. *Journal of Visual Impairment & Blindness, 84*(1), 11–15.

Guzzetta, A., D'Acunto, G., Rose, S., Tinelli, F., Boyd, R., & Cioni, G. (2010). Plasticity of the visual system after early brain damage. *Developmental Medicine & Child Neurology, 52*, 891–900.

Hatton, D. D., Bailey, D. B., Burchinal, M. R., & Ferrell, K. A. (1997). Developmental growth curves of preschool children with vision impairments. *Child Development, 68*(5), 788–806.

Hodgdon, L. (Ed.). (1997). *Visual strategies for improving communication: Vol. 1.* Troy, MI: QuirkRoberts Publishing.

Hooks, B. M., & Chen, C. (2007). Critical periods in the visual system: Changing views for a model of experience-dependent plasticity. *Neuron, 56*(2), 312–326.

Howe, D. (2006). Disabled children, parent-child interaction and attachment. *Child & Family Social Work, 11*(2), 95–106.

Jakobson, L. S., Frisk, V., & Downie, A. L. (2006). Motion-defined form processing in extremely premature children. *Neuropsychologia, 44*(10), 1777–1786.

Jan, J. E., & Groenveld, M. (1990). Visual behaviors and adaptations associated with cortical and ocular impairment in children. *Journal of Visual Impairment & Blindness, 87,* 101–105.

Kekelis, L. S., & Prinz, P. M. (1996). Blind and sighted children with their mothers: The development of discourse skills. *Journal of Visual Impairment & Blindness, 90*(5), 423–436.

Kelly, J. F., & Barnard, K. E. (2000). Assessment of parent-child interaction. In J. P. Shonkoff & S. M. Meisels (Eds.), *Handbook of early intervention* (2nd ed., pp. 258–289). New York: Cambridge University Press.

Lane, G. M. (1996). The effectiveness of two strategies for teaching students with blindness and mental retardation. *Journal of Visual Impairment & Blindness, 90*(2), 125–133.

Levtzion-Korach, O., Tennenbaum, A., Schnitzer, R., & Ornoy, A. (2000). Early motor development of blind children. *Journal of Paediatrics and Child Health, 36*(3), 226–229.

Loots, G., & Devisé, I. (2003). An intersubjective developmental perspective on interactions between deaf and hearing mothers and their deaf infants. *American Annals of the Deaf, 148*(4), 295–307.

Loots, G., Devisé, I., & Sermijn, J. (2003). The interaction between mothers and their visually impaired infants: An intersubjective developmental perspective. *Journal of Visual Impairment & Blindness, 97*(7), 403–417.

Lueck, A. H., Chen, D., Kekelis, L. S., & Hartmann, L. E. (2008). *Developmental guidelines for infants with visual impairment: A guidebook for early intervention* (2nd ed.). Louisville, KY: American Printing House for the Blind.

Malekpour, M. (2007). Effects of attachment on early and later development. *The British Journal of Developmental Disabilities, 53*(105), 81–95.

McCollum, J. A., & Hemmeter, M. L. (1997). Parent-child interaction intervention when children have disabilities. In M. J. Guralnick (Ed.), *The effectiveness of early intervention* (pp. 549–576). Baltimore: Paul H. Brookes.

McDaid, G., & Dutton, G. (2007). *Cerebral visual impairment in children: The development of optimum management strategies.* Glasgow, UK: Glasgow Caledonian University, Research and Education Department.

Mercuri, E., Baranello, G., Romeo, D. M., Cesarini, L., & Ricci, D. (2007). The development of vision. *Early Human Development, 83*(12), 795–800.

Minter, M. E., Hobson, R. P., & Pring, L. (1991). Recognition of vocally expressed emotion by congenitally blind children. *Journal of Visual Impairment & Blindness, 85*, 411–415.

Morgan, P. (2004). Instructional strategies for students with cortical visual impairment. In A. H. Lueck (Ed.), *Functional vision: A practitioner's guide to evaluation and intervention* (pp. 325–328). New York: AFB Press.

Morse, M. T. (1992). Augmenting assessment procedures for children with severe multiple handicaps and sensory impairments. *Journal of Visual Impairment & Blindness, 86,* 73–77.

Neisser, U. (1991). Two perceptually given aspects of the self and their development. *Developmental Review, 11*(3), 197–209.

Neisser, U. (Ed.). (1993). *The perceived self: Ecological and interpersonal sources of self knowledge.* New York: Cambridge University Press.

Ortibus, E. L., De Cock, P. P., & Lagae, L. G. (2011). Visual perception in preterm children: What are we currently measuring? *Pediatric Neurology, 45*(1), 1–10.

Pavlova, M., Sokolov, A., & Krägeloh-Mann, I. (2007). Visual navigation in adolescents with early periventricular lesions: Knowing where, but not getting there. *Cerebral Cortex, 17*(2), 363–369.

Pérez-Pereira, M., & Conti-Ramsden, G. (Ed.). (1999). *Language development and social interaction in blind children.* Hove, UK: Psychology Press.

Pérez-Pereira, M., & Conti-Ramsden, G. (2001). The use of directives in verbal interactions between blind children and their mothers. *Journal of Visual Impairment & Blindness, 95*(3), 133–149.

Prechtl, H. F. (2001). General movement assessment as a method of developmental neurology: New paradigms and their consequences.

The 1999 Ronnie MacKeith lecture. *Developmental Medicine & Child Neurology, 43*(12), 836–842.

Preisler, G. (1991). Early patterns of interactions between blind infants and their sighted mothers. *Child: Care, Health and Development, 17*, 45–52.

Preisler, G. (1993). *Developing communication with blind and with deaf infants* (Report No. 761). Stockholm University, Department of Psychology.

Pring, L., & Tadic, V. (2010). The cognitive and behavioral manifestations of blindness in children. In R. D. Nass & Y. Frank, *Cognitive and behavioral abnormalities of pediatric diseases* (pp. 531–543). New York: Oxford University Press.

Prusky, G. T., Silver, B. D., Tschetter, W. W., Alam, N. M., & Douglas, R. M. (2008). Experience-dependent plasticity from eye opening enables lasting, visual cortex-dependent enhancement of motion vision. *The Journal of Neuroscience, 28*(39), 9817–9827.

Pueyo, V., Garcia-Ormaechea, I., Gonzale, I., Ferrer, C., de la Mata, G., Dupla, M., . . . Andes, E. (2014). Development of the preverbal visual assessment (PreViAs) questionnaire. *Early Human Development, 90*, 165–168.

Ricci, D., Cesarini, L., Romeo, D. M., Gallini, F., Serrao, F., Groppo, M., . . . Mercuri, E. (2008). Visual function at 35 and 40 weeks' postmenstrual age in low-risk preterm infants. *Pediatrics, 122*(6), 193–198.

Rogers, S. J., & Puchalski, C. B. (1984). Social characteristics of visually impaired infants' play. *Topics in Early Childhood Special Education, 3*, 52–56.

Rogers, S. J., & Puchalski, C. B. (1986). Social smiles of visually impaired infants. *Journal of Visual Impairment & Blindness, 80*, 863–865.

Rogers, S. J., & Puchalski, C. B. (1988). Development of object permanence in visually impaired infants. *Journal of Visual Impairment & Blindness, 82*, 137–142.

Roman, C. A. (1996). Validation of an interview instrument to identify behaviors characteristic of cortical visual impairment in infants. *Dissertation Abstracts International, 57*(07), 2968A. (UMI No. 9637846)

Roman-Lantzy, C. A. (2007). *Cortical visual impairment: An approach to assessment and intervention*. New York: AFB Press.

Rossi, A., Gritti, M., Mattei, P., Alessandrini, A., Tansini, F., Chirico, G., . . . Fazzi, E. (2013, April). *Neurovisual function in preterms: Early marker for developmental risk?* Poster session presented at the 41 Ème Congrès SENP of the Société Européenne de Neurologie Pédiatrique.

Sale, A., Putignano, E., Cancedda, L., Landi, S., Cirulli, F., Berardi, N., & Maffei, L. (2004). Enriched environment and acceleration of visual system development. *Neuropharmacology, 47*(5), 649–660.

Scali, M., Baroncelli, L., Cenni, M. C., Sale, A., & Maffei, L. (2012). A rich environmental experience reactivates visual cortex plasticity in aged rats. *Experimental Gerontology, 47*(4), 337–341.

Shaman, D. (2009). A team approach to cortical visual impairment (CVI) in schools [Electronic version]. Louisville, KY: American Printing House for the Blind. Retrieved from http://www.aph.org/cvi/articles/shaman_1.html

Smith, D. W., & Kelley, P.A. (2007). A survey of the integration of assistive technology knowledge into teacher preparation programs for individuals with visual impairments. *Journal of Visual Impairment & Blindness, 101*(7), 429–433.

Sonksen, P. M., & Dale, N. (2002). Visual impairment in infancy: Impact on neurodevelopmental and neurobiological processes. *Developmental Medicine & Child Neurology, 44*(11), 782–791.

Spitz, R. A. (1946). The smiling response: A contribution to the ontogenesis of social relations. *Genetic Psychology Monographs, 34*, 57–125.

Spolidoro, M., Sale, A., Berardi, N., & Maffei, L. (2009). Plasticity in the adult brain: Lessons from the visual system. *Experimental Brain Research, 192*(3), 335–341.

Stiers, P., van den Hout, B. M., Haers, M., Vanderkelen, R., de Vries, L. S., van Nieuwenhuizen, O., & Vandenbussche, E. (2001). The variety of visual perceptual impairments in pre-school children with perinatal brain damage. *Brain and Development, 23*(5), 333–348.

Strickling, C. A., & Pogrund, R. L. (2002). Motor focus: Promoting movement experiences and motor development. In R. L. Pogrund & D. L. Fazzi (Eds.), *Early focus: Working with young children who are blind or visually impaired and their families* (2nd ed., pp. 287–325). New York: AFB Press.

Swift, S. H., Davidson, R. C., & Weems, L. J. (2008). Cortical visual impairment in children: Presentation, intervention, and prognosis in educational settings. *TEACHING Exceptional Children Plus, 4*(5).

Tadic, V., Pring, L., & Dale, N. J. (2008). *Strengths and difficulties in language of children with congenital visual impairment.* Presented at the annual British Psychological Society Conference, Oxford Brookes University.

Tadic, V., Pring, L., & Dale, N. (2010). Are language and social communication intact in children with congenital visual impairment at school age? *Journal of Child Psychology and Psychiatry, 51*(6), 696–705.

Trevarthen, C., & Aitken, K. J. (2001). Infant intersubjectivity: Research, theory, and clinical applications. *Journal of Child Psychology and Psychiatry, 42*(1), 3–48.

Tröster, H., & Brambring, M. (1992). Early social-emotional development in blind infants. *Child: Care, Health and Development, 18*(4), 207–227.

Tröster, H., Brambring, M., & Beelmann, A. (1994). Prevalence and situational causes of stereotyped behaviors in blind infants and preschoolers. *Journal of Abnormal Child Psychology, 19*(5), 569–590.

Volpe, J. (1996). Subplate neurons—Missing link in brain injury of the premature infant? *Pediatrics, 97*(1), 112–113. Retrieved from http://pediatrics.aappublications.org/content/97/1/112.full.pdf

Warren, D. H. (1994). *Blindness & children: A developmental differences approach.* New York: Cambridge University Press.

Warren, S. L., Huston, L., Egeland, B., & Sroufe, L. A. (1997). Child and adolescent anxiety disorders and early attachment. *Journal of the American Academy of Child & Adolescent Psychiatry, 36*(5), 637–644.

# 5

# Brain Plasticity and Development

*Zaira Catteneo and Lotfi B. Merabet*

A remarkable feature of the human brain is its natural capacity to change. The ability of the brain to continuously reorganize itself as it develops and to learn from experience is called *plasticity*, from the Greek *plaistikos*, meaning to mold or form. Just as a piece of plastic can be molded and formed into a new shape, so can the brain progressively change its structure and the way it functions in response to the surrounding environment. Although this plasticity is a normal intrinsic property of the brain, the first insights into this property have come from studying the outcomes of brain injury, and from experimental work.

Much of what is known comes from investigating visual deprivation and blindness because the way the brain adapts to the loss, the potential for recovery and its limitations, and the underlying mechanisms, can all be studied. The visual brain develops and changes rapidly during early life, when the brain is most capable of growing in response to sensory input. This window for development of vision and hearing is known as the "critical," or "sensitive," period because interference with sensory input at this time—for example, as a result of congenital cataract—leads to lifelong visual impairment from amblyopia if not treated within two or three months of birth (Gelbart, Hoyt, Jastrebski, & Marg, 1982). However, plasticity is a dynamic property of the brain that continues throughout an individual's lifetime and has important implications for rehabilitation and learning following a brain injury.

## Plasticity: The Dynamic Brain

### Types and Mechanisms of Brain Plasticity

Some of the earliest ideas about how the brain is organized come from the work of Hebb (1949), who suggested the idea that "cells that fire together, wire together." In the act of repeatedly exchanging information among themselves, clusters of brain cells or neurons progressively change, enhancing their ability to communicate with one another. This occurs at the junction sites between neurons, called *synapses,* where the transfer of chemical and electrical information takes place. This ability to enhance communication between neurons through synaptic efficacy is essential to learning and memory, as well as recovery of sensory and motor functions following brain damage.

Plasticity is a process that takes place at all structural levels in the brain, from the molecular processes of communication at synapses, to neural network systems (how different regions of the brain are organized in terms of structure and function), to behavior (how regions of the brain interact to improve skills or bring about compensatory strategies) (Shaw & McEachern, 2001). Therefore, the overall concept of plasticity includes changes in both brain structure and function, as well as behavior.

The senses of sight, sound, smell, and touch are processed and represented in the brain, with each representation considered a "mode." The processes of plasticity can be divided into those taking place within a sense, or "intramodal," and those taking place between senses, or "crossmodal" (for reviews, see Grafman, 2000; Röder & Neville, 2003). A dramatic example of crossmodal plasticity is the phenomenon of the occipital, or visual, cortex learning to process touch and sound in individuals who are blind. This finding has led to the intriguing idea that the occipital cortex may be the source of compensatory behaviors (such as higher tactile discrimination abilities or better sound localization) exhibited by people who are blind, in response to loss of sight (Bavelier & Neville, 2002).

How the brain generates such dramatic neuroplastic changes is the subject of intense investigation and debate. There is evidence that two mechanisms play a role: (1) the formation of new neural pathways, and (2) the unmasking and strengthening of existing pathways.

Evidence for the first mechanism, the formation of new neural pathways, has been found in animal studies. In these studies, new connections in effect rewiring the neural pathways between the thalamus (a structure deep in the brain that processes input from the senses) and the cerebral cortex have resulted from experimental manipulation (Sur, Garraghty, & Roe, 1988). Similar processes in the human brain have not yet been conclusively demonstrated.

In humans, there is more evidence for the second mechanism, strengthening of existing pathways. Tactile and auditory information are known to reach the occipital cortex via existing brain pathways between cortical areas (Leclerc, Segalowitz, Desjardins, Lassonde, & Lepore, 2005; Wittenberg, Werhahn, Wassermann, Herscovitch, & Cohen, 2004). In the case of sensory deprivation, these neural pathways may be reinforced through practice and lead to the observed compensatory behaviors just described.

## The Timing of Plasticity

Children demonstrate a greater facility for learning and memory skills, such as learning a new language or a musical instrument, than do adults. It is also known that the brain is more sensitive to developmental disruption early rather than later in life (Hubel, Wiesel, & LeVay, 1977; Teuber, 1975). This early "critical period" refers to a specific time window during which exposure to a particular stimulus or experience, such as vision or speech, was necessary for the normal development of brain processes supporting that particular function or skill. At first, it was thought that the brain's capacity for plasticity beyond this early critical period was very limited, that outside this time window, the same experiences would not lead to the same outcomes, and the lack of such experience could have potentially devastating effects on development (Michel & Tyler, 2005).

However, more recent studies have shown that this time window is much more flexible than previously thought and depends on the unique experience of each individual (Michel & Tyler, 2005). It is now recognized that the brain maintains the capacity to rewire itself throughout life. Although this ability declines with advancing age (Singer, Lindenberger, & Baltes, 2003), there is consistent evidence that the aging brain maintains a considerable degree of plasticity (Jones et al., 2006). In light of these more recent findings, the concept of the critical period has now been largely replaced with the more apt "sensitive period," reinforcing the idea that the time window of plasticity is broader than previously thought and does not have an abrupt beginning or end.

Sensitive periods may vary depending on the brain function in question (Armstrong et al., 2006). There are three different sensitive periods relating to the development of the visual system (Lewis & Maurer, 2005):

1. The period in which normal visual experiences lead to the development of adult-level visual processing.
2. The time window during which injury to the visual system leads to permanent deficits.
3. The period during which the visual system has the capacity to recover function following damage.

These three periods underline the important notion that the timing of development, plasticity, and recovery from damage may differ for specific visual functions—a crucial concept that needs to be considered when developing both habilitation and rehabilitation programs for the visually impaired (see Cattaneo & Vecchi, 2011).

## Tools for Studying Human Brain Plasticity

Careful observation of patients with brain damage, as well as well-designed experimental animal studies, have greatly informed professional knowledge of the interplay between brain structure, function, and behavior. More recently, modern brain imaging methods have allowed for the safe and noninvasive study of the human brain (Figure 5.1). Each technique has advantages and disadvantages. A brief overview of each technique is presented here. (For a more comprehensive discussion, see Logothetis, 2008; Walsh & Pascual-Leone, 2003.)

***Magnetic resonance imaging (MRI)*** shows the anatomical features of the brain in great detail and can be used to study brain structure following injury, or after the learning of a new skill.

***Diffusion tensor imaging (DTI)*** allows for the study of how structures within the brain are interconnected. Movement of water molecules in the brain is tracked with a high degree of precision, which allows the complex organization of nerve fibers that connect different brain areas to be determined and studied. This is particularly useful in studying how the brain rewires itself following sensory deprivation (Obretenova, Halko, Plow, Pascual-Leone, & Merabet, 2010) or damage to the brain.

***Functional MRI (fMRI)*** and ***positron emission tomography (PET)*** permit observation of the brain in action when performing a particular task. This is done by tracking changes in brain metabolism, such as oxygen

FIGURE 5.1
## Techniques Used to Investigate Brain Plasticity

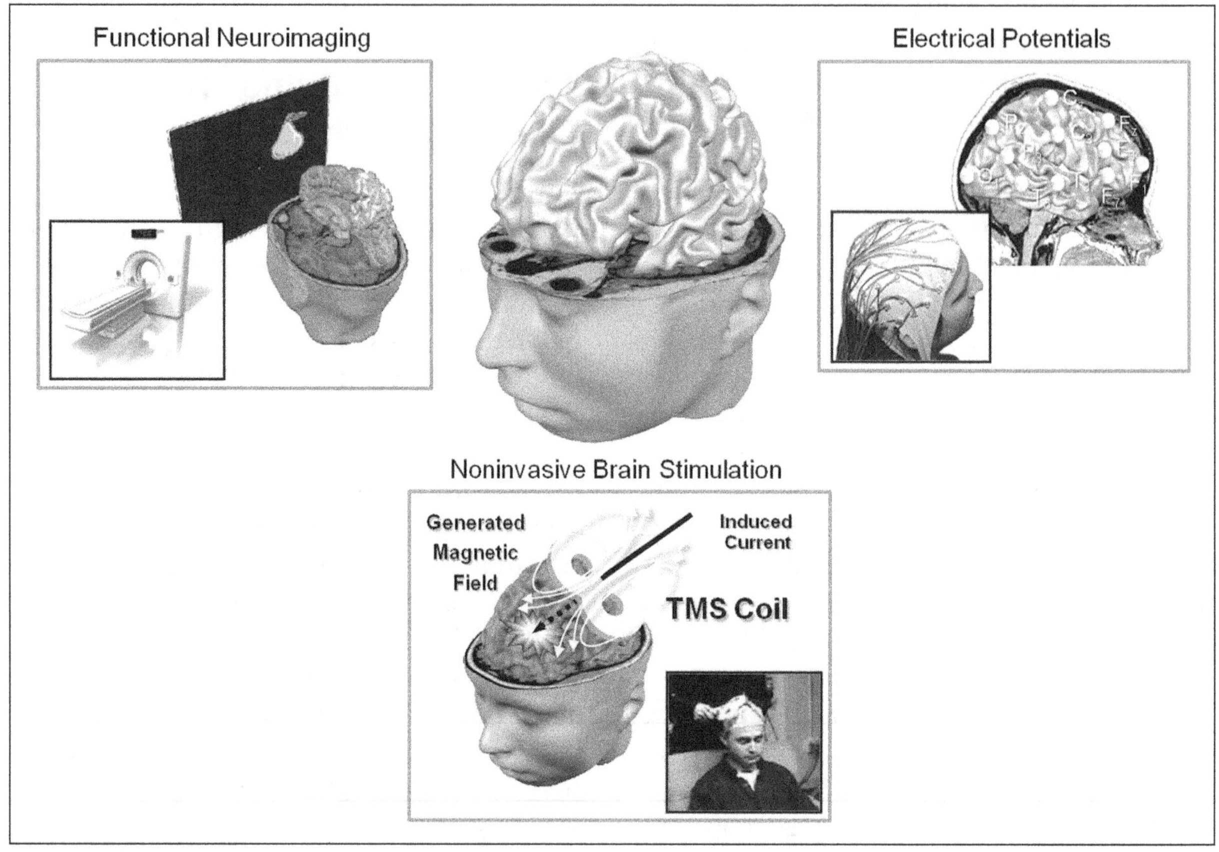


Methods of studying the human brain illustrated here include functional neuroimaging (functional magnetic resonance imaging or fMRI), which measures levels of oxygen consumption in different parts of the brain; direct measurement of electrical potentials, through electroencephalography; and noninvasive brain stimulation, to temporarily interfere with the activity of a brain region using transcranial magnetic stimulation (TMS).

consumption, hemoglobin levels, or blood flow, that are known indicators of brain activity. Foci of enhanced activity observed on the brain scan while a task is being carried out allow for extrapolation of the principal anatomical areas related to that particular task.

***Electroencephalography (EEG),*** and its magnetic counterpart, *magnetoencephalography (MEG),* noninvasively record brain activity from the surface of the scalp. This provides direct measure of brain function.

***Visual evoked potentials (VEPs)*** work with weak but detectable electrical currents that carry information from one nerve cell to another. When neighboring neurons work together during a specific task, the resulting brain activity can be detected and accurately timed. Electrical signals measured in the occipital lobe in response to flashing lights or reverse checkerboard patterns are known as visual evoked potentials (VEPs). VEPs can be used to investigate vision and visual perception, to assist in diagnosis, and to classify cerebral and ocular visual disorders (Betsuin, Mashima, Ohde, Inoue, & Oguchi, 2001).

***Transcranial magnetic stimulation (TMS)*** emits electrical pulses to trigger brain activity. Low-frequency pulses (about one per second) of electrical stimulation, delivered to the surface of the scalp with a specially designed coil, inhibit brain activity directly underneath the coil. On the other hand, electrical pulses delivered at a high frequency (10–20 per second) can actually enhance the activity of the underlying brain region (Merabet, Theoret, & Pascual-Leone, 2003; Walsh & Pascual-Leone, 2003). In a sense, TMS is like a bladeless knife that can cut both ways, inhibiting or activating a particular brain area depending on the stimulus delivered. In this way, the role of a region of the brain can be probed directly. Unlike functional brain imaging that aims to relate the site of brain activity to a particular task, TMS seeks a causal relationship between a specific brain area and the specific task (Walsh & Pascual-Leone, 2003). By temporarily interfering with the activity of a specific brain region and observing its effect on a person's behavior, the contribution that area makes to the task can be better understood.

## Features of Brain Plasticity

### Adaptive Plasticity

Plasticity of the parts of the brain that control movement has been studied in detail. For example, the activated area in the part of the brain's cortex serving skilled movement gets bigger as the skill improves, following four weeks of repeated practice (Karni et al., 1995). This change persists for several months after training (Karni et al., 1995), suggesting that the ability to acquire and retain new motor skills as an adult is underpinned by reorganization of the brain's cortex. With time, these functional changes often lead to more permanent structural changes in the brain (Landi, Baguear, & Della-Maggiore, 2011).

Musical abilities also serve as a good model for studying plasticity related to learning. Most musicians learn to play an instrument during childhood, and continue learning by means of a highly focused and dedicated practice routine throughout their lives. It is therefore not surprising that the brains of musicians show a different organizational structure from that of nonmusicians. For example, auditory regions of the cortex, sensitive to tones of the musical scale (as compared to pure tones—those consisting of a single frequency), are enlarged in skilled musicians (Pantev et al., 2003). Similarly, mathematicians show structural changes within the parietal cortex, the part of the brain associated with spatial information processing (Aydin et al., 2007; Draganski et al., 2006).

Licensed London taxi drivers go through extensive training to develop their navigational skills. Remarkably, the posterior hippocampus (the part of the brain responsible for memory and spatial learning) is significantly larger than that of similarly aged Londoners who are not taxi drivers (Maguire et al., 2000). The longer the experience of driving a taxi, the larger the posterior hippocampus becomes (Maguire et al., 2000). These studies signify that practice, learning, and experience lead to functional and structural neuroplastic changes within the brain.

### Maladaptive Plasticity and the Effects of Rehabilitation

Plasticity is not always a positive and adaptive phenomenon. Two well-known examples of "maladaptive plasticity" are focal dystonia (Pujol et al., 2000) and phantom limb pain.

### Focal Dystonia

*Focal dystonia* (also called "musician's cramp") may result from the highly repetitive and synchronous movements of the fingers required to play a stringed musical instrument, such as a violin. In some cases, the pain and loss of hand function related to this condition may even curtail a musician's career. Studies using MEG imaging have demonstrated that the inability to move the affected fingers independently can be the outcome of vigorous and frequent musical practice, and is related to a disordered and "smeared" representation of the fingers in the associated somatosensory or motor cortex (Quartarone, Siebner, & Rothwell, 2006). Fortunately, rehabilitation therapy can restore both hand function and brain activity back to normal.

### Phantom Limb Pain

Another example of maladaptive plasticity is *phantom limb pain,* which typically follows amputation of a limb. The phantom sensations have been related to changes in activity in the primary somatosensory cortex (Flor, 2008; Schwenkreis et al., 2000). Remarkably, the act of looking at the intact limb, using a mirror system in such a way that it appears to the amputee that the amputated limb is still present, can help reverse both the symptoms and the maladaptive changes in the brain (Ramachandran & Altschuler, 2009).

## Plasticity in Cases of Ocular Blindness

Blindness presents considerable challenges when living in a world heavily reliant upon vision, but compensatory and adaptive behaviors develop that rely heavily on nonvisual senses such as hearing and touch. This is accompanied by dramatic parallel plastic changes in the brain.

People who are totally blind can identify sounds and tactile stimuli more quickly than typical individuals. These faster responses result from faster brain processing, and may be related to enhanced selective attention (Röder, Kramer, & Lange, 2007; Röder, Rosler, Hennighausen, & Nacker, 1996). The areas of the brain responsible for touch (somatosensory cortex) and hearing (auditory cortex) also exhibit plastic changes in blind individuals, with expansion of the parts of the auditory cortex that serve the ability to hear different tones (Elbert et al., 2002; Hamilton, Pascual-Leone, & Schlaug, 2004). Similarly, fingers used to read braille are served by an enlarged cortical brain area (Burton, Sinclair, & McLaren, 2004; Pascual-Leone & Torres, 1993; Sterr, Muller, Elbert, Rockstroh, & Taub, 1999). Highly proficient braille readers can develop changes in the brain areas serving the reading fingers. These areas can appear "fused" together as a result of repetitive simultaneous stimulation of the fingers during reading. This change in brain mapping may explain how braille patterns are processed more holistically and at a greater speed in proficient readers (Sterr, Green, & Elbert, 2003; Sterr et al., 1998).

Even brain areas responsible for smell undergo plastic changes in cases of early-onset blindness. Using MRI, it has been shown that the part of the brain that serves smell (the olfactory bulb) is larger in individuals with early-onset blindness as compared to sighted individuals. This enlargement is accompanied by enhanced olfactory abilities (Rombaux et al., 2010). Similarly, fMRI studies have shown that, unlike in people

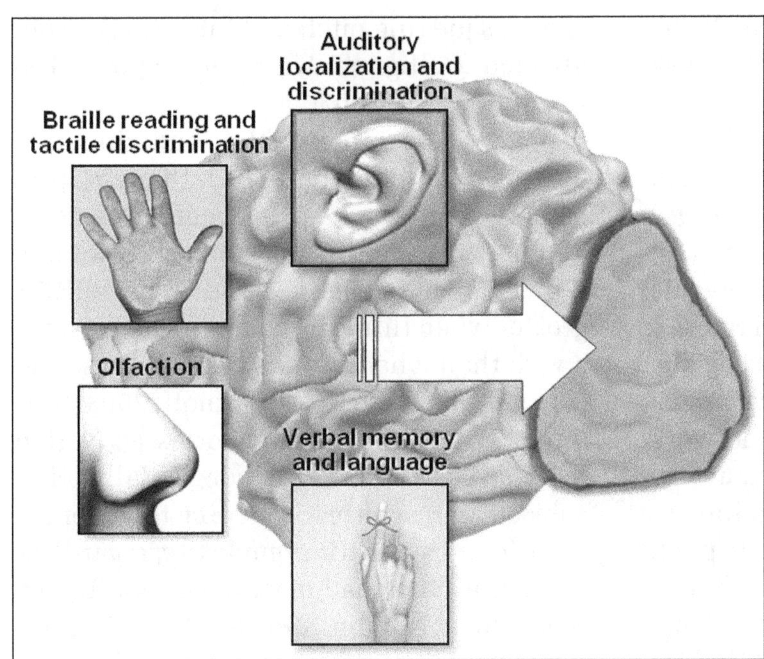


FIGURE 5.2
**Crossmodal Changes Following Blindness**

The brain can compensate for a severe sensory loss by reorganizing itself in order to more efficiently process information in the available sensory modalities. Here, the occipital cortex, responsible for processing visual information in normally sighted individuals, is shown being recruited to process information from other sensory modalities—hearing, touch, olfaction—also active during cognitive tasks, for instance in language production and memory.

with typical sight, odor activates the occipital cortex in congenitally blind subjects, as well as having a greater effect on activating the olfactory areas (Kupers et al., 2011).

Intermodal cortical plasticity based on increased use of a particular sensory modality, as demonstrated in these examples, may underpin the compensatory behaviors observed in blind individuals. A key question that deserves attention, then, is, What is the fate of brain regions normally associated with processing visual information? The answer is that intermodal or crossmodal plastic changes take place in these areas as well (see Figure 5.2). Neuroimaging studies suggest that the same occipital areas that serve visual processing in sighted individuals are employed for tactile and auditory processing, and even for olfaction and memory tasks, in blind individuals. This crossmodal engagement of the occipital cortex in blind individuals was first discovered in the late 1980s (Veraart et al., 1990; Wanet-Defalque et al., 1988). The level of brain metabolic activity—specifically, glucose utilization—was higher in the occipital cortical regions of early blind subjects as compared to sighted individuals, both at rest and during tactile object manipulation and auditory tasks. Nonvisual tasks have repeatedly been shown to increase occipital brain activity in people who are blind. For example, braille reading activates the occipital cortex when studied by EEG (Uhl, Franzen, Lindinger, Lang, & Deecke, 1991; Uhl, Franzen, Podreka, Steiner, & Deecke, 1993). In addition, braille reading and other tactile tasks, such as estimating angles and identifying embossed letters, activate the occipital cortex in both early and late blind participants when studied by PET or fMRI scans (see, for example, Burton, McLaren, & Sinclair, 2006; Burton et al., 2002; Sadato & Hallett, 1999; Sadato et al., 1996).

Listening tasks also activate the visual cortex in blind individuals (for a review, see

Collignon, Voss, Lassonde, & Lepore, 2009), but like tactile discrimination, the task needs to be sufficiently demanding. The occipital visual areas are not activated by the mere presence of sound, but are involved in paying attention to changes in the auditory environment that may serve detection of important or potentially dangerous events (Kujala et al., 2005). In blind musicians, absolute pitch—the rare ability to identify the pitch of a musical note without a reference tone—is related to a different brain network than in sighted individuals, and may explain why a greater proportion of blind individuals have an aptitude for absolute pitch as compared to sighted musicians (Gaab, Schulze, Ozdemir, & Schlaug, 2006; Pring, Woolf, & Tadic, 2008). The ability of blind individuals to localize sound sources has been found to activate cortical areas typically associated with dorsal stream visual processing (Weeks et al., 2000; see also Collignon et al., 2011).

Some blind individuals are able to use sound echoes to perceive certain aspects of their surroundings, an ability known as *echolocation*. Echolocators have learned to sense and even identify the presence and movement of objects in their environment simply by generating clicks with their tongues and mouths and listening to the reflecting echoes. These echoes facilitate mobility and can provide a skilled echolocator with information regarding the position, distance, size, shape, and texture of objects; and there is evidence that the data provided by these echoic sounds are analyzed in the visual cortex (Thaler, Arnott, & Goodale, 2011). This concept is supported by the finding that TMS delivered to the occipital cortical areas, specifically the right hemisphere, interferes with these auditory spatial location tasks, whereas other auditory tasks (such as judging pitch and intensity) are not affected (Collignon, Lassonde, Lepore, Bastien, & Veraart, 2007).

The visual cortex of blind individuals is also involved in high-level thought processing such as language comprehension and memory. For instance, the activation of the visual cortex as observed on an fMRI is greater when thinking about the meaning of a verb than when thinking about the sound (Burton, Diamond, & McDermott, 2003; Burton et al., 2002). Occipital cortex activation has also been observed in congenitally blind subjects in response to listening to sentences of different syntactic complexity, regardless of whether they had meaning or not (Röder, Stock, Bien, Neville, & Rosler, 2002). In addition, verbal memory tasks bring about visual cortex activity (Amedi, Raz, Pianka, Malach, & Zohary, 2003; Raz, Amedi, & Zohary, 2005). The greater the activation, the larger the number of words recalled. Delivery of TMS to the occipital lobes impairs the ability to generate verbs in people who are blind, but not in sighted individuals (Amedi, Floel, Knecht, Zohary, & Cohen, 2004).

## Variables that Affect Plasticity in People with Ocular Blindness

Changes in plasticity have been found to be most robust in those with congenital or early-onset blindness, with altered tactile and auditory capacities of the visual cortex most pronounced (Gougoux et al., 2004; Theoret, Merabet, & Pascual-Leone, 2004; Wan, Wood, Reutens, & Wilson, 2010a, 2010b). However, the brain's ability to develop cross-modal neuroplastic adaptation is drastically reduced after puberty.

Braille reading is impaired when repetitive TMS, or rTMS, is used to deactivate the primary visual cortex, but only in those who lost vision before the age of 14 (Cohen et al.,

1999). For touch discrimination tasks, a similar cutoff has been found before age 16 (Sadato, Okada, Honda, & Yonekura, 2002). This suggests that there may be an age window from 14–16 for the development of crossmodal reorganization in the brain. (However, this finding may relate to technical issues and should not be taken as definitive.) The development of intramodal plasticity is also likely to be less robust in late-onset blindness when compared to early-onset blindness (Gougoux et al., 2009).

Crossmodal engagement of the occipital cortex during tactile tasks can be identified even after a few days of visual deprivation (Merabet et al., 2008). Sighted adults who underwent an intensive tactile training program and were then blindfolded for five days to simulate sudden and complete visual deprivation exhibited an enhanced ability to discriminate braille when compared to a group that had not been blindfolded. Moreover, fMRI scanning revealed increased levels of activity in the occipital visual cortex in response to tactile stimulation in the blindfolded group, indicating that the occipital cortex was engaged in tactile processing. This result was confirmed using TMS on the occipital cortex on the fifth day, when impaired braille character recognition was observed in the blindfolded group but not in the group that had not been blindfolded, suggesting that activation of the visual cortex in the blindfolded group became critical for recognizing braille characters. However, this effect was not detectable one day after removing the blindfold. This "blindfold study" is important because it shows that the occipital cortex becomes engaged in processing nonvisual information through neuroplastic change, even in normally sighted adults after a short period of sudden and complete visual deprivation, but is rapidly reversed when sight is restored (Merabet et al., 2008).

Partial visual deficits can also lead to functional compensatory mechanisms. Myopia (nearsightedness or short-sightedness) can lead to greater spatial auditory sensitivity (Despres, Candas, & Dufour, 2005; Dufour & Gérard, 2000) and enhanced tactile discrimination capacities (Alary et al., 2008; Goldreich & Kanics, 2003). On the other hand, residual vision is associated with lower performance in auditory localization tasks in people with partial vision as compared to individuals who are totally blind (Lessard, Pare, Lepore, & Lassonde, 1998), possibly as a result of competing inputs of sound and degraded vision.

The visual brain itself adapts in response to low vision. For example, the parts of the visual cortex that usually process information from the central visual field adapt and become activated by peripheral visual stimuli in individuals who have lost central vision, following longstanding damage to the center of the retina resulting from macular degeneration (Baker, Peli, Knouf, & Kanwisher, 2005). Such changes in the brain appear to be affected by the age of onset and duration of the visual deficit (Baker et al., 2005; Smirnakis et al., 2005; Sunness, Liu, & Yantis, 2004), although a few years of partial visual deprivation may not be sufficient to produce significant changes at the cortical level (Sunness et al., 2004).

## Plasticity in Cerebral Visual Impairment

Studies examining the neuroplasticity changes associated with CVI are still in the early stages. Since one of the most common causes of CVI is brain injury following lack of oxygen delivery, the related neuroplastic changes are rarely limited to a single brain area or function. Additionally, many children with CVI also have cerebral palsy, seizure disorders, and communication disorders, making vision assessment more challenging.

Plasticity phenomena associated with recovery of visual functions, whether spontaneous or induced by behavioral training, have been observed in children with CVI. For example, one type of behavioral training that has been studied frequently involves visual field training consisting of systematic stimulation of the blind area with a target such as a concentrated spot of light, which has been successful in expanding the size of the visual field in some individuals with CVI. However, the study of plasticity phenomena in children with CVI is limited by some methodological constraints that need to be considered when evaluating spontaneous or training-induced recovery of visual function and associated plasticity reorganization (Werth, 2008):

1. Instructions about the tests used to measure visual functions (see Chapter 12) may be too difficult to understand and follow; accordingly, testing methods typically used to assess visual functions in adults and to determine improvements cannot be employed with infants or brain-damaged young children, and training protocols developed for adults—such as visual field training—are not suitable for young children.
2. Children may be unable to describe their visual experiences with sufficient detail.
3. Neuroimaging techniques such as fMRI cannot be easily carried out, as young children have to be anesthetized during the procedure; this limits the number of possible investigations and in effect precludes testing behavioral performance.

Werth and Seelos (2005) analyzed the effect of a specific visual field training procedure on a number of children who had complete or partial blindness resulting from CVI and who had been blind for at least one year without any sign of spontaneous recovery. The training consisted of stimulating the visual field by slowly moving a light on a dark background every day for approximately half an hour. Many of the children developed evidence of detectable visual function within weeks or months, but this was observed only when very bright stimuli were used. The training-related gains in visual functions observed in these children were higher than those for adults (as reported in other studies), once again showing that children have a greater capacity to gain or recover certain visual functions (Werth & Seelos, 2005). This difference between children and adults may depend on a series of factors:

1. The type of training used may have played a role. With children, brighter stimuli were used, which may have made the training more effective.
2. The type and extent of the damage may be responsible for greater success in training children. In particular, damage to the brain around the time of birth may be partly reversible, with visual field training enhancing recovery of function in neuronal networks and enlarging the intact visual field.
3. The higher efficacy of training in children may relate to a greater inherent plastic capacity of the young brain.

In light of these issues, the authors also investigated whether younger children have a greater capacity to recover than older children, but this was not found to be the case. Specifically, after 1 year of age, the age of the children at the onset of training had no influence on either the duration of the training needed to gain visual function or the extension of the visual field following training (Werth & Seelos, 2005).

Mechanisms leading to visual recovery in children with CVI are likely to be similar to those in adults, but enhanced by potentially greater brain plasticity (Werth, 2008), balanced against the severity and extent of the damage. Recovery of visual functions may relate to still functioning brain tissue in the visual cortex, or to intact areas in the damaged hemisphere that support new functions, or by an undamaged hemisphere potentiating visual development (Werth, 2008). Interestingly, Werth (2006) has reported the case of a child who required one cerebral hemisphere to be removed (hemispherectomy) at the age of 4 months, but who by the age of 6 years was able to see stimuli with full awareness in her whole visual field, despite missing one hemisphere. These visual functions in both hemifields (both halves of the visual field) may be produced either by the intact hemisphere, the brain stem, or most likely, a combination of the two.

Other researchers have reported the case of a girl born without the right cerebral hemisphere (Muckli, Naumer, & Singer, 2009), whose left hemisphere not only maps the visual field on the opposite side (for both eyes) as expected, but also maps the visual field on the same side. A possible role of the brain stem in this process is supported by studies showing that children lacking both hemispheres are able to respond to diffuse illumination of their eyes, fixate, and visually track objects (see Werth, 2008 for a review). Support for this idea also comes from imaging evidence by DTI that there are brain connections running from the deep brain subcortical structures to the visual areas in the intact hemisphere (Leh, Johansen-Berg, & Ptito, 2006).

As described in Chapter 3, children with CVI may also have impaired visual functions related to recognizing objects. In one published case, a child with a brain infection (encephalitis) occurring at 8 weeks of age was reported to have impaired object recognition. Despite the infection occurring early in development, with time, she was able to recognize objects by their alignment and by studying them up close, but was unable to use color and shape effectively as a means of recognition. This unique case shows that the capacity for recognizing shapes can emerge, albeit slowly, after such early-onset damage (Funnell & Wilding, 2011). This contrasts with previous reports on visual agnosia developing in children as young as 3 years of age (reviewed in Funnell & Wilding, 2011) who have shown no recovery of visual functions over several years, which suggests a lack of plasticity for recovery of visual recognition when damage affects a fully developed visual system and takes place after the "sensitive period" for the development of this function (Lewis & Maurer, 2005).

Gillen and Dutton (2003) discuss the case of a 10-year-old child who suffered damage to the left and right parietal and occipital lobes, which led to the inability to perceive more than one or two objects at once, as well as impairment in reaching for objects resulting from lack of visual guidance of movement (Balint's syndrome, described in Chapter 3).

A rehabilitation approach of teaching the child how to make best use of his available functions was applied. One year later, he had learned to manage his disability much better. Moreover, his self-esteem and confidence as well as his school performance also improved. Although this study does not provide direct evidence for any plastic changes occurring at the cortical level as a result of training, it does demonstrate that it is possible to compensate for high-level visual deficits, and suggests that compensatory mechanisms are likely to be associated with changes at the level of the brain.

Further research is needed to fully understand the potential for plasticity in the brains of young children with CVI, but available evidence suggests that children affected by CVI can successfully undergo intensive behavioral training to gain increased visual capabilities. It is important to keep in mind that the specific nature of the deficit, the age at the time of onset, and the specific training paradigm all need to be considered when evaluating rehabilitation and habilitation protocols for children with CVI.

Brain stimulation techniques may also prove useful, by enhancing the effects of behavioral training. TMS has been used in healthy children to probe motor cortex function, thus providing insights into typical neuromotor maturation. (For a review, see Garvey & Mall, 2008.) TMS has also proven to be useful in detecting abnormal motor function and delayed neuromotor development in children, abnormalities possibly connected to neurological and neuropsychiatric disorders (Garvey & Mall, 2008). In some disorders, TMS has been sensitive to changes that occur after treatment, and its potential as a tool to investigate plasticity is now receiving increased attention (Oberman, Horvath, & Pascual-Leone, 2010).

## Habilitation, Rehabilitation, and Neuroplasticity

An important factor that deserves consideration when embarking on rehabilitation programs for individuals with visual impairments is motivation. Motivation is a critical component of all the major theories of learning (Green & Bavelier, 2008) and needs to be tailored to the specific context. For example, a program that may be suitable for the adult population may prove to be unappealing to children, which, in turn, may diminish the overall efficacy of the treatment. Therefore, the development of specific training protocols needs to identify motivational factors that are important for the individual in question, and incorporate these into the program.

In this regard, skills training based on video games is a promising option that has received attention in brain plasticity research. Video game play has demonstrated positive gains in children's visual skills (for reviews, see Achtman, Green, & Bavelier, 2008; Bavelier, Green, & Dye, 2010; Green & Bavelier, 2008). For instance, fMRI scans of 6–7-year-old children, who played a grapheme-to-phoneme (letter-to-sound) game, exhibited enhanced maturation of the visual word form area, a region of the brain critical for literacy. When 4- and 6-year-old children were studied while playing video games designed to train attention skills, their patterns of brain activity related to executive attention became more like that of adults (Rueda, Rothbart, McCandliss, Saccomanno, & Posner, 2005). In addition, action video game training may significantly improve aspects of visual attention, such as the ability to effectively distribute attention, as well as the number of stimuli that can simultaneously be attended to (Achtman et al.,

2008). Adult studies have shown that action video game training leads to enhanced visual performance, with enhanced contrast sensitivity (Li, Polat, Makous, & Bavelier, 2009) and faster visual processing (Li, Polat, Scalzo, & Bavelier, 2010).

Playing video games can stimulate plasticity in what was previously thought to be the immutable visual system of adults with a lazy eye or amblyopia. In particular, playing video games (both action and nonaction games) for a short period of time (40–80 hours, 2 hours per day) using the amblyopic eye led to substantial improvements in a wide range of fundamental visual functions, from low level to high level, including visual acuity, Vernier acuity (ability to discern misalignment among two line segments), and stereopsis (Li, Ngo, Nguyen, & Levi, 2011). Even greater improvements in visual function were attained in amblyopic children over the age of 7 who participated in a visual perceptual learning task (based on a simple computer game) for five one-hour sessions over the course of one week (Knox, Simmers, Gray, & Cleary, 2012). These results are important because they suggest the feasibility of a binocular approach to the treatment of childhood amblyopia (Knox et al., 2012), and indicate that visual training has the potential to be successful even after the sensitive period of visual development in children. It is important to recognize, however, that not all video games have beneficial effects on vision. To obtain gains in visual learning, it has been suggested that video games need to be fast-paced and unpredictable to promote a high level of active engagement and learning. Such factors would be different with children with CVI and would need to be matched to their speed of visual and intellectual processing. Moreover, such games need to be motivating, and their level of difficulty graded and adjusted to be consistently challenging for children, but not overwhelming.

Video games need not be "visual" per se. Video game–based learning also enhances spatial cognition abilities in profoundly blind adults and children (Merabet & Sanchez, 2009). Verbal instructions and auditory spatial cues are used to describe and characterize a particular environment, and to identify objects and their locations (for example, the sound of a door knock in the right ear signifying a door on the right). In this way, a blind player can actively interact with the virtual environment and objects within it. For instance, AudioDoom is an auditory-based computer game specifically developed to enhance spatial navigation skills and problem-solving abilities in blind children (Sanchez & Lumbreras, 1999). The player navigates through a series of virtual corridors and rooms, and performs a series of actions, such as opening doors and picking up objects. To succeed, the player has to generate and maintain a mental spatial map of the explored space. Blind children trained with AudioDoom have improved spatial cognition, enhanced cognitive abilities, and greater self-confidence, all developed while enjoying playing the game (Sanchez & Lumbreras, 1999). Evidence from fMRIs indicates these games activate brain regions serving navigation in the real world (Merabet & Sanchez, 2009). The creative use of such software should be taken into consideration when developing training protocols for children with CVI.

One website with online games that involve visual training tasks for students with visual impairments is called EVIN (http://siea.ia.uned.es). The games on this and similar sites should be carefully selected to match the precise training needs of children with CVI, and used alongside additional activities infused in real-world tasks that address the same or similar skill sets. Once a basic skill has been acquired, instruction can move away from learning exercises in a particular game and focus primarily on children's real-world application of that basic skill (A. Lueck, personal communication, October 20, 2014; see also Chapter 19). These games can be used for independent leisure time activities by children once some degree of skill mastery has been achieved so they can experience success in their independent performance.

There is sufficient evidence to encourage educators to develop and incorporate carefully selected motivational games that train visual and visual-motor skills into the curriculum of children with CVI, along the lines of exercises outlined in Chapter 24. These software applications and games are gaining increased attention in education programs and can be used with standard computers, touch tablets, and some smartphones. (Some applications matched to a child's age and processing level are discussed in more detail in Chapter 18 and its Appendix.)

## Conclusion

Current and future approaches to habilitation and rehabilitation of children with CVI need to take into account the potential for brain plasticity in restoring visual functioning. Both normal and damaged brains adapt, and can change in structure and function, in response to experience, training, and self-motivated learning, an ability that is known to persist for life. These neuroplastic changes, as a consequence of impairment or loss of vision, demonstrate the capacity for redeploying parts of the brain to serve a range of alternative functions, particularly in young people who have received structured, highly motivational habilitation or rehabilitation. With this conceptual framework in mind, it is highly likely that in children with damage to the visual brain, training that is carefully matched to the child's profile, and that the child enjoys, wishes to join in, and is spontaneously driven to complete, will enhance intact functions and redeploy other higher functioning brain areas to adopt additional compensatory abilities through neuroplasticity. The challenge for the future is to apply these fundamental ideas in the delivery of all habilitation and rehabilitation strategies, both old and new.

An important issue that often arises in educational programs for children with CVI concerns the age at which dedicated training in visual skills should be started or discontinued. It is safe to say that training in potentially responsive visual skills needs to begin as early as possible. The age at which training can be discontinued must take into account the skills targeted by the training and the nature of the visual disorder. It has generally been assumed that dedicated visual skills training sessions should be discontinued as children get older (see Lewis & Maurer, 2005, for a discussion on "sensitive" periods for effective interventions), although no precise age limit has been recommended in research studies or best practice literature. However, research demonstrating neuroplastic changes occurring well beyond the period of early development (Jones et al., 2006) suggests the need to reexamine this assumption more carefully with regard to children with visual impairments.

New research and knowledge is still needed to provide detailed guidelines about what visual skills to train (alone, or in conjunction with other sensory skills), the ages at which to begin and end training for these skills, and what types of brain damage can affect these skills. Our recent knowledge that the brain is not fixed in nature but is in a constant state of flux, particularly in children, will no doubt inspire leaders in the field to innovatively expand the range of available habilitation approaches, while auditing and researching the outcomes to provide the requisite evidence base.

## References


Achtman, R. L., Green, C. S., & Bavelier, D. (2008). Video games as a tool to train visual skills. *Restorative Neurology and Neuroscience, 26*(4–5), 435–446.

Alary, F., Goldstein, R., Duquette, M., Chapman, C. E., Voss, P., & Lepore, F. (2008). Tactile acuity in the blind: A psychophysical study using a two-dimensional angle discrimination task. *Experimental Brain Research, 187*(4), 587–594.

Amedi, A., Floel, A., Knecht, S., Zohary, E., & Cohen, L. G. (2004). Transcranial magnetic stimulation of the occipital pole interferes with verbal processing in blind subjects. *Nature Neuroscience, 7*(11), 1266–1270.

Amedi, A., Raz, N., Pianka, P., Malach, R., & Zohary, E. (2003). Early "visual" cortex activation correlates with superior verbal memory performance in the blind. *Nature Neuroscience, 6*(7), 758–766.

Armstrong, V. L., Brunet, P. M., He, C., Nishimura, M., Poole, H. L., & Spector, F. J. (2006). What is so critical? A commentary on the reexamination of critical periods. *Developmental Psychobiology, 48*(4), 326–331.

Aydin, K., Ucar, A., Oguz, K. K., Okur, O. O., Agayev, A., Unal, Z., . . . Ozturk, C. (2007). Increased gray matter density in the parietal cortex of mathematicians: A voxel-based morphometry study. *American Journal of Neuroradiology, 28*(10), 1859–1864.

Baker, C. I., Peli, E., Knouf, N., & Kanwisher, N. G. (2005). Reorganization of visual processing in macular degeneration. *The Journal of Neuroscience, 25*(3), 614–618.

Bavelier, D., Green, C. S., & Dye, M. W. (2010). Children, wired: For better and for worse. *Neuron, 67*(5), 692–701.

Bavelier, D., & Neville, H. (2002). Cross-modal plasticity: Where and how? *Nature Reviews Neuroscience, 3*(6), 443–452.

Betsuin, Y., Mashima, Y., Ohde, H., Inoue, R., & Oguchi, Y. (2001). Clinical application of the multifocal VEPs. *Current Eye Research, 22*(1), 54–63.

Burton, H., Diamond, J. B., & McDermott, K. B. (2003). Dissociating cortical regions activated by semantic and phonological tasks: A fMRI study in blind and sighted people. *Journal of Neurophysiology, 90*(3), 1965–1982.

Burton, H., McLaren, D. G., & Sinclair, R. J. (2006). Reading embossed capital letters: An fMRI study in blind and sighted individuals. *Human Brain Mapping, 27*(4), 325–339.

Burton, H., Sinclair, R. J., & McLaren, D. G. (2004). Cortical activity to vibrotactile stimulation: An fMRI study in blind and sighted individuals. *Human Brain Mapping, 23*(4), 210–228.

Burton, H., Snyder, A. Z., Conturo, T. E., Akbudak, E., Ollinger, J. M., & Raichle, M. E. (2002). Adaptive changes in early and late blind: A fMRI study of Braille reading. *Journal of Neurophysiology, 87*(1), 589–607.

Cattaneo, Z., & Vecchi, T. (2011). *Blind vision: The effect of blindness on visuospatial cognitive abilities.* Boston, MA: The MIT Press.

Cohen, L. G., Weeks, R. A., Sadato, N., Celnik, P., Ishii, K., & Hallett, M. (1999). Period of susceptibility for cross-modal plasticity in the blind. *Annals of Neurology, 45*(4), 451–460.

Collignon, O., Lassonde, M., Lepore, F., Bastien, D., & Veraart, C. (2007). Functional cerebral reorganization for auditory spatial processing and auditory substitution of vision in early blind subjects. *Cerebral Cortex, 17*(2), 457–465.

Collignon, O., Vandewalle, G., Voss, P., Albouy, G., Charbonneau, G., Lassonde, M., et al. (2011). Functional specialization for auditory-spatial processing in the occipital cortex of congenitally blind humans. *Proceedings of the National Academy of Sciences of the United States of America, 108*(11), 4435–4440.

Collignon, O., Voss, P., Lassonde, M., & Lepore, F. (2009). Cross-modal plasticity for the spatial processing of sounds in visually deprived subjects. *Experimental Brain Research, 192*(3), 343–358.

Despres, O., Candas, V., & Dufour, A. (2005). Auditory compensation in myopic humans: Involvement of binaural, monaural, or echo cues? *Brain Research, 1041*(1), 56–65.

Draganski, B., Moser, T., Lummel, N., Ganssbauer, S., Bogdahn, U., Haas, F., et al. (2006). Decrease of thalamic gray matter following limb amputation. *NeuroImage, 31*(3), 951–957.

Dufour, A., & Gérard, Y. (2000). Improved auditory spatial sensitivity in near-sighted subjects. *Cognitive Brain Research, 10*(1–2), 159–165.

Elbert, T., Sterr, A., Rockstroh, B., Pantev, C., Muller, M. M., & Taub, E. (2002). Expansion of the tonotopic area in the auditory cortex of the blind. *The Journal of Neuroscience, 22*(22), 9941–9944.

Flor, H. (2008). Maladaptive plasticity, memory for pain and phantom limb pain: Review and suggestions for new therapies. *Expert Review of Neurotherapeutics, 8*(5), 809–818.

Funnell, E., & Wilding, J. (2011). Development of a vocabulary of object shapes in a child with a very-early-acquired visual agnosia: A unique case. The *Quarterly Journal of Experimental Psychology, 64*(2), 261–282.

Gaab, N., Schulze, K., Ozdemir, E., & Schlaug, G. (2006). Neural correlates of absolute pitch differ between blind and sighted musicians. *NeuroReport, 17*(18), 1853–1857.

Garvey, M. A., & Mall, V. (2008). Transcranial magnetic stimulation in children. *Clinical Neurophysiology, 119*(5), 973–984.

Gelbart, S. S., Hoyt, C. S., Jastrebski, G., & Marg, E. (1982). Long-term visual results in bilateral congenital cataracts. *American Journal of Ophthalmology, 93*(5), 615–621.

Gillen, J. A., & Dutton, G. N. (2003). Balint's syndrome in a 10-year-old male. *Developmental Medicine & Child Neurology, 45*(5), 349–352.

Goldreich, D., & Kanics, I. M. (2003). Tactile acuity is enhanced in blindness. *The Journal of Neuroscience, 23*(8), 3439–3445.

Gougoux, F., Belin, P., Voss, P., Lepore, F., Lassonde, M., & Zatorre, R. J. (2009). Voice perception in blind persons: A functional magnetic resonance imaging study. *Neuropsychologia, 47*(13), 2967–2974.

Gougoux, F., Lepore, F., Lassonde, M., Voss, P., Zatorre, R. J., & Belin, P. (2004). Neuropsychology: Pitch discrimination in the early blind. *Nature, 430*, 309.

Grafman, J. (2000). Conceptualizing functional neuroplasticity. *Journal of Communication Disorders, 33*(4), 345–355.

Green, C. S., & Bavelier, D. (2008). Exercising your brain: A review of human brain plasticity and training-induced learning. *Psychology and Aging, 23*(4), 692–701.

Hamilton, R. H., Pascual-Leone, A., & Schlaug, G. (2004). Absolute pitch in blind musicians. *NeuroReport, 15*(5), 803–806.

Hebb, D. (1949). *The organization of behavior.* New York: John Wiley & Sons.

Hubel, D. H., Wiesel, T. N., & LeVay, S. (1977). Plasticity of ocular dominance columns in monkey striate cortex. *Philosophical Transactions of the Royal Society B: Biological Sciences, 278*(961), 377–409.

Jones, S., Nyberg, L., Sandblom, J., Stigsdotter Neely, A., Ingvar, M., Magnus Petersson, K., et al. (2006). Cognitive and neural plasticity in aging: General and task-specific limitations. *Neuroscience Biobehavioral Reviews, 30*(6), 864–871.

Karni, A., Meyer, G., Jezzard, P., Adams, M. M., Turner, R., & Ungerleider, L. G. (1995). Functional MRI evidence for adult motor cortex plasticity during motor skill learning. *Nature, 377*(6545), 155–158.

Knox, P. J., Simmers, A. J., Gray, L. S., & Cleary, M. (2012). An exploratory study: Prolonged periods of binocular stimulation can provide an effective treatment for childhood amblyopia. *Investigative Ophthalmology & Visual Science, 53*(2), 817–824.

Kujala, T., Palva, M. J., Salonen, O., Alku, P., Huotilainen, M., Jarvinen, A., et al. (2005). The role of blind humans' visual cortex in auditory change detection. *Neuroscience Letters, 379*(2), 127–131.

Kupers, R., Beaulieu-Lefebvre, M., Schneider, F. C., Kassuba, T., Paulson, O. B., Siebner, H. R., et al. (2011). Neural correlates of olfactory processing in congenital blindness. *Neuropsychologia, 49*(7), 2037–2044.

Landi, S. M., Baguear, F., & Della-Maggiore, V. (2011). One week of motor adaptation induces structural changes in primary motor cortex that predict long-term memory one year later. *The Journal of Neuroscience, 31*(33), 11808–11813.

Leclerc, C., Segalowitz, S. J., Desjardins, J., Lassonde, M., & Lepore, F. (2005). EEG coherence in early-blind humans during sound localization. *Neuroscience Letters, 376*(3), 154–159.

Leh, S. E., Johansen-Berg, H., & Ptito, A. (2006). Unconscious vision: New insights into the neuronal correlate of blindsight using diffusion tractography. *Brain, 129*(Pt 7), 1822–1832.

Lessard, N., Pare, M., Lepore, F., & Lassonde, M. (1998). Early-blind human subjects localize sound sources better than sighted subjects. *Nature, 395*(6699), 278–280.

Lewis, T. L., & Maurer, D. (2005). Multiple sensitive periods in human visual development: Evidence from visually deprived children. *Developmental Psychobiology, 46*(3), 163–183.

Li, R. W., Ngo, C., Nguyen, J., & Levi, D. M. (2011). Video-game play induces plasticity in the visual system of adults with amblyopia. *PLoS Biology, 9*(8), e1001135.

Li, R., Polat, U., Makous, W., & Bavelier, D. (2009). Enhancing the contrast sensitivity function through action video game training. *Nature Neuroscience, 12*(5), 549–551.

Li, R., Polat, U., Scalzo, F., & Bavelier, D. (2010). Reducing backward masking through action game training. *Journal of Vision, 10*(14):33, 1–13.

Logothetis, N. K. (2008). What we can do and what we cannot do with fMRI. *Nature, 453*(7197), 869–878.

Maguire, E. A., Gadian, D. G., Johnsrude, I. S., Good, C. D., Ashburner, J., Frackowiak, R. S., et al. (2000). Navigation-related structural change in the hippocampi of taxi drivers. *Proceedings of the National Academy of Sciences of the United States of America, 97*(8), 4398–4403.

Merabet, L. B., Hamilton, R., Schlaug, G., Swisher, J. D., Kiriakopoulos, E. T., Pitskel, N. B., . . . Pascual-Leone, A. (2008). Rapid and reversible recruitment of early visual cortex for touch. *PLoS One, 3*(8), e3046.

Merabet, L. B., & Sanchez, J. (2009). Audio-based navigation using virtual environments: Combining technology and neuroscience. *AER Journal: Research and Practice in Visual Impairment and Blindness, 2*(3), 128–137.

Merabet, L. B., Theoret, H., & Pascual-Leone, A. (2003). Transcranial magnetic stimulation as an investigative tool in the study of visual function. *Optometry and Vision Science, 80*(5), 356–368.

Michel, G. F., & Tyler, A. N. (2005). Critical period: A history of the transition from questions of when, to what, to how. *Developmental Psychobiology, 46*(3), 156–162.

Muckli, L., Naumer, M. J., & and Singer, W. (2009). Bilateral visual field maps in a patient with only one hemisphere. *Proceedings of the National Academy of Sciences of the United States of America*, 106(31), 13034–13039.

Oberman, L. M., Horvath, J. C., & Pascual-Leone, A. (2010). TMS: Using the theta-burst protocol to explore mechanism of plasticity in individuals with Fragile X syndrome and autism. *Journal of Visualized Experiments*, (46), e2272.

Obretenova, S., Halko, M. A., Plow, E. B., Pascual-Leone, A., & Merabet, L. B. (2010). Neuroplasticity associated with tactile language communication in a deaf-blind subject. *Frontiers in Human Neuroscience, 3,* 60.

Pantev, C., Ross, B., Fujioka, T., Trainor, L. J., Schulte, M., & Schulz, M. (2003). Music and learning-induced cortical plasticity. *Annals of the New York Academy of Sciences, 999,* 438–450.

Pascual-Leone, A., & Torres, F. (1993). Plasticity of the sensorimotor cortex representation of the reading finger in Braille readers. *Brain, 116*(Pt 1), 39–52.

Pring, L., Woolf, K., & Tadic, V. (2008). Melody and pitch processing in five musical savants with congenital blindness. *Perception, 37*(2), 290–307.

Pujol, J., Roset-Llobet, J., Rosines-Cubells, D., Deus, J., Narberhaus, B., Valls-Sole, J., . . . Pascual-Leone, A. (2000). Brain cortical activation during guitar-induced hand dystonia studied by functional MRI. *NeuroImage, 12*(3), 257–267.

Quartarone, A., Siebner, H. R., & Rothwell, J. C. (2006). Task-specific hand dystonia: Can too much plasticity be bad for you? *Trends in Neurosciences, 29*(4), 192–199.

Ramachandran, V. S., & Altschuler, E. L. (2009). The use of visual feedback, in particular mirror visual feedback, in restoring brain function. *Brain, 132*(Pt 7), 1693–1710.

Raz, N., Amedi, A., & Zohary, E. (2005). V1 activation in congenitally blind humans is associated with episodic retrieval. *Cerebral Cortex, 15*(9), 1459–1468.

Röder, B., Kramer, U. M., & Lange, K. (2007). Congenitally blind humans use different stimulus selection strategies in hearing: An ERP study of spatial and temporal attention. *Restorative Neurology and Neuroscience, 25*(3–4), 311–322.

Röder, B., & Neville, H. (2003). Developmental functional plasticity. In J. Grafman & I. H. Robertson (Eds.), *Handbook of neuropsychology: Plasticity and rehabilitation* (pp. 231–270). Amsterdam: Elsevier Science.

Röder, B., Rosler, F., Hennighausen, E., & Nacker, F. (1996). Event-related potentials during auditory and somatosensory discrimination in sighted and blind human subjects. *Cognitive Brain Research, 4*(2), 77–93.

Röder, B., Stock, O., Bien, S., Neville, H., & Rosler, F. (2002). Speech processing activates visual cortex in congenitally blind humans. *European Journal of Neuroscience, 16*(5), 930–936.

Rombaux, P., Huart, C., De Volder, A. G., Cuevas, I., Renier, L., Duprez, T., et al. (2010). Increased olfactory bulb volume and olfactory function in early blind subjects. *NeuroReport, 21*(17), 1069–1073.

Rueda, M. R., Rothbart, M. K., McCandliss, B. D., Saccomanno, L., & Posner, M. I. (2005). Training, maturation, and genetic influences on the development of executive attention. *Proceedings of the National Academy of Sciences of the United States of America, 102*(41), 14931–14936.

Sadato, N., & Hallett, M. (1999). fMRI occipital activation by tactile stimulation in a blind man. *Neurology, 52*(2), 423.

Sadato, N., Okada, T., Honda, M., & Yonekura, Y. (2002). Critical period for cross-modal plasticity in blind humans: A functional MRI study. *NeuroImage, 16*(2), 389–400.

Sadato, N., Pascual-Leone, A., Grafman, J., Ibanez, V., Deiber, M. P., Dold, G., et al. (1996). Activation of the primary visual cortex by Braille reading in blind subjects. *Nature, 380*(6574), 526–528.

Sanchez, J., & Lumbreras, M. (1999). Virtual environment interaction through 3D audio by blind children. *Cyberpsychology, Behavior, and Social Networking, 2*(2), 101–111.

Schwenkreis, P., Witscher, K., Janssen, F., Dertwinkel, R., Zenz, M., Malin, J. P., et al. (2000). Changes of cortical excitability in patients with upper limb amputation. *Neuroscience Letters, 293*(2), 143–146.

Shaw, C. A., & McEachern, J. C. (Eds.). (2001). *Toward a theory of neuroplasticity.* Hove, England: Taylor & Francis.

Singer, T., Lindenberger, U., & Baltes, P. B. (2003). Plasticity of memory for new learning in very old age: A story of major loss? *Psychology and Aging, 18*(2), 306–317.

Smirnakis, S. M., Brewer, A. A., Schmid, M. C., Tolias, A. S., Schuz, A., Augath, M., . . . Logothetis, N. K. (2005). Lack of long-term cortical reorganization after macaque retinal lesions. *Nature, 435*(7040), 300–307.

Sterr, A., Green, L., & Elbert, T. (2003). Blind Braille readers mislocate tactile stimuli. *Biological Psychology, 63*(2), 117–127.

Sterr, A., Muller, M. M., Elbert, T., Rockstroh, B., Pantev, C., & Taub, E. (1998). Perceptual correlates of changes in cortical representation of fingers in blind multifinger Braille readers. *The Journal of Neuroscience, 18*(11), 4417–4423.

Sterr, A., Muller, M., Elbert, T., Rockstroh, B., & Taub, E. (1999). Development of cortical reorganization in the somatosensory cortex of adult Braille students. *Electroencephalography and Clinical Neurophysiology Supplement, 49*, 292–298.

Sunness, J. S., Liu, T., & Yantis, S. (2004). Retinotopic mapping of the visual cortex using functional magnetic resonance imaging in a patient with central scotomas from atrophic macular degeneration. *Ophthalmology, 111*(8), 1595–1598.

Sur, M., Garraghty, P. E., & Roe, A. W. (1988). Experimentally induced visual projections into auditory thalamus and cortex. *Science, 242*(4884), 1437–1441.

Teuber, H. L. (1975). Recovery of function after brain injury in man. In R. Porter & D. W. Fitzsimons (Eds.), *Ciba Foundation Symposium 34—Outcome of severe damage to the central nervous system* (pp. 159–190). Chichester, UK: John Wiley & Sons, Ltd.

Thaler, L., Arnott, S. R., & Goodale, M. A. (2011). Neural correlates of natural human echolocation in early and late blind echolocation experts. *PLoS One, 6*(5), e20162.

Theoret, H., Merabet, L., & Pascual-Leone, A. (2004). Behavioral and neuroplastic changes in the blind: Evidence for functionally relevant cross-modal interactions. *Journal of Physiology - Paris, 98*(1–3), 221–233.

Uhl, F., Franzen, P., Lindinger, G., Lang, W., & Deecke, L. (1991). On the functionality of the visually deprived occipital cortex in early blind persons. *Neuroscience Letters, 124*(2), 256–259.

Uhl, F., Franzen, P., Podreka, I., Steiner, M., & Deecke, L. (1993). Increased regional cerebral blood flow in inferior occipital cortex and cerebellum of early blind humans. *Neuroscience Letters, 150*(2), 162–164.

Veraart, C., De Volder, A. G., Wanet-Defalque, M. C., Bol, A., Michel, C., & Goffinet, A. M. (1990). Glucose utilization in human visual cortex is abnormally elevated in blindness of early onset but decreased in blindness of late onset. *Brain Research, 510*(1), 115–121.

Walsh, V., & Pascual-Leone, A. (2003). *Transcranial magnetic stimulation: A neurochronometrics of mind*. Cambridge, MA: MIT Press.

Wan, C. Y., Wood, A. G., Reutens, D. C., & Wilson, S. J. (2010a). Early but not late blindness leads to enhanced auditory perception. *Neuropsychologia, 48*(1), 344–348.

Wan, C. Y., Wood, A. G., Reutens, D. C., & Wilson, S. J. (2010b). Congenital blindness leads to enhanced vibrotactile perception. *Neuropsychologia, 48*(2), 631–635.

Wanet-Defalque, M. C., Veraart, C., De Volder, A., Metz, R., Michel, C., Dooms, G., et al. (1988). High metabolic activity in the visual cortex of early blind human subjects. *Brain Research, 446*(2), 369–373.

Weeks, R., Horwitz, B., Aziz-Sultan, A., Tian, B., Wessinger, C. M., Cohen, L. G., . . . Rauschecker, J. P. (2000). A positron emission tomographic study of auditory localization in the congenitally blind. *The Journal of Neuroscience, 20*(7), 2664–2672.

Werth, R. (2006). Visual functions without the occipital lobe or after cerebral hemispherectomy in infancy. *European Journal of Neuroscience, 24*(10), 2932–2944.

Werth, R. (2008). Cerebral blindness and plasticity of the visual system in children. A review of visual capacities in patients with occipital lesions, hemispherectomy or hydranencephaly. *Restorative Neurology and Neuroscience, 26*(4–5), 377–389.

Werth, R., & Seelos, K. (2005). Restitution of visual functions in cerebrally blind children. *Neuropsychologia, 43*(14), 2011–2023.

Wittenberg, G. F., Werhahn, K. J., Wassermann, E. M., Herscovitch, P., & Cohen, L. G. (2004). Functional connectivity between somatosensory and visual cortex in early blind humans. *European Journal of Neuroscience, 20*(7), 1923–1927.

# 6

# The Role of Attention and Executive Brain Functions in Seeing and Behavior in Children with CVI

*Sander Zuidhoek*

The visual system cannot function in isolation. It needs an outside world to trigger visual processing and an inside world to guide the processing. This chapter discusses the cognitive processes that make it possible for us to use the visual system, which, for the purposes of this chapter, is considered in the context of a tool for us to use. Among the cognitive processes, attention plays a vital part; different types of attentional processing turn sensory processing into conscious perception. Without giving attention to the visual system, we do not truly consciously see. Only when we consciously see can we use our visual "tool" the way we see fit.

There are essentially two ways in which attention can be allocated to the visual system. The first is via so-called "bottom-up" processing, which is initiated by the outside world. Visual stimuli in the outside world are processed to a certain extent, but only those that automatically stand out draw attention to themselves, bringing them into consciousness. This process is unsupervised by any conscious process. It is called bottom-up processing because it starts from the midbrain and brain stem at the bottom of the brain's functional hierarchy and works its way up to the higher levels of the frontal lobes (see Chapter 2).

The second way in which attention can be allocated to the visual system is when an individual chooses to pay attention to what the visual surroundings have to offer, in which case the attention is consciously controlled. This kind of processing—which starts at the top and influences the processes lower in the hierarchy—is called "top-down" processing. In normal visual situations, both types of processing are constantly functioning. So far in this book, the detrimental effects of disorders in bottom-up processing have been considered—that is, the effects of impairment in visual processing on what is consciously seen. In this chapter, the focus is on a top-down approach to the visual system, in which it is considered more as a servant of the conscious mind. This chapter considers how deficits in higher-order brain functioning, such as allocating attention to information from the visual sense, may contribute to the behaviors and characteristics found in cerebral visual impairment (CVI).

## Hierarchy in Brain Function

The brain performs many functions. The functions performed by the visual sense allow for the experience of a rich visual world. However, the visual functions cannot do the job of presenting the visual world to us all by themselves; they need to be governed and guided. Like all brain functions, they are subject to hierarchy. Arguably, the most important functions the brain performs are the so-called *executive functions*—those that control and orchestrate cognitive abilities and behaviors to achieve a particular goal. Together, these functions form the *executive system,* sometimes called the *executive committee* (Faw, 2003). Among other things, these functions allow a person to decide which information to pay attention to (Hart & Jacobs, 1993). By controlling attentional processes, the executive system allows for the selection, at will, of information from the outside world, as well as the "inside world" of the mind. By controlling attention, the executive system rules the sensory systems (which provide information from the outside world), our urges—emotional, visceral, cognitive (forming the content of the "inside world"), and our motor systems (allowing for interaction with the outside world).

There is considerable debate about the nature of executive functions and how and when they develop. Barkley (1997) proposes that the executive system consists of four central elements, each with its own time of onset. These central elements are separate, but hierarchically integral to, a general behavioral inhibition system which is active from birth; they provide an intuitive grasp of what is needed to take control of our brain's functions, and thus, our behavior:

1. Working memory (from about 5 months)
2. Self-regulation of affect (feelings), motivation, and arousal (from about 5 months)
3. Internalization of speech (verbal working memory, from about 3 years)
4. Reconstitution (behavioral analysis and synthesis, from about 6 years)

In essence, these four core executive processes allow an individual to rise above reflexive behavior in the here and now to exercise control, at multiple levels of functioning. Without them, we would always be giving in to our environment and our urges.

At the most basic level, attentional control allows a person to inhibit reactions to salient stimuli (stimuli that "stand out") in the outside world (*behavioral inhibition*), and to shape our behavior by suppressing socially unacceptable impulses and urges (*self-regulation* of affect, motivation, and arousal). Exerting control and not being subject to our urges paves the way for attending to nonverbal and verbal thinking (*nonverbal working memory* and *verbal working memory,* respectively), allowing behavior based on reasoning, memory, and prediction.

*Reconstitution,* which starts to develop at about 6 years of age and is not fully mature until the mid-twenties, is the fourth and most elaborate and advanced central element of executive functioning. It involves reflecting on and planning one's own behavior in relation to that of others. As such, its development depends on the other central elements, and more. Paying attention to, thinking about, and interpreting emotions, urges, and motivations is crucial for forming (and changing) long-term and short-term goals accordingly. As the executive system, in principle, has access to and tries to control emotions from early on, and also has access to a growing amount of declarative knowledge (factual information) at will, it is perfectly suited for setting goals and breaking them down into subgoals and concrete plans. In addition, access to all kinds of knowledge, and the capacity to combine that information, allows for flexibility and creativity. Due to their access to detailed visual and other sensory information, social knowledge, and social rules, the executive functions allow us to monitor and interpret our own behavior and that of others with respect to our—and their—goals and plans (reconstitution).

From the aforementioned, it is clear that executive functions play a determining role in behavior. With respect to vision, the executive system rules the other functional systems by controlling attentional processes. By shifting and employing attention, information can be accessed and functions operated by the other functional systems can be utilized to form and attain goals. Attention can be thought of as the door through which different databases of information—of which vision is one—can be entered.

## Attention and Attentional Control

### The Brain's Visual Subsystems: Processing Depends on Attention

Seeing encompasses more than just the eyes; it requires visual processing by the brain's visual processing areas. Processing of visual information by the brain is what allows us to understand and use the visual information. Visual information is processed by several visual subsystems that answer questions about the identity of objects and subjects (what is it?), their emotional value (what is it to me?), and their spatial arrangement (where is it?), often before these questions have even been consciously addressed. These subsystems allow for swift and efficient interaction with the world (via the "how" pathway [see Chapter 2]).

However, to actually see, a lot more than just the eyes and these different visual processing pathways are needed. For one, paying attention to the visual sensory modality is a prerequisite for consciously seeing. Since our daily lives are experienced as a constant stream of visual information, it may seem that attention is paid to visual information all the time. However, there are degrees of visual awareness that depend upon the amount of attention paid to the visual modality; sometimes vision is hardly used for perception. For example, when engaged in an animated telephone conversation, people tend to move their eyes around a lot, but do not thoroughly process the visual information falling on their retinae. Consequently, they are not fully, if at all, aware of their visual surroundings. Most of their attention is paid to the verbal input to one ear, thoughts on what is being said, and on mentally formulating an input to the conversation. As a result of a decreased level of attention to the visual domain, the activity in the visual processing areas is low, and not much attentional reserve is left to fully, consciously see. If during or after the conversation that person was asked to answer questions about visual events that happened during the conversation, they would likely perform poorly. Does this mean the person has a visual processing disorder? No, it just means they weren't paying enough attention to the visual modality. Thus, the eyes and the visual system in the brain do not result in "seeing" when no attention is paid to the visual information.

## Attention to the Visual Modality: Controlling External Pulling and Internal Pushing

In essence, all attention is about survival: forming goals and achieving those goals in order to promote survival. Arguably, the visual modality provides greater and richer information about the outside world than other sensory modalities. Therefore, our primary attention is often with the visual modality because it is most appropriate for achieving our goals. Indeed, vision often seems to be the favorite sensory system.

Evolution has shaped our brains to process information in two ways: Either it starts from the outside world, resulting in processing from lower brain centers to higher ones (bottom-up processing, with the executive system on top), or from within, starting at an emotional level and feeding the executive system, which in turn employs lower systems (such as the sensory and motor systems) to gather information in order to make and execute decisions (top-down processing).

Both the outside and the inside worlds make use of attention to take control of the brain's systems. The brain allows attention to be seized by the outside world through the visual and/or other sensory systems as stimuli are brought into consciousness: a bright flash of light in a dark night will pull our attention to the visual modality; an uncommon sound will allow auditory information "to flow" (bottom-up) to the brain's auditory processing areas, and will probably utilize vision as well, in order to visually confirm or further identify the origin and cause of the sound.

On the other hand, evolution provided individuals with a brain that allows us to decide whether we want to see or not. To a certain extent, we decide for ourselves whether to look, listen, do both at the same time, or engage in some other cognitive activity. When the burst of light does not appear to represent a threat, we are able to turn our attention back to issues that are more important to us, and even if it does represent a threat, our attention will have to be redirected in order to make plans to escape that threat.

Seen in this light, the brain is in a constant tension between impending stimuli from the outside world (*exogenous attention*) pulling attention, and possible threats, and our own emotions, motivations, and urges (*endogenous attention*), which try to push attention in order to achieve or satisfy our basic needs.

In order to be able to exert control over the constant demands of the present moment, both exogenous attentional pulling and endogenous attentional pushing need to be balanced and controlled. This control is exercised by the mind's executive system. Using Barkley's (1997) terminology, instinctive reactions to external events need to be controlled (behavioral inhibition), as well as the urges and impulses from within that are socially unacceptable or otherwise unfit for the situation at hand (self-regulation of affect). This clears the way for the pursuit of higher goals, which are formed using nonverbal working memory, internalization of speech, and reconstitution (analysis and synthesis of behavior).

Attentional pushing and pulling are controlled by the executive system. Without the executive system, a person would not be able to form higher goals, select and coordinate behavioral patterns to achieve these goals, or shape behavior in a socially accepted manner; they would be at the complete mercy of their environment and their own impulses. The executive system allows a person to inhibit attentional pushing and pulling, to interpret and prioritize some feelings and motivations over others, to set goals accordingly, to break them down into parts, and to monitor and control their own behavior by matching it to these goals. The key tool to perform any of the steps for the achievement of goals and subgoals is to control the directing of attention.

By setting goals based on urges and emotional needs, the executive system allows individuals to set priorities and exercise free will. In the ideal case, when a person decides there are no impending threats, they are able to, at will, direct attention to one or more modalities (for example, to seeing, listening, or both at the same time), to a component within a modality (for example, to only a small part of the visual scene or to all red things in the visual scene), or to any cognitive process, and are able to retain the attention there as long as is needed, regardless of any environmental exogenous pulling of attention. Whether attention is paid to the visual modality, and thus whether, and to what extent, an individual sees or not, depends on whether the battle between exogenous pulling and endogenous pushing of attention is decided in favor of the visual modality over other modalities and other cognitive processes. If the battle is in favor of directing attention toward the visual modality, we see; if it is not, we do not (consciously) see, or we do so to a lesser extent. (It should be noted that the outcome is hardly ever all or none. Attention is almost always divided over multiple cognitive processes: at the same time that we are consciously seeing, thoughts are also being formed about what is seen, as well as planning the next step.)

To summarize:

- Processing in the brain's visual systems, and thus seeing, depends on attention.
- Attention is controlled according to prioritizing processes performed by the executive system. As such, it both forms and exercises free will.
- These prioritizing processes are driven by the inside world (urges, emotions, and motivations), but take into account possible environmental threats and social factors.
- The decision about whether or not to pay attention to the visual input, and by how much, is the first role of executive functions in seeing.

## The Brain Mechanisms of Attention

The executive decision to pay attention to the visual modality leads to activation in the cortical brain areas involved in the processing of visual information (Newman, 1997). Attention to the visual and some other sensory systems is brought about via the two thalami, which are relatively large structures near the center on each side deep in the brain, one for information coming from the right, and one for information coming from the left (see Sidebar 6.1 and Figure 6.1). The thalami function as a relay station: information from the senses (except olfactory and taste information) is gathered by the thalami before being processed or not processed in the cortical areas, depending on whether or not attention is paid to the particular sensory system. This implies that the thalami are at the core of decisions involving attentional direction (Vuilleumier, Chiche-

SIDEBAR 6.1

## Control of Seeing through Higher Brain Functions

Seeing depends not only on activity in the cortical visual pathways, but also the amount of attention paid to the visual modality (see Figure 6.1). The prefrontal cortex (PFC) connects to the thalami (T) (via the basal ganglia, not depicted) to control this process. At the thalamus, the "flow" of visual information to the cortical visual pathways ("what," "where," and "how") is modulated by altering the amount of attention paid to the visual modality (models of this process are referred to as "attentional gating" or "attentional attenuation"). The prefrontal cortex connects to the limbic system of the brain, which together interpret and inhibit emotions, motivations, and urges. The interpretation of these elements determines our goals. The prefrontal cortex changes the amount of attention paid to the visual modality at will, while the superior colliculi (SC) on top of the brain stem affect thalamic gating and attenuation by reflexively reacting to salient (potentially hazardous) visual stimuli in the outside world. These reactions and related eye movements are inhibited and controlled by the frontal eye fields (FEF), which are connected to the prefrontal cortex. Both the left and the right temporoparietal areas (TP) connect to the thalami; they play a role in visual selective attention by decreasing and increasing the size of the attended visual area, which determines what is selected in the visual field and processed further in the visual pathways. Working memory (WM) is a functional system in the prefrontal cortex. It is controlled by the executive functions and allows for mental imagery and mental manipulation of visual information that is stored in the "what" and "where" pathways (ventral and dorsal streams).

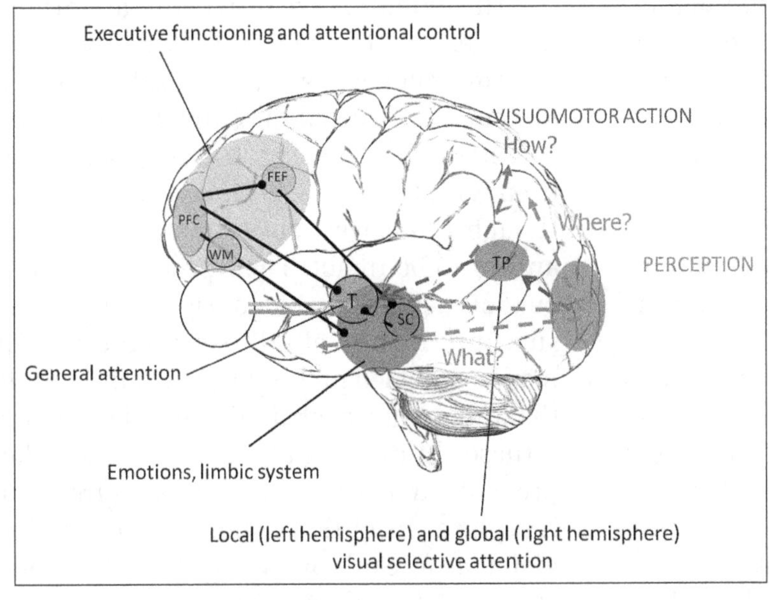


FIGURE 6.1
**Simplified Schematic Overview of the Visual Pathways and the Executive, Attentional, and Emotional Systems**

rio & Assal, 2001). Each thalamus can be thought of as a sort of sensory filter (Saalmann & Kastner, 2009); if a person decides to look, or impending stimuli in the environment make the decision that he or she looks, the thalami "open up" more to allow visual information "to flow" to the cortical areas, resulting in further and more active processing in the visual processing streams, such as the "what" pathway (ventral stream) and "where" pathway (dorsal stream), which start at the primary visual cortex (see Chapter 2).

The exogenous pulling of attention to the visual modality is most likely brought about through the superior colliculi, located in the midbrain at the top of the brain stem, and their projections to the thalami (Shipp, 2004; see Figure 6.1). The superior colliculi make us react reflexively to peripheral visual stimulation by pulling attention to the visual modality and to the most salient stimulus or location in space (Trappenberg, Dorris, Munoz, & Klein, 2001), and are responsible for the accompanying eye movements directed at that spatial location. Calling upon the brain's executive control allows for the inhibition of most of these reflexive eye movements; the inhibition is produced by the frontal eye fields ("FEF" in Figure 6.1), located in the frontal cortex close to the (dorsolateral) prefrontal executive control areas. Such inhibition of eye movements is arguably one of the most basic forms of what Barkley (1997) meant by behavioral inhibition.

## Disorders in Visual Attention

Children (and adults) vary in their executive control over attentional processes. In practice, children are observed to be easily distracted from their visual tasks because it is hard for them to retain visual attention. Therefore, it is possible that some children who perform poorly on visual tasks do so not because of a disorder in the visual processing areas, but as a result of an attentional disorder that makes it hard for them to pay attention to the visual modality. In addition, children who do have control over the direction of their attention (for example, to the visual modality) may have a disorder in maintaining their attention once directed. Thus, it is important to understand the attentional capacities of a child before determining whether any visual functions are disturbed. In many children, poor performance on visual tasks results from a complex interaction of executive, attentional, visual, and other functions. (This is discussed in more detail later in this chapter.) As a result, an extensive neuropsychological examination is often needed to determine the actual cause of failure on different tasks. This may not be possible, however, for children who are not able to access current neuropsychological tests used for this purpose as a result of their visual or cognitive constraints. (Neuropsychology studies the functions of the brain and how they relate to particular brain structures both clinically and experimentally. Neuropsychological tests are specifically designed tasks used to assess a cognitive function or ability.)

The extent of executive and attentional disorders can be so profound that the visual information never seems to reach the visual system. As reported in clinical practice and literature (see Chapters 1 and 3), some children with CVI seem, at times, to be blind although their eyes, optic tracts, and nerves appear to be intact. Their problem seems to be that they are unable to pay attention to visual information at all. Based on the information provided in this chapter, damage to the thalami may be contributing to this outcome. If these children's thalami are "closed," they prevent further visual processing from taking place. In children born with very low vision as a result of damage to the occipital lobes, the likelihood of improvement in vision is lower in those who also have sustained damage to the thalami (Ricci et al., 2006), presumably because they lack the intrinsic drive to gain and maintain visual attention. It seems that visual stimuli do not appear to attract attention to the visual modality. In addition, affected children appear to be unable to push attention to the visual modality, or "open up" their thalami on their own, by executive decision. As a result, they do not seem to know that the visual modality even exists.

One may want to consider a type of visual intervention treatment, in which different kinds of carefully selected salient visual stimuli are used to try to draw the child's attention to the visual modality (See Chapters 19 and 21). This systematic exogenous pulling may result in children becoming aware of their visual sense. In addition, it appears to have allowed slowly progressive but limited development of their visual processing areas, resulting in a gradual growing of understanding of visual information and its use for goal-directed behavior (Steendam, 2007).

## Visual Selective Attention Processes

When a child's thalami have facilitated access of visual information to the occipital lobes, other attentional processes await. While the first attentional processes are of a general nature, employed to choose and switch among sensory modalities, thought processes, and determining to what extent visual information is processed, the next level of attentional processing is specifically visual. The brain needs to select specific visual information from among all the visual information in the visual field. As such, it determines what is perceived from the visual scene.

The visual field is processed in the occipital lobes, creating a mapped representation of the outside world (see Chapter 2), which can be seen as an "improved" version of the information on the retina. The visual representation is not a projection like that of a camera. Different types of fibers carry different types of visual information, depending on their retinal location. (In addition, the amount of information has been reduced and the quality improved in the transition from the retina to the visual cortex, in which the transfer of information to ganglion cells enhances contrast. Moreover, the representation is binocular, giving rise to binocular depth perception.)

In most normal situations, the abundance of information in the visual field is too much to take in at once, the amount of information needs to be reduced again, but this time within the set of visual information. Different processes play a role in achieving this, some of which are under executive control; others depend on the saliency of the objects and the spatial characteristics of the visual information. The processes involved in attentional selection within the visual field form the first group of higher visual functions: the visual selective attentional functions.

### Locus of Attention and the Size of the Attended Area

As previously mentioned, a burst of light in a dark night will attract attention to the visual modality, but it will do more than that because it also pulls visual selective attention toward the location of that burst in the visual field. General attention and visual selective attention cooperate to bring salient stimuli into consciousness. Visual selective attention cannot come into play unless there is general attention to the visual modality, and this cannot be used efficiently without visual selective attentional processes, and the requisite eye movements.

Most of the time the eyes move to look toward the location where visual attention becomes directed, or the *locus of attention*, but the accompanying eye movements contribute only part of the story. While the eyes can only be directed to one point in space per each fixation, visual selective attention can cover an area as large as the whole visual field.

In other words, the size of the attentional "spotlight" (La Berge, 1983) or "zoom lens" (Eriksen & St. James, 1986) may vary from being very small to very large. The size of the object or scene capturing our attention largely dictates the size of the attended area. In visual scenes with multiple visual components without clear differences in saliency, it may not be so straightforward. The visual system is tuned to uncovering possible relationships between the components of the scene. When there are multiple parts to the visual information making up a meaningful whole, the initial size of the attended area is large. After initially devoting attention to "the whole," specific parts of the scene may then be selected, according to a smaller attended area (global visual selective attention versus local visual selective attention [Navon, 1977]). For example, parts making up a car attract attention to the car, but not to a specific element, such as a headlight. However, an observer may decide to take a closer look at the headlights, the doors, or any other part, and are able to do so at will, whenever it suits them and fits their goals.

When our eyes are fixed on a particular location in a visual scene, the size of the attended area determines what is visually perceived. While in most cases the initial size of the attended area will be large, the size of the attended area also depends on our expectations and goals, and the executive system, which monitors them. In addition, this process depends on how the exogenous attentional processes react to a specific stimulus, and the extent to which the brain areas responsible for the change in size of the attentional field are intact and developed.

It has been suggested that within the brain, the left temporoparietal area is involved in decreasing the size of the area being attended to, and the right temporoparietal area in increasing its size (Weissman & Woldorff, 2005; see Figure 6.1). Another brain area called the anterior cingulate cortex (not depicted) is proposed to boost attention to relevant stimuli (Weissman, Gopalakrishnan, Hazlett, & Woldorff, 2005). The actual changing of the size of the selected area is performed by connections between the thalamus and the visual cortex (Rees, 2009).

Clinical practice suggests that both functions, decreasing and increasing the size of the attended area, can be disturbed. For example, some children, when presented with the image in Figure 6.2 (similar to those described by Navon, 1977), are unable to see the letter *P* that is composed of smaller letter *A*'s; they report "A, A, A" to the question "What do you see?" Similarly, they are unable to identify pictures like the one of the cat in Figure 6.3. This suggests that they have difficulty selecting a large visual area, or "zooming out." Other children are able to identify pictures like the cat, mentally completing the picture to do so (*Gestalt closure*, or the ability to perceive incomplete visual images as a whole object, pattern, or configuration [Kaufman & Kaufman, 1983]), but are unable to report the "P," suggesting that they are visually able to attend to a large area, but do not do this automatically when confronted with details that are meaningful to them. It is as if the default size of their visually attended area is small, and they only en-

FIGURE 6.2

**Stimulus for Evoking Global Visual Selective Attention and Local Visual Selective Attention**

```
A A A A A
A       A
A        A
A       A
A A A A A
A
A
A
A
```

Stimuli such as this (similar to that described by Navon, 1977) are used to assess the child's ability to attend to the whole (global visual selective attention) and its parts (local visual selective attention). The normal response to the question "what do you see?" is to report seeing the *P* before mentioning the multiple *A*'s, or at least mentioning both in the same utterance. A disorder in global visual selective attention causes an inability to attend to the whole, which leads to the perception of the *A*'s, but not perception of the *P*.

large it when the details are not informative to them. Children who have a disorder in adopting a large visually attended area have trouble seeing the relationship between details; they lack overview and often fail to see "the larger picture." (This may not be restricted to the visual modality; some children have a more general tendency to pay attention to detail.)

FIGURE 6.3

**Gestalt Closure Stimulus**

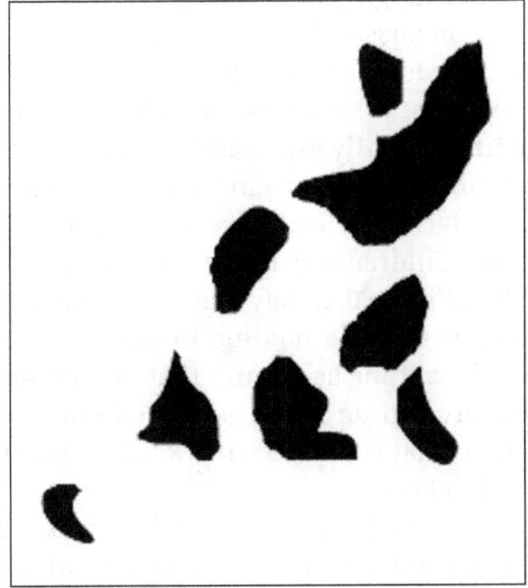

The stimulus pictured here is similar to those on the Gestalt Closure subtest from the Kaufman Assessment Battery for Children (K–ABC; Kaufman & Kaufman, 1983). Global visual selective attention to the whole of the picture allows parallel processing of its components, which is required to perceive the cat.

These children in particular may be trained to increase the size of the visually attended area at will, by employing executive functions. Eventually, they may gain a greater overview in situations where they would have normally lost track. Another option would be to restrict their workspace to a smaller area and present them with smaller stimuli. For example, one mother reported that her son was unable to identify the number on the diving block in a swimming pool when close to it, but had no trouble identifying it from about 20 yards away, when it was smaller. While it is generally thought that enlarging materials always helps visually impaired persons, observations have shown that this is not the case in children who have trouble enlarging the visually selected area.

As discussed in Chapter 3, simultanagnosia is generally described as an inability to see more than a small number of things at a time, usually associated with lack of visual guidance of movement and damage in the posterior parietal lobes of the brain. Although children may not initially see the letter *P* in Figure 6.2, they may see it when the stimulus is made smaller. In clinical practice, the author has found that simultanagnosia in children can be explained as a result of the visual selective attentional functions described here.

In contrast, there are children who, despite normal visual acuity and normal oculomotor abilities, have difficulty finding small elements in visually crowded stimuli. They report seeing a blur, or detest looking at crowded visual scenes (which they usually express by looking away), and may shorten their viewing distance in order to compensate for these experiences. Affected children seem to be unable to select a small area of the visual field; they appear to have a limited ability to decrease the size of the selected area, and have difficulty "zooming in" on details. As a result, by selecting too large an area of a crowded visual field, they access multiple details at once, which makes it hard for them to see these details clearly and independently of one another, resulting in the experience of blur, or details that appear to "dance." In some children, this effect of *central crowding* (experiencing crowdedness as blur, and being unable to select details in the center of their visual field) appears only after a period of viewing, suggesting they have a difficulty decreasing the visually selected area, which only increases with fatigue, and thus do not have the ability to adopt a small visual area. These children may have a disorder in decreasing the size of the visually selected area.

Children with central visual crowding typically have difficulty finding information in crowded visual scenes, and have difficulty reading small text. Children who experience central crowding can be aided by limiting the amount of visual information and by spacing text or pictures more widely. In addition, highlighting the start of a new paragraph using the same color, helping children organize their workspace, and assigning fixed locations for books, along with their writing, drawing, and reading tools, can also be very helpful.

Some children exhibit difficulty with both crowded visual stimuli and Gestalt stimuli, suggesting that they are unable to increase or decrease the visually attended area enough. This implies that the size of their attended area is relatively stationary, and that both functions (increasing or decreasing the area of attention), or a common mechanism, are disrupted.

Since the mechanism by which the size of the attended area is changed is housed in the thalami, it precedes visual processing in the visual cortex. As this cortical brain area represents the start of the three visual processing pathways, this mechanism seems to determine what is processed in the "what" and "where" pathways, and may also precede visual-motor actions brought about by the "how" pathway (Pardhan, Gonzalez-Alvarez, Subramanian, & Cheng, 2012). As such, it has a large impact on visual development. How can a child learn what a triangle is if he or she is unable to attend to the whole item at once, seeing only several lines, without their relationship being instantly clear? How can we identify differences between different triangles, when what we see comprises multiple sets of unrelated lines? How can we learn to pick up a cup by its handle when we are unable to identify the handle?

## Visual Selective Attention and Visual Features: Visual Search and Visual Imagery

The ability to flexibly increase and decrease the attended area is also a critical function in search tasks, allowing one to zoom out for overview, zoom in to see detail, and be able to identify whether what is being seen matches what is being looked for.

Sometimes we attend visually to a location or object in the periphery of our visual fields, without moving the eyes to use central vision to look at it. This kind of visual attention is called *covert attention*. It can also be brought about exogenously by fixating on a point in front of us and having someone move their hand in the periphery of the visual field. The movement is likely to capture visual selective attention, but it should be fairly easy to suppress the eye movements to shift gaze to the hand, partly because the movement is expected and partly by using the covert attention system.

Covert attention requires effort, however. Since visual acuity in the periphery is low, it is hard to accurately position attention, especially to objects or features that are not very salient. To do so, a sort of visual anchor is needed, a somewhat salient visual object to lock one's attention on to. In other words, when endogenously trying to push attention into the peripheral visual field, focusing on a somewhat salient object in the periphery helps direct our attention to the periphery by pulling it exogenously. This shows that exogenous and endogenous attentions, in addition to competing with one another, also cooperate. Especially in search tasks, attention often seems to be drawn toward salient or potentially interesting stimuli in the periphery.

Visual attention is all about limiting the amount of visual information processing. In addition to being able to select on the basis of the location and size of the visually attended area, visual information can be attended to based on specific visual properties, such as color, shape, or class of object. This can be done at will, by employing executive functions. For example, when seeking something red, attention can be devoted to red objects only, while filtering out all other colors, thus making all red objects in the visual field stand out.

For search tasks, the process is more complex. Many children in the author's clinic have been observed to experience trouble with searching and finding. Too often it is assumed that this is caused by some kind of visual disorder. Before considering this, however, it should be taken into account that many of the executive functions come into play in what may appear to be "just" visual tasks, including the following functions:

- Paying sustained attention to the visual modality
- Inhibiting salient objects (that is, those that do not match the target) from being (re)attended to (a more-or-less automatic process helps us not to attend to the same salient objects or locations again, the so-called *inhibition of return* [Posner & Cohen, 1984])
- Adopting a systematic search strategy, which greatly improves the chances of a successful finding
- Moving the eyes and zooming out at will to get an overview
- Moving attention around without moving the eyes all the time and, when

something is detected in the periphery of the visual field, using covert attention or a large visually attended area to match the target
- Zooming in at will
- Consciously using knowledge of the world to preselect locations where the target may be

In addition to these executive abilities, at least one important cognitive process in which executive functioning is involved is missing: the ability to form visual imagery. In addition to being size-based, visual selective attention can be feature-based, and as such, it can depend on an active mental visual representation of one or more features of the search target.

## The Role of Executive Functions in Visual Perception: Visual Working Memory

### Visual Imagery, Visual Closure, and Mental Visual Manipulation

Deciding whether visual stimuli that are encountered while searching are indeed the target implies that there is a database of something to match these stimuli to. In other words, in order to look for something, one or more active representations or visual images are needed in the mind, to which visual stimuli can be matched. Although representations of objects, features of objects, and faces in the "what" pathway are used to provide the image of the target, the ability to call on the visual images and to keep them active in the visual working memory is considered an executive function (Baddeley, 1986; Cornoldi & Vecchi, 2003). According to Barkley's (1997) model, nonverbal working memory allows children to represent and visually think about objects and places in the outside world even when the objects are not visually present. When a vivid mental image has been successfully created in the mind's eye, so much attention may be paid to it that no other events taking place before one's eyes are visually perceived, even though one's eyes are open. The outside visual world may interfere with mental imagery abilities. This is why, when engaged with visual mental imagery, people generally prefer to look up or at another location where the surrounding visual information is less distracting.

A topic related to visual imagery is visual closure, the ability to mentally fill in gaps of incomplete visual objects or pictures. Figure 6.4 shows typical visual closure tasks (inspired by those used in assessment instruments like RAKIT, a Dutch intelligence test for children whose name freely translates into "Figure Recognition," although "Name the picture" is a more apt description [Bleichrodt, Resing, Drenth, & Zaal, 1987], and the Test of Visual Perception Skills [TVPS-3; Martin, 2006]).

Regardless of how this ability is described, it is important to distinguish two higher visual functions that are required to perform this sort of task. First, the child should be able to attend to the whole stimulus area (global visual selective attention). Attending to just the details is not likely to lead to the right identification, which—if this is not automatically triggered by the stimulus—depends on executive functions. Second, the child should be able to engage in the formation of mental visual images to actively fill in large gaps in visual objects or pictures, again involving the executive system. From a clinical perspective, if a child is unable to complete visual closure tasks, it is necessary to know which of these functions—if not both—causes the trouble.

In addition to forming visual images, filling in gaps in visual stimuli, and keeping visual images active by sustaining attention to them, individuals are also able to actively, mentally manipulate their own visual images. Baddeley (1986) suggested that, to be able to do this, our visual working memory contains some sort of mental "visuospatial sketchpad," in addition to an executive component. To mentally manipulate an image requires active mental imagery. The image needs to be changed into different forms according to the desired manipulation. Typically, it needs to be mentally rotated or reshaped. Although visuospatial processing areas in the parietal cortex are involved in these kinds of actions in the visuospatial sketchpad, the actual changing, manipulation, and updating of the image in the mind's eye requires sustained attention and mental action based on will, implying executive control (Cornoldi & Vecchi, 2003).

In the author's clinic, there are children who appear to have trouble with only one or two types of visual working memory tasks, such as mentally rotating an image, without having other visual dysfunctions. Within the executive system, there may be different functions involved, for example, recruiting an image in the "what" pathway, keeping it active by sustaining attention, and manipulating the image.

The clinical consequences of dysfunction in executive mental vision include being unable to create good quality images or manipulate images in the mind, which has major consequences for issues such as the ability to draw from memory, find missing objects, solve jigsaw puzzles, and retrace a route by remembering landmarks or creating a mental map of the environment. Although visual processing areas are employed in order to achieve these goals, the initiative and the coordination required to recruit or form, maintain, and change the mental images is in the hands of the prefrontal areas housing the executive functions, not the visual cortex. Thus, when a child has difficulty with any of these or related visual tasks, it is possible that the cause may not be a purely visual one, and that the child may also have trouble mentally manipulating

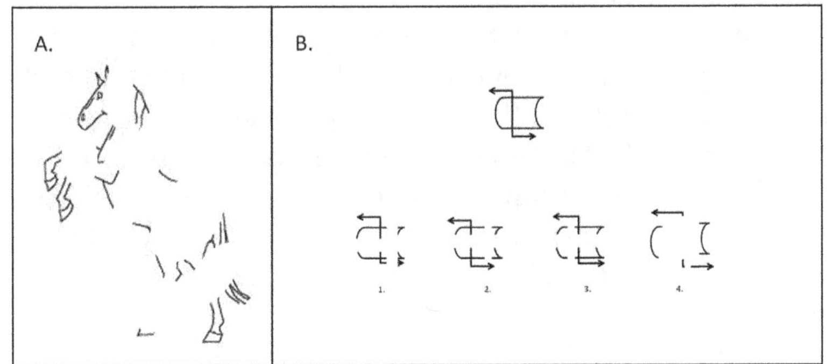


FIGURE 6.4
**Typical Visual Closure Tasks**

In visual closure tasks such as these, children are assessed on the ability to mentally fill in gaps of incomplete visual objects or pictures. **(A)** A stimulus similar to those of the *Figuur Herkennen* (figure recognition) subtest of RAKIT (a Dutch intelligence test for children). **(B)** A stimulus similar to those of the Visual Closure subtest of the TVPS-3 (Test of Visual Perception Skills).

the information. Such difficulties may therefore result from more general working memory disorders that affect visual task performance.

FIGURE 6.5
**Context in Visual Closure: THE CAT**

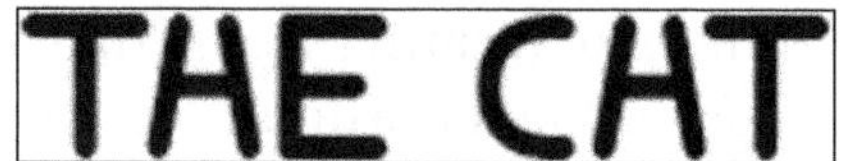


Most people will read this image as "THE CAT," even though the *H* in "The" and the *A* in "Cat" are the same. The perceived difference is a result of the context and the initial visual selective attention to the whole, not the individual letters.

## Executive Functions and Perception: Knowledge about the World Influences Perception by Creating Expectations and by Dealing with Ambiguity

Executive functions, in addition to having a huge impact on visual perception by controlling general and visual attentional processes—which determine what is being processed in the "what," "where," and "how" pathways—and active mental imagery and manipulation of visual images also play a role in providing a contextual background against which the visual input is interpreted. Expectations based on knowledge about the world influence our perception. A well-known example involves the images shown in Figure 6.5. Most people will look at this image and read "THE CAT," even though the *H* in "The" and the *A* in "Cat" are actually the same. They are perceived differently, however, by virtue of their context (in this case, provided by knowledge of the English language), and because initial visual selective attention is given to the whole—giving global attention to the words, not the individual letters.

Another example of how knowledge of the visual world influences perceptions is a cat owner's perceiving a coat draped on a dark staircase as his or her cat, if the owner knows from experience that is her favorite spot. Those who do not keep a cat as a pet would probably never experience this misperception.

In these examples, however, the contextual effect is quite automatic; without noticing it, our knowledge about the world and our former experiences determine how we interpret ambiguous visual information. Written language is a well-known territory to most adults; therefore, the example of "THE CAT" does not pose any problems for them, whereas to an inexperienced reader, it is likely to do so. Consider an example in which the image of the *A* or *H* is not ambiguous, like "THE CHT" or "TAE CAT." Would this pose a problem for us? Maybe so. To be able to decipher the information, we might need to do some problem solving by asking ourselves some questions, such as "What could this mean?" or "Does the rest of the text provide clues about what this should say?" At this point, there is clearly a role for the executive functions to play in perception.

The same goes for the interpretation of scenes. In the author's clinic, RAKIT Vertelplaten ("Storytelling Pictures" from the Dutch Revision Amsterdam Children's Intelligence Test [Bleichrodt, Resing, Drenth, & Zaal, 1987]) is used to test children's interpretations of scenes. The test comprises two colorful, semi-realistic scenes, created with aquarelle paint and pen. The first depicts a girl on a ladder picking apples from a tree on the left side of the picture, with a dog fastened to the ladder by a leash. Also in the scene, more to the right, are a cat (middle right) that is sneaking up on a chicken and her chicks (far right). The scene thus contains the storyline that the cat will attack the chicken and chicks, the dog will chase the cat, pulling the ladder from under the girl, and the girl will fall down. Children are asked to report everything they see in the picture, and after a minute or so, are asked explicitly about the story in the scene. From clinical practice, children who have difficulty adopting a large selective attentional area (resulting from a disorder in global visual attention) experience a big disadvantage in discovering the story line. While most people select larger parts of the scene and understand it almost at once, affected children select only small parts and see just the details. As a consequence, the only way for them to discover the story line is by serial and effortful reasoning. Moreover, their knowledge about the world and their access to it through executive functions helps them in their reasoning. Children with a disorder in global visual attention, who actively use their knowledge and actively try to discover the story line, may eventually succeed, although it will take them more time and effort. In contrast, children with the same disorder who do not or cannot employ their executive functions will probably never discover the story line.

In addition, missing the bigger picture may also result in misperceiving the smaller details. More than once, the author has seen children who tend to focus on details, mistaking the cat in the picture for a fox. On the other hand, children who use their executive functions and actively reason about the relationships between the elements, often change their perception of the fox to that of a cat after they have understood the story line, because cats fit in better with the scene and dogs are typically expected to chase cats, not foxes.

In visuospatial perception tasks, an active approach to discovering visuospatial features (for example, estimating the distance between a couch and a wall by dividing the distance into a series of more manageable known units such as meters, or appraising the elements of a picture instead of their relationships) will aid the perceptual analysis, and thus, the accuracy of visual spatial perception. Such active visual analysis, especially visuospatial analysis, requires involvement of the executive system.

In sum, the executive system is involved in visual problem solving, which is required in cases of ambiguous visual information and other reasoning-based visual perceptual tasks, such as the understanding of complex visual scenes and difficult visuospatial estimation tasks. Most of the time we are unaware that our knowledge of the world influences and supplements our perceptions, but when our sensory systems give us ambiguous information, or we are faced with a challenging visual task, our executive system can help us gain access to knowledge and solve inconsistencies more easily. It provides us with contextual information to get a grip on a task, it may warn us when our initial perceptions contradict what we would expect, and it allows us to more actively access information from memory in order to unravel and solve ambiguity by reasoning.

## The Role of Executive Functions in Task Behavior

While the ways in which executive functions influence the processing of visual information have been explained to this point, this is not where their role ends when it comes to the assessment and interpretation of a child's visual abilities. We tend to judge children's visual abilities and disabilities by their performance on visual tasks and observation of their visual behavior. However, as suggested earlier in this chapter, executive functions play a crucial role in task and test performance, as well as behavior. They do so by setting goals based on emotions and needs and knowledge of the world, through the orchestration of attentional processes. Children's performances on tasks reflect their emotional state because this largely determines their goals, as well as the quality of their executive and attentional functions. This, in turn, influences the potential quality of response to the visual function we intend to assess. This can be illustrated by sketching out the cognitive functions that a child needs to be able to orchestrate to provide valid test results.

The following simplified sequence shows that, before the visual functions come into play, the child needs to achieve a number of emotional, executive, and attentional prerequisites before he or she can show valid evidence of visual processing abilities. The child needs to:

- Understand what is being asked using attentional, selective auditory attentional functions, and verbal working memory, in which the verbal elements are decoded and interpreted.
- Interpret his or her own emotions and motivations (How do I feel? How do I feel about what this person is asking me to do? Do I want to do this, or do I feel like doing something else? Do I trust this person? Can I do this? What does he think of me?).
- Make socially acceptable plans accordingly (Shall I comply? How can I do this? Will I cheat? Will he notice?).
- Keep these plans in mind and break them down into manageable subplans (What is the sequence in which I am going to do this? Can I manage these substeps, or do I have to do something more?).
- Control attention to select the required perceptual, cognitive, or motor systems ("tools") at the right time.
- Control attentional processes within one or more selected modalities or cognitive systems, using working memory to keep the right information and knowledge active (by sustaining attention), and manipulating the information if necessary.
- Control attentional processes to accurately perform motor functions.
- Check the progress and execution of the sequence of subplans to work toward the initially set goal.
- Interpret the test leader's reaction to his or her behavior by using social knowledge.
- Decide to what extent his or her goals and the test leader's are met.
- Decide whether he or she is satisfied by the result.
- Decide whether to change the goal, or to change the plan to reach the goal.

The complex nature of factors influencing the performance of a visual task, as shown in the sequence just presented, demonstrates how difficult it is to isolate the cause of any particular dysfunction when trying to assess higher visual functions, or any brain function. The emotional sublayer and its interpretations by the executive system determine the extent to which the child will be motivated to perform the task, or even listen to the task instructions. Often, the emotional or motivational aspects do not need executive interpretation, as they surface without the need for the executive system to clarify them. In these cases, however, the executive system is primarily needed to suppress emotions and urges, so as to succumb to the investigator's wishes.

Consider the following examples in which emotions negatively affect task performance. If a child has had multiple experiences of failure with tasks similar to the one at hand—as is often the case with children with one or more visual processing disorders—the child may decide not to cooperate or not to do his or her best to avoid the pain of failing, resulting not only in a poor but invalid performance on the test. If the child is afraid of the examiner, the child will be stressed and will pay attention to the examiner instead of the task, which is likely to significantly hamper performance. Moreover, stress negatively affects attentional processes and executive functioning. Alternatively, the child may actually like the examiner and, as a consequence, would prefer to play with him rather than do "stupid and difficult" tasks. Or, the child may be so thrilled by making the examiner laugh at jokes that the child decides to act like a clown. Maybe the child is tired because he or she did not have a good night's sleep. Hunger, thirst, and distracting thoughts can all interfere with a test session. A child can have any reason not to want to comply, or have difficulty complying. A functioning executive system is necessary to overcome these difficulties and to suppress emotions and urges, and hence, is a crucial prerequisite for reliable test performance.

In short, a child's task-related visual performance always reflects his or her emotional state and the state of the different components of his or her executive system. Moreover, once the emotional foundations for reliable task performance have been met, the child needs to monitor his or her own behavior and take appropriate, well-timed actions by shifting between and within sensory and motor systems, and by controlling different attentional processes in order to accomplish his or her goals.

## Conclusion

The visual system is a complex tool with many features that have hierarchical and parallel relationships that interact and work together. However, vision is not an independent entity; it is part of a complex organism in its own personal social environment, whose performance depends on a number of functional systems and subsystems that are hierarchically related to each other, with the visual system and the other sensory systems playing an integrated, supportive role. Figure 6.6 presents a graphic summary of the model of visual perception presented in this chapter.

Without control over the visual and other sensory systems, we would be ruled by salient stimuli in the environment, as well as by our urges and emotions. We would react to stimuli and impulses only at the present moment. The executive system helps us to expand our scope beyond what is in front of us by controlling attention. Through the orchestration of attentional processes, the executive system allows us to gain access to different sources of information in both the outside world via the different senses, and the inside world by accessing emotional and memory systems. It allows

FIGURE 6.6
## Hierarchical Model of Visual Perception and Behavior

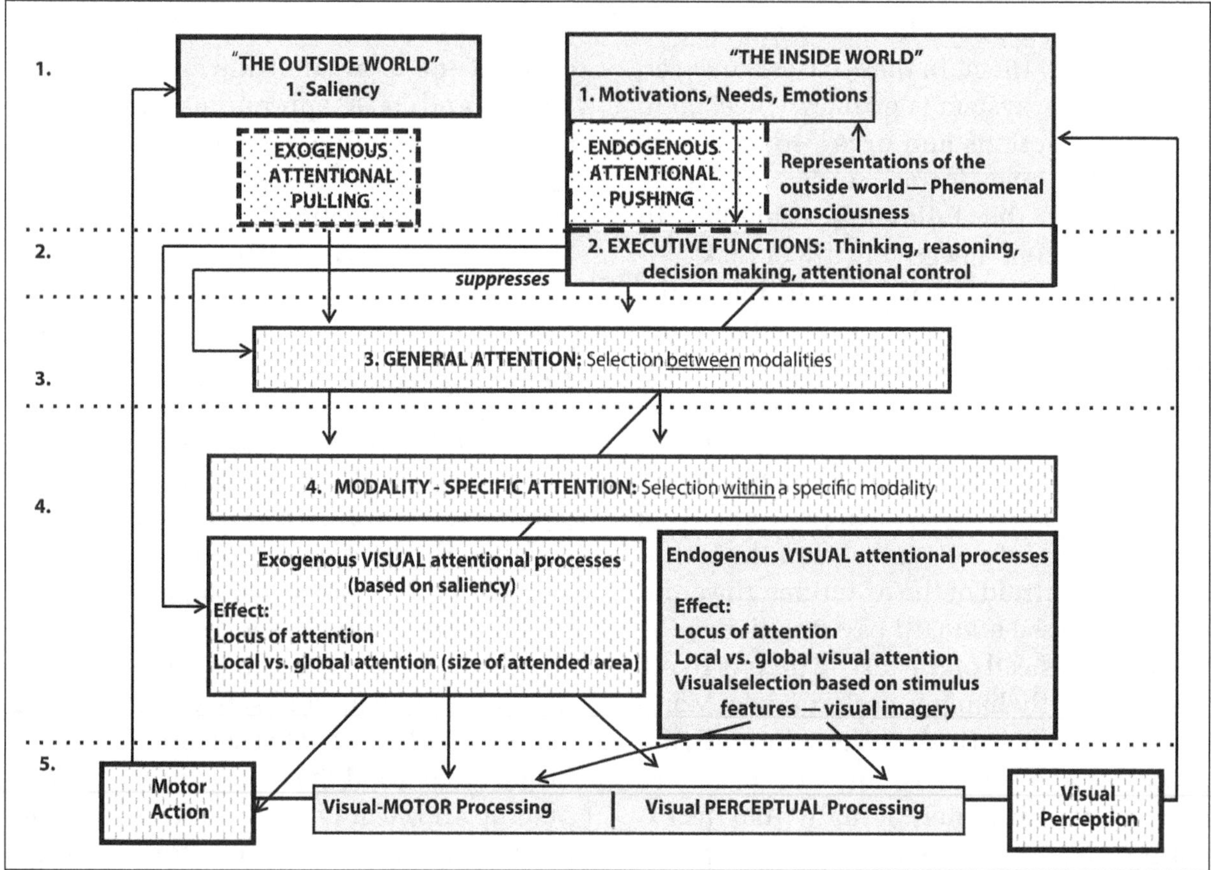


Visual perception and behavior are part of a never-ending loop of bottom-up and top-down processes that are performed in order to continuously form input to both the emotional and executive systems. Both our visual-motor behavior affecting the physical environment and the outcome of all the visual perceptual processes form new input to the emotional and executive systems. This information functions as the basis for new goals and subgoals, which are again performed by the visual-motor system and monitored by the visual perceptual system, creating an ever-ongoing process.

us to determine whether we want to pay attention to the visual or another modality, whether we want to pay attention to details and their spatial relationships, when and what we want to think about, as well as to form goals based on our emotions and urges, but censored by our reasoning and knowledge.

To be able to find out to what extent a child experiences problems and restrictions in daily life as a result of visual dysfunctions, the exact nature of the tasks and circumstances need to be specified, and alternative causes to problems and limitations need to be explored. The causes may be visual, but can be manyfold, including attentional or executive in nature. Often it turns out that difficulties result from complex interactions among visual and attentional, executive, or other dysfunctions, plus possible effects from the emotional consequences of a history of failure and reaction from the social environment. Thus, to uncover the causes of specific problems and limitations, a complete understanding of the person is needed. This requires the gathering and integration of a lot of information by multiple disciplines and employing different data collection methods such as observation and interviews with parents, teachers, and the child (discussed in Part 3 of this book). It also requires the assessment of visual and attentional functions, as well as executive, motor, and other cognitive and sensory functions, and connecting this information to medical records. The reliability of assessment of any function depends heavily on the person's executive and attentional abilities. Since in children these abilities are not yet fully developed, their performance on tasks is difficult to interpret.

In addition to understanding the roles of nonvisual brain functions in task performance, professionals need to understand which visual functional units are meaningful in visual task performance, to be able to properly assess them. Furthermore, professionals need to identify the functional units a specific test requires in order to be able to interpret which functional units may be disrupted. Approaches to this type of assessment are considered in Chapter 13.

In summary, understanding visual behavior requires a functional model of visual processing, which acknowledges that processing of visual information is part of a hierarchy of functions that incorporates the visual system's relationships with the outside world, as well as its relationships to the rich and complex inside world. The executive functions play a central role in this hierarchy, primarily by controlling attentional processes.

## References


Baddeley, A. D. (1986). *Working memory.* New York: Oxford University Press.

Barkley, R. A. (1997). Behavioral inhibition, sustained attention, and executive functions: Constructing a unifying theory of ADHD. *Psychological Bulletin, 121*(1), 65–94.

Bleichrodt, N., Resing, W. C. M., Drenth, P. J. D., & Zaal, J. N. (1987). *Intelligentie-meting bij kindere: Empirische en methodologische verantwoording van de gereviseerde Amsterdamse kinder intelligentie test.* Lisse, The Netherlands: Swets & Zeitlinger.

Cornoldi, C., & Vecchi, T. (2003). *Visuo-spatial working memory and individual differences.* Hove, England: Psychology Press.

Eriksen, C. W., & St. James, J. D. (1986). Visual attention within and around the field of focal attention: A zoom lens model. *Perception & Psychophysics, 40*(4), 225–240.

Faw, B. (2003). Pre-frontal executive committee for perception, working memory, attention, long-term memory, motor control, and thinking: A tutorial review. *Consciousness and Cognition, 12*(1), 83–139.

Hart, T., & Jacobs, H. E. (1993). Rehabilitation and management of behavioral disturbances following frontal lobe injury. *Journal of Head Trauma Rehabilitation, 8*(1), 1–12.

Kaufman, A. S., & Kaufman, N. L. (1983). *Kaufman assessment battery for children.* Circle Pines, MN: American Guidance Service.

La Berge, D. (1983). Spatial extent of attention to letters and words. *Journal of Experimental Psychology: Human Perception and Performance, 9*(3), 371–379.

Martin, N. (2006). *Test of visual perceptual skills* (3rd ed.). Novato, CA: Academic Therapy Publications.

Navon, D. (1977). Forest before trees: The precedence of global features in visual perception. *Cognitive Psychology, 9*(3), 353–383.

Newman, J. (1997). Putting the puzzle together. Part I: Toward a general theory of the neural correlates of consciousness. *Journal of Consciousness Studies, 4*(1), 47–66.

Pardhan, S., Gonzalez-Alvarez, C., Subramanian, A., & Cheng, S. (2012). How do flanking objects affect reaching and grasping behavior in participants with macular disorders? *Investigative Ophthalmology & Visual Science, 53*(10), 6687–6694.

Posner, M. I., & Cohen, Y. (1984). Components of visual orienting. In H. Bouma & D. G. Bouwhuis (Eds.), *Attention and performance X: Control of language processes* (pp. 531–556). Hillsdale, NJ: Erlbaum.

Rees, G. (2009). Visual attention: The thalamus at the centre? *Current Biology, 19*(5), 213–214.

Ricci, D., Anker, S., Cowan, F., Pane, M., Gallini, F., Luciano, R., . . . Mercuri, E. (2006). Thalamic atrophy in infants with PVL and cerebral visual impairment. *Early Human Development, 82*(9), 591–595.

Saalmann, Y. B., & Kastner, S. (2009). Gain control in the visual thalamus during perception and cognition. *Current Opinion in Neurobiology, 19*(4), 408–414.

Shipp, S. (2004). The brain circuitry of attention. *Trends in Cognitive Sciences, 8*(5), 223–230.

Steendam, M. (2007). *Weet jij wat ik zie?: Cerebrale visuele stoornissen bij kinderen, een handleiding voor professionals* [Do you know what I see? Cerebral visual impairment in children, instructions for professionals]. Huizen, Netherlands: Koninklijke Visio.

Trappenberg, T. P., Dorris, M. C., Munoz, D. P., & Klein, R. M. (2001). A model of saccade initiation based on the competitive integration of exogenous signals in the superior colliculus. *Journal of Cognitive Neuroscience, 13*(2), 256–271.

Vuilleumier, P., Chicherio, C., & Assal, F. (2001). Functional neuroanatomical correlates of hysterical sensorimotor loss. *Brain, 124*, 1077–1090.

Weissman, D. H., Gopalakrishnan, A., Hazlett, C. J., & Woldorff, M. G. (2005). Dorsal anterior cingulate cortex resolves conflict from distracting stimuli by boosting attention toward relevant events. *Cerebral Cortex, 15*(2), 229–237.

Weissman, D. H., & Woldorff, M. G. (2005). Hemispheric asymmetries for different components of global/local attention occur in distinct temporo-parietal loci. *Cerebral Cortex, 15*(6), 870–876.

# 7

# Considerations in the Behavioral Diagnosis of CVI: Issues, Cautions, and Potential Outcomes

*Terese Pawletko, Sylvie Chokron, and Gordon N. Dutton*

Cerebral visual impairment (CVI) may go undiagnosed because the variety of behaviors and characteristics exhibited by affected children may be unrecognized or misconstrued as behavioral or developmental disorders. The focus of this chapter, therefore, is threefold: (1) to explain how childhood CVI may go undetected owing to its many possible presentations; (2) to highlight the potential for CVI to contribute to, or masquerade as, a developmental or behavioral disorder (such as attention deficit/hyperactivity disorder [ADHD] or autism spectrum disorders); and (3) to outline the potential impact of an undetected or hidden disability resulting from CVI on the child, the family, and the community at large. To illustrate these points, the chapter will focus on several conditions whose symptoms and manifestations overlap with those of CVI, including ADHD, developmental dyslexia, and autism spectrum disorders. The aim is to highlight the possibility of unrecognized CVI among at-risk children, and to facilitate its detection and habilitation.

## Behavioral Responses to CVI

Cerebral visual impairment affects behavior. This, in turn, can affect a child's responses to environmental, educational, academic, interpersonal, and physical situations. Moreover, associated damage to other brain areas can compound the clinical picture. At the same time, parents' and service providers' prior experiences with children can influence their expectations and interpretation of behaviors resulting from CVI. Thus, if the contributory impact of visual dysfunction goes unrecognized, the child's behaviors may be considered "inappropriate," or "within the child's ability to control," or the child may be given inaccurate alternative behavioral diagnoses.

## Children's Behavioral Responses as a Result of CVI

When children are affected by any of the visual disorders that result from CVI, they may exhibit unexpected responses to their physical and social environment in a variety of ways (as described in Chapter 3), depending on the type of damage to the brain. Children's unusual behavioral responses as a result of these visual disorders may be categorized as one of the following:

- lack of response, due to lack of vision
- reactive responses
- adaptive responses

### *Lack of Response*

A child with low visual acuity, limited visual field, prosopagnosia (inability to recognize faces), or a combination of these, may be unable to respond to social cues such as gestures and facial expressions because they are not seen by the child. As a result, the child may ignore friends or family, or react to them in an unusual way. This may even be manifested during the first year of life, when parents sometimes report their child's lack of reaction to them when they approach or smile at the child—almost as if they were strangers. If the visual impairment is not recognized, such responses may be misinterpreted as features of autism spectrum disorders, such as lack of anticipation, joint attention, and eye contact.

### *Reactive Responses*

A child with simultanagnostic visual difficulties (inability to see more than a few items at a time) may be overwhelmed by the people, sights, and sounds in a crowded environment, and the resulting stress may lead to withdrawal, an angry outburst, or anxiety. If undiagnosed, this type of reactive response may incorrectly be interpreted as oppositional (e.g., a refusal) or noncompliant behavior.

Children with simultanagnostic visual dysfunction may also exhibit apparently contradictory behaviors. Details such as a tiny shape or a small letter may be recognized, but not larger shapes or objects (see Chapter 6). This behavior can be misinterpreted as faking.

Some children with unrecognized CVI can have panic attacks that may be ignored or misunderstood by close relatives. For example, children with visual field defects may fixate on their mother's face, but when the mother's face moves into the blind area in the visual field, the children experience that as a loss because they can no longer see her. An affected infant may thus experience a visual world in which people and objects appear and disappear without warning. This experience can be associated with behaviors indicative of fear and anxiety.

### *Adaptive Responses*

Adaptive responses result when a child with CVI uses an alternative way to accomplish a task. For example, holding on to another person to help find someone in a crowded area may compensate for simultanagnosia, optic ataxia, or dyskinetopsia (difficulty seeing things that move). Some children with CVI close their eyes when holding their parent's hand in the street, probably to avoid the need to process details of the visual scene. Another adaptive strategy is to ask for food items on a plate to be separated to help identify them (McKillop et al., 2006). Such adaptive strategies enable the child to succeed at otherwise difficult tasks.

### Adults' Responses to the Child's Behaviors

The way adults label a child's responses to visual or motor impairments, whether known or unknown, may affect the way the adult interacts with the child, as well as the child's sense of self-worth and competence. If the origin of the child's visual behaviors is not recognized, the adult may assume that the child "should know better" or "behave better." For example, distress or anger in a crowd can be misinterpreted as disobedience, and the parent may become frustrated or embarrassed. Or if a child trips and breaks something because of a narrow visual field, a parent may chastise the child for not taking sufficient care. In these examples, the adults' reactions are likely to be different if the child's behavior is recognized as a result of a diagnosed condition, not simply as misconduct.

## Difficulties in Identifying CVI

Every child has a unique biological, temperamental, and developmental makeup. They respond to their environment and the people and objects within it in a wide variety of ways (verbally, nonverbally, socially, and motorically, for example). This is no different for the child with visual, physical, or learning disabilities, whether or not they have been identified. Unexpected behaviors and responses to specific tasks or environments may sometimes require the attention of medical, psychological, or developmental professionals. The nature, setting, duration, and frequency of these observable behaviors tend to determine which professional sees the child (such as an ophthalmologist, psychologist, teacher of the visually impaired, or physical therapist). Each professional applies his or her specialized training to understand the underlying mechanisms of the child's behavioral presentation, but may not be aware of the full range of causes for a behavior, including those that result from CVI. While assessment outcomes and recommended interventions reflect the expertise of each professional evaluating the child, there is still the chance that CVI will be overlooked.

In addition, parents and teachers may not be aware that dysfunctional vision is causing difficulties for the child. Moreover, if assessment of vision is primarily focused on ocular visual impairments, then CVI may go undiagnosed, with resulting behaviors being attributed to other causes.

### CVI Behaviors Identified with Alternative Labels

As already noted, children's behaviors associated with CVI are often attributed to other conditions, such as developmental delay, and personality, adjustment, or behavioral issues.

#### *Developmental Delay*

Children may suffer brain damage from a range of causes (as described in Chapter 3). The resulting damage may lead to developmental delays in motor, language, cognitive, physical, and visual functions. While intellectual or cognitive impairments impact development, the possibility that CVI also exists and can have an impact (Stiers, De Cock, & Vandenbussche, 1999) may not be taken into account. The same applies to the existence of ophthalmological disorders such as strabismus and amblyopia, which are, in some cases, also associated with CVI (Cavezian et al., 2013), and can go unidentified.

### *Personality, Adjustment, and Behavioral Issues*

A child without physical disabilities or other major conditions, but with undetected CVI as the primary cause of unusual behaviors, may be misunderstood. For example, parents or teachers may be confused by a child with impaired dorsal stream functions (see Chapter 3) who can read large, well-spaced text and recognize people and objects, yet has great difficulty reading smaller text, finding objects, copying text or pictures, moving through space, or accurately reaching for objects. They may incorrectly think the child must be trying to feign difficulty or get out of doing something. Associated peripheral lower visual field impairment can lead to tripping, fear of jumping into a swimming pool, and refusal to jump off a bench. These reactions can mistakenly be interpreted as the child being clumsy and anxious.

Impaired dorsal stream functions tend to cause fatigue, so as it gets later in the day, the affected child cannot find things, becomes clumsy, and gets easily distressed in crowded environments. This may cause parents or caregivers to wonder why the child started behaving badly later in the day, leading to the incorrect assumption that this conduct is related to a behavior problem.

Children with ventral stream damage (see Chapter 3) have an inability to recognize text and objects in the context of negotiating complex environments, and have a tendency to get lost. This can lead to difficulty on the part of adults in understanding the inconsistencies of the child's behavior. They think, "If he can see well enough to move around, how can he not see other things? He just needs to try harder."

Some children with unidentified CVI may be labeled as "noncompliant," "oppositional," or "irritable" when they avoid or refuse to do a task, when in fact they have become visually fatigued or may be experiencing fluctuations in visual function and need better scheduling of activities and regular rest periods to optimize functioning, rather than a behavioral reinforcement plan. Other children with CVI may be described as continuing a specific activity and being "perseverative," rather than being recognized as having difficulty shifting visual attention. They may be considered "inattentive," rather than having difficulty picking out an object or individual from a cluster, or "disrespectful," "withdrawn," or "autistic-like" because they do not look people in the eye or respond to facial expressions (Freeman, 2010).

The diagram in Figure 7.1 presents a graphic illustration of how failure to recognize a child's visual difficulties can result in adverse behavioral, social, and emotional outcomes. It outlines potential scenarios for the child whose CVI has yet to be identified and acted upon (McKillop & Dutton, 2008), with the potential outcomes of criticism or punishment, leading to emotional reactions of anxiety, depression, stress, embarrassment, frustration, and fear. Children with undiagnosed CVI who are otherwise able-bodied are particularly at risk for such misdiagnoses and their adverse consequences. The consequences of undiagnosed CVI are discussed in more detail at the end of this chapter.

## Other Impairments are Given Priority

Children with CVI frequently have other conditions, including cerebral palsy, seizure disorders, and cognitive and hearing impairments (Freeman, 2010; Matsuba & Soul, 2010; Whiting et al., 1985). Neurological health may be affected, influencing sleep, feeding,

FIGURE 7.1

**Potential Interactions between Undetected Visual Difficulties, the Environment, and Social Demands in Children with Undiagnosed CVI**

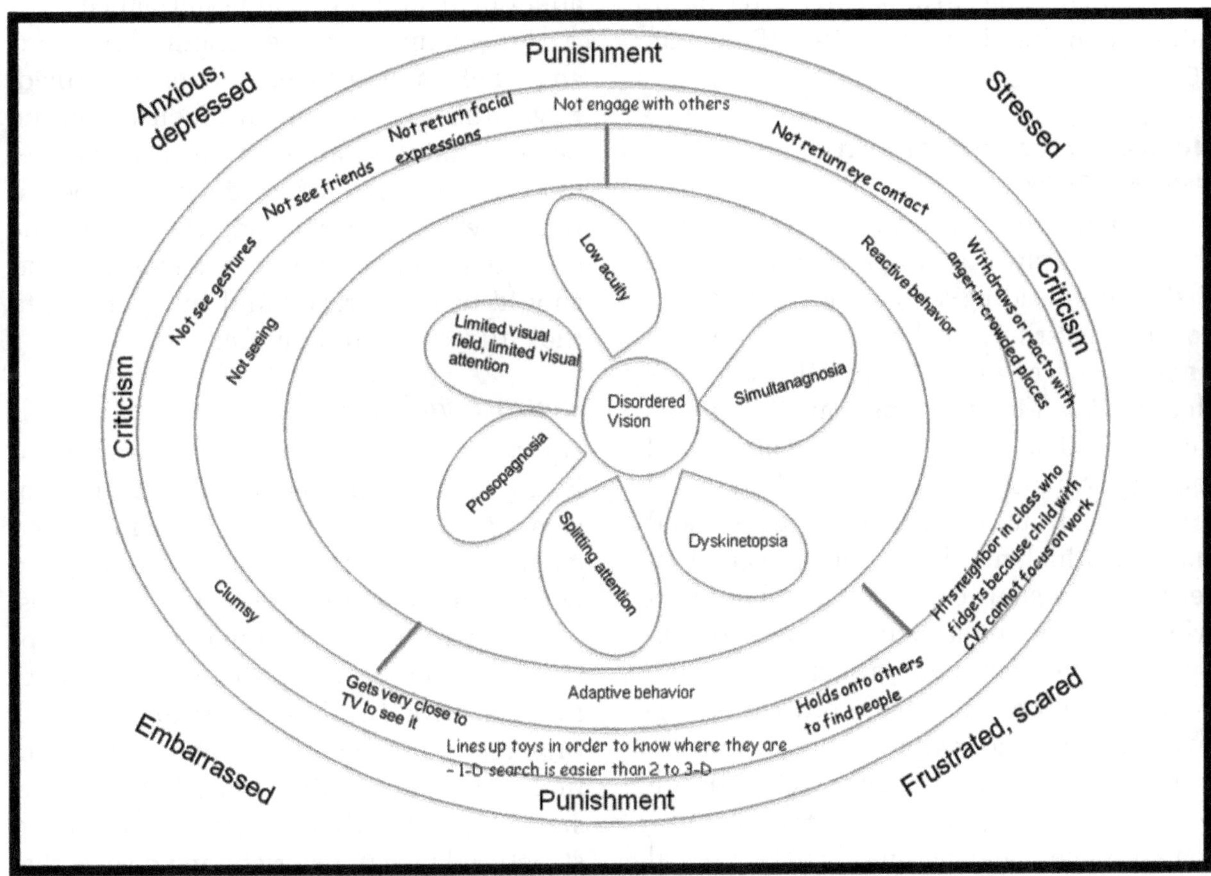


Undiagnosed visual impairment is shown in the center of the diagram, with the child's natural adaptive and reactive behaviors surrounding it. Moving toward the outside of the diagram, the text represents the child's behaviors that may not be understood and may be inappropriately criticized, or even punished, particularly outside the home. Potential emotional outcomes for the child are illustrated in the outermost ring.

and emotion. Additional orthopedic impairments may need surgery with ongoing physiotherapy and occupational therapy. Premature infants may need extended hospital stays and multiple procedures, including laser eye treatment. When attention is focused on all these issues, CVI can go unrecognized because it is not as evident (see Chapter 23). The following sections describe some considerations to be alert for when working with children who have these conditions.

### *Cerebral Palsy*

The definition of cerebral palsy (which was recently revised in recognition of increasing knowledge about the condition) highlights that motor and visual impairments are integral components of the same disorder (Bax, Flodmark, & Tydeman, 2007;

Rosenbaum et al., 2007). Children with cerebral palsy may have any of the visual disorders typical of CVI, but the resulting behaviors may be attributed to the physical, rather than the visual, disability (Freeman, 2010).

#### NONAMBULATORY CHILDREN WITH CEREBRAL PALSY

The visibility of a child in a wheelchair and the child's physical impairments can be distractors, leading adults and peers to incorrectly attribute behaviors to impaired physical or cognitive capabilities, rather than to CVI. Motor and orthopedic impairments limit a child's access, control, and mastery of his or her world. The child exerts effort to maintain and control posture and stability, which may leave limited mental reserve for visual engagement. The child whose CVI goes undetected may miss out on opportunities for intervention to promote communication, hand-eye coordination, active learning, and reciprocal social interaction. Teachers and caregivers of children with cerebral palsy need to carry out ongoing assessment and monitoring of functional vision and be vigilant in documenting the child's case history.

#### MOBILE CHILDREN WITH CEREBRAL PALSY

While children with spastic diplegia are able to move around, they face vulnerabilities in all aspects of vision and perception (Fazzi, Signorini, & Bianchi, 2010; Jacobson & Dutton, 2000). Yet, the very fact that they are free to walk around and to engage with their environment may cause these associated visual challenges to go unrecognized. The wide-ranging difficulties caused by lower visual field impairment and dorsal and ventral stream dysfunction (Fazzi et al., 2004, 2010; see also Chapter 3) may become more evident by school age, owing to increasing demands on vision, as well as increasing expectations of educational, attentional, and physical performance.

For example, if peripheral lower visual field impairment is not identified, physiotherapists—who are focused on the need to maintain an erect posture, may require the child not to look down while walking. However, intermittent viewing of the ground ahead facilitates safe mobility and should be encouraged and integrated into the child's overall program.

### *Hydrocephalus*

Hydrocephalus is a result of impaired circulation of cerebral spinal fluid causing increased intracranial pressure, with increased cerebral spinal fluid volume expanding the water spaces in the brain (the ventricles) (Andersson, 2010). A common visual symptom associated with hydrocephalus is refractive error (Andersson, 2010), but it is important to assess more than just refraction and visual acuity, to get a better understanding of the whole system. Detailed and structured visual history taking reveals that more than one-half of affected children show evidence of cognitive, visual, and perceptual problems (Houliston, Taguri, Dutton, Hajivassiliou, & Young, 1999; Andersson et al., 2006; see Chapter 3). (This is less frequent among those with associated spina bifida.) Therefore, ongoing assessment and monitoring of visual function and neurodevelopmental status is important.

### *Prematurity*

When a child is born preterm, the initial focus is on the child's survival and, later, on management of associated conditions. However, preterm children are also at risk of underdeveloped brain structures and periventricular white matter damage that can impair vision, but these conditions may be overlooked because the focus is on other priorities. Retinopathy of prematurity may also occur and need treatment, but the focus on that condition can lead to CVI being missed (Jacobson & Dutton, 2000). In addition, preterm children with low birth weight can have impaired visual attention as a result of perceptual visual impairment (Dutton 2013; Macintyre-Béon et al., 2013), but this may be incorrectly ascribed to an attention deficit disorder (see Chapter 23). Long-term follow-up of prematurely born children should include refraction and monitoring of vision and visual perception, especially since perceptual disorders related to dorsal stream dysfunction may only become apparent at 5 or 6 years of age (Dutton et al., 2004; Macintyre-Béon et al., 2013).

## Children with Behavioral Challenges of Undetermined Origin

Some children have perceptual visual impairment despite having no manifest additional impairments. Their development may appear normal, but there may be a history of early neurological insult. Even children with normal obstetric or medical histories may have slightly impaired visual acuities associated with perceptual visual impairment (Cavezian et al., 2010, 2013; Saidkasimova, Bennett, Butler, & Dutton, 2007; Williams et al., 2011). These findings indicate the importance of seeking evidence of visual impairment resulting from brain damage as a potential explanation of a child's behavioral presentation. Behaviors to consider include the following:

- The possibility of refractive error or lack of accommodation
- An "emotional meltdown" associated with being in an overstimulating environment
- Refusal to do schoolwork related to excess near or distant visual clutter
- Difficulties in social situations resulting from the inability to identify faces or facial expressions
- Problems identifying people in a crowd or objects in an array, with variability in performance

If CVI is not correctly diagnosed and the underlying reason for the behavior not understood, such behaviors may lead teachers and other caregivers to question whether the student is being lazy (Cavezian et al., 2010). (See Chapter 23 for additional examples and suggested solutions.) Parents are keen observers and experts in their children's functioning over time and in different environments, and, if asked the right questions, such as the following, will usually lead the physician, teacher, or other professional to the correct explanation for a child's behavior. If a child is frequently observed to have two or more of the difficulties described in these questions, then CVI warrants consideration as a possible cause of the child's difficulties (Dutton et al., 2010).

- Does your child have difficulty walking down stairs?
- Does your child have difficulty seeing things that are moving quickly, such as small animals?
- Does your child have difficulty seeing something that is pointed out in the distance?
- Does your child have difficulty locating an item of clothing in a pile of clothes?
- Does your child find copying words or drawings time consuming and difficult?

Once the nature and origins of the child's visual difficulties are properly understood and diagnosed, then it becomes possible to tailor a child's environment and habilitation to match his or her identified needs.

## Overlapping Diagnoses

Three common diagnoses—attention deficit / hyperactivity disorder (ADHD), dyslexia, and autism spectrum disorder—have been selected to illustrate how behaviors resulting from unrecognized CVI might be given one of these diagnoses instead, and how additional visual perceptual components of these diagnoses may go unrecognized (Das, Bennett, & Dutton, 2007). The diagnostic criteria and features published in the *Diagnostic and Statistical Manual of Mental Disorders,* 5th Edition (DSM–5; American Psychiatric Association, 2013), by the International Dyslexia Association (2008, 2012, 2014), and in the *International Statistical Classification of Diseases and Related Health Problems*, 10th Edition (ICD–10; World Health Organization, 1992) are highlighted, and explanations are provided on how CVI has the potential to cause behaviors that may be ascribed to one of these three conditions.

### ADHD vs. Cerebral Visual Impairment

The diagnosis of ADHD is based on the presence or absence of clusters of certain behaviors. It is divided into two categories: 1) inattention and 2) hyperactivity and impulsivity, that include behaviors such as failing to pay close attention to details, difficulty organizing tasks and activities, excessive talking, fidgeting, or an inability to remain seated in appropriate situations. It is associated with deficits in various executive functions. Typically developing young children improve over time in their ability to mobilize, direct, and sustain their attention, and ignore extraneous environmental stimuli. Children who are assumed to have normal vision, who forget what they have been taught, who have difficulties attending to tasks and working to completion, and who have additional difficulties organizing their approach across time and locations, may have ADHD. However, it is also possible that these observed behaviors are, in fact, reactive or adaptive responses to a visual impairment. Table 7.1 presents areas of potential overlap in behavioral characteristics between ADHD and CVI.

For example, one diagnostic criterion of ADHD reads "often fails to give close attention to details or makes careless mistakes in schoolwork, at work, or during other activities" (American Psychiatric Association, 2013, p. 59). These are behaviors that may also be exhibited by children with CVI. Similarly, low visual acuities and visual field impairments can affect children's ability to keep track of items, organize their approach, and detect and correct errors, while dorsal stream dysfunction can lead to difficulty splitting attention between multiple stimuli, as well as difficulty simultaneously looking and listening.

Children typically monitor their peers' nonverbal cues (such as how many classmates have their hands up) and those of their teacher (for example, "the look" that indicates that what a child is doing is not acceptable). When playing a game, they know when it is their turn by watching the movement of their peers' game pieces. ADHD, combined with impulsivity, presents difficulty for the child in waiting his or her turn. At the same time, children with CVI who have difficulty processing the visual scene can also miss these cues. These children may not see when it is their turn in a board game or discussion. Adults, not aware that the child has a problem seeing and processing the information, may remind the child to pay better attention, or ask, "Aren't you watching what is going on around you?" For the child, this can lead to embarrassment and, over time, lowered self-esteem or more marked reactions. Some children with CVI may also have ADHD, but regardless of the potential combination of conditions, the primary focus should be on understanding the full range of underlying causes and taking appropriate action.

## Developmental Dyslexia vs. Cerebral Visual Impairment

Reading involves many brain regions, including the visual, visual perceptual, and eye movement control areas, as well as the auditory processing and language systems.

TABLE 7.1

### Potential Overlap in Behavioral Characteristics between Attention Deficit/Hyperactivity Disorder and CVI

| *Diagnostic Label and Criteria: DSM–5 Criteria for ADHD 314*[a] | *Source of Similar Behaviors in Children with CVI* | *Explanation* |
|---|---|---|
| **A. A persistent pattern of inattention and/or hyperactivity-impulsivity that interferes with functioning or development as characterized by (1) and/or (2) below:**<br><br>1. Inattention: Six or more of the following symptoms have persisted for at least six months, to a degree that is inconsistent with developmental level and that negatively impacts social and academic/occupational activities. | | |
| Fails to give close attention to details or makes careless mistakes in schoolwork, work, or other activities | Difficulty splitting attention as part of dorsal stream dysfunction | Child may miss key visual and auditory information because of difficulty looking, listening, and shifting attention<br>Child has difficulty checking work if he or she is unable to shift visual attention |
| | Simultanagnosia | Child may miss visual information and is unable to correct mistakes that are not seen |
| | Hemianopia and other visual field impairments | Fatigue causes problems of sustained attention, with selective attentional deficits |

(continued on next page)

**TABLE 7.1** *(continued from previous page)*

| *Diagnostic Label and Criteria: DSM–5 Criteria for ADHD 314*[a] | *Source of Similar Behaviors in Children with CVI* | *Explanation* |
|---|---|---|
| Has difficulty sustaining attention in tasks or play activities | Visual field deficits | Child has difficulty attending to activities he cannot see |
| | Constricted visual fields | Child has a tendency to move head and eyes a lot to compensate |
| | Simultanagnosia | Child has difficulty attending and shifting attention as needed |
| | Visual fatigue | Child may have difficulty attending if he is fatigued |
| | Difficulty splitting attention as part of dorsal stream dysfunction | Child may have difficulty with multiple simultaneous demands involved in play or other tasks (e.g., looking, moving, shifting between visual, motor, social, and language demands) |
| | Impaired visual guidance of movement as a result of dorsal stream dysfunction | Child may appear "inattentive" owing to limited or no response, resulting from an inability to use vision to guide movements and respond to environmental and social demands |
| Appears not to listen when spoken to directly | Difficulty splitting attention as part of dorsal stream dysfunction | Child may not be able to look and listen at the same time |
| Does not follow through on instructions and fails to finish schoolwork, chores, or duties in the workplace (not resulting from oppositional behavior or failure to understand instructions) | Difficulty splitting attention as part of dorsal stream dysfunction | Child may not be able to look and listen at the same time |
| | Simultanagnosia | Child has difficulty with complex visual scenes (at near and at a distance) |
| | Visual field impairments | Child cannot finish a task that he does not see |
| | Ventral stream dysfunction | If specific steps are required to accomplish a task, the child may have difficulty completing them |
| Has trouble organizing tasks and activities | Inaccurate visually guided movements (related to dorsal stream dysfunction) | Child has difficulty organizing or taking direction because he is unable to follow a demonstration or use vision to accurately guide movement |
| | Simultanagnosia | Child has difficulty with visual clutter and shifting visual attention |
| | Visual field and acuity impairments | Child has difficulty organizing because he cannot see the objects |

*(continued on next page)*

**TABLE 7.1** *(continued from previous page)*

| *Diagnostic Label and Criteria: DSM–5 Criteria for ADHD 314*[a] | *Source of Similar Behaviors in Children with CVI* | *Explanation* |
|---|---|---|
| Avoids, dislikes, or is reluctant to engage in tasks that require sustained mental effort (e.g., schoolwork, homework, completing forms) | Cumulative effect of dorsal and/or ventral stream dysfunctions | A lot of effort is required to process visual information and cope with a mismatch between visual abilities and functions and the environment, resulting in significant fatigue and decreased visual function |
| Loses things necessary for tasks or activities (e.g., school materials, pencils, books, tools) | Low visual acuities<br>Simultanagnosia<br>Visual field impairments<br>Inaccurate visually guided movements (associated with dorsal stream dysfunction) | A child struggles to keep track of things if he has difficulty scanning his environment (at near and at a distance)<br>Organization is difficult if a child cannot use vision to guide organization and retrieval |
| Easily distracted by extraneous stimuli | Difficulty splitting attention as part of dorsal stream dysfunction | A child may be distracted by environmental sounds and may be "fixated" on something at the exclusion of the important stimuli as a result of difficulties shifting attention |
| Forgetful in daily activities (e.g., doing chores, running errands) | Dorsal and ventral stream dysfunctions | A child being "forgetful" may be associated with visual fatigue and difficulties splitting attention and recognizing location |
| **2.** Hyperactivity and impulsivity: Six or more of the following symptoms have persisted for at least six months, to a degree that is inconsistent with developmental level and that negatively impacts social and academic/occupational activities. | Children with CVI commonly have difficulty maintaining proactive behaviors as a result of limited attentional capacity | |
| Fidgets with hands or feet, or squirms in seat | May fidget, squirm | These movements may be related to associated features of brain abnormalities, such as cerebral palsy |
| Leaves seat when expected to remain in seat | Difficulty splitting attention as part of dorsal stream dysfunction<br>Dyskinetopsia | Child may incorrectly assume instruction has been completed, so she gets up<br>Child may miss teacher's nonverbal cues indicating when it is time to stand up |

*(continued on next page)*

**TABLE 7.1** *(continued from previous page)*

| *Diagnostic Label and Criteria: DSM–5 Criteria for ADHD 314*[a] | *Source of Similar Behaviors in Children with CVI* | *Explanation* |
|---|---|---|
| Runs about or climbs in situations where it is inappropriate (Note: adolescents and adults may feel restless) | Children with lower visual field impairment | Child may run, perhaps to get to the ground further ahead that she can see, while it is still in her subconscious memory |
| | Possible accompanying frontal pathology | Child has an inability to perceive risk |
| Unable to play or engage in leisure activities quietly | Difficulty splitting attention as part of dorsal stream dysfunction | Child has difficulty simultaneously regulating movements, vision, and affect |
| Appears "on the go" or acts as if "driven by a motor" (e.g., unable to be still for extended periods of time, as in restaurants, meetings) | Not a feature in children with CVI | |
| Is talkative | Difficulty splitting attention as part of dorsal stream dysfunction | Child may have trouble shifting attention between listening, looking, and engaging her motor system, and monitoring the reactions of the teacher or peers |
| | High functioning children with periventricular leukomalacia, causing reduced vision, can often become adept and frequent talkers[b] | Child may miss nonverbal cues from teachers or peers regarding verbalizations |
| Blurts out answers before a question has been completed | Frontal dysfunction associated with CVI | This condition can be associated with disinhibition |
| Has difficulty waiting his or her turn | Low visual acuities<br>Dyskinetopsia | Child may miss nonverbal cues from teachers or peers |
| | Simultanagnosia<br>Visual field impairment | Child may not be able to process the visual scene or materials to know when it is her turn in a board game or discussion |
| Interrupts or intrudes on others | Low visual acuity<br>Dyskinetopsia | Child may miss nonverbal cues from teachers or peers to know whether she is welcome or if there is an open space |
| | Simultanagnosia | Child may not be able to process the visual scene or materials to know when it is her turn in a board game or discussion |

*(continued on next page)*

**TABLE 7.1** *(continued from previous page)*

| *Diagnostic Label and Criteria: DSM–5 Criteria for ADHD 314*[a] | *Source of Similar Behaviors in Children with CVI* | *Explanation* |
|---|---|---|
| | Difficulty splitting attention as part of dorsal stream dysfunction | Child may not be able to look and listen, and so may blurt out a comment, fearing that she will forget what she wants to say; may have difficulties with social timing |

[a]*Additional criteria for ADHD diagnosis (314.0—attention deficit disorder in DSM–5):*

**I.** Several inattentive or hyperactive-impulsive symptoms were present prior to 12 years of age.

**II.** Several inattentive or hyperactive-impulsive symptoms are present in two or more settings (e.g., at home, school, work, with friends or relatives).

**III.** There is clear evidence that the symptoms interfere with, or reduce the quality of, social, academic, or occupational functioning.

**IV.** The symptoms do not occur exclusively during the course of schizophrenia or another psychotic disorder, and are not better explained by another mental disorder (e.g., mood disorder, anxiety disorder, dissociative disorder, personality disorder, substance intoxication, or withdrawal).

Specify whether:

**314.01 (F90.2) Combined presentation:** if both Criterion A1 (inattention) and Criterion A2 (hyperactivity-impulsivity) are met for the past 6 months

**314.00 (F90.0) Predominantly inattentive presentation:** if Criterion A1 is met but Criterion A2 is not met for the past 6 months

**314.01 (F90.1) Predominantly hyperactive-impulsive presentation:** if Criterion A2 is met but Criterion A1 is not met for the past 6 months

[b]The reason for the observation by the authors and their colleagues that some children with periventricular leukomalacia and poor vision can become competent frequent talkers is not known. Possible explanations can include the use of language as a way for young children with visual impairments to establish joint attention (Bigelow, 2003), or that these children show a lack of executive control (see Chapter 6). Use of language as a means of communication can be a strength to be capitalized upon and developed, particularly since a wide and meaningful vocabulary affords enhanced understanding for learning.

*Source*: American Psychiatric Association. (2013). *Diagnostic and statistical manual of mental disorders* (5th ed.). Washington, DC: Author.

Therefore, it is not surprising that children with CVI may struggle with reading. The challenge for service providers is to differentiate children whose impaired reading, spelling, and writing result from CVI from those with developmental dyslexia. (See Chapter 15 for an in-depth discussion of the processing systems involved in reading, math, and writing, as well as assessment and intervention.)

While developmental dyslexia may be a common cause of difficulty in reading, reading difficulties can also result from low visual acuities, refractive error, impaired accommodation, eye movement disorders, impaired visual fields, or perceptual visual impairment, all of which can contribute to CVI (Cavezian et al., 2010). Figure 7.2 illustrates how an acquired right hemianopic visual field defect can cause a child to miss the right-hand part of each viewed word as the eyes scan across the line of print (the visual field impairment moving with the eyes).

Features common to both dyslexia and CVI are presented in Table 7.2. (Note that this is not a detailed list of all features and findings associated with dyslexia, but rather a framework for beginning to consider some additional explanations for a child's difficulties in the area of reading.) Both children

TABLE 7.2

## Potential Overlap in Characteristics between Dyslexia and CVI

| *Diagnostic Label and Criteria: Dyslexia* | *Source of Similar Behaviors in Children with CVI* | *Explanation* |
|---|---|---|
| Poor decoding abilities | Ventral stream dysfunction<br>Alexia and anomias<br>Simultanagnosia | Poor information capture<br>Impaired naming of letters and words and of objects<br>Impaired recognition of letters and words<br>Difficulty with visual clutter |
| Difficulty with accurate and fluent word recognition, automatic recall of words, and visual images | Ventral stream dysfunction, anomias<br>Simultanagnosia<br>Visual field deficit or visual neglect on one side<br>Ocular motor dysfunction | Language center involved<br>Difficulty with crowded text, such as insufficient gaps between words and lines<br>Cannot read what is not evident<br>Impacts saccades |
| Poor spelling | Simultanagnosia<br>Visual field impairments<br>Dorsal stream dysfunction | Difficulty shifting attention between letters (when reading, learning, writing)<br>Difficulty encoding words and recognizing if letters are missing when writing or proofreading<br>Inaccuracy in visually guided movements may result in poor letter formation |
| Deficit in phonological component of language (Shaywitz, 2003) | Manifest slow auditory and attentional processing[a] | |
| Problems in reading comprehension | Low visual acuity<br>Visual field impairments<br>Visual fatigue<br>Ocular motor dysfunction<br>Ventral stream dysfunction<br>Simultanagnosia | Factors that contribute to reading fluency and accuracy will impact a child's ability to make sense of what he or she reads<br>Slow or hesitant reading resulting from visual difficulties leads to less time to learn reading skills |

[a]In the authors' experience, many children with profound CVI manifest slow auditory and attentional processing. This processing difficulty must be verified by slowing and chunking the presentation of elements of speech and noting if this makes a difference in children's ability to understand.

*Source:* International Dyslexia Association. (2008). Definition of dyslexia. Baltimore: Author. Retrieved from www.interdys.org/ewebeditpro5/upload/Definition.pdf; International Dyslexia Association. (2012). Dyslexia basics. Baltimore: Author. Retrieved October 14, 2014, from www.interdys.org/ewebeditpro5/upload/DyslexiaBasicsREVMay2012.pdf; International Dyslexia Association. (2014). *IDA dyslexia handbook: What every family should know.* Retrieved October 14, 2014, from www.interdys.org/ewebeditpro5/upload/IDADyslexiaHandbookWhatEveryFamilyShouldKnow.pdf

FIGURE 7.2

**Impact of a Right Hemianopic Visual Field Defect on Reading**

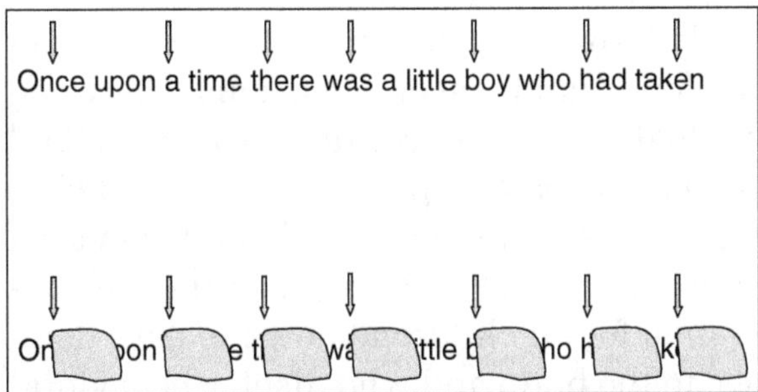


The vertical arrows indicate the position of the saccades (the movement of the eyes between fixation points), while the shapes superimposed on the bottom set of words simulate the visual field defect, which moves with the eyes as they scan across the line of print.

with dyslexia and those with CVI demonstrate difficulties with decoding text, but for different reasons. For children with CVI, low visual acuities and contrast sensitivities (frequently related to unrecognized refractive errors or poor focusing) can prolong the reading process. Ventral stream dysfunction with associated letter or shape agnosias, as well as deficits in form constancy, can lead to difficulties in letter and word recognition or "naming" of letters or words (*alexia*) (O'Hare, Dutton, Green, & Coull, 1998). Dorsal stream dysfunction can impair word finding and copying. Combinations of these difficulties impair word retrieval, decoding, fluency, and comprehension. In children with dyslexia, difficulties in decoding script result from weak connections between sound and symbol. There is also recent evidence that visual crowding of letters may also be a contributing factor (Callens, Whitney, Tops, & Brysbaert, 2013). In children with CVI, however, these difficulties result from problems seeing and visually decoding the printed material (Goldstein, 2011; Ramus et al., 2003; Shaywitz, 2003; Tallal, 2012). In addition, poor control of saccadic eye movements and eye tracking related to CVI can contribute to dysfluent reading. Poor spelling abilities are also common to both groups of children, but the approaches to teaching a child with dyslexia are different from those required to habilitate a child with a visual impairment (see Chapter 15).

If reading problems resulting from a visual impairment go undetected and are not addressed, these children may experience a sense of fatigue and failure, and feel misunderstood (Cavezian et al., 2010) as they progressively fall behind their peers. It is therefore important to seek a detailed history for dyslexia.

## Autism Spectrum Disorder vs. CVI

Cerebral visual impairment and autism spectrum disorder are both brain-based conditions that are complex and multifaceted in presentation. Neither can be fully characterized by objective tests such as EEGs, MRIs, or blood tests, and both can exhibit behavioral patterns typical of dorsal stream dysfunction (Das et al., 2007). Diagnoses for both conditions are founded on specific clusters of behaviors, as well as often complex medical and developmental histories.

Autism spectrum disorder is a neurodevelopmental disorder that can include disturbances in the areas of social interaction and communication, along with restricted, repetitive, and stereotyped patterns of behavior (including motor mannerisms), interests and activities, as well as rigid adherence to nonfunctional routines. Autism spectrum disorders are diagnosed on the basis of clusters of behaviors. It is therefore possible to consider behaviors typical of CVI, such as averting eye gaze, difficulties with social interaction, and stereotypic mannerisms, as being primarily related to autism spectrum disorder, rather than CVI.

The potential for overlap between CVI and autism spectrum disorders raises the question of whether a child who has behaviors that are characteristic of both disorders might have one of the following combinations of characteristics:

- Autism spectrum disorder with perceptual anomalies as an integral element
- Both autism spectrum disorder and CVI related to damage to the brain
- CVI with features resembling autism spectrum disorder

This type of ambiguity has led to the argument that a new classification warrants future consideration that provides a diagnostic code for cerebral dysfunction, with subcodes for each of the specific functions that are impaired, such as cerebral palsy and CVI (Jacobson, 2014).

The overlap in behaviors between CVI and autism spectrum disorder can potentially lead to different interpretations of behaviors, and even tensions between evaluation teams, service providers, and parents. A balanced approach is needed to ensure that potential visual and behavioral consequences of CVI are taken into consideration for all children known to have damage to the brain and who display behavioral features suggestive of autism spectrum disorder. Table 7.3 offers additional mapping for the diagnosis of childhood autism—based on the International Classification of Diseases (ICD–10; World Health Organization, 1992)—and indicates how a child with CVI may demonstrate similar behaviors.

It is important that the behaviors cited in Table 7.3 for considering a classification of

TABLE 7.3

## Potential Overlap in Behavioral Characteristics between Childhood Autism and CVI

| *Diagnostic Label and Criteria ICD–10 Criteria for Childhood Autism F84.0* | *Source of Similar Behaviors in Children with CVI* | *Explanation* |
|---|---|---|
| **Social Impairment**<br>Manifested in at least one of the following areas: | | |
| Failure to adequately use eye-to-eye gaze, facial expression, body posture, or gesture to regulate social interaction | Low visual acuities | Faces are not seen clearly beyond the maximum distance at which facial expressions can be seen and interpreted |
| | Delayed visual maturation | Possibly less opportunity at an early stage to learn language conveyed by facial expression and gesture (Guellai & Streri, 2011) |
| | Lower visual field impairment | Hand gestures in the blind area are not seen |
| | Prosopagnosia | Faces are not recognized, and expressions may not be either |

(continued on next page)

**TABLE 7.3** *(continued from previous page)*

| ***Diagnostic Label and Criteria ICD–10 Criteria for Childhood Autism F84.0*** | ***Source of Similar Behaviors in Children with CVI*** | ***Explanation*** |
|---|---|---|
| | Dyskinetopsia<br><br>Simultanagnosia (as part of dorsal stream dysfunction)<br>Difficulty splitting attention as part of dorsal stream dysfunction | Fast facial expressions and gestures are not seen<br>Person in a group or crowded scene may not be identified<br>May preclude looking at a face and listening at the same time |
| Failure to develop—in a manner appropriate to mental age, and despite ample opportunities—peer relationships that involve a mutual sharing of interests, activities, and emotions | Low visual acuities<br>Visual field deficits<br>Simultanagnosia<br>Prosopagnosia<br>Dyskinetopsia | All these visual deficits conspire to prevent a child's engagement with others, and learning how to interact socially using his or her vision |
| Lack of social-emotional reciprocity exhibited by an impaired or aberrant response to other people's emotions; lack of modulation of behavior according to social content; or a weak integration of social, emotional, and communicative behaviors | Poor vision resulting from any manifestation (poor visual acuity, simultanagnosia, dyskinetopsia, field restrictions, etc.) | Items that are not seen cannot be shown, brought, or pointed out; facial expressions that cannot be processed (to read or imitate) prevent a child from modulating or responding in kind, and affect verbal and nonverbal communication |
| **Communication Impairment**<br>Manifested in at least two of the following areas: | | |
| Delay in, or total lack of, the development of spoken language (not accompanied by an attempt to compensate through the use of gesture or mime as alternative modes of communication); often preceded by a lack of communicative babbling | Possible agnosias that may be associated with ventral stream dysfunction<br><br>Lower visual field impairment<br><br>Simultanagnosia (as part of dorsal stream dysfunction)<br><br>Left-sided cerebral damage | Impairment in the language area may impact word finding and retrieval<br><br>Hand gestures in the blind area are not seen<br><br>Difficult to develop a gesture if the child cannot observe and imitate it; cannot shift attention easily<br><br>Often accompanied by developmental language difficulties, right-sided motor impairment (hemiplegia), and mild right-sided inattention (hemianopia) |
| Relative failure to initiate or sustain conversational interchange (at present level of language skills), in which there is reciprocal responsiveness to the communications of the other person | Simultanagnosia | Difficulty arises if part of a conversation is dependent on tracking the nonverbal cues of the speaker and responding accordingly |

*(continued on next page)*

**TABLE 7.3** *(continued from previous page)*

| *Diagnostic Label and Criteria ICD–10 Criteria for Childhood Autism F84.0* | *Source of Similar Behaviors in Children with CVI* | *Explanation* |
|---|---|---|
| | Dyskinetopsia | Difficulty looking and listening at the same time |
| | Difficulty splitting attention (as part of dorsal stream dysfunction) | Children may experience difficulty with communication that exceeds the aural threshold |
| Stereotyped and repetitive use of language, or idiosyncratic use of words or phrases; abnormalities in pitch, stress, rate, rhythm, and intonation of speech | Delayed auditory and auditory attentional processing | Children with brain damage cannot process information at the rate that most people generate it (i.e., faster than their temporal thresholds can perceive it) Pedagogy in the field of visual impairment has historically suggested professionals "describe all the visual information that a child is missing by virtue of their limited sight," which may, in some instances, result in echolalia (automatic repetition of vocalizations spoken by another person) |
| **Restricted, Repetitive, and Stereotyped Patterns of Behavior, Interests, and Activities** | | |
| Preoccupation with one or more stereotyped and restricted patterns of interest that are abnormal in content or focus; or one or more interests that are abnormal in their intensity and circumscribed nature, although not abnormal in their content or focus | Simultanagnosia | If a child has difficulty with clutter and shifting attention from object to object, or taking in the whole field, the resulting behavior may be viewed as a "perseveration" |
| | Ventral stream dysfunction | If a child has trouble processing quickly moving visual information, it may be hard to encode different play scenarios or scenes that occur in real life, in books, or on TV, for use in pretend play |
| | Visual fatigue | Repetitive behaviors may also be associated with stress or fatigue |
| Compulsive adherence to specific, nonfunctional routines or rituals | Dorsal and ventral stream dysfunction<br>Balint's syndrome | If a child cannot use vision to guide movement, cannot shift attention to take in a whole scene and understand where objects and people are in relation to one another, and cannot see objects unless they are moving, the world may feel unpredictable and frightening to such an extent that a child will cling to something routine and predictable |

*(continued on next page)*

**TABLE 7.3** *(continued from previous page)*

| *Diagnostic Label and Criteria ICD–10 Criteria for Childhood Autism F84.0* | *Source of Similar Behaviors in Children with CVI* | *Explanation* |
|---|---|---|
| Need to keep possessions and furniture in the same fixed locations | Visual field deficits<br><br>Simultanagnosia<br>Optic ataxia | If objects are not in their fixed location, the child has a difficult time finding them<br>Impaired visual search<br>Increased risk of collision with furniture that has been moved |
| Stereotyped and repetitive motor mannerisms (e.g., hand or finger flapping or twisting, or complex whole-body movements) | | These repetitive behaviors may be seen in a number of children with cognitive, developmental, and neurological challenges; they are not specific to autism spectrum disorder |
| Persistent preoccupation with parts of objects or nonfunctional elements of play materials, such as odor, feel of the surface, or noise and vibration they generate | Simultanagnosia<br>Dorsal stream dysfunction<br><br>Lack of visual field | Difficulty shifting attention<br>Difficulty with visually guided movements<br>May not be aware of all the parts, or the relationship of the parts to the whole |
| Distress over changes in small, nonfunctional details of the environment | Ventral and dorsal stream dysfunction | When a child depends on the visual, physical, and aural world to follow predictable patterns and it does not, or there is cumulative stress and fatigue, small changes may result in larger than expected reactions |

*Source*: Based on World Health Organization. (1992). *International Statistical Classification of Diseases and Related Health Problems* (10th ed.). Geneva, Switzerland: Author.

CVI rather than autism spectrum disorder do not lead to dismissal of a diagnosis of autism spectrum disorders or result in the explaining away of behaviors (for example, eliminating them by attributing their presence to something else, or separating out the characteristics rather than looking at the cluster of characteristics present). It is appropriate to diagnose an autism spectrum disorder when a child with a visual impairment meets all of the criteria based on the presentation of a cluster of associated behaviors, rather than the presence of just one. Under these circumstances, CVI may be considered a contributory cause of the behaviors and may mean that the child meets the criteria for a dual diagnosis. In addition, it is important to avoid using descriptors such as "the child is exhibiting autistic-like behaviors" or "blindisms." Describing repetitive behaviors as "autistic-like" does not help clarify whether autism is suspected (in conjunction with the child demonstrating other characteristics) or whether shorthand is being used to describe repetitive behaviors. If the child is engaged in repetitive behaviors (such as flapping or spinning), they may be described as stereotypic, perseverative, or repetitive. To call these behaviors "blindisms" is also inaccurate, as such stereotypic behaviors are not only exhibited by children with visual impairments or autism (Cunningham & Schreibman, 2008). It is incumbent on all professionals to keep an open mind and maintain curiosity regarding observable patterns of responses (educational, visual, behavioral, social, communicative, etc.), and to consider any underlying brain-related causes that may lead to these manifestations.

A full review of the complexity of vision and visual processing in individuals with autism spectrum disorder is beyond the scope of this chapter. (See Simmons et al., 2009 for a detailed review.) However, given the challenge of teasing out whether an autism spectrum disorder is present—or whether observed behaviors relate to dysfunctional vision, or both—the following sections discuss in more detail the links between perception, particularly visual perception, social interaction as manifest in CVI and autism spectrum disorder, and the ways these conditions overlap.

### *Role of Vision in the Development of Social Interaction*

Social interaction in typical children involves the exchange of both verbal and visual information, expressed through body language, the eyes, and facial expressions. During early life, the visual system is recruited as an essential tool to interact with others. Visual communication and joint attention underpin the development of what is known as "theory of mind" (ToM) (Itier & Batty, 2009), which allows individuals to understand the behavior of others (Mitchell & Lacohée, 1991). Visual deficits resulting from CVI may interfere with the development of relationships, the skills needed to interact socially, as well as theory of mind (see Chapter 4), and thus may be a cause of disturbance in social interaction that might otherwise be diagnosed as autism spectrum disorder.

### *Visual and Visual Perceptual Disorders in Individuals with Autism Spectrum Disorder*

Visual and visual perceptual disorders are well defined in people with autism spectrum disorder, including abnormalities of visual acuity, contrast sensitivity, color discrimination, visual form processing, orienting attention, and disorders of oculomotor control (see Dakin & Frith, 2005; Milne, Griffiths, Buckley, & Scope, 2009; Simmons et al., 2009). Dorsal stream dysfunction has been raised as a possible contributing factor (Das et al., 2007; Macintyre-Béon et al., 2010). The ability to imitate others' actions may also be limited (Williams, Whiten, & Singh, 2004), which may be associated with impaired detection and analysis of visual motion, a disordered ability to interpret facial expressions, as well as difficulties judging socially acceptable distances for communication (Atkinson, 2000; Kaplan, 2006; Simmons et al., 2009). These visual disorders are also features of CVI (Chapter 3; Dutton & Bax, 2010).

Some people with autism spectrum disorder have superior perception of details with enhanced central visual functions (Kéïta, Mottron, & Bertone, 2010; Tavassoli, Latham, Bach, Dakin, & Baron-Cohen, 2011), but their integration of information across space may be limited (Shah & Frith, 1983). This capacity for detailed visual information processing may relate to the way visual attention is distributed (Robertson, Kravitz, Freyberg, Baron-Cohen, & Baker, 2013), the visual system maturing in a different way (Goodman & Ashby, 1990; Kaplan, 2006), disturbed visual processing (Evers et al., 2014), or possibly to a type of visual spatial neglect (Vakalopoulos, 2007).

### *Visual and Visual Perceptual Disorders Associated with CVI that May be Viewed as Indicative of Autism Spectrum Disorder*

CVI can impede attention, recognition, and exploration, interfering not only with learning, but also with global social and affective interaction with the external world. Visual perceptual problems can strain social interactions because they affect many aspects of communication and engagement.

The development of social relationships requires a child to read and use verbal and nonverbal cues, share interests, shift attention, and engage in various play behaviors, including sports, constructive play, and pretend play. Flexibility of thought and the ability to shift perspective are also needed. Imitative play requires the child to be able to observe, track, and shift gaze, as well as plan and execute motor performance. Make-believe play assumes that a child can imagine a scene, use an object to represent something else—such as using a wooden spoon to represent a magic wand—and actively respond to others' gestures and scripts, as well as attend to, and shift attention among, the features of the scene. Children with CVI may experience challenges in all these areas, leading them to exhibit behaviors similar to autism spectrum disorder. For example, the inability to identify a person in a group as a result of posterior parietal brain damage makes it difficult to engage with that person socially. Such limitations may also lead to a preoccupation with clearly visible parts of objects, such as brightly colored red or yellow knobs against a high-contrast background, and can lead to repetitive play or restricted interest as a reactive behavior. Difficulty finding possessions can lead to the adaptive behavior of lining them up or storing them in fixed locations. Interference with these strategies, for example when an adult tidies up, can lead to anxiety, or even anger on the part of the child.

Children with CVI may have difficulty recognizing and labeling objects, people, toys, locations, emotions, or actions. This makes it difficult to engage in joint or imitative play, or participate in a conversation about a referenced object.

Temporal lobe damage can lead to difficulty in recognizing faces (prosopagnosia) (see Chapter 3), making it challenging to differentiate people. Strangers can look the same as friends. The result may be that a child with impaired facial recognition copes by acting as if everyone is a friend, or on the contrary, the child does not react to family members and friends since he or she does not recognize them.

An alternative strategy for some children with CVI is to avoid being in groups. The inability to see the language of facial expression that can accompany prosopagnosia can further impede social engagement. An additional complication in the interpersonal world for children with CVI is that social interactions demand both visual and auditory attention, but giving simultaneous attention to both the face and voice can be difficult for children with dorsal stream dysfunction, which may contribute to the child not looking someone in the eye. All these behaviors can affect a child's friendships and may be interpreted as signs of autism spectrum disorder.

Children with autism spectrum disorder, as well as those with CVI, can experience weaknesses in processing and using language. For some, this may lead to stereotypical and repetitive use of language. Some children with CVI also have difficulties processing auditory signals (both verbal and environmental).

Visual processing problems may have such profound effects on social skills that some children with CVI have been diagnosed with Asperger syndrome, autism, or pervasive development disorder (PDD, prior to the DSM–5) because their visual problems caused them to miss social cues and struggle to make friends (see Chapter 23) (Freeman, 2010).

In the authors' experience, several patients have presented with features associated with autism, likely related to undiagnosed CVI. When the families of these children have understood and acted on the visual difficulties, and the children were provided with specific neurovisual habilitation (such as visual stimulation, detection, localization, pointing, and training to look into the blind visual field) and environmental modifications, a dramatic diminution of the "autistic" features was observed (see Chapter 21).

### *Dual Diagnosis of Autism Spectrum Disorder/CVI*

The behavioral features of autism spectrum disorder may lead to a primary diagnosis of autism spectrum disorder, despite the obvious presence of cerebral damage with clear features of CVI. Jambaqué, Mottron, Ponsot, & Chiron (1998) describe the case of a girl who, at 1 month of age, experienced epilepsy as a result of damage to the right temporo-occipital region of her brain. At 5 years, a left homonymous hemianopia and signs of left-sided neglect became evident. The right occipital lobe was removed at 7 years to treat the epilepsy. At 13 years, left homonymous hemianopia and a visual agnosia for objects and faces (prosopagnosia) were evident. She also had deficits of planning and mental flexibility. The results of the Autism Diagnosis Interview (Rutter, LeCouteur, & Lord, 2003) at the age of 4–5 years were positive for the diagnosis of autism. At that time, she showed wandering gaze, inability to point to objects or people, and little interest in interacting with others or playing with children of the same age. The authors suggested that her lack of interest and difficulties in interacting with others could be explained by her visual disorder, while her stereotyped and ritualized behavior could stem from a secondary disorder of executive function.

A dual diagnosis of autism spectrum disorder and CVI may be warranted in some cases when features of both conditions are present. As a result of overlapping areas of brain dysfunction, affected children may benefit from strategies used to address both neurodevelopmental challenges.

Given the complex link between perception and social interaction, there is a need to systematically screen children with social, intellectual, or behavioral disabilities for evidence of contributory visual disorders, particularly visual perceptual deficits. This is done in the hope that by appropriately managing the visual dysfunction, both at home and at school, it could prevent the development of features that could be suggestive of autism in at-risk children (Dammeyer, 2012; see Chapters 20–23).

### *Case Study: Ian*

**Ian, a 4-year-old boy, was referred for an evaluation** for a possible diagnosis of autism spectrum disorder. Ian was described as exhibiting "autistic-like" behaviors. His presentation included repetitive behaviors (such as flapping and hand posturing), as well as repetitive play and restricted interests. He perseverated on letters and numbers, and toys with letters and numbers, such as a toy cash register, microwave, and push-button alphabet toy, to the exclusion of anything else. He reportedly had difficulty communicating, relied on routines, and engaged in somewhat repetitive language. Ian's parents reported that he repeated a lot of what he heard and talked most often about letters and numbers.

At school, during group instruction in his physical education class, Ian would stand in the middle of the group and spin his body, pivoting on one foot. Staff noted that Ian had difficulty interacting with peers. He neither made eye contact, nor was he responsive to classmates' overtures to join them in play or when greeted. He was protective and somewhat possessive of his toys when his peers tried to touch them. Staff also noted some finger posturing (positioning his fingers in a nonfunctional manner) and facial grimacing. A review of his records revealed a medical diagnosis of periventricular leukomalacia (bilateral marked damage to the white matter surrounding the lateral ventricles in the brain) following a premature birth, complicated by stage 2 bleeding into the lateral ventricles, spastic diplegia with left hemiparesis, variable muscle tone, delayed motor milestones, binocular visual acuities estimated as 20/200 (or 6/60), mild myopic astigmatism corrected with glasses, variable esotropia, and mild optic nerve hypoplasia. The binocular visual field was not assessed, but it was thought to be "relatively full."

The psychologist spent three hours at Ian's home. Upon arrival, she observed him outside the house repeatedly sifting dirt through his fingers. Once inside, after his mother introduced Ian to the psychologist, he went to play on his musical keyboard. Shortly afterward, he invited the psychologist (referring to her by name) to come and watch him play his piano keyboard. Ian would strike a key and state, "This is the letter C, this is the letter D."

After about 20 minutes, Ian joined his mother and the psychologist at the table, sitting in a chair that provided excellent support for his feet, back, and arms, enabling him to be at eye level with the psychologist. He alternated between looking at a familiar book and spontaneously sharing information, again using the psychologist's name to gain her attention—for example, "Miss Betsy, I love bubbles"—puckering his lips as if to blow, making a puffing sound, and repeating, "I love bubbles." Later, he said, "Miss Betsy, I love dinosaurs," and shared the names of about eight of them; and still later, said the number "26." The psychologist asked if his mother thought he was trying to talk about his day at school, and she commented that, "Ian repeats everything." Despite his mother's report, the psychologist's impression was that Ian's comments were communicative and deliberate, since Ian gained attention by using the psychologist's name, shared something specific, invited her to join him at the keyboard, and used gestures. At school the next day, the teacher confirmed that the children had played with bubbles, had been studying dinosaurs all month, and that Ian's reference to "26" was the result of his being the "calendar boy" the day before on March 26. Ian had indeed been purposefully sharing information about his day at school!

The psychologist observed Ian in school, spoke to staff, and performed further assessments. Two staff members had suspected that Ian had an inability to recognize faces, and tested it by going into rooms other than where they worked with Ian. Ian could not identify either of them unless they spoke, despite their being within the requisite distance to recognize a face with his level of visual acuity. The nurse independently "tested" whether he could detect objects that were not moving. She stood perfectly still in the middle of the hallway one day, and he walked right into her. In the gym, seated among peers in a circle, Ian walked to the middle of the circle and pivoted repeatedly on one foot, almost oblivious to the children seated around him (perhaps suggesting a lower field deficit as well), but stopped and moved to retrieve a slow-moving ball that crossed his visual field.

Given Ian's love of letters and numbers, the psychologist wanted to examine how he dealt with letters and numbers that were cluttered rather than organized. Ian was given a cluster of

Scrabble letter tiles. He recognized they were letters, stating, "Let's find the letter M," which was among the eight tiles presented. However, he could not locate it until the tiles were lined up in a row with a space between each one. As noted earlier, Ian's preferred toys were a cash register and alphabet letter boards. This is not surprising since the keys on each toy are distinct (one letter or number per key, following a logical order). The toys in his classroom also had highly contrasting colors that made them stand out more and be more visible to Ian. Ian's love of letters served him well when changing between classrooms in the school hallway. He knew he had arrived at the correct room when he reached the wall that displayed rainbow paintings and each child's name in large block letters (which he could easily read) that were opposite his classroom.

The information collected at home and in school suggested that Ian was not on the autism spectrum, but rather had CVI (with low visual acuities, impaired perception of movement, possible lower visual field impairment, and dorsal and ventral stream dysfunctions; findings that were subsequently validated). Without the introduction of modifications and habilitation to address his visual perceptual and motor challenges, Ian would have continued to experience difficulties organizing and responding to the information within his world. Ian's repetitive behaviors (similar to children with autism spectrum disorder) may have served a coping function, a way to keep his environment the same (that is, predictable and consistent), or as a means of distraction. His propensity to move may improve his vision by enhancing his perception in the context of his apparent dyskinetopsia. It is likely that additional challenges will become evident as Ian's academic and social worlds expand beyond his preschool years, but recognition of the proper diagnosis will facilitate appropriate adaptations, interventions, and habilitation.

Teaching a child such as Ian, with a significant visual processing disorder, is markedly different from teaching a child with autism spectrum disorder alone. If he is not provided with resources and instruction appropriate to his condition, the outcome could be very different. For example, Ian's social development would likely be compromised, not as a consequence of autism spectrum disorder, but because his visual needs would not have been addressed to support and encourage his natural social interests. His family and school staff members were confused by his ability and interest in reading letters and numbers, while at the same time, failing to recognize faces or engage directly with familiar individuals. They also did not understand his limited interest in a variety of toys. Failing to identify, understand, and address each of Ian's visual needs would deprive him of the resources and adaptations he needs to thrive in the world around him.

In controlled, physically supportive, visually quiet settings, with clearly organized presentation of materials, Ian became interested in and engaged with others. Professionals and staff working with Ian needed to provide him with a means to communicate across settings. This was accomplished by providing him with specific objects that represented the activities he engaged in on a daily basis, along with written materials for family members engaging with him. Once his needs had been addressed, Ian was no longer viewed as a child with autism who repeated everything he heard.

## Consequences of Undetected Cerebral Visual Impairment

When a child's visual condition as the result of CVI goes undiagnosed or behaviors are misdiagnosed as the result of another condition, inappropriate intervention strategies may be used, and there may be negative effects on the child's academic and social progress, and psychological adjustment, as illustrated earlier in Figure 7.1.

## Inappropriate Habilitation Strategies

Misunderstanding the behaviors of a child with CVI can lead to inappropriate interventions rather than "best fit" interventions and support, such as those described in Chapters 19–24.

## Academic Attainment

A child with CVI whose condition goes undetected may experience significant difficulty reading, which is unlikely to be ameliorated if appropriate measures are not put in place (see Chapter 15).

## Social Attainment

Play is the universal language of children. Through play, children learn to problem solve, negotiate, and try out various roles, as well as to develop fine and gross motor skills. Children with undetected CVI face a multitude of social challenges in these areas. These children cannot play effectively because they may not be able to pick out a toy from a toy box, may struggle to get the attention of a particular child on the playground because they cannot locate them, and may not be able to read the facial expressions of other children. They have difficulty participating in sports and athletics because they may not be able to identify team members, use vision to guide movement, or track a ball moving at a fast speed, or generally move freely around a field or ball court. Children with CVI, who may perform inconsistently because of variability in what they see, may feel rejected as a result of behaviors that could have been prevented with a correct diagnosis and appropriate interventions.

## Psychological Reactions

There is little information about CVI in the psychological literature, and care must be taken when attributing a child's behavior to this condition without a "normative group" to serve as comparison for determining typical behavior (Freeman, 2010). Nevertheless, when there is a mismatch between a child's skills or abilities and the environment (or expectations of parents or teachers), a range of behavioral and psychological reactions is possible. It may be distressing for a child when he or she is experiencing difficulties whose sources are unknown and that go undetected by family members, teachers, or caregivers. In addition, the authors have seen a number of children with previously undiagnosed CVI who demonstrated a severe phobia for different objects or situations that may have been related to a misunderstanding of their visual environment. For example, a child may refuse to go to the toy store—or even get into a car to go to the store—despite loving certain toys, because he associates the car ride and toy store with the mall, which he found to be scary, confusing, and overwhelming. Or, a child may become fearful when certain reassuring landmarks are removed, such as a rainbow painting on the wall outside a classroom that helped her identify the classroom. In this case, the child might get lost in the hallway or assume she is being taken to a different room, so refuses to go into the room with the staff. (See Freeman [2010] and Chapter 23 of this text for a detailed discussion of this subject.)

## Conveying and Handling the Diagnosis of CVI

Professionals need to be aware that the reaction of the identified child and his or her parents to the diagnosis of CVI may vary, depending on whether this is a new diagnosis in a very young child, a change in diagnosis in an older child, or a new diagnosis later in a child's life. In the case of a new diagnosis in a young child, parents and interventionists may feel more in control because they now have a specific direction in which to go to further the child's social, cognitive, academic, motor, and visual development. For the older individuals (child, adolescent, young adult), a variety of reactions are possible. The older the individual is at the time of diagnosis, the more difficulties may have accumulated, and been reinforced and ingrained. Parents may feel a mixture of relief (at receiving an explanation), guilt (for not having recognized the difficulties earlier), and even blame (from their child, if the child had been treated as not trying hard enough). Professionals need to be understanding and supportive of the child and family during this challenging time (see Chapter 23 for an additional discussion).

## Conclusion

CVI may often go unidentified, and it is therefore crucial to recognize the telltale signs in order to set in motion the processes leading to formal identification and characterization of the condition through collaborative and comprehensive assessment. Without proper identification and intervention, children with CVI may struggle in the school system and fail to reach their full potential.

## References

American Psychiatric Association. (2013). *Diagnostic and statistical manual of mental disorders* (5th ed.). Washington, DC: Author.

Andersson, S. (2010). Visual dysfunction associated with hydrocephalus. In G. N. Dutton & M. Bax (Eds.), *Visual impairment in children due to damage to the brain* (pp. 35–40). London: Mac Keith Press.

Andersson, S., Persson, E. K., Aring, E., Lindquist, B., Dutton, G. N., & Hellström, A. (2006). Vision in children with hydrocephalus. *Developmental Medicine & Child Neurology, 48*(10), 836–841.

Atkinson, J. (2000). *The developing visual brain.* Oxford, UK: Oxford University Press.

Bax, M. C., Flodmark, O., & Tydeman, C. (2007). Definition and classification of cerebral palsy. From syndrome toward disease. *Developmental Medicine & Child Neurology Supplement, 109,* 39–41.

Bedwell, J. S., Chan, C. C., Cohen, O., Karbi, Y., Shamir, E., & Rassovsky, Y. (2013). The magnocellular visual pathway and facial emotion misattribution errors in schizophrenia. *Progress in Neuro-Psychopharmacology & Biological Psychiatry, 44,* 88–93.

Bigelow, A. E. (2003). The development of joint attention in blind infants. *Development and Psychopathology, 15,* 259–275.

Callens, M., Whitney, C., Tops, W., & Brysbaert, M. (2013). No deficiency in left-to-right processing of words in dyslexia but evidence for enhanced visual crowding. *Quarterly Journal of Experimental Psychology, 66*(9), 1803–1817.

Cavezian, C., Vilayphnh, M., de Agostini, M., Vasseur, V., Watier, L., Kazandjian, S., . . . Chokron, S. (2010). Assessment of visuo-attentional abilities in young children with or without visual disorder: Toward a systematic screening in the general population. *Research in Developmental Disabilities, 31*(5), 1102–1108.

Cavezian, C., Vilayphonh, M., Vasseur, V., Caputo, G., Laloum, L., & Chokron, S. (2013). Ophthalmic disorder may affect visuo-attentional performance in childhood. *Child Neuropsychology, 19*(3), 292–312.

Cunningham, A. B., & Schreibman, L. (2008). Stereotypy in autism: The importance of function. *Research in Autism Spectrum Disorders, 2*(3), 469–479.

Dakin, S., & Frith, U. (2005). Vagaries of visual perception in autism. *Neuron, 48*(3), 497–507.

Dammeyer, J. (2012). Children with Usher syndrome: Mental and behavioral disorders. *Behavioral and Brain Functions, 8,* 16.

Das, M., Bennett, D. M., & Dutton, G. N. (2007). Visual attention as an important visual function: An outline of manifestations, diagnosis and management of impaired visual attention. *British Journal of Ophthalmology, 91*(11), 1556–1560.

Dutton, G. N. (2013). The spectrum of cerebral visual impairment as a sequel to premature birth: An overview. *Documenta Ophthalmologica, 127*(1), 69–78.

Dutton, G. N., & Bax, M. (Eds.). (2010). *Visual impairment in children due to damage to the brain.* London: Mac Keith Press.

Dutton, G. N., Calvert, J., Ibrahim, H., MacDonald, E., McCulloch, D. L., Macintyre-Béon, C., et al. (2010). Structured clinical history taking for cognitive and perceptual visual dysfunction and for profound visual disabilities due to damage to the brain in children. In G. N. Dutton & M. Bax (Eds.), *Visual impairment in children due to damage to the brain* (pp. 117–128). London: Mac Keith Press.

Dutton, G. N., Saaed, A., Fahad, B., Fraser, R., McDaid, G., McDade, J., . . . Spowart, K. (2004). The association of binocular lower visual field impairment, impaired simultaneous perception, disordered visually guided motion and inaccurate saccades in children with cerebral visual dysfunction—A retrospective observational study. *Eye, 18,* 27–34.

Evers, K., Panis, S., Torfs, K., Steyaert, J., Noens, I., & Wagemans, J. (2014). Disturbed interplay between mid- and high-level vision in ASD? Evidence from a contour identification task with everyday objects. *Journal of Autism and Developmental Disorders, 44*(4), 801–815.

Fazzi, E., Bova, S. M., Uggetti, C., Signorini, S. G., Biahchi, P. E., Maraucci, I., & Lanzi, G. (2004). Visual-perceptual impairment in children with periventricular leukomalacia. *Brain & Development, 26*(8), 506–512.

Fazzi, E., Signorini, S. G., & Bianchi, P. E. (2010). Visual impairment in cerebral palsy. In G. N. Dutton & M. Bax (Eds.), *Visual impairment in children due to damage to the brain* (pp. 194–203). London: Mac Keith Press.

Freeman, R. D. (2010). Psychiatric considerations in cortical visual impairment. In G. N. Dutton & M. Bax (Eds.), *Visual impairment in children due to damage to the brain* (pp. 174–180). London: Mac Keith Press.

Goldstein, S. (2011). Attention-deficit/hyperactivity disorder. In S. Goldstein & C. Reynolds (Eds.), *Handbook of neurodevelopmental and genetic disorders in children* (2nd ed., pp. 131–150). New York: Guilford Press.

Goodman, R., & Ashby, L. (1990). Delayed visual maturation and autism. *Developmental Medicine & Child Neurology, 32*(9), 814–819.

Guellai, B., & Streri, A. (2011). Cues for early social skills: Direct gaze modulates newborns' recognition of talking faces. *PLoS One, 6*(4), e18610.

Houliston, M., Taguri, A., Dutton, G. N., Hajivassiliou, C., & Young, D. (1999). Evidence of cognitive visual problems in children with hydrocephalus: A structured clinical history-taking strategy. *Developmental Medicine & Child Neurology, 41*(5), 298–306.

International Dyslexia Association. (2008). Definition of dyslexia. Baltimore: Author. Retrieved from www.interdys.org/ewebeditpro5/upload/Definition.pdf

International Dyslexia Association. (2012). Dyslexia basics. Baltimore: Author. Retrieved October 14, 2014, from www.interdys.org/ewebeditpro5/upload/DyslexiaBasicsREVMay2012.pdf

International Dyslexia Association. (2014). *IDA dyslexia handbook: What every family should know.* Retrieved October 14, 2014, from www.interdys.org/ewebeditpro5/upload/IDADyslexiaHandbookWhatEveryFamilyShouldKnow.pdf

Itier, R. J., & Batty, M. (2009). Neural bases of eye and gaze processing: The core of social cognition. *Neuroscience & Biobehavioral Reviews, 33*(6), 843–863.

Jacobson, L. (2014). Cerebral dysfunction in children: Should this be the central tenet for a new system of classification? *Developmental Medicine & Child Neurology, 56*(2), 102.

Jacobson, L., & Dutton, G. N. (2000). Periventricular leucomalacia: An important cause of visual and ocular motility dysfunction in children. *Survey of Ophthalmology, 45*(1), 1–13.

Jambaqué, I., Mottron, L., Ponsot, G., & Chiron, C. (1998). Autism and visual agnosia in a child with right occipital lobectomy. *Journal of Neurology, Neurosurgery & Psychiatry, 65*(4), 555–560.

Kaplan, M. (2006). *Seeing through new eyes: Changing the lives of children with autism, Asperger syndrome and other developmental disabilities through vision therapy.* London: Jessica Kingsley Publishers.

Kéïta, L., Mottron, L., & Bertone, A. (2010). Far visual acuity is unremarkable in autism: Do we need to focus on crowding? *Autism Research, 3*(6), 333–341.

Macintyre-Béon, C., Ibrahim, H., Hay, S., Cockburn, D., Calvert, J., Dutton, G. N., et al. (2010). Dorsal stream dysfunction in children: A review and an approach to diagnosis and management. *Current Pediatric Reviews, 6*(3), 166–182.

Macintyre-Béon, C., Young, D., Dutton, G. N., Mitchell, K., Simpson, J., Loffler, G., et al. (2013). Cerebral visual dysfunction in prematurely-born children in mainstream school. *Documenta Ophthalmologica, 127*(2), 89–102.

Matsuba, C., & Soul, J. (2010). Clinical manifestations of cerebral visual impairment. In G. N. Dutton & M. Bax (Eds.), *Visual impairment in children due to damage to the brain* (pp. 41–49). London: Mac Keith Press.

McKillop, E., Bennett, D., McDaid, G., Holland, B., Smith, G., Spowart, K., et al. (2006). Problems experienced by children with cognitive visual dysfunction due to cerebral visual impairment—And the approaches which parents have adopted to deal with these problems. *British Journal of Visual Impairment, 24*(3), 121–127.

McKillop, E., & Dutton, G. N. (2008). Impairment of vision in children due to damage to the brain: A practical approach. *British & Irish Orthoptic Journal, 5*, 8–14.

Milne, E., Griffiths, H., Buckley, D., & Scope, A. (2009). Vision in children and adolescents with autistic spectrum disorder: Evidence for reduced convergence. *Journal of Autism and Developmental Disorders, 39*(7), 965–975.

Mitchell, P., & Lacohée, H. (1991). Children's early understanding of false belief. *Cognition, 39*(2), 107–127.

O'Hare, A. E., Dutton, G. N., Green, D., & Coull, R. (1998). Evolution of a form of pure alexia without agraphia in a child sustaining occipital lobe infarction at 2 1/2 years. *Developmental Medicine & Child Neurology, 40*(6), 417–420.

Ramus, F., Rosen, S., Dakin, S. C., Day, B. L., Castellote, J. M., White, S., et al. (2003). Theories of developmental dyslexia: Insights from a multiple case study of dyslexic adults. *Brain, 126*(4), 841–865.

Robertson, C. E., Kravitz, D. J., Freyberg, J., Baron-Cohen, S., & Baker, C. (2013). Tunnel vision: Sharper gradient of spatial attention in autism. *Journal of Neuroscience, 33*(16), 6776–6781.

Rosenbaum, P., Paneth, N., Leviton, A., Goldstein, M., Bax, M., Damiano, D., . . . Jacobsson, B. (2007). A report: The definition and classification of cerebral palsy April 2006. *Developmental Medicine & Child Neurology, 46*(Suppl. 109), 8–14.

Rutter, M., LeCouteur, A., & Lord, C. (2003). *Autism diagnostic interview, revised.* Torrance, CA: WPS.

Saidkasimova, S., Bennett, D. M., Butler, S., & Dutton, G. N. (2007). Cognitive visual impairment with good visual acuity in children with posterior periventricular white matter injury: A series of 7 cases. *Journal of American Association for Pediatric Ophthalmology and Strabismus, 11*(5), 426–430.

Shah, A., & Frith, U. (1983). An islet of ability in autistic children: A research note. *Journal of Child Psychology and Psychiatry, 24*(4), 613–620.

Shaywitz, S. (2003). *Overcoming dyslexia: A new and complete science-based program for reading problems at any level.* New York: Alfred A. Knopf.

Simmons, D. R., Robertson, A. E., McKay, L. S., Toal, E., McAleer, P., & Pollick, F. E. (2009). Vision in autism spectrum disorders. *Vision Research, 49*(22), 2705–2739.

Stiers, P., De Cock, P., & Vandenbussche, E. (1999). Separating visual perception and non-verbal intelligence in children with early brain injury. *Brain & Development, 21*(6), 397–406.

Tallal, P. (2012). Neuroscience, phonology and reading: The oral to written language continuum [Online interview]. Retrieved from http://www.childrenofthecode.org/interviews/tallal.htm

Tavassoli, T., Latham, K., Bach, M., Dakin, S. C., & Baron-Cohen, S. (2011). Psychophysical measures of visual acuity in autism spectrum conditions. *Vision Research, 51*(15), 1778–1780.

Vakalopoulos, C. (2007). Unilateral neglect: A theory of proprioceptive space of a stimulus as determined by the cerebellar component of motor efference copy (and is autism a special case of neglect). *Medical Hypotheses, 68*(3), 574–600.

Whiting, S., Jan, J. E., Wong, P. K., Flodmark, O., Farrell, K., & McCormick, A. Q. (1985). Permanent cortical visual impairment in children. *Developmental Medicine & Child Neurology, 27*(6), 730–739.

Williams, C., Northstone, K., Sabates, R., Feinstein, L., Edmond A., & Dutton, G. N. (2011). Visual perceptual difficulties and under-achievement at school in a large community-based sample of children. *PLoS One, 6*(3), e14772.

Williams, J. H. G, Whiten, A., & Singh, T. (2004). A systematic review of action imitation in autistic spectrum disorder. *Journal of Autism and Developmental Disorders, 34*(3), 285–299.

World Health Organization. (1992). *International statistical classification of diseases and related health problems* (10th ed.). Geneva, Switzerland: Author.

# PART II

## Related Visual Issues

# 8

# Eye Movement Disorders in Children with Cerebral Visual Impairment

*Gordon N. Dutton*

A range of eye movement disorders commonly accompanies cerebral visual impairment (CVI) in children (Salati, Borgatti, Giammari, & Jacobson, 2002). This chapter describes these conditions and the ways in which they may contribute to the overall visual impairment. The greater the degree of visual impairment, the more frequently these disorders are observed and the greater their severity. Children who also have cerebral palsy are more likely to be affected. These disorders are a concern because if a child's eyes cannot be held steady to look at a target, or if the eyes cannot move to look toward a new event or follow a moving target, then that child is likely to miss out on what is happening around him or her.

The medical diagnosis of an eye movement disorder entails an understanding of the brain systems that bring about eye movements, as well as characterization of the site, and possible cause of, any disorder. However, it is important for caregivers and teachers of children with CVI to be able to observe eye movement disorders, and to recognize and understand the potential impact these may have upon the ability to see, so that appropriate accommodations can be made. This chapter describes a number of conditions related to disorders of eye movement, including how to recognize them and specific considerations in working with children experiencing these conditions.

## Misalignment of the Eyes: Strabismus

In *strabismus,* also referred to as *squint,* one eye is looking straight ahead, while the other eye is pointing in a different direction. If the child is able to choose to look with either eye, then the vision in each eye is likely to be equal. However, if one eye is constantly turned and not used to look as much as the other eye, it is likely to have poorer vision.

A major benefit of having two eyes is that the slightly different pictures they form in the mind are combined to afford a sense of three dimensions. This has been recognized since Victorian times, when pictures from two horizontally separated cameras focused on the same target provided graphic three-dimensionality when viewed separately by the two eyes.

The ability to see in three dimensions involves several processes or mechanisms, only one of which, stereopsis, is impaired by strabismus:

- ***Stereopsis:*** Steropsis is the innate capacity to see in three dimensions brought about by the disparity between the pictures provided by both eyes being computed by the brain as a percept of depth. It results in fine depth perception.
- ***Parallax:*** Parallax refers to the perception of the relative alignment of objects in relation to the position of viewing. When the forefinger of each hand is held up, one in front of the other in front of you, and the head is moved from side to side, the apparent movement of the fingers tells the viewer which one is in front. This relative movement of targets is a major clue to their relative distance away from the viewer. This viewing strategy can compensate for lack of stereopsis.
- ***Size:*** The further away things are, the smaller they appear. The knowledge of what size they should be at different distances contributes to overall three-dimensional perception.
- ***Moving targets:*** The relative position of moving targets as they move with respect to the environment indicates their distance away.

Misalignment of the eyes is common in children with CVI. Most commonly the eyes are misaligned horizontally. When the eyes are turned in, this is called convergent strabismus or *esotropia*. When they are turned out, this is called divergent strabismus or *exotropia*. Both these types of strabismus can be constant or intermittent, but when the eyes are misaligned in this way, the affected person does not have stereopsis.

Strabismus that occurs during late childhood or adulthood commonly causes double vision. Early-onset strabismus, on the other hand, does not cause double vision because the developing brain ignores the central part of the picture coming from the deviated eye and mentally realigns the periphery of the picture from that eye, as if it were looking straight ahead. For some, when the nondeviated eye is covered, the ignored central image is immediately switched on in the deviating eye, which realigns itself (while the eye that is covered becomes misaligned instead). For others, however, the effect of turning off the picture becomes permanent, and central vision becomes impaired even when the "good" eye is covered. This poor vision in the strabismic (misaligned) eye has no obvious cause that can be found when the eye is examined, and is called *amblyopia*.

Amblyopia is usually treated in young children, typically under the age of 7 years, by covering (or occluding) the good eye. Spectacles need to be worn by many children with strabismus because they play a major part in helping to realign the eyes. Children with CVI who have a persistent turn in the eye (strabismus or squint) despite wearing a patch and spectacles, may benefit from surgery to correct the misalignment. Often, though, strabismus surgery is deferred because in some children with cerebral damage, the angle of strabismus can diminish or the strabismus can even reverse on its own, from turning in to turning out, or vice versa.

The following are some issues for caregivers and teachers to bear in mind with regard to strabismus:

- Lack of stereopsis means that fine hand-eye coordination tasks are difficult because subtle differences in depth cannot be seen, and the child appears to be clumsy. Recognition that the ability to guide hand movement is only impaired in depth, but not in the transverse plane (going from side to side), means that children can be taught alternative methods to accomplish certain tasks, for example, to thread a needle by viewing the eye of the needle directly and inserting the thread by forward movement. However, if the task is carried out in the usual way, with the eye of the needle viewed from the side, depth perception is required, and the task becomes much more difficult.
- Two automatic actions allow the eyes to see a single clear image of a nearby target. The lenses in the eyes become more convex (this is called *accommodation*), and the eyes turn in, or converge, to look at the target. In children who are farsighted (hyperopic or long-sighted), the eyes compensate by focusing, and in some, especially those with damage to the brain, this extra accommodation is accompanied by associated turning in of the eyes (convergent strabismus). Correcting the hyperopia with spectacles diminishes or eliminates the convergence. Similarly, nearsightedness (myopia or short-sightedness) in children with CVI can be associated with divergent strabismus. Spectacle wear for myopia also helps correct misalignment of the eye in such cases.
- The development of optimal vision requires the eyes to focus well to produce clear images in the eyes, and for the eyes to be aligned. Poor image clarity and lack of eye alignment can result in impaired visual development for affected eyes. This is known as amblyopia. Treatment includes appropriate spectacle wear and patching of the better eye.
- When spectacle wear and patching are implemented in a child with strabismus, it is important that spectacles are worn at all times, and patching is carried out as prescribed, if optimal visual correction is to be achieved.
- When an eye is turned out, the field of view is widened, but when the eye is turned in, it is narrowed. (Such narrowing of the visual field resulting from convergent strabismus can lead, for example, to a child with cerebral palsy being startled by someone approaching from the side affected by the strabismus, because they appear to pop into view. This observation may influence where such a child is positioned in a classroom.)

## Deviations of Both Eyes in One Direction

Another type of eye movement disorder involves both eyes turned in the same direction. The deviation can be constant (*tonic*) or intermittent (*paroxysmal*).

### Constant, or Tonic, Deviations

In children with tonic deviations, both eyes, and often the head as well, are constantly turned in the same direction—to the left, right, up, or down. The eyes may be constantly turned in one direction in children with extensive damage to the brain, which usually causes both cerebral palsy and CVI. The eyes can be deviated horizontally or vertically. When the eyes, and often the head as well, are constantly turned to the left or to the right, it usually results from damage to the front of the brain on the same side toward which the eyes are turned, while weakness of the body (resulting from cerebral palsy) is greater on the opposite side. Gradual improvement tends to take place.

Tonic downward deviation of the eyes is more commonly seen in children with cerebral palsy in association with premature birth, but the condition slowly improves in the majority of cases (Yokochi, 1991).

Rarely, if ever, are the eyes turned by an individual as a coping mechanism with the intention of seeing better, as the deviation of the eyes is a disorder of eye movement, not an intentional or adaptive strategy.

The following are some issues for caregivers and teachers to bear in mind with regard to tonic deviation:

- When giving a child one-to-one attention, it is best done from the side of the head that is turned toward the caregiver or teacher, since it is easier for the child to see the person, and attention tends to be better on that side as well.
- When teaching in a group, the child with horizontally deviated eyes needs to sit so that the head and eyes are looking toward the focus of attention.
- For prolonged, involuntary (tonic) downward deviation of the eyes, the focus of attention is again best placed in the direction of view.
- Children with tonic deviation commonly have additional significant dorsal stream dysfunction (see Chapter 3), therefore removing clutter and pattern, combined with affording optimal comfort and diminishing background sound, serves to optimize attention in many cases.

## Intermittent, or Paroxysmal, Deviations

In intermittent (paroxysmal) deviation, both eyes turn together in one direction for a variable duration, often with an accompanying head turn.

Children whose CVI is associated with cerebral palsy severe enough to necessitate the use of a wheelchair commonly experience intermittent involuntary rapid-onset head and eye movements. They are commonly upward and to one side, and interfere with the capacity to use vision both to access information and to communicate. On the other hand, some children with quadriplegic cerebral palsy, who are cognitively intact but have involuntary, "dyskinetic" (jerky) body movements, may have remarkably good vision when given a structured opportunity to demonstrate their abilities. In the author's experience, a small proportion of such children are thought to have poor vision and limited comprehension, but when their communication methods are put to the test, they function much better than anyone had anticipated. They may not even have any additional visual difficulties apart from not being able to capture information when precluded from doing so by their paroxysmal involuntary head and eye movements.

The following are issues for caregivers and teachers to bear in mind with respect to intermittent (paroxysmal) deviation:

- Vision is limited during paroxysmal head and eye movements.
- Some children with dyskinetic cerebral palsy, which can include these head and eye movements, may have very limited

opportunity for communication, but may be seeing and functioning at significantly higher levels than thought (although the parents of these children usually recognize this inner capability).

## To and Fro Movement of the Eyes: Nystagmus

In nystagmus, both eyes are constantly moving to and fro in harmony. The movements may resemble a pendulum (*pendular nystagmus*), or take place quickly in one direction and slowly in the other (*jerk nystagmus*).

To-and-fro oscillatory movement of the eyes, or nystagmus, can occur in children whose CVI results from periventricular white matter damage (Jacobson & Dutton, 2000) or maternal drug abuse during pregnancy (Hamilton et al., 2010). Nystagmus is also seen in children who have very low or no vision as a result of damage to the eyes or optic nerves. In children with damage to the brain, this type of nystagmus is associated with additional damage to the optic nerves, rendering them very small (*optic nerve hypoplasia).* Visual acuities are degraded by the eye movements, which are more pronounced when looking into the distance than when looking at objects nearby. This means that the distance visual acuity is commonly worse than the near visual acuity.

The following are issues for caregivers and teachers to bear in mind with regard to nystagmus:

- There is commonly an eye position in which nystagmus is minimized (called the null point); a particular head position may facilitate achieving the null point and minimizing the nystagmus in order to attain clearer vision. Therefore, children with nystagmus should not be told to straighten their heads, because they are optimizing their vision by the head turn, especially when viewing details.
- The use of digital cameras and iPad-type devices with built-in cameras enables distant images to be seen up close. Since people with nystagmus have better near vision, images in the distance can be focused upon and even enlarged so that the child does not miss out when viewing distant events, like team sports or animals in the zoo. (Pictures can also be taken for the child to review the experience.)

## Difficulty Keeping the Eyes Steady: Impaired Fixation

In children with impaired fixation, the eyes do not stay on target for long and drift off to look in another direction in a manner that appears aimless, since the eyes do not appear to be looking at a particular target.

The ability to keep the eyes steady and on target requires the visual system to provide the requisite level of vision and that all the computing systems in the brain keep the eyes steady despite head and body movement; all must be intact and functioning normally. It is, therefore, not surprising that some children with CVI are unable to maintain steady fixation upon a visual target, and their gaze moves or drifts off target, requiring the eyes to readjust. Part of the assessment of the child with CVI is to look closely at the eyes of the child while testing near visual acuity, to check whether gaze is maintained or whether fixation is impaired because of difficulty keeping the eyes steady.

The following are issues for caregivers and teachers to bear in mind with respect to impaired fixation:

- Children with impaired fixation need more time to carry out tasks that require prolonged effort at near.
- Apparent lack of attention can, in fact, be a result of difficulty maintaining fixation or can be due to eccentric viewing (also known as eccentric fixation), described later in this chapter.

## Difficulty Turning the Eyes in to Look at Something Close: Impaired Convergence

When looking at a nearby object, the eyes typically turn in (known as *convergence*), so that both eyes receive almost the same picture (the small horizontal disparity between the images produces stereo perception). As an associated condition, many children with CVI experience impairment of the ability to turn the eyes inward. This can be observed when a visual target is brought toward a child's eyes and the child attempts to follow the approaching target, but the eyes do not turn in in the normal way. Either the eyes do not turn in at all, or they begin to turn in, but one eye then drifts out as the target is brought closer. (This can be seen normally when a target is closer than about 2½ inches [6 cm]). Impaired convergence of the eyes may also be accompanied by impaired focusing of the eyes, referred to as lack of accommodation.

The following are issues for caregivers and teachers to bear in mind with regard to impaired convergence:

- If the child appears to see better in the distance than at near, there may well be poor focusing for near (accommodation), usually accompanied by a diminished ability to turn the eyes in to look at a nearby target, like a pencil or a picture up close.
- Lack of ability to turn the eyes in is often accompanied by poor constriction of the pupils of the eyes when looking at a near target. This too needs to be observed in any child whose near vision is suspected as being poor.
- All children with CVI need to have an assessment of focusing (or accommodation) (Saunders, Little, McClelland, & Jackson, 2010) as part of their vision test for eyeglasses. This is not routinely carried out in children and needs to be requested for any child who:
    - does not see well at near
    - does not converge his or her eyes well, or
    - has poor pupil constriction for a near target (Saunders, McClelland, Richardson, & Stevenson, 2008).

## Disorders of Fast Eye Movement: Disorders of Saccades

The eyes are constantly making small, fast movements to look at new aspects of the visual scene. (The mind takes in the resultant series of scenes, and blends them together to give the sensation of visual continuity.) Larger fast eye movements are also made when our attention is caught by something of interest and our eyes rapidly move to look. We can also choose to move our eyes by fast eye movements in any direction. These fast eye movements are called *reflex saccades* and *voluntary saccades,* respectively.

If a finger is first held up with one hand in front of a child's eyes, then a toy is held up to the side with the other hand, rapid (saccadic) movement of the eyes from the finger to the toy usually takes place. This can be done for left, right, upward, and downward eye movements. Failure of movement may be a result of a target being located in a non-seeing area of the visual field (visual field defect), or may be a result of disordered saccades. Consistent incomplete movements, accompanied by an extra jerk as the eyes move toward a target, are common in children with CVI.

The most common disorder of saccades is that they are not sufficient to get to the target in one move; therefore, a smaller, second "catch up" saccade is needed, thus slightly prolonging the time it takes to gain and give attention to a new target.

Another disorder of saccades is a difficulty making saccades at all, known as *saccadic initiation failure,* with the most common form called *oculomotor apraxia* (also known as Cogan's oculomotor apraxia). It is usually thought to be associated with an abnormality of the cerebellum, which sorts out the timing of actions and thoughts (Schmahmann, 2010). Oculomotor apraxia is not currently considered to be a form of CVI. However, some children with cerebral palsy and CVI also have anomalies in the cerebellum, which can interfere with the generation of fast eye movements. Affected children often carry out intermittent rapid shakes of the head. These rapid shakes are thought to recenter the eyes by using the automatic balance system.

The following are issues for caregivers and teachers to bear in mind with respect to saccades:

- Difficulty in generating fast eye movements can interfere with the capacity to shift attention from one thing to another, particularly when witnessing fast-moving events like team sports, with the affected children missing key elements because they are unable to keep up with the events.
- Children with intermittent rapid head-shakes may have saccadic initiation failure as part of the clinical picture.

## Disorders of Eye Movements to Follow a Target: Impaired Pursuit

Lack of ability to pursue a target with the eyes usually means that visual acuity or visual attention is poor. However, if a target can be pursued with the eyes when moving to the left, but not when moving to the right, and this behavior is consistent and vision is adequate, then the child probably has impaired visual pursuit. If a moving target is followed poorly, then instead of the eye movements being smooth, they are broken up with intermittent, small, fast eye movements of "catch up" saccades.

The ability to follow a moving target with the eyes is a remarkable process. First, a moving target, such as a car, is perceived in the occipital lobes. It is located within the three-dimensional virtual map of the surroundings provided by the posterior parietal lobes. This map provides the location for the eyes to move to. Next, a smooth pursuing set of eye movements is generated by processing systems in the lower part of the brain that send out a message along 6 nerves, to the 12 muscles that move the eyes to the target. The whole process takes place with almost no delay, and is facilitated by predictive systems that estimate where the car will move next. This allows the eyes to lock on and follow the target, accompanied by matching head movements. It is a truly remarkable piece of "engineering," but with such complexity, it is not surprising that this system can also be dysfunctional.

If one occipital lobe is damaged, and this damage extends into the parietal lobe, then pursuit eye movements to the same side as the damage can be impaired. Jerky pursuit eye movements are observed if the damage is not extensive, but the movement can be absent in more severe (but rare) cases.

The following are issues for caregivers and teachers to bear in mind with regard to impaired pursuit:

- Jerky pursuit eye movements may not have a significant impact on perception, but this has yet to be studied.
- Absent pursuit eye movement in one horizontal direction may sometimes accompany lack of vision in the other direction (hemianopia). This means that the affected child is not able to see on one side, as well as unable to follow moving targets in the other direction. When working with an affected child, teachers and caregivers are best positioned on the sighted side, but they also need to recognize that the child is unable to pursue targets moving toward the side where they are sitting. Vertical eye movements tend to be intact, and this is the facility to use if eye pointing is required as a means of communication.

## Impairment of Eye Movements for Reading: Visual Tracking

Although tracking generally applies to maintaining fixation on a moving object, it is also commonly used to refer to the jerky eye movements used to move along a line of print when reading, known as saccadic movements. A more specific term to describe saccadic eye movements along a line of print is *tracing* (Lueck, 2004). In typical readers, the eyes flick across the text with 4 or 5 flicks per line, they then give a single fast flick back to the beginning of the next line. Some children with CVI who are able to learn to read have difficulties harmonizing eye movements with the act of reading, or they have disordered pursuit, disordered saccadic eye movements, or both. If one holds a chosen text up in front of them while looking at the child's eyes as he or she is reading, their eye movements may appear to stutter, often with a number of return movements. The child with impaired visual tracking tends to make a number of return movements, as if wanting to look back at a word again.

Printed material on a transparent overhead projector sheet, held so that a child sees the print against a plain background and the observer can also see the child's eyes as they move across the page, can help the observer see whether the eyes are moving in harmony with the words being read (Hyvärinen & Jacob, 2011). If this is not available, watching from behind the book the child is reading can also provide a good observation.

There is a wide array of literature on the subject of eye movements and reading difficulties in academically able children, with the main question concerning "the chicken and the egg." That is, it is difficult to know whether "stuttering" eye movements lead to hesitant reading, or whether the reverse is the case, in which reading difficulty leads to apparent faulty eye movements as the eyes return to words that have been difficult to decode or understand.

The following are issues for caregivers and teachers to bear in mind with respect to visual tracking:

- If the eyes are not tracking well while reading, enlarge the words to be at least twice the measured visual acuity, space the words further apart, separate the lines, remove peripheral clutter, and try again. If the eyes start to track normally, and this is accompanied by improvement in reading, it is likely that the cause is visual crowding rather than a motor eye movement problem.
- As demonstrated throughout this chapter, there are many ways in which eye movements may be impaired, and many of these can affect a child's ability to read. If the disorders of eye movement are severe, consideration could be given to using software programs which present words sequentially on a computer screen, thereby eliminating the eye movement disorder from being a barrier to accessing the information (see Chapter 18). It is important to recognize that although such software may be marketed to increase reading speed (because eye movements present a major rate limiting factor to access the printed word), a considerable amount of training time is needed. Without necessary training, this reading technique will be considered inadequate, which could well be a lost opportunity.

## Disorders of Attention and Their Effect on Eye Movements: Apraxia of Gaze

*Apraxia* is the inability to execute learned purposeful movements, and *apraxia of gaze* refers to inability or difficulty in moving the eyes from one visual target to another. This disorder of eye movement is a result of bilateral damage to the posterior parietal (dorsal stream) area of the brain. It is associated with simultanagnostic visual dysfunction and impaired visual guidance of movement (optic ataxia).

The condition may be identified by asking the child with CVI to look at different large, clear targets (whose locations are not already known) around the room. Children with apraxia of gaze are likely to accomplish this task for only a small percentage of the targets within their intact field of vision. Performance tends to be worse when the child is tired (see Chapter 3). The combination of apraxia of gaze and simultanagnosia limits the number of entities that can be attended to and seen at once, thus impairing visual search (discussed in Chapter 6) and visual attention. In its severe form (Balint's syndrome), bilateral posterior parietal brain damage also results in severe inability to use vision to guide movement (despite intact stereopsis in some cases), accompanied by the disability of only being able to be aware of and identify a very limited number of items at once. Although eye movements are intact, the eyes can only move from one item that the individual has seen to another. This may be the cause of inability to elect to move the eyes from one visual target to another, despite the potential for normal eye movements that can be seen when the affected person is simply asked to move the eyes in different directions. (This condition was first called psychic paralysis of gaze [Rizzo & Vecera, 2002].) Despite having the motor capacity to do so, the affected person cannot move his or her eyes to something that has not been registered, because there is insufficient image processing capacity in the mind to handle all the visual information in the surroundings (i.e., simultanagnosia).

The following are issues for caregivers and teachers to bear in mind with regard to apraxia of gaze:

- If a child who is looking at a single object on a desk is unable to look across at something else, but is able to do so when the object on the desk is removed and there is nothing on the desk, it suggests that the child could have simultanagnostic visual difficulties. Children with this condition may also be unable to move their eyes from one item to another (especially when there is clutter), as a result of their accompanying apraxia of gaze, despite having normal eye movements when they are asked to follow a moving target or to look from one item to another when there is a plain background and no clutter. They are unable to find things easily and may be clumsy because of impaired visual guidance of movement. In the author's experience, taking the actions recommended for developmental simultanagnostic visual dysfunction is likely to reap dividends. (See Table 19.4 for suggested interventions.)

## Looking to the Side: Eccentric Viewing

In *eccentric viewing,* the child looks away to the side when reaching for things or talking to people. Instead of looking directly at what is being picked up, the arm reaches out to the side to pick up the object, and instead of looking people in the eye when talking to them, the child may look upward and to the side. This is a common characteristic of children with CVI that many parents and professionals are likely to recognize.

The cause of this behavior is unknown, but in most cases, it is accompanied by evidence of dorsal stream dysfunction. Therefore, it is possible that the "wiring" of the system that brings about visually guided reach has identified that the peripheral visual field proves a more effective input for guiding reach than the central visual field.

Other children with CVI will choose to look away from people's faces when talking to them. Although this is not technically an eye movement disorder, it is a form of behavior that accompanies both dorsal and ventral stream dysfunction. When one wants to raise a complex topic, it is nearly universal behavior not to look at the person while formulating what to say, but then turning toward them to say it. The reason for looking away could be to liberate thought capacity by looking at a blank area, so as not to be distracted by having to interpret the language on the other person's face. In this way, children with dorsal stream dysfunction may simply be performing a more pronounced version of what everyone else does.

In the context of ventral stream dysfunction, lack of ability to recognize faces, along with inability to see language in facial expressions, means that faces may hold little interest for the affected child.

Another reason for eccentric viewing is when a child has lack of central vision in both eyes. Such children consistently look slightly off to the side to use their best vision.

The following are issues for caregivers and teachers to bear in mind with respect to eccentric viewing:

- The tendency to reach for things in the peripheral visual field diminishes, except in the most profoundly impaired children, in whom it persists long term.

Minimizing clutter and background noise may reduce the frequency of this behavior in a young child who has just started to exhibit it, as well as reducing the likelihood of the behavior becoming habitual.
- It does not help to tell a child to "look at me when I am talking to you," because when these children look, they describe having difficulty remembering what is said. In the author's experience, an approach in which the child is taught to look and smile, after having spoken, or having been spoken to, has often proven to be an effective social strategy.

## Assessment and Interpretation of Eye Movements

Observation of the child and the way the eyes move to appraise the scene provides most of the requisite information about eye movements. The following are issues to have in mind when observing visual behaviors:

- Are the eyes aligned or is there strabismus present? If so, which eye is turned? (This is often the eye with amblyopia.)
- Are spectacles worn?
  - Usually, if the eyes are turned in, the child is farsighted (long-sighted) and the spectacles magnify the face.
  - If the eyes are turned out, the overall disability is likely to be greater, and the child may be nearsighted (short-sighted). The spectacles, if worn, diminish the apparent size of the face behind the glasses.
- Are the eyes deviated in any particular direction, and is this present all the time or is it intermittent?
- Are there to-and-fro eye movements (nystagmus) present? If so, is there a typical head posture, and is the nystagmus least in this position? Is vision better for near than for distance?
- Do the eyes stay steady and on target, or do they wander off target as a result of poor fixation?
- Do the eyes turn in adequately when looking at a nearby target?
- Is the child able to make fast eye movements? If so, are they normal or inaccurate (*dysmetric*), and are supplementary eye movements needed?
- Are pursuit eye movements accurately matched to the rate of a moving target? If not, do they catch up?
  - Absence of pursuit in one direction can accompany a hemianopic visual field on the opposite side. If pursuit to one side is absent, hemianopia should be suspected on the other side.
- If the child is a poor reader, carefully watch how his or her eyes move across a printed page, and see whether there are any small backward movements. These may indicate the need to modify the presentation of the text.
- Determine whether a child has apraxia of gaze by asking him or her to look at large surrounding targets that have not previously been encountered in these positions. This condition indicates that profound dorsal stream dysfunction is also present.
  - Difficulty may be exhibited when moving the eyes to look at targets on only one side.
  - If there is evidence of intact vision on one side when gaze is not being attracted centrally, but the eyes do not move to that side when they are being

attracted centrally, lack of attention to that side needs to be considered.

- The tendency to not look at what is being picked up and not look at people's faces when communicating with them indicates that perceptual visual impairment is likely.

## Conclusion

The full effects of the various eye movement disorders that accompany CVI on vision and perception have yet to be determined. However, it is well understood that misalignment of the eyes leads to diminished depth perception; nystagmus diminishes visual acuity, particularly in the distance; and lack of ability to fixate on a target, whether static or moving, limits the ability to access information. Recognition of the adverse effects these disorders have on vision allows the skilled practitioner to minimize their impact by optimizing the surrounding environment and presentation of educational material. (See Chapters 19 and 21 for methods to optimize learning environments for children who have CVI.)

It is important to recognize that in the context of CVI, underlying vision and perception disorders are compounded by additional eye movement disorders that limit access to information. The two sets of conditions effectively augment one another, as they are not separate, but are inextricably intertwined.

## References

Hamilton, R., McGlone, L., MacKinnon, J. R., Russell, H. C., Bradnam, M. S., & Mactier, H. (2010). Ophthalmic, clinical and visual electrophysiological findings in children born to mothers prescribed substitute methadone in pregnancy. *British Journal of Ophthalmology, 94*, 696–700.

Hyvärinen, L., & Jacob, N. (2011). *WHAT and HOW does this child see?* Helsinki, Finland: VISTEST Ltd.

Jacobson, L. K., & Dutton, G. N. (2000). Periventricular leukomalacia: An important cause of visual and ocular motility dysfunction in children. *Survey of Ophthalmology, 45*, 1–13.

Lueck, A. H. (2004). Overview of intervention methods. In A. H. Lueck (Ed.), *Functional vision: A practitioner's guide to evaluation and intervention* (pp. 257–275). New York: AFB Press.

Rizzo, M., & Vecera, S. P. (2002). Psychoanatomical substrates of Bálint's syndrome. *Journal of Neurology, Neurosurgery & Psychiatry, 72*, 162–178.

Salati, R., Borgatti, R., Giammari, G., & Jacobson, L. (2002). Oculomotor dysfunction in cerebral visual impairment following perinatal hypoxia. *Developmental Medicine & Child Neurology, 44*, 542–50.

Saunders, K. J., Little, J. A., McClelland, J. F., & Jackson, A. J. (2010). Profile of refractive errors in cerebral palsy: Impact of severity of motor impairment (GMFCS) and CP subtype on refractive outcome. *Investigative Ophthalmology & Visual Science, 51*, 2885–2890.

Saunders, K. J., McClelland, J. F., Richardson, P. M., & Stevenson, M. (2008). Clinical judgement of near pupil responses provides a useful indicator of focusing ability in children with cerebral palsy. *Developmental Medicine & Child Neurology, 50*, 33–37.

Schmahmann, J. D. (2010). The role of the cerebellum in cognition and emotion: Personal reflections since 1982 on the dysmetria of thought hypothesis, and its historical evolution from theory to therapy. *Neuropsychology Review, 20*, 236–260.

Yokochi, K. (1991). Paroxysmal ocular downward deviation in neurologically impaired infants. *Pediatric Neurology, 7*, 426–428.

# 9

# Refractive Errors, Impaired Focusing, and the Need for Eyeglasses in Children with CVI

*Kathryn J. Saunders*

Many people wear eyeglasses or contact lenses to enable them to see more clearly. This is because they have a focusing inaccuracy, known as *refractive error*, within the eye. Refractive errors and poor focusing are more prevalent among children with developmental disabilities and cerebral visual impairment (CVI), and many such children will benefit from wearing eyeglasses in order to allow their vision to achieve its full potential.

If refractive errors or deficits in focusing are not identified and managed, whether through spectacle correction or other strategies, children with CVI will be disadvantaged in terms of their visual development, visual performance, and in accessing information about the world around them. This is likely to have adverse implications for their social, general, and educational development.

The first part of this chapter reviews general information about the different types of refractive errors and how they affect visual functioning, as well as *ocular accommodation,* the process by which the typical eye changes focus from distance to near. Then the greater incidence of refractive errors and impaired focusing among children with developmental disabilities, including many children with CVI, is discussed, along with the need to monitor this population for these common eye conditions. The final section of the chapter examines how to manage the treatment of refractive errors and impaired focusing among children, including those with CVI, as well as strategies for encouraging compliance with spectacle wear.

## Refractive Error and Its Measurement

Chapter 2 describes how we see, starting with light entering the eye and then being focused on the retina by the cornea and crystalline lens (see Figure 2.2). If light is not adequately focused on the retina, the quality of the retinal image is poor, and optimal visual functioning will not be achieved. When this occurs and continues during infancy and early childhood, the developing

FIGURE 9.1
**Emmetropic Focus**

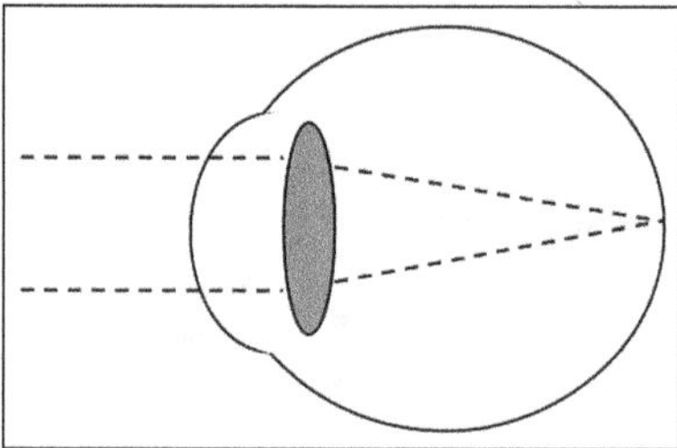

In emmetropia, or perfect focus, the light rays are focused exactly on the retina at the back of the eye.

FIGURE 9.2
**Retinoscopy Procedure to Determine Refractive Error**

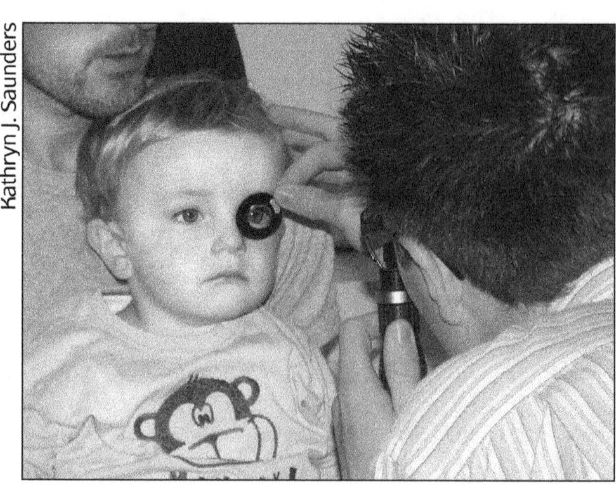
Kathryn J. Saunders

brain does not get the opportunity to "learn to see" properly. The result may be long-term impairment of vision. Although identification of refractive error and the prescription of spectacle correction to ensure that the image received by the retina is in focus are very important parts of the visual care of the child, poor vision may not be eliminated if the visual pathways and higher levels of visual processing are also impaired. It is not obvious just from looking at a child or observing the child's behavior whether or not he or she needs eyeglasses. It is important, therefore, that all children with a developmental disability or suspected CVI have an accurate assessment of refractive error and focusing ability, so that the need for eyeglasses is taken into consideration when creating a treatment plan for each child (Das, Spowart, Crossley, & Dutton, 2010).

Light entering the eye is bent, or refracted, as it passes through the cornea and the crystalline lens (see Chapter 2). The term *refractive error* is used to describe a condition in which this light is focused inaccurately on the retina, forming a blurred image. An eye that perfectly refracts the light coming from a distant object to create a crisp, focused image on the retina does not have a refractive error. This is referred to as an *emmetropic* eye by eye care professionals (Figure 9.1). The majority of people are emmetropic.

Eye care professionals measure refractive error by shining a light into the eye and observing how the light is reflected out from the back of the eye. In this retinoscopy procedure, lenses held in front of the eye allow the examiner to measure how far the eye is from perfect focus, and to determine the correct lens needed to attain focus (see Figure 9.2). Eye drops are often instilled prior to this measurement, to ensure that an accurate result is obtained. These drops increase the size of the pupil and reveal the full extent of any refractive error present. This has the added benefit of allowing the examiner a good view inside the eye to assess eye health.

## Types of Refractive Error and Their Impact on Vision

### *Hyperopia (Long-sightedness or Farsightedness)*

If light coming into the eye is not bent sufficiently to focus on the retina, and instead would focus behind the eye (if this were possible), the image on the retina would be blurred (Figure 9.3a). This is known as *hyperopia* (long-sightedness or farsightedness). In this scenario the eye is usually able to bring the image into focus by changing the shape of the crystalline lens using internal eye muscles (ciliary muscles) (Figure 9.3b). This process is called *ocular accommodation,* and it can only happen if the ciliary muscles are functioning normally and if the crystalline lens is intact and flexible. If the crystalline lens has been removed, is not positioned correctly, is rigid, or if the muscles are not functioning optimally, the eye may not be able to change focus to correct a hyperopic refractive error. Even when the crystalline lens and muscles are functioning properly, some children cannot focus accurately or sustain accurate accommodation. These children require eyeglasses to maintain good focus and quality vision (Figure 9.3c).

Hyperopia is often associated with strabismus (a misalignment of the eyes, with one eye usually turning in toward the nose; see Chapter 8). In most of these cases, correcting the hyperopia with spectacle lenses also helps to keep the eyes straight. A spectacle lens for correcting hyperopia is convex in shape. This type of lens is thicker in the center and magnifies the image viewed through it. When worn in spectacles a convex lens also magnifies the contours of the wearer's face (Figure 9.4).

### *Myopia (Short-sightedness or Nearsightedness)*

A myopic eye has a blurred image on the retina when viewing objects in the distance (Figure 9.5a). The eye itself cannot sharpen the image, therefore eyeglasses are needed to bring this distant image into focus on the retina (Figure 9.5b). However, a myopic eye is naturally focused for objects viewed

FIGURE 9.3
**Hyperopic Focus**

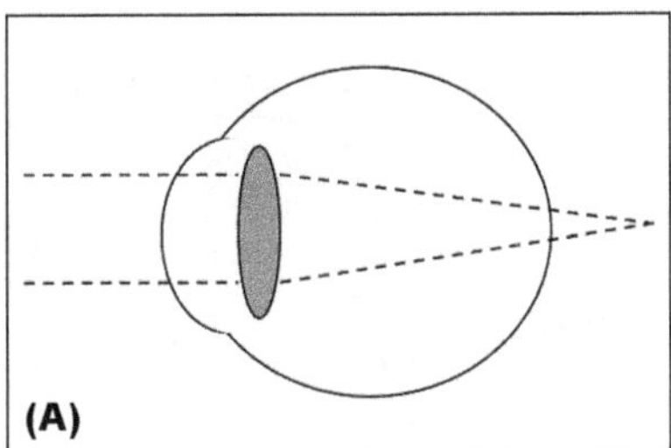


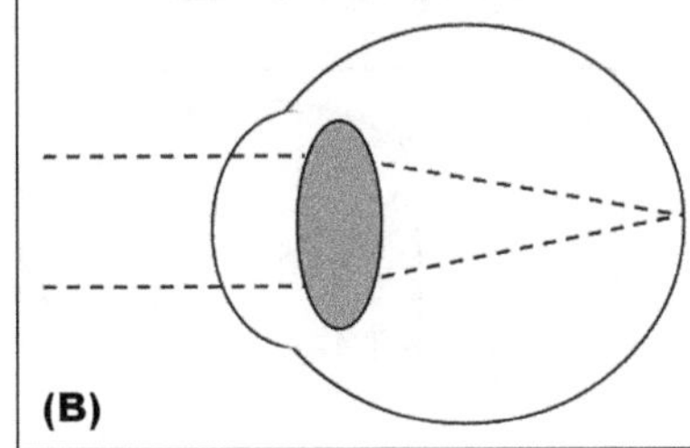


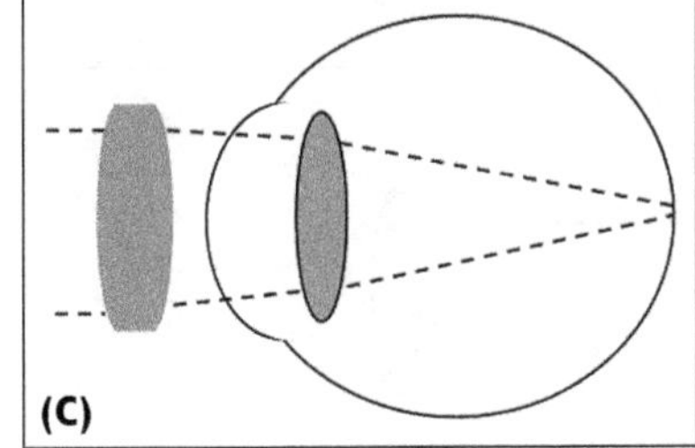


**(A)** In hyperopia (long-sightedness or farsightedness) the image is blurred because the light rays are in focus behind the retina, not on it. **(B)** Muscular effort by the ciliary muscles is used to change the shape of the crystalline lens (ocular accommodation) and bring the light rays into focus on the retina. **(C)** A convex spectacle lens may also be used to focus light rays on the retina of a hyperopic eye.

at close range (Figure 9.5c). The distance from the eye at which vision is sharpest is related to the degree of myopia—the more myopic the eye, the closer the object needs to be in order to be seen clearly without eyeglasses. People who have myopia but do not wear prescription lenses have to get up close to objects to see them clearly. This type of close focus also provides magnification.

The lenses used to correct myopia are concave; they are thicker at the edges than in the center of the lens, and they make objects viewed through them appear smaller. This type of lens makes the face of the individual wearing spectacles appear smaller behind the lenses (Figure 9.6).

FIGURE 9.4
**Convex Lens for Hyperopia**

Nigel McDowell

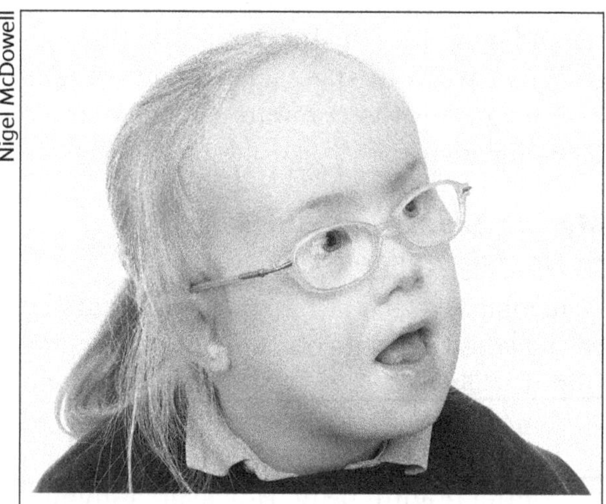

The magnification of the child's face by the convex lenses used to correct hyperopia can be seen through her left spectacle lens.

### *Astigmatism*

A hyperopic or myopic eye can also be astigmatic. This type of refractive error focuses light at different points, and results in reduced clarity of vision for both distant and near objects. Astigmatism is usually due to subtle asymmetry in the shape of the cornea and is sometimes referred to as "football-shaped eyes" in the United States, or "rugby ball-shaped eyes" in other countries, in reference to the non-spherical shape of the cornea. Eyeglasses are normally required to correct astigmatism in children.

### *Anisometropia*

The visual system usually develops in a relatively balanced fashion, with both eyes having the same, or similar, refractive er-

FIGURE 9.5
**Myopic Focus**

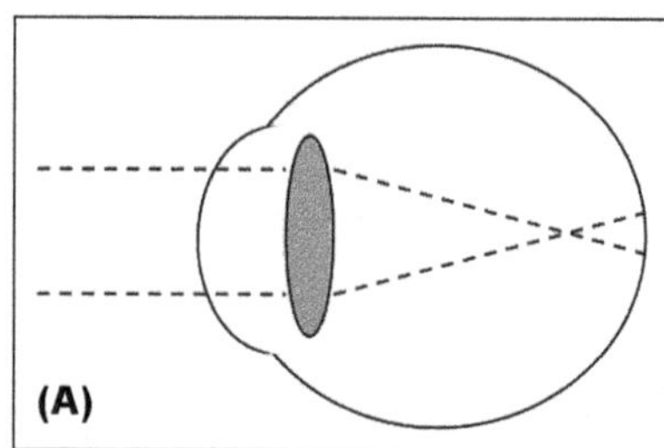


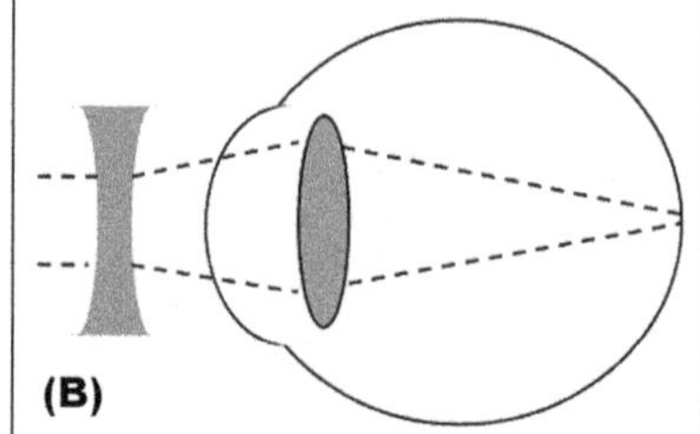


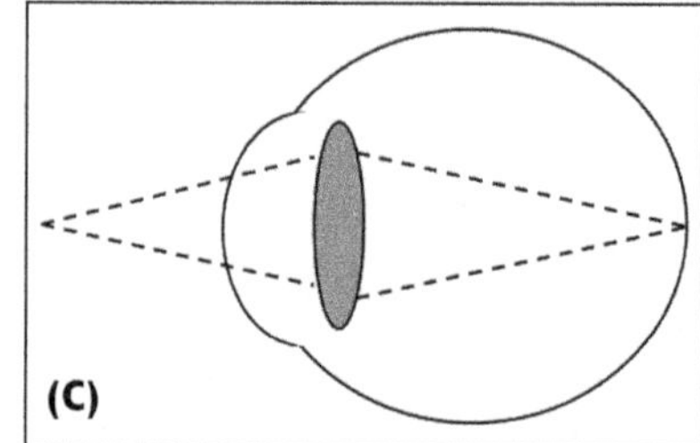


**(A)** In myopia (short-sightedness or nearsightedness) the image of distant objects is blurred because the light rays are in focus in front of the retina, not on it. **(B)** Distant objects can only be brought into focus if a concave spectacle lens is used to focus light rays on the retina of a myopic eye. **(C)** Objects viewed at near distance are usually in focus without spectacles.

FIGURE 9.6
**Concave Lens for Myopia**

Nigel McDowell

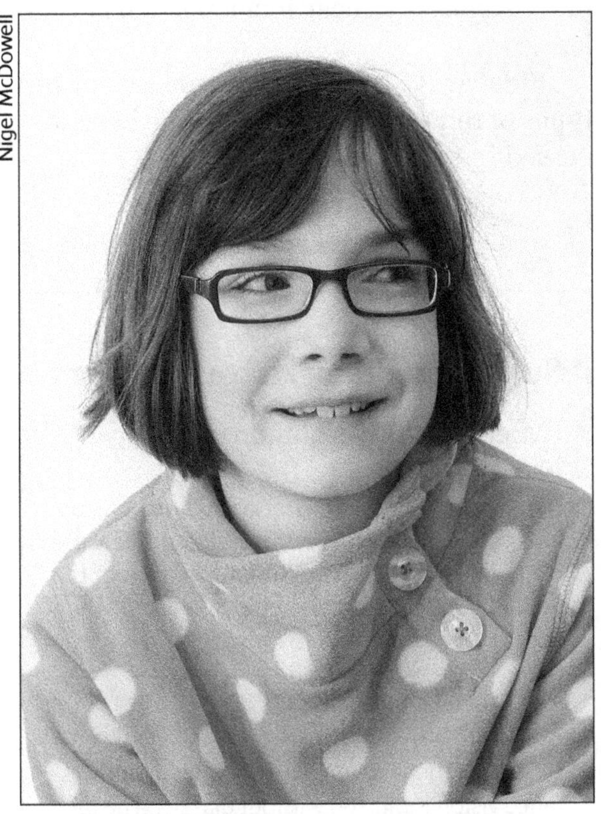

The concave lenses used to correct myopia make this child's face appear smaller behind the lenses, as can be seen through the lens to the side of her left eye.

rors. However, a difference in refractive error between the two eyes can occur, called *anisometropia*. One of the consequences of anisometropia is that, when spectacles are not worn, only one eye is able to focus images on the retina at a time. This has implications for visual development and for depth perception. Anisometropia is often associated with strabismus (squint) and amblyopia (lazy eye).

In most cases, correction with spectacles is relatively straightforward and restores balance, but when anisometropia is large, full correction of the different refractive errors with eyeglasses may not be tolerated or be visually beneficial. This is because the spectacle correction may result in very different image sizes on the two retinae, and this size disparity is not compatible with comfortable vision, because the mind cannot join the two images together to create a single picture. In such cases it may be suitable for only one eye to be fully corrected using spectacle lenses, with the other eye given a "balance" lens of matching strength. The balance lens may not provide optimal vision in one eye, but it does allow for comfortable vision when both eyes are viewing together. Alternatively, depending on the child's needs, visual function, and level of disability, contact lenses may be considered an appropriate form of treatment for anisometropia, since they do not result in such a large difference in image size.

## Impairment of Ocular Accommodation

*Ocular accommodation* is the process by which the ciliary muscle in the eye can change the shape of the crystalline lens to alter focus. This change in focus occurs in an automatic, reflexive manner and involves a complex neurological pathway within and beyond the eye. Ocular accommodation plays an important role in maintaining clear vision for objects at a distance, as well as close by. When accommodation does not function properly, it has a severe impact on visual performance. If the visual system cannot accommodate, a person cannot see objects clearly at different distances.

In the typical eye, the effectiveness of ocular accommodation decreases as age increases. Consequently, most people begin to struggle with near vision tasks during their fifth decade of life, and often require reading glasses, or the introduction of a bifocal or progressive lens into their existing pair of eyeglasses. A bifocal lens is a spectacle lens with two separate areas, each with a different strength or power of lens. The upper portion of the lens (or upper segment) focuses the eye for distance vision; the smaller, lower portion of the lens (or lower segment) comprises the near, or reading, portion of the lens. The line dividing the upper and lower segments is visible when looking at the lens (Figure 9.7). A progressive lens also provides correction for distance and near vision in a single lens, but unlike a bifocal lens, it has a continuous, invisible change in lens power and no abrupt separation or line between the distance and near focus portions of the lens.

Sidebar 9.1 provides a summary of the types of refractive errors that have been discussed in this section.

FIGURE 9.7
**Child Wearing Bifocal Lenses**

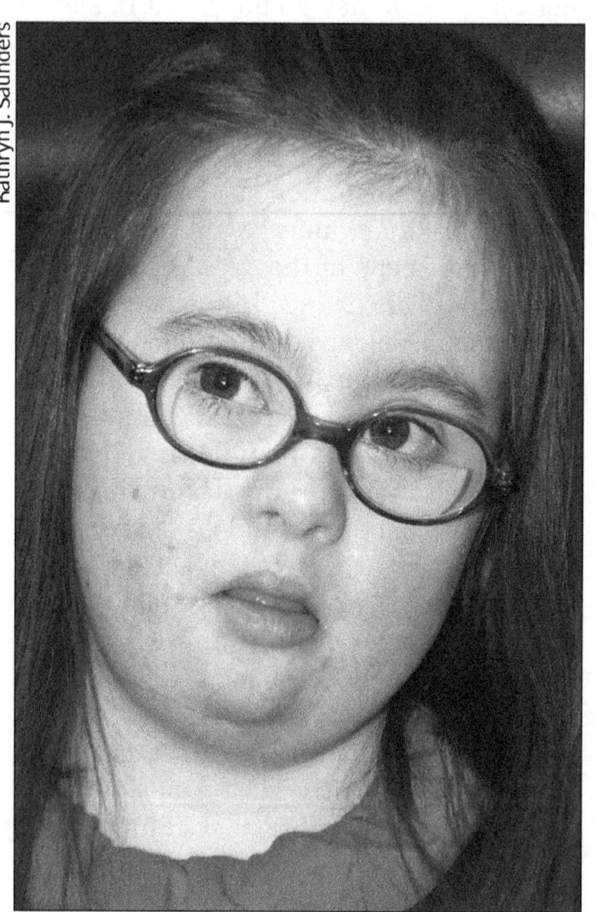

Kathryn J. Saunders

SIDEBAR 9.1

## Summary of Refractive Disorders

### Hyperopia (long-sightedness or farsightedness)

Hyperopia can affect distance and near vision, but ocular accommodation may compensate for hyperopia in some children. The face of the person wearing eyeglasses is magnified when spectacles are worn for hyperopia.

### Myopia (short-sightedness or nearsightedness)

In myopia, near vision is usually good, but distance vision is blurred without glasses. The face of the person wearing eyeglasses appears smaller (or "minified") when spectacles are worn for myopia.

### Astigmatism

Astigmatism reduces the quality of vision at all distances and can occur in combination with other refractive errors.

### Anisometropia

Anisometropia is a difference in refractive error between the two eyes. One eye may look larger or smaller than the other when spectacles are worn.

### Impairment of Ocular Accommodation

Ocular accommodation is the ability to change focus from distance to near, and vice versa. When this function is impaired, a person cannot see objects clearly at different distances.

## Developmental Disability, Refractive Error, and Focusing Ability

### Refractive Error and the Need for Spectacles

The visual system has a dynamic nature during infancy and early childhood. Refractive errors change in response to the eyes' growth and the quality of the visual environment to which an infant or young child is exposed. Typically, most infants are a little farsighted (long-sighted), astigmatic, or both, but grow out of these refractive errors as they age. By the time most children enter formal education, they have little or no refractive error. A 2010 UK study reported that the number of children in elementary (primary) school who require spectacle correction is 12.8 percent (approximately one in eight children) (O'Donoghue et al., 2010). Young children who are still significantly farsighted or astigmatic beyond the first few years of life are at increased risk of an eye turn (squint or strabismus) and poor vision (Atkinson, Braddick, Nardini, & Anker, 2007). In such cases, spectacle correction improves the child's visual prognosis. There is also evidence that improved visual performance resulting from appropriate spectacle correction benefits cognitive skills and educational attainment (Atkinson et al., 2007; Leone, Mitchell, Morgan, Kifley, & Rose, 2010; Williams, Latif, Hannington, & Watkins, 2005). The number of nearsighted (short-sighted) children increases during adolescence; approximately 25 percent of UK schoolchildren wear spectacles at 12–13 years of age (O'Donoghue et al., 2010).

The pattern of refractive error development for typical children is in marked contrast to that described for children who have a developmental disability, as many children with CVI do. Where evidence exists, it is clear that a developmental disability often has a marked impact on the development of refractive error, to the extent that infants do not grow out of them, as typical children might do. These refractive errors are either retained or increase throughout childhood. For example, approximately 60 percent of children with Down syndrome need spectacles at elementary school age (Saunders, 2009). A study of children and young adults with cerebral palsy reports 30 percent with significant refractive errors requiring spectacle correction (Saunders, Little, McClelland, & Jackson, 2010). The prevalence of refractive error is high among infants born preterm, or with very low birth weights. These infants tend to retain high refractive errors beyond infancy and require spectacles during childhood (O'Connor et al., 2006; Saunders, McCulloch, Shepherd, & Wilkinson, 2002).

### Ocular Accommodation and Impaired Focusing

From about 3 months of age, the typical infant will be able to change focus rapidly and accurately from objects held at distance to those close to his or her face, and vice versa. This process of accommodation and relaxation of accommodation occurs reflexively. Relatively few typically developing children have deficits in ocular accommodation during school years (Sterner, Gellerstedt, & Sjöström, 2004). Change in focus is usually accompanied by a change in pupil size. While focusing ability can, and should, be measured formally by an eye care professional, an indication of focusing ability may be obtained by observing the eye's pupil as a child switches attention from a distant object (such as a parent's face at several yards' distance) to a near one (for example, a small toy with detail big enough to be seen, as determined from the measured binocular visual acuity, held at about 8 inches [20 cm] from the child's face). A child with typical vision will exhibit a marked reduction or constriction in the diameter of the pupil as he or she changes attention and focus from a distant object to a near one. If this change in pupil diameter is not apparent, it may indicate that accommodation is impaired (Saunders, McClelland, Richardson, & Stevenson, 2008).

While the typical eye exhibits good ocular accommodation during childhood, increased awareness in recent years has indicated that children with a developmental disability are often unable to produce or sustain accurate focus. For example, Woodhouse, Meades, Leat, & Saunders (1993) report that 80 percent of children with Down syndrome in their study failed to focus accurately, even when wearing appropriate spectacle correction. In another study, 57 percent of children with various types and severities of cerebral palsy were found to have reduced focusing ability (McClelland, Parkes, Hill, Jackson, & Saunders, 2006).

Children with these conditions are in an analogous position to typically sighted adults in middle age who experience increasing difficulty with near vision. However, adults in middle age have experienced normal focusing and are generally able to understand and articulate the perceived change in their visual function, in order to seek help. Children whose vision has always been impaired by poor focusing do not have this advantage. Since much of a child's learning occurs at near, failure to focus accurately up close for sustained periods of time will have important implications, and may compound the effects of both CVI and other underlying developmental difficulties.

Among children with a developmental disability, the number of children with focusing difficulties is further increased by the use of scopolamine (hyoscine) skin patches to control drooling. Excessive salivation, poor control of salivation, and drooling are common problems for children with developmental disabilities. A common approach is to use skin patches that provide a slow release of medication to reduce the production of saliva. However, in addition to the beneficial effect on salivation, the side effects of these patches include an increase in pupil size and reduction in the focusing capacity of the eyes (Firth & Walker, 2006; Saeed, Henderson, & Dutton, 2007). The latter is likely to blur vision considerably, and the large pupil may also result in discomfort for the child when exposed to bright sunshine, as he or she is unable to restrict the amount of light entering the eyes.

In summary, not only do more children with a developmental difficulty need spectacles, but they often have larger refractive errors than are commonly observed among typically developing populations, and therefore need stronger spectacles than their peers. Children with a developmental difficulty are at increased risk of having difficulty changing focus from distance to near. It is important, therefore, that in addition to a measure of refractive error, a measure of accommodative function is carried out on all children with, or suspected of having, CVI.

## Treating Refractive Error and Focusing Difficulties in Children with CVI

It is straightforward to recommend that all children have their refractive error measured so that significant refractive errors are identified. However, decisions regarding the management of such errors (such as the appropriateness of spectacle correction, the strength of the eyeglasses, and when the eyeglasses should be used) will depend on the individual child's circumstances—his or her physical, developmental, and visual needs and abilities. The eye care team working with each child will need to consider both visual and nonvisual issues when deciding whether spectacles are appropriate, and if so, when they should be worn.

Some children who have not received optimal eye care early in life and who have a significant refractive error that has never previously been corrected with spectacles may be considered too old to benefit from eyeglasses. However, age and previous vision care should not preclude consideration of each child's needs and visual status on a case-by-case basis. While the best visual outcome may generally be expected when spectacles are prescribed at a young age, during the early years when the visual system is undergoing its most rapid period of development and is most sensitive to treatment, older children may also benefit from intervention. Myopia, for example, is often successfully treated with spectacles in older childhood, resulting in improved distance vision and enhanced quality of life. However, the eye care team should also be sure to consider the child's focusing ability and the effect of the prescription on the child's perception of the surrounding world.

## When to Wear Spectacles

If spectacles are required to improve vision, they are usually prescribed for full-time wear, but clear instructions should be provided to the child, parents, and caregivers about when and where the spectacles should be worn. For a child who is myopic, and therefore can naturally focus at short distances, it may be useful to remove eyeglasses when viewing objects up close because the child is able to take advantage of this natural magnification. Conversely, when the child is trying to see a distant object clearly (for example, when the teacher is demonstrating something at a distance, or when the child is watching television or a film at the cinema), the spectacles must be worn because they improve focus and function. Spectacles worn to correct hyperopia and astigmatism are likely to be most beneficial if worn full-time.

Keeping track of eyeglasses that may be removed for some tasks but worn for others can be troublesome. When eyeglasses are required only for near or distance vision, it is helpful to mark the purpose of the spectacles on the side of the frames, so educational support workers and others can readily check whether they are being used correctly. In general, it is a good idea to mark children's names on their spectacle frames to make sure they are wearing their own eyeglasses and not one of their classmate's pairs accidentally. After a particularly fun session in the soft play area, one teacher described how a pile of spectacles was found among a play pool of balls. It was difficult to distribute the correct eyeglasses to the correct student since all the eyeglasses looked similar and none were marked with a name.

Contact lenses may be an appropriate form of refractive error correction for a child with CVI who has had cataracts removed, or who has a considerable degree of anisometropia or myopia, but this is a rare scenario.

## Management When Spectacles Are Not Appropriate

Although spectacle correction is an important therapy in many cases, there are some situations where spectacle wear may not be appropriate, even with the presence of a significant refractive error. Spectacles will improve the clarity of the image produced on the retina, but if CVI is particularly severe, the extent of the damage to the brain may limit the improvement in image clarity perceived by the child. Although it is important not to raise false hopes regarding possible improvements in visual performance, it may be appropriate to try spectacle correction of refractive error and monitor for effectiveness, even if there is no guarantee that vision will improve. There may not be immediate measurable or noticeable benefits from correction of significant refractive error because in some cases, visual performance improves over the long term. It may take weeks or months to fully realize the improvement in vision that can be achieved with spectacle correction of a young child's refractive error.

## Treatment of Focusing Difficulties

Regardless of a child's cognitive ability or interest in reading formal text, near vision functioning should be taken into consideration for all children, not just those utilizing reading material. The importance of clarity of near vision when accessing information about the world around us (such as faces, pictures, or food) is not limited to written information. Impaired ocular accommodation and poor near focus, once identified, must be addressed. This can be done in several ways, with the optimal method likely to differ for each child, depending on factors such as physical abilities and disabilities, head and eye control, and visual status. The strength of the lenses required in the spectacles, and the additional cost of a bifocal or progressive lens, may also inform management decisions. The following are some of the considerations:

- A child with emmetropia (no refractive error) who does not require spectacle correction for optimal distance vision, but has focusing difficulties, will require only a near vision or reading spectacle correction. The challenge in this case is that spectacles that are only needed for near viewing are easily misplaced or forgotten. It may also be more difficult to encourage compliance and familiarization with part-time spectacle wear rather than full-time. A more successful approach is often to prescribe bifocal lenses, with the distance portion of the lens essentially plain, allowing for good near and distance vision without the need to remove and replace spectacles for different tasks.
- A child with myopia (short-sightedness or nearsightedness) will need spectacles for clear distance vision, but may remove the eyeglasses to take advantage of the natural near focus of his or her eyes. Removal of distance spectacles should provide clear near vision and some additional and beneficial magnification. Children may discover this on their own, and parents may notice children looking over or under their spectacles when viewing near objects. In such cases, it may be reasonable (after discussion with a child's eye care provider) to encourage removal of spectacles for close observation of objects.
- A child with a focusing difficulty who normally wears spectacles for distance vision, but is not simply myopic, will need two different strengths of spectacle lenses: one to see clearly at a distance and another (usually stronger) to see clearly at near. This can be provided with two separate pairs of glasses, bifocals, or progressive lenses.

- If two separate pairs of spectacles are prescribed, it is essential that the chosen frames be visibly different, to ensure that each pair is worn for the correct task. Incorrect use will result in blurred vision. In the author's experience, many children, schools, and families find the use of separate pairs of spectacles confusing and unsuccessful, as the eyeglasses are misplaced or worn for the wrong task.

Bifocals and progressive lenses have been shown to be a successful method to manage accommodative dysfunction (inadequate ocular accommodation) in children with Down syndrome and other developmental disabilities, including CVI (Al-Bagdady, Stewart, Watts, Murphy, & Woodhouse, 2009; Nandakumar & Leat, 2010; Ross, Heron, Mackie, McWilliam, & Dutton, 2000).

The choice between separate pairs of spectacles, bifocals, and progressive lenses also depends on the child's eye and head control. Correctly utilizing the different portions of a bifocal or progressive lens for proper viewing distance requires the child to position his or her eyes and head in the appropriate location. While this is often done in a reflexive manner by children in order to access the clearest image, it may not be physically possible for children who are severely impaired.

## Fitting and Adjustment of Spectacles

When spectacles are prescribed, plastic lenses are generally the most appropriate, since they are lighter and safer than glass lenses. (Lenses can be made from different types of plastics and glass. In North America, the preferred material—because of safety considerations for children—is a polycarbonate resin because it is not only stronger than typical plastics, it is also thinner and lighter.) The choice and careful adjustment of frames is critical, so that the child is able to easily and comfortably view through the lenses. The side "arms" of the frames may need to be shortened or converted to ones that curl around the ear to help keep the spectacles in place. A child with an unusual posture may require extra manipulation of the frames, to ensure that they are looking through the lenses correctly, despite their individual head or eye position. Parents are encouraged to keep returning to their child's spectacle provider for adjustments, since eyeglasses become misaligned very easily, especially during the early phases of learning to wear them. The frequency of visits to the eye care provider for readjustments and replacements is likely to decrease as the child's compliance improves and the eyeglasses spend more time on the child's nose, and less time being pulled off his or her face. For some very young children or children with motor impairments, soft, pliable, plastic frames may be recommended. If these children fall or move their head into objects, they are less likely to get hurt by the soft frames. For more information on ensuring that spectacles fit well and are tolerated, see Sidebar 9.2.

## Effects of Clearer Vision on Simultanagnosia

One common issue in CVI is simultanagnosia (see Chapters 3 and 8), in which cluttered or busy visual scenes can reduce a child's ability to perceive what is in front of him or her. Children with hyperopia who experience simultanagnosia may remove their spectacles to deliberately blur the cluttered scene, particularly when they are tired or under stress. This effectively reduces the amount of confusion they experience since

SIDEBAR 9.2

## Ensuring that Spectacles Fit Well and Are Tolerated

*Barry S. Kran and D. Luisa Mayer*

Successful spectacle wear depends on a correct prescription, good frame selection and fit, and tolerance of the child, family, and school staff toward full-time spectacle use. The following are some issues to bear in mind when fitting children with eyeglasses:

- Frame selection may be limited for young children.
- Frames need to be comfortable, fit well, and have the lowest possible weight. Proper fit cannot be emphasized enough. The child should be present for both the fitting and the dispensing. Adjustable nose pads are often helpful. It is important to be sure that eyelashes do not touch the rear lens surface.
- Polycarbonate lenses mounted in full frame eyeglasses are robust and provide eye protection.
- In children with tactile defensive issues around their face (who cannot tolerate a hat or having their face touched by someone else, for example), spectacle wear may be deferred until this issue has been successfully addressed by the child's therapists. A stepwise approach to improving the tolerance of eyeglasses should be considered. This can range from using nonprescription sun eyewear outdoors to simply putting on the prescription eyeglasses first thing in the morning. A good time to consider having the child wear the eyeglasses is when the child is engaged in a preferred manual activity, such as eating, or otherwise engaged in a task. Positive reinforcement is needed as well. The child's school staff can assist in helping the child tolerate eyeglasses, often because they are able to enforce wear and because the child is occupied with interesting activities during the day. If the child is somewhat light sensitive, photochromic lenses that dim outdoors and lighten indoors may be considered.
- Children with dual sensory loss (vision and hearing) can have a difficult time simultaneously accepting both spectacles and hearing aids. Practitioners, parents, and therapists need to collaborate throughout this process.
- Some children may have medical issues, such as cerebral palsy or seizure control, that the family considers a higher priority than the need to wear eyeglasses. Manifest improvement of vision with eyeglasses provides significant incentive for their use; if the family sees no benefit from them, they tend to be less motivated to encourage use of eyeglasses.
- Failure by the child to accept eyeglasses at one point in time is not a reason to permanently dismiss them. Sometimes, when the child is more mature or when medical issues have become resolved, eyeglasses will be accepted more easily.

the blurred visual picture that results removes detail from the scene and makes the amount of available visual information less overwhelming. While this may be more comfortable for the child, it is also likely to reduce his or her ability to access visual information.

The solution may be to keep the spectacles on to maintain clarity of vision, but reduce the amount of information presented at one time (see Chapter 19) in order to maximize visual performance. Reduction in the amount of information presented at one time can be achieved by masking or removing extraneous material, or by magnifying pertinent information, either through the use of optical devices (see the following section on the use of magnifiers), enlarging material with a photocopier, or utilizing large print resources.

## The Use of Optical Magnifiers

Children whose CVI reduces their ability to see fine detail may benefit from the use of optical devices, such as magnifiers (in addition to, or instead of, spectacles or contact lenses), to increase the size of what they are viewing.

A magnifier can be a useful tool for a child with CVI and simultanagnosia whose visual performance suffers when the amount of visual information presented increases. Magnification reduces the field of view, thereby decreasing the amount of visual information available at one time.

Magnification of near objects can be achieved using simple, robust magnifiers such as dome, stand, or handheld magnifiers (see Figure 9.8). Dome and stand magnifiers are placed directly on the material to be magnified, making them stable, easy to manage, and appropriate for young children or those with physical impairments. The magnifier naturally frames the material under observation, and many simple magnifiers also contain an indicator that can be used to help children maintain their place when following text.

FIGURE 9.8
**Child Using Dome Magnifier**

L. Penny Rosenblum

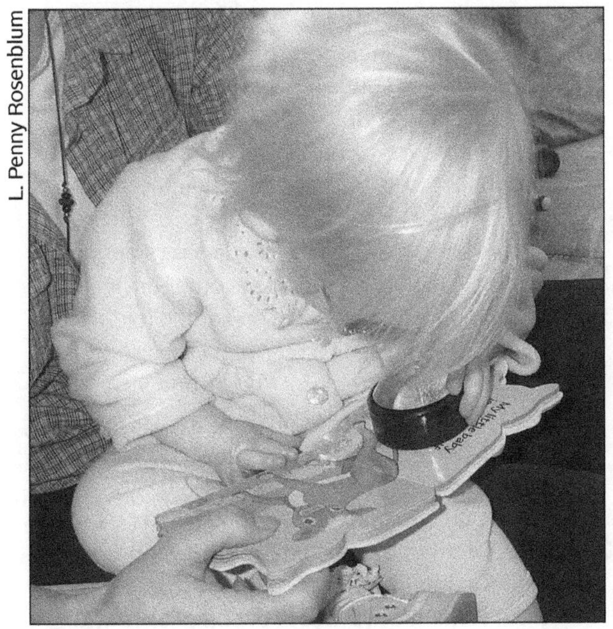

Dome magnifiers like this one are placed directly on the material to be magnified, making them stable, easy to manage, and appropriate for young children or those with physical impairments.

## Encouraging a Child to Wear Eyeglasses

With most children, encouraging spectacle wear and achieving good compliance requires perseverance. The child may not like the new and challenging feel of the spectacles on his or her face, or the child may not immediately appreciate the benefit of the spectacles to improve vision. In addition, the child's vision may be altered radically by the new spectacles, and the sudden change in how the world looks may be alarming and require adaptation. Many children with a developmental disability are stressed by new or different experiences; the impact of new eyeglasses should be treated with sensitivity. In the author's experience, gentle perseverance and reward for compliance with wearing spectacles pay off in the end. It may take weeks, months, or in extreme cases, years, for full-time wear (if that is the goal) to be achieved, but it is possible. Some parents find that compliance begins with wearing the eyeglasses for a favorite activity (such as eating, watching a special movie, or playing a game). The activity should be short at first and stopped when the spectacles come off. The length of time the spectacles are worn can be extended through positive reinforcement, such as compliments on the look of the spectacles and praise for keeping the eyeglasses on during a specific activity. The process should not be turned into a battle, because in all likelihood the child will win. A more successful approach is for the child to understand that it is a treat when the eyeglasses are on and a disappointment when they are off.

Concurrent with parental and school support and encouragement, the fit and adjustment of the spectacles should be monitored and reevaluated. Parents should be encouraged to visit the eye care provider on an ongoing basis to ensure that this is the case.

Although middle-aged adults may report difficulties adapting to the use of bifocal and progressive lenses, it is the author's experience that most children who already wear spectacles and need to switch to bifocal or progressive lenses make the transition to the new lenses easily. For some children, it may be appropriate to suggest that bifocals initially be worn in school and for homework, and then gradually ex-

SIDEBAR 9.3

## Points to Remember: Treatment of Refractive Error and Focusing Difficulties in Children with CVI

- All children with CVI need thorough and regular eye examinations, including assessment of refractive error and focusing.
- Children with myopia (short-sightedness or nearsightedness) should wear their spectacles for distance viewing (such as blackboard work, television, and movies), but may find it beneficial to remove them for viewing near objects.
- Children with hyperopia (long-sightedness or farsightedness) and astigmatism usually need to wear their spectacles for all tasks.
- Bifocal or progressive lenses have been shown to be beneficial where focusing problems exist. Parents should be encouraged to ask the eye care provider about possible use of these lenses for their child's focusing problems.
- When spectacles are required for a specific task, this should be indicated on the frames so that all caregivers and therapists know whether they are being used appropriately.
- It may be helpful to mark spectacle frames with the child's name, particularly when they are to be worn in large-group settings.
- When simultanagnosia is present, spectacle correction may reduce visual performance, as the improved visual clarity increases the amount of visual information available and increases the visual clutter.
- Performance may be improved by retaining clarity through spectacle wear, but reducing the amount of visual detail presented for children who have difficulty with visual clutter.
- Magnifiers can be helpful in reducing visual clutter, and many are simple and easy to use.
- It may take some time for a child to accept spectacle wear.
- Praise and compliment the child when he or she is wearing the eyeglasses, to encourage their continued use.
- Avoid turning the process of compliance with spectacles into a fight.
- Make sure the fit and condition of the eyeglasses is well maintained.

tended to full-time use, with the child leading the way.

## Conclusion

Sidebar 9.3 summarizes key points to remember about treatment of refractive error and focusing difficulties in children with CVI. Children with developmental disabilities and CVI are more likely to have refractive error and difficulties with accurate focusing. It is important to thoroughly investigate these aspects of visual functioning early in a child's life, and review them regularly, as refractive status is likely to change with development and visual maturation. Unless detected and appropriately managed, refractive errors and poor focusing will compound other visual impairments and limit a child's visual potential.

## References


Al-Bagdady, M., Stewart, R. E., Watts, P., Murphy, P. J., & Woodhouse, J. M. (2009). Bifocals and Down's syndrome: Correction or treatment? *Ophthalmic and Physiological Optics, 29*(4), 416–421.

Atkinson, J., Braddick, O., Nardini, M., & Anker, S. (2007). Infant hyperopia: Detection, distribution, changes and correlates—Outcomes from the Cambridge infant screening programs. *Optometry and Vision Science, 84*(2), 84–96.

Das, M., Spowart, K., Crossley, S., & Dutton, G. N. (2010). Evidence that children with special needs all require visual assessment. *Archives of Diseases in Childhood, 95*(11), 888–892.

Firth, A. Y., & Walker, K. (2006). Visual side-effects from transdermal scopolamine (hyoscine). *Developmental Medicine & Child Neurology, 48*(2), 137–138.

Leone, J. F., Mitchell, P., Morgan, I. G., Kifley, A., & Rose, K. A. (2010). Use of visual acuity to screen for significant refractive errors in adolescents: Is it reliable? *Archives of Ophthalmology, 128*(7), 894–899.

McClelland, J. F., Parkes, J., Hill, N., Jackson, A. J., & Saunders, K. J. (2006). Accommodative dysfunction in children with cerebral palsy: A population-based study. *Investigative Ophthalmology & Visual Science, 47*(5), 1824–1830.

Nandakumar, K., & Leat, S. J. (2010). Bifocals in children with Down syndrome (BiDS)—Visual acuity, accommodation and early literacy skills. *Acta Ophthalmologica, 88*(6), e196–204.

O'Connor, A. R., Stephenson, T. J., Johnson, A., Tobin, M. J., Ratib, S., & Fielder, A. R. (2006). Change of refractive state and eye size in children of birth weight less than 1701 g. *British Journal of Ophthalmology, 90*(4), 456–460.

O'Donoghue, L., McClelland, J. F., Logan, N. S., Rudnicka, A. R., Owen, C. G., & Saunders, K. J. (2010). Refractive error and visual impairment in school children in Northern Ireland. *British Journal of Ophthalmology, 94*(9), 1155–1159.

Ross, L. M., Heron, G., Mackie, R., McWilliam, R., & Dutton, G. N. (2000). Reduced accommodative function in dyskinetic cerebral palsy: A novel management strategy. *Developmental Medicine & Child Neurology, 42*(10), 701–703.

Saeed, M., Henderson, G., & Dutton, G. N. (2007). Hyoscine skin patches for drooling dilate pupils and impair accommodation: Spectacle correction for photophobia and blurred vision may be warranted. *Developmental Medicine & Child Neurology, 49*(6), 426–428.

Saunders, K. J. (2009). Optometric assessment and management of patients with developmental disability. In M. Rosenfield & N. Logan (Eds.), *Optometry: Science, Techniques and Clinical Management* (2nd ed., pp. 513–530). Philadelphia: Butterworth Heinemann, Elsevier.

Saunders, K. J., Little, J. A., McClelland, J. F., & Jackson, A. J. (2010). Profile of refractive errors in cerebral palsy: Impact of severity of motor impairment (GMFCS) and CP subtype on refractive outcome. *Investigative Ophthalmology & Visual Science, 51*(6), 2885–2890.

Saunders, K. J., McClelland, J. F., Richardson, P. M., & Stevenson, M. (2008). Clinical judgement of near pupil responses provides a useful indicator of focusing ability in children with cerebral palsy. *Developmental Medicine & Child Neurology, 50*(1), 33–37.

Saunders, K. J., McCulloch, D. L., Shepherd, A. J., & Wilkinson, G. (2002). Emmetropization following preterm birth. *British Journal of Ophthalmology, 86*(9), 1035–1040.

Sterner, B., Gellerstedt, M., & Sjöström, A. (2004). The amplitude of accommodation in 6–10-year-old children—Not as good as expected! *Ophthalmic and Physiological Optics, 24*(3), 246–251.

Williams, W. R., Latif, A. H., Hannington, L., & Watkins, D. R. (2005). Hyperopia and educational attainment in a primary school cohort. *Archives of Disease in Childhood, 90*(2), 150–153.

Woodhouse, J. M., Meades, J. S., Leat, S. J., & Saunders, K. J. (1993). Reduced accommodation in children with Down syndrome. *Investigative Ophthalmology & Visual Science, 34*(7), 2382–2387.

# PART III

## Assessment of Children with CVI

# 10

# Assessment of Children with CVI: Introduction and Overview

*Amanda Hall Lueck and Gordon N. Dutton*

This chapter presents an overview of elements in a comprehensive assessment for children who have cerebral visual impairment (CVI). More detailed information on this topic is provided in the chapters that follow in Part 3 of this book.

The focus of a comprehensive assessment for children with CVI is to elicit and understand the behavioral manifestations of this condition and their origin (Dutton, 2003; Hyvärinen, 2003). Through the careful evaluation of a child's behaviors and visual reactions, an understanding of the reasons behind the behaviors, and the impact of CVI on the individual child can be established. Such an understanding, in turn, forms the basis for identifying a student's strengths and the development of appropriate interventions and environmental adaptations to promote academic, daily living, and social success in school, at home, and in the community. Recent investigations have shown that behaviors associated with CVI tend to fall into predictable patterns tied to neurological correlates that can provide guidance for interventionists and families (see, for example, Macintyre-Béon et al., 2010). To determine these patterns, a range of behaviors must be evaluated. This chapter provides an overview of the areas that need to be assessed, along with a model of the assessment process, and a framework for the organization of assessment findings. The early part of this chapter details the steps involved in the assessment process, after which a three-tier model is presented of the specific areas that need to be evaluated.

The assessment of children with CVI includes and extends beyond the components of the assessment process for children who have ocular visual impairments. (Details about the assessment of ocular visual impairment can be found in Chapter 12 and in texts that discuss evaluation of children's vision, including those with low vision; see, for example, Corn & Erin, 2010; Duckman, 2006; Lueck, 2004a). It is critical to assess the effects of any ocular visual impairment in children who have CVI. It is also imperative that assessment protocols for these children address the intricate functional ramifications of damage to the visual brain, including impairments of both lower- and higher-order visual functions (see Chapter 2).

The concepts of assessment and screening are applied in this book from an educational perspective. Some useful definitions come from Salvia, Ysseldyke, and Bolt (2013). "Assessment is the process of collecting data for the purpose of (1) specifying or verifying problems and (2) making decisions about students" (Salvia et al., 2013, p. 371). Screening is an "initial stage of assessment in which those who may evidence a particular problem, disorder, disability or disease are discriminated from the general population" (Salvia & Ysseldyke, 2013, p. 378). Screening helps to identify problems early and is a process in which evaluators actively look for specific conditions such as impaired hearing or vision. Screening helps to identify hitherto unrecognized issues, which can then be evaluated in greater depth and managed accordingly (Ysseldyke, Salvia, & Bolt, 2009).

## Multidimensional Assessment Requirements

Assessment for children with CVI must meet the needs of children who fall into three general groups (see Chapter 1):

- those with profound visual impairment, many of whom have additional disabilities
- those with functionally useful vision and cognitive challenges
- those who have functionally useful vision who work at or near the expected academic level for their age group

Comprehensive assessment for all these children with CVI is multidimensional. A variety of functional domains may need to be evaluated in individual children:

- Both *visual functions* (measurable components of the way in which the eyes and visual system operate, including visual acuity, visual fields, contrast sensitivity, and so forth) and *functional vision* (the ways in which a person uses visual skills and abilities binocularly in typical tasks of daily life) need to be assessed. (For more information, see Chapter 1.)
- *Visual processing concerns,* related to damage to the visual brain, need to be addressed. This requires gathering information about higher-order brain functions through history taking, brain imaging, observation, interviews, and performance on key assessment tasks.
- *Motor function* and *knowledge of abilities and disabilities in verbal and performance tasks* must be analyzed, so that their effects can be taken into account in the design of appropriate intervention strategies (Dutton & Jacobson, 2001).
- The *social and emotional ramifications of the child's condition and behaviors* must be considered so that evaluators are aware of the ways in which the child, family, and other caregivers have addressed and adapted to the child's CVI.
- *Auditory processing* needs to be assessed, as disorders can be associated with CVI in children (Morse, 2012). Parents of children with dorsal stream dysfunction have commonly reported to one chapter author (GD) that their child does not know where voices are coming from, particularly when there are other background voices. This corresponds with recent concepts about the functioning of the hearing system (Rauschecker, 2011). Consequently, sound localization may not be a substitute for visual search when this occurs. Thus it is important to consider the evaluation of auditory processing as well as visual processing for

children who have CVI. (See Chapter 15 for more information on auditory processing related to reading.)

- *Evaluation of the influence of a child's environment on performance* is critical, since the performance of children who have CVI can be particularly sensitive to the way the environment is structured, and to the effects of competing sensory stimuli. This will lead to recommendations about ways in which each setting can be structured to support a child's growth and learning.

Sidebar 10.1 presents four principles of assessment of visual functioning for children with CVI that have been formulated by Hyvärinen, Jacob, and Henriksen.

## Role of Professionals on the Evaluation Team

Given all the areas in which assessment is needed for a child with CVI, cross-disciplinary, collaborative assessment is necessary to obtain a meaningful, integrated, multidimensional evaluation of the outcomes of CVI. No one profession may have sufficient knowledge to tap the range of behavioral manifestations of damage to the visual brain in children. A team assessment

SIDEBAR 10.1

### Four Principles in Assessment of Visual Functioning

*Lea Hyvärinen, Namita Jacob, and Anne Henriksen*

In the assessment of visual functioning of infants and children with damage to the visual brain, children at all developmental and communication levels are seen. Four principles related to assessment, planning of therapies and instruction, and execution of intervention plans can be applied to these children, especially to those with severe and multiple involvements. These principles are generalizations and need to be adapted to the specific needs of each child and his or her family.

#### 1. *Always look for the potential all children have for learning, including children with severe and multiple involvements.*

About 80 percent of children with manifest damage to the visual brain have at least one other disability that may affect the use of vision (Hatton, Schwietz, Boyer, & Rychwalski, 2007). Many children with very severe multiple disabilities have had minimal assessment and intervention because many practitioners find it hard to imagine the child's potential for development in the context of the severity of multiple impairments.

All children have the right to assessment and intervention that maximizes their ability to communicate and obtain information from the environment. While these children represent a challenge, we must strive to think creatively about ways to elicit information about their visual and other capacities and about ways to promote the development of these capacities. Increasing children's access to information by advancing their sensory capacities can have a tremendous positive impact on their development and quality of life. Many children may look disinterested and passive as a result of conditions such as face blindness or partial facial paralysis, when, in fact, they are deeply

*(continued on next page)*

engaged and curious. Children with multiple impairments are easily misunderstood so professionals need to take time to listen to those who interact closely with them and act accordingly.

### 2. *Use tests and testing situations creatively and formulate recommendations relevant to the child's reality.*

The poor integration of sensory input of children with multiple disabilities makes it difficult for them to organize their responses to new environments and people. Since they must often marshal most of their capacity to understand and orient to their surroundings, they may not be able to participate fully in typical test situations in the way that their counterparts with isolated visual impairments can. When testing is done in a clinic or in another center, it should become regular practice to ask the family and teachers to bring along the child's familiar possessions, for his or her comfort, such as the child's naptime mat or items the child likes to hold or view. The child's teacher, therapist, or parent can be partners in testing, ready in the background to take cues from evaluators for help when needed.

Suggestions for intervention should be strongly tied to the abilities and the activities of the child and take into consideration the other adaptations that are used to enable participation in life. For example, when planning spectacle correction, consider correction to enable the use of the best visual image *at a distance relevant to the child.* Ask for reading correction for a very close distance for infants and children with a limited visual sphere or, infrequently, at the distance from the eye to the foot for those rare older children who use their feet to type. Also consider the typical position of the child's head and the supports used to maintain these positions when selecting spectacle frames. Frames should be large enough, but not too large, and well fitted so that the part of the lens that is used for close observation is at the correct height in the frame.

### 3. *Consider the strong relationship between motor development and vision when testing and planning recommendations.*

The development of the motor and visual systems is deeply intertwined in all children. Motor functions can serve to activate vision for children who have multiple impairments. For example, body position and maintenance of position are related to the ability to direct and maintain visual attention. In addition, vision can often be the impetus for novel motor performance, as in cases where children reach for desired items that they see, or try new motor functions to achieve a goal motivated by vision. Before testing begins, make sure to enlist the help of the child's therapists, O&M specialist, family, and/or teacher to ensure that the child is positioned in a way that enables optimal attention and best ability to respond. As the most effective positions are discovered, make sure to incorporate them into suggestions for intervention. Ask the therapist, O&M specialist, and teacher to observe visual functioning in other positions/postures that are used during the day so that the variation of visual functioning in a variety of positions is carefully documented.

### 4. *Do not expect children with brain damage to follow normal developmental sequences in their visual development.*

This is a very important principle. If brain damage occurs early in development, visual functions may unfold in unusual ways. It has been documented that after brain damage, even in adults at 60 years of age, visual functions may relocate from the damaged neural area to the corresponding area in the other hemisphere (Henriksson, Raninen, Näsänen, Hyvärinen, & Vanni, 2007). Similar large changes are likely to happen in the very plastic brains of infants and young children.

*(continued on next page)*

**SIDEBAR 10.1** *(continued from previous page)*

These changes may not show in an MRI. This group of children may have poor visual fixation, impaired accommodation, and impaired following (pursuit) and saccadic eye movements. Yet some of these children can read—a task that places high demands on the entire visual system. They have learned to use compensatory strategies to overcome the lack of some basic visual functions. Some children's saccadic functions or fixation may improve slowly over the years as their overall motor spasticity decreases and all motor functions improve as a sequel to medical and educational interventions. Their functioning therefore needs to be assessed regularly so that changing educational and communication needs are met by updated instructional strategies. These children demonstrate the importance of enhancing visual capacity based on each child's individual abilities, not using typical visual training schedules that assume a certain pattern of development.

requires a compilation of results from various fields of expertise and a group consensus about the ways in which all the parts of the assessment results fit together to form a profile that guides the habilitation or rehabilitation of a particular child with CVI.

Clinical judgment in the assessment of students with CVI is critical in determining what to assess, how to assess it, and how to interpret the findings. Working as a team throughout the assessment process ensures an integrated approach to such decisions. Parents and other caregivers are a vital part of the assessment team since they know their children's behaviors and needs so well. In some instances, children can also participate in assessment team meetings. The role of different specialists will vary depending on the issues presented by each child, as well as on the availability and roles of evaluators in a particular country or region. The evaluation team for a comprehensive assessment can include, but is not limited to, the following:

- caregivers, parents, and students
- neuroradiologists
- occupational therapists
- ophthalmologists
- optometrists
- orthoptists
- orientation and mobility (O&M) specialists
- pediatric neurologists
- pediatricians
- physical therapists
- psychologists/neuropsychologists
- regular education teachers
- speech-language pathologists
- teachers of students with visual impairments

Not all the evaluators listed are required for every child. The composition of the assessment team depends on each child's known and emerging unique needs.

The ways in which children with CVI use their vision in their home, school, and community is a major concern; therefore, teachers of students with visual impairments and O&M specialists are often intimately involved in the processes of both assessment and intervention. Their expertise is especially valuable when applied to children with CVI who have a range of vision capabilities that affect their ability to access educational materials and instruction using vision. Whether or not these specialists should be the case managers for a particular child with CVI and what roles they and other professionals assume in the assessment process need to be determined on a case-by-case basis. They can, however, contribute their expertise as part of the team to help determine appropriate instructional strategies, educational materials, assistive technology, environmental adaptations, and educational goals that address the child's core curriculum and expanded core curriculum needs. How goals are implemented will depend on team recommendations, which, in turn, are determined from assessment results and available resources.

Table 10.1, which is presented later in this chapter and provides an overall guide to assessment of children with CVI, shows possible roles for the various professionals in different areas of the assessment process. How teams operate will vary depending on the organization of services in a particular country or region. Some teams will be centralized within a medical facility, agency, or school. Others will be more spread out, working for a variety of medical or educational services. The key to "teaming" is not that everyone works under the same roof, but that good leadership and planning lead to everyone working in a coordinated and collaborative way as information is gathered, interpreted, and reported, so that intervention recommendations based on team decisions are compiled in a way that promotes optimal strategies for children with CVI (Lueck, 2004b).

## Steps in the Evaluation Process

Since CVI can affect many behavioral areas in addition to vision, evaluation methods must be expanded to ensure that the full range of effects of CVI are appraised and subsequently addressed. Since each CVI case is unique, the nature of the planned assessment should match the child's condition and needs. If additional needs are identified as the assessment process evolves, the assessment plan and team may require modifications that target those additional needs. Initial efforts are guided by a comprehensive review and summary of medical and educational records in order to understand the range of behaviors that may be affected for a particular child. For example, the ability to read regular print may be compromised in a child with CVI, even though the child's visual acuity may be close to 20/20. With a firm foundation in medical findings (for example, ophthalmological, neurological, pediatric), the following steps need to be taken to formulate comprehensive evaluation protocols for children who have CVI.

### Step 1: Preparations for the Comprehensive Evaluation[1]

***Assign a case manager who will coordinate the evaluation process.*** Case managers will need to have knowledge of the condition and its ramifications in order to bring together appropriate personnel for the assessment process and guide the compilation of findings that leads to coordinated written and verbal reports of assessment results and recommendations.

***Work in tandem with medical practitioners to ensure that eye examinations and other medical examinations are current and complete.*** For children with CVI, it is important to seek out services from ophthalmologists, optometrists, or orthoptists familiar with CVI. Other medical specialists should be included, based on recommenda-

[1] This section was adapted in part from Lueck, 2004b, pp. 93–85.

tions from attending clinicians. If possible, a member of the educational evaluation team (often the teacher of the visually impaired or O&M specialist) as well as caregivers should be present during eye examinations (including the general eye examination and the low vision evaluation) to gather salient information from the assessments, as well as provide information and feedback to the eye care providers as needed.

***Review existing records***. Be sure to review the full range of medical reports, educational records, and functional areas that may be affected in a child with CVI. If videotapes of the child are available, they can be helpful in gaining an understanding of a child's performance in various settings. A review of associated visual and visually based behaviors that are linked to each child's medical, visual, and behavioral conditions can contribute valuable information to the design of the assessment plan. Appendix 3B in Chapter 3, which reviews the visual consequences of CVI that are associated with a range of medical conditions and presenting behaviors, is designed to assist in this process and is discussed in more detail later in this chapter.

***Recruit the initial multidisciplinary assessment team based on a review of records***. This team may need to be amended as the assessment process progresses. Typically, an education system assigns an individual to be the case manager for a child with disabilities. If a child is first seen in a medical context, appropriate referrals for other medical and educational evaluations are often built into follow-up procedures.

***Have the necessary optical prescription in place during evaluations***. Any required spectacle corrections for nearsightedness (myopia), farsightedness (hyperopia), and astigmatism, as well as any near prescription for impaired accommodation, to aid in close viewing, should be worn by the child with CVI in order to provide a picture of optimum performance. (See Chapter 9 for more information.)

***Establish rapport with the child and family***. Caregivers of children with CVI are able to provide a wealth of information about how their children function, but may be confused about the cause and adaptive purpose of any atypical behaviors since the condition may be new to them. An approach that welcomes and respects the insights afforded by the caregivers' knowledge and understanding of their children promotes rapport and provides valuable assessment information. Children can be quite sensitive to the emotional needs of their caregivers; therefore, it is important to put family members at ease and to seek their input and advice prior to, and during, the assessment process. In addition, efforts to make children comfortable with an examiner in a test situation are likely to result in assessment responses that more accurately represent their optimal performance. Taking the time to establish rapport is well worth the effort.

***Include family members and key professionals throughout the evaluation process***. It is best to work in tandem with the child and family, involving them as active participants in the assessment process. Caregivers can provide valid and accurate reports about how a child functions at home and in the community with a variety of people. They can also help practitioners interpret behavioral responses during testing. For children who have cognitive challenges, caregivers can provide input to practitioners about ways to present assessment items so that children fully understand what is expected of them. The presence of caregivers during testing may also create a secure environment and lead to more typical response patterns on the part of the child.

It is up to the evaluators to determine how best to facilitate family participation during assessment procedures. Some physical layouts may be more conducive to active participation by family members than others. (For example, there may be a one-way mirror for viewing so that a large group can observe. Examination rooms that are crowded with equipment and only have room for one family member should be avoided.) There may be certain times during the assessment process when more active participation by family members is sought. (For example, during a visual acuity assessment, a family member may be able to clarify the types of symbols that a child is best able to identify, such as letters, numbers, or pictures.) The best ways to work with family members so that they provide welcome support and advice without distracting the child will be specific to each situation, but it is helpful to set ground rules right away during an assessment session (such as explaining where to sit, how an assessment procedure will be performed, and at what moments during the procedure assistance will be sought). When caregivers are present, it is also important to pause occasionally during the assessment process to summarize for them what has just happened and what will happen next.

As family members participate in the evaluation process, they may raise questions and concerns about their child's present status and about their future expectations. Evaluators will need to be sensitive to these queries and provide information that helps the child and family understand the child's visual condition and its implications as the evaluation process unfolds. In addition to providing information, evaluators must also be skilled and respectful listeners in order to learn about a child's skills, abilities, preferences, and needs. This two-way communication can improve the quality of evaluation outcomes for the evaluator, the children, and their families.

***Conduct assessments when children are best able to respond.*** Some children's performance will vary greatly when conditions are not optimal for them. For example, they may be taking medications with side effects, need quiet time after eating, require frequent naps, need time to adjust to new environments, respond best after their arousal level has been heightened through specific motor activity, or respond best in a particular body position. It is important to ensure that the necessary conditions for optimal performance are taken into account when scheduling a time for formal testing. Evaluators may learn that a particular child's best performance time is one hour after taking a certain medication, early morning in the classroom, two hours after eating meals in a familiar environment, or positioned in a stander after swinging for five minutes. Information about situations that promote maximum performance, gained from interview and observation, can also be used to guide the design of intervention programs to ensure success.

***Understand the communication input and response modes for each child.*** For children who have communication challenges, it is critical to obtain a valid evaluation of their skills and abilities in this area prior to any formal or informal testing. This can be determined from observation and prior reports, as well as input from caregivers and key staff who know the child well. For example, the child may use alternative communication channels to respond, such as with a smile, a head turn, gestures, vocalizations, pointing with the hand or foot, or changes in posture. Additionally, the child's condition may require evaluators to devise a special response system, such as a system with only two choices, when presenting test items. What each child requires will vary, and introducing test items that take into account individual receptive and expressive communication needs will ensure that indicators of optimum performance are obtained.

## Step 2: Gather Information

Once preparations for the comprehensive assessment have been made, the evaluation team will need to use a variety of methods to gather information to determine a child's abilities, skills, and behaviors. Hyvärinen (2003) calls for repeated assessment to get a full picture of how a child functions over time. It is also helpful to check functional performance outcomes across a child's typical environments. Evaluation data may be collected through special testing in clinical settings, in the home, at school, and in the community. All children with functional vision should have a low vision evaluation by an eye care specialist who specializes in children with low vision. (Specific areas for evaluation are discussed later in this chapter in the section "A Comprehensive Model of Assessment for Children with CVI.") Additional recommended assessment methods include the following:

***Administration of an open-ended interview and, if needed, a structured interview, to discover functional concerns from the perspectives of the child and caregivers as well as others in close contact with the child.*** This information is pivotal to characterizing visual difficulties and plays a central role in the assessment process. An open-ended interview starts with general questions and does not provide response options (for example, "Tell me about your child's vision"), while a structured interview provides response-specific options (such as "Does your child recognize you when you are in a crowd of people nearby?" (See Chapter 11 for more detailed information on history taking.)

***Observation of the child's behavior.*** Direct observation of the child can inform, verify, and expand findings from interviews and formal testing situations. Observations made during a testing session help inform how a child approaches or responds to specific assessment tasks, while observations made in a child's typical environment reveal the impact of the visual impairment on daily activities. Many evaluators find that recording videos of children in different settings provides a way to gather valuable information about a child's performance capabilities. Steendam recommends that teachers or the family provide video recordings of the child in different circumstances and states of mind to view the range of visual behaviors, from the least to the most efficient (M. Steendam, personal communication, July 2012).

***Testing of functional vision involving observation during activities that require vision.*** Evaluators administer formal or informal tests in typical environments to determine how a child functions on specific visual tasks. They may also evaluate the child's use of vision in critical activities in order to design optimal interventions. For children with CVI, performance may vary depending on the setting, and this variable performance may be highly instructive for the design of interventions and optimal environments.

***Testing in other areas***. Recommended testing in other areas includes assessment of hearing and auditory processing, assessment of motor and O&M skills (see Chapter 17), and assessment of executive functions by a psychologist or neuropsychologist. Since basic literacy and mathematics skills form the foundation for learning in all areas of both the core curriculum and the expanded core curriculum (which addresses the unique skills and information needed by students with visual impairments to live independently, exercise personal decision making, and access the general curriculum), the impact of CVI on these areas may also require more formal and informal assessment. (See Chapters 15 and 16 for further information.)

***Structured play or learning situations designed to elicit specific target behaviors that might shed light on a child's functional needs.*** Specially designed "real-world" situations provide excellent opportunities to learn how a child operates using vision and other senses during structured play situations or when completing typical tasks. An example of a structured learning situation for assessment is a play environment including a child's favorite toys with meaningful visible elements matched to the child's visual abilities, and designed to elicit reaching behavior based on visual cues. Additional examples can be found in Chapter 16.

### Step 3: Integration of Information, Report Writing, and Intervention Recommendations

The information gathered during the assessment process needs to be compiled and integrated by the multidisciplinary team (including family members and the children themselves, whenever possible) into a report that presents a picture of how a child functions visually, along with recommendations for interventions matched to the evaluation findings. Coordination between school and home is important at this stage to ensure that recommendations are understood, accepted, and implemented in the same way by both caregivers and professional staff (Walthes, Hyvärinen, & Petz, 2011). Written and verbal reports need to be conveyed using language that all team members, including the family, fully understand. (Writing of reports is discussed in more detail in the section on "Assembling and Reporting Assessment Results" later in this chapter.) Methods that tie evaluation findings to instruction can be found throughout Parts 3 and 4 of this book.

### Step 4: Ongoing Assessment for Children with CVI: Observation and Diagnostic Teaching

As children grow and develop, their vision, the adaptations they make, their visual requirements, their other skills, and their typical environments all change. The impact of these changes requires regular and timely review. Therefore, another step in the assessment process is to determine the frequency and nature of any formal or informal follow-up assessments required to meet changing needs and situations.

Although the next formal comprehensive assessment process may be scheduled at some time in the future, assessment by means of observation within a diagnostic teaching model can provide a continuous stream of information about the needs of a child. In the diagnostic teaching approach, individualized assessment data that inform the teaching and learning process are gathered, analyzed, and used to determine the next steps in intervention. Diagnostic teaching methods have been adapted to meet varying needs of students in regular and special education (see, for example, Fahsi & McAndrews, 2012; Gregory & Kuzmich, 2004). Assessment and instruction are considered interactive and continuous processes where student performance and understanding is monitored before, during, and after each lesson. While the details of the methods may vary depending on the type of instruction implemented, the learner, and the learning situation, the overarching principles of diagnostic teaching can be applied to a range of students who have CVI.

Diagnostic teaching requires instructors to

1. gather key information from records, interviews, assessments, and observations,
2. make intervention decisions about what and how to teach based on these initial data (these interventions are hypotheses about what will work best for a particular student),
3. determine how students manifest their learning,
4. evaluate learning within the context of the actual teaching environment and the teaching strategies employed, and then
5. formulate the next steps in the teaching-learning process based on outcomes noted for the individual student.

With this approach, immediate feedback informs the next steps in instruction. Activities and strategies can be progressively modified based on student performance (International Reading Association, 2006). Modifications in teaching strategies are made regularly by teachers who "reflect consciously on student learning and then connect their conclusions to the most effective next steps" (Gregory & Kuzmich, 2004, p. 52). In the context of assessment, this method makes it possible to maintain a record of learning over time for a particular child, and relate any changes in learning outcomes to specific intervention strategies or other factors that may have led to them. Diagnostic teaching methods are discussed in Chapter 15 in relation to the assessment of literacy and math instruction, in Chapter 16 with respect to independent living skills, and in Chapter 21 in relation to the instruction of young children and children with multiple disabilities.

## Use of Available Assessment Tools with Children Who Have CVI

Since the multidimensional effects of CVI overlap numerous areas of professional specialization, a comprehensive evaluation requires the assessment findings from a variety of disciplines to be assembled and collated. Furthermore, the need to individualize assessment for each child is critical due to the wide-ranging behavioral expressions of the condition. There are a number of assessment tools available that are not specifically devised for children who have CVI, but which can be recruited for use with this population. Materials developed to evaluate vision or visual performance issues specifically associated with CVI are beginning to emerge.

Assessment tools that are currently available are discussed in the chapters that follow in Part 3 and in Chapter 24. It must be emphasized that a firm understanding of CVI is critical when administering any formal tests to children with CVI. Only then can evaluators make sound clinical judgments about ways to administer the tests, interpret the results, and translate these results into appropriate intervention strategies. It must also be stressed that any test items requiring vision must be well within a specific child's visual capabilities. Additional assessment material will likely be developed in the coming years as understanding about CVI increases.

## Knowing What to Look for: An Initial Guide for the Evaluation Process

The visual consequences of brain damage cover a broad range of visual behaviors as well as behaviors in other associated domains. Since CVI can vary significantly from child to child, identification of potential behaviors related to a specific presenting condition at the start of the evaluation process will help guide members of the evaluation team as they formulate a plan to pinpoint and characterize a child's atypical visual behaviors that are brain-based. To this end, Appendix 3B in Chapter 3 presents various features that children with CVI may exhibit; Tables 3.2–3.9 provide additional information about behavioral manifestations. The informed practitioner can be on the lookout for these behavioral manifestations in the clinic or in the classroom in children who have been diagnosed with CVI, as well as in children who may have been overlooked for the CVI diagnosis. Evaluators can seek evidence for their presence or absence as the assessment process unfolds, as in the following example:

**Ricardo is a bright high school junior with cerebral** palsy affecting the right side of his body (right hemiplegia), who has moved to a new school district. His visual acuity was reported to be 20/80 in each eye by his eye doctor. No visual field limitations were noted in his eye reports. He uses a wheelchair to get around and has very limited use of his right hand. In his class, his new teacher found that even though he must move quite close to view them, Ricardo prefers to have a limited number of smaller icons clustered toward the middle and left side of the computer screen rather than large icons spread evenly over his entire computer screen. During mobility lessons designed to familiarize Ricardo with his new school site, his O&M instructor noted that Ricardo was often not aware of students walking on his right side in crowded hallways or on school grounds, and he also had problems negotiating curbs. Using the information in Appendix 3B, the team found that, for children with right hemiplegia, there may be lack of vision or impaired visual attention on the right side. The team needed to determine whether the following visually related behaviors were present:

- Intermittent lack of attention for sights and sounds on the right side, when distracted, tired, or angry.
- Lack of visual attention on the right, and possibly peripheral lower visual field impairment as well. (The best vision may be in the left upper quadrant of the visual field.)
- Inaccuracy when drawing on the right side of the page (but not on the left side).

The education team will incorporate evaluation methods that pay particular attention to the presence or absence of these visual consequences associated with right hemiplegia, as well as investigate, through a comprehensive assessment, other issues that might arise and that characterize Ricardo's visual and other needs.

## A Comprehensive Model of Assessment for Children with CVI

### Three Tiers of Assessment

Children with CVI display an array of behaviors that require evaluation by a variety of professionals with different areas of expertise. As mentioned earlier, vision assessments must consider the examination of vision functions, functional vision, and higher-order visual functions that result from damage to the visual brain. Other assessments may also be necessary when additional disabilities are present or suspected. As such, the evaluation process for children with CVI can be approached from a variety of perspectives. The model proposed in this chapter is one way to conceptualize a holistic evaluation process for children with CVI.

Comprehensive assessment for children with CVI can be a complicated process that may seem overwhelming at first. It can, however, be understood in terms of a process composed of three tiers. The results from each tier of assessment provide the basis for evaluation questions to be addressed at the next tier. Figure 10.1 provides a graphic overview of the process, and a detailed explanation of each tier of assessment is provided in the following sections.

FIGURE 10.1

**Tiers of Assessment for Vision and Visual Processing of Children with CVI**

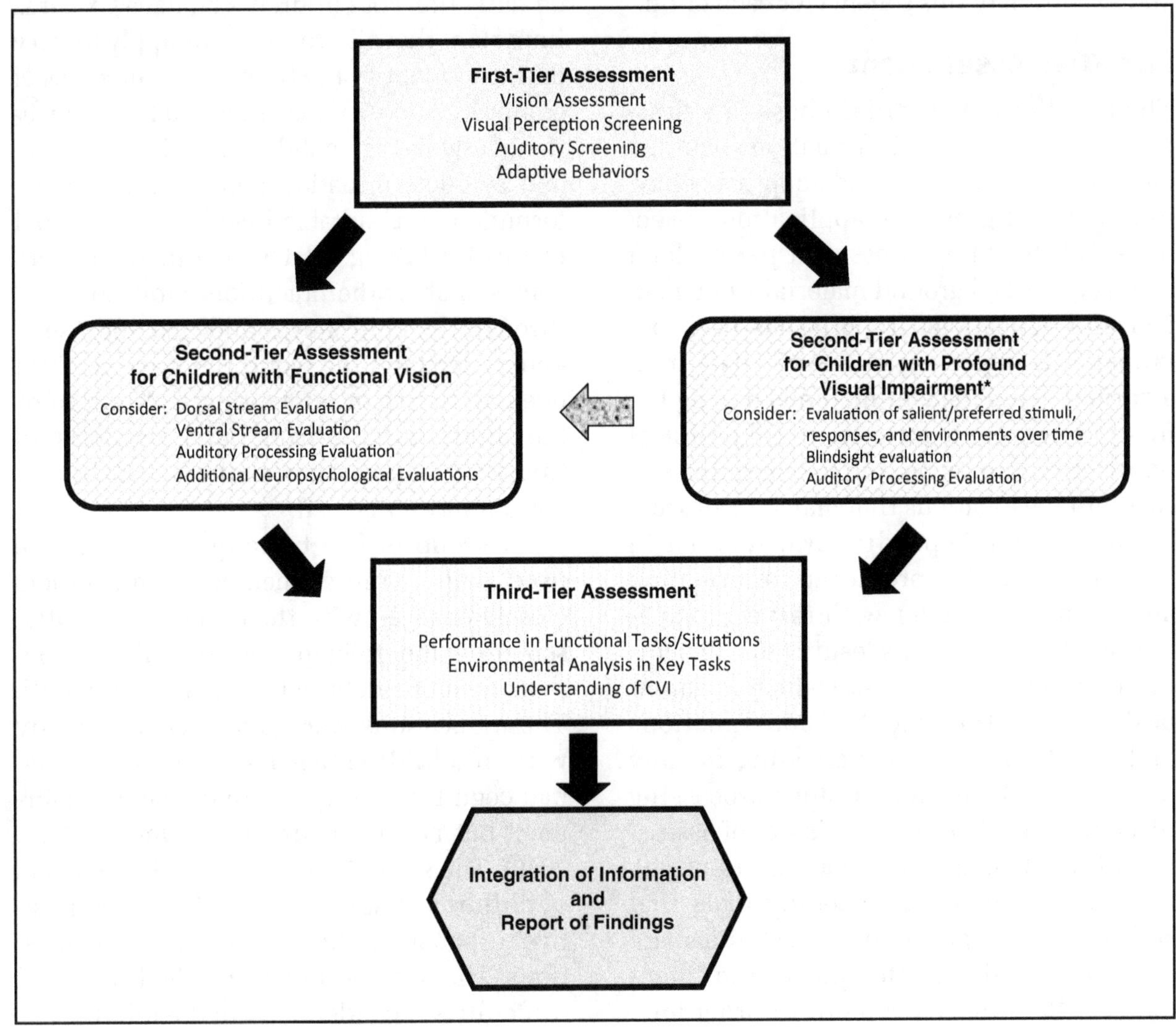


*Note: For children with profound visual impairment whose vision improves over time, additional Second Tier evaluation methods related to children with functional vision can be conducted.

Table 10.1 summarizes information about the tiers of assessment, listing specific areas for evaluation in each tier, behavioral indicators that may suggest that an area requires a more in-depth evaluation, and practitioners who can potentially conduct these evaluations. It is designed to provide a starting point for practitioners in selecting the assessments that need to be performed for a particular child; however, practitioners must use their clinical judgment about the application and extension of this schema for each child.

## First-Tier Assessment

The first tier is the initial phase of assessment for preliminary information about the child's vision, hearing, and adaptive behaviors that will guide the application of second- and third-tier assessment protocols. It begins once background material from medical and educational reports has been obtained. It is important to compile data from a variety of assessment methods during the first tier in order to form an initial profile of how a child functions, and to determine any further investigations that may be required. Chapter 3 and Appendix 3B can assist in this endeavor by providing information about what to look for with respect to specific medical conditions leading to CVI. During first-tier assessments, evaluators gather basic information about vision functions and functional vision. Screening for any hearing problems and auditory processing difficulties is also part of this tier of assessment (see Chapter 15 for more information). Formal and informal screening tools that address visual processing capabilities are administered during this phase (see Chapters 12, 13, and 14 for more information). In addition, screening for visual processing problems is undertaken through interviews that involve open-ended questions and structured history taking (see Chapter 11). Observation and interviews play a large role during the first-tier assessment phase, guiding subsequent formal and informal testing, as well as observations made later in the assessment process.

### *Taking a Visual History*

Every child with a visual impairment needs to have an in-depth history elicited that addresses the impact of the visual impairment on daily life. For children who have CVI, it is important that all professionals apply history taking to identify the functional outcomes of compromised vision as they relate to education, daily living, mobility, social interaction, and self-determination and to assist in the formulation of suitable interventions. A goal of history taking related to functional outcomes enables the practitioner to "look out" through the child's eyes and imagine, "see," and understand the world the way the child does, rather than attempting to "look into" the child's mind to work out a diagnosis. In this way, intervention methods can be immeasurably enhanced.

A group of five basic questions can be used with family members and others closely engaged with the child, as an initial screening tool to help identify children who require more detailed evaluation for CVI. These questions were generated in a study with 40 children, aged 4 to 16 years, who had cognitive and perceptual visual impairment but no motor disability (Dutton et al., 2010). The study found that family members of children diagnosed with CVI gave positive responses to three or more of these questions. The five questions, and the functional difficulties they identify, are the following:

1. How does your child handle stairs? (Difficulty walking down stairs)

## TABLE 10.1

# Assessment Model for Vision and Visual Processing Tied to Behavioral Indicators

This set of tables provides a quick assessment guide for children with CVI. The sample behaviors are not exhaustive of those that may need careful evaluation, but represent ones that are commonly seen. Evaluators, listed in alphabetical order, are potential practitioners and will vary by country or region.

Any assessments conducted with children who have CVI must identify ways in which the environment may affect test results (such as background noise, pattern, and clutter). Ideally, outcomes can be examined under varying environmental conditions that may have an impact on performance. The evaluation areas are separated into tiers to ensure that they are all accounted for during the design of assessment protocols. Evaluation areas can often overlap across Tiers (for example, examining near viewing during an eye examination [Tier 1] and during a reading assessment [Tier 3]; examining visual guidance of movement for the upper limbs in the performance of formal tests [Tier 2] and during an O&M assessment [Tier 3]). Observational assessments can occur across all three tiers.

| *Evaluation Areas* | *Sample Behavioral Indicators of a Potential Difficulty* | *Possible Evaluators* | |
|---|---|---|---|
| **First-Tier Assessment: To Determine Initial Information about Vision and Hearing Capabilities** | | | |
| **Part 1**<br>**Vision (for children with low vision)**<br>Note: All children with potential visual impairments require all vision assessments listed in Part 1 | | **Visual Functions** | **Functional Vision** |
| Refraction/eyeglass provision | Narrowing the eyelids to see in the distance, getting up close to see, missing information, taking longer to carry out tasks that require vision, and not seeing facial expressions | Ophthalmologist<br>Optometrist | |
| Accommodation/near eyeglass provision | Better vision for distance than near<br>Near vision seems worse at age 7 or 8 as print size gets smaller<br>All children with cerebral palsy need to be checked, in particular, dyskinetic types of cerebral palsy (with involuntary movements of arms, legs, face, and trunk) in which child has high intelligence and good vision | Ophthalmologist<br>Optometrist | Pediatrician (in some countries)<br>Teacher of students with visual impairments (to identify reading problems at near) |
| Visual acuity | Difficulty distinguishing details at near and/or distance | Ophthalmologist<br>Optometrist | Occupational therapist<br>O&M specialist<br>Pediatrician (in some countries)<br>Teacher of students with visual impairments |

*(continued on next page)*

**TABLE 10.1** *(continued from previous page)*

| *Evaluation Areas* | *Sample Behavioral Indicators of a Potential Difficulty* | *Possible Evaluators* | |
|---|---|---|---|
| Visual field | Bumping into things and missing things in certain consistent areas<br>It may be difficult to distinguish visual field and visual neglect<br>Bruises on both legs (lower field), or one leg (left or right field or neglect on one side) | Ophthalmologist<br>Optometrist | Occupational therapist<br>O&M specialist<br>Pediatrician (in some countries)<br>Teacher of students with visual impairments |
| Contrast sensitivity | Low-contrast items difficult to see, such as human faces, stairs, drop-offs<br>More prominent in poor lighting or with low-contrast materials such as poor photocopies | Ophthalmologist<br>Optometrist | Occupational therapist<br>O&M specialist<br>Pediatrician (in some countries)<br>Teacher of students with visual impairments |
| Oculomotor | Obvious eye movement abnormalities, head turns | Ophthalmologist<br>Optometrist | Occupational therapist<br>O&M specialist<br>Pediatrician (in some countries)<br>Teacher of students with visual impairments |
| **Part 2 (consider for all children with all levels of vision)**<br>**Hearing/Auditory Screening** | Difficulty hearing, locating, and interpreting the spoken word or environmental sounds, especially in noisy situations | Ear, nose, and throat physician<br>Psychologist/neuropsychologist<br>Speech-language pathologist | |
| **Part 3**<br>**Vision Perception Screening through History Taking and Informal Screening Tests of Visual Perceptual Skills** | Parent, caregiver, or teacher concerns about difficulties with:<br>• Changes in floor height (e.g., steps, curbs)<br>• Seeing moving targets<br>• Seeing a distant person or object<br>• Finding clothes in a pile<br>• Copying at normal speed<br>Difficulty with visual matching, identifying pictures when parts are missing, distinguishing a form from its background, remembering a form or its dominant features, identifying a form when it is changed in size, orientation, or embedded into other forms, inability to make equal bisection of lines | Diagnostic history taking:<br>Ophthalmologist<br>Optometrist<br>History taking (open-ended and structured) to characterize the visual difficulties and to develop intervention strategies:<br>Occupational therapist<br>O&M specialist<br>Psychologist/neuropsychologist<br>Teacher of students with visual impairments | |

*(continued on next page)*

**TABLE 10.1** *(continued from previous page)*

| *Evaluation Areas* | *Sample Behavioral Indicators of a Potential Difficulty* | *Possible Evaluators* |
|---|---|---|
| **Part 4**<br>**Adaptive Behaviors** | Unusual behaviors accompany task performance (e.g., eye turn, hand-waving, close-viewing) or tasks are performed in an unusual manner (e.g., stacking objects into a pile and taking them one by one to identify them rather than loosely spreading them out on a table), or unusual reactive behaviors (e.g., anger, distress, or disruptive behavior in a busy, crowded environment) | All evaluators |
| **Second-Tier Assessment:**<br>**A. To Determine Dorsal Stream Function for Children with Functional Vision** | | |
| Visual search | Difficulty finding items in background pattern and/or foreground clutter | Occupational therapist<br>O&M specialist<br>Psychologist/neuropsychologist<br>Teacher of students with visual impairments |
| Visual guidance of movement | Inaccurate grasp using wide thumb finger gap or whole hand<br>Probing floor boundaries with foot; inaccurate movement of foot up/down step while looking at it | Occupational therapist<br>O&M specialist<br>Psychologist/neuropsychologist<br>Teacher of students with visual impairments |
| Visual attention<br>Maintaining/splitting visual attention | Looks away when talking<br>Difficulty copying | Occupational therapist<br>O&M specialist<br>Psychologist/neuropsychologist<br>Teacher of students with visual impairments |
| Intersensory attention | Bumping into obstacles when walking and talking | Occupational therapist<br>O&M specialist<br>Psychologist/neuropsychologist<br>Speech-language pathologist<br>Teacher of students with visual impairments |
| Auditory processing assessment, including knowledge of where sounds and speech are coming from and auditory search | Not knowing where voice is coming from; worse with background sound | Psychologist/neuropsychologist<br>Speech-language pathologist<br>Audiologist |
| Dysfunction of lower field of vision<br>• Lower visual field impairment | Difficulty going down steps and slopes<br>Missing nearest food, toys, or images<br>Opening mouth for food on a spoon presented in upper but not lower visual field | Occupational therapist<br>O&M specialist<br>Psychologist/neuropsychologist<br>Teacher of students with visual impairments |



*(continued on next page)*

**TABLE 10.1** *(continued from previous page)*

| *Evaluation Areas* | *Sample Behavioral Indicators of a Potential Difficulty* | *Possible Evaluators* |
|---|---|---|
| • Neglect of lower visual field | Walking over obstacles without being aware of them | Occupational therapist<br>O&M specialist<br>Psychologist/neuropsychologist<br>Teacher of students with visual impairments |
| Visual guidance of movement of lower limbs | Looking directly at floor boundaries, yet probes with foot to identify if a step is present | Occupational therapist<br>O&M specialist<br>Psychologist/neuropsychologist<br>Teacher of students with visual impairments |
| Visual guidance of movement of upper limbs and hands | Misreaching for items or misplacing them on a table (or even missing the table) unless part of the body locates the table by touching it<br>Reaching with wider gap between fingers and thumb than is typical<br>Reaching with extended hand, to touch item or gather it up in order to identify its correct location | Occupational therapist<br>O&M specialist<br>Psychologist/neuropsychologist<br>Teacher of students with visual impairments |
| Estimation of speed of moving targets | Walking out in front of traffic with wrong timing despite perceiving risks | Occupational therapist<br>O&M specialist<br>Psychologist/neuropsychologist<br>Teacher of students with visual impairments |
| **B. To Determine Ventral Stream Function for Children with Functional Vision** | | |
| Identification of people, facial expressions, objects, shapes, pictures, words | Not recognizing known people, wrongly recognizing unknown people<br>Not seeing language in facial expression<br>Not recognizing objects, shapes, pictures, and words | Occupational therapist<br>O&M specialist<br>Psychologist/neuropsychologist<br>Teacher of students with visual impairments |
| Orientation in surrounding environment related to topographic agnosia | Easily getting lost in uncrowded places that should be known<br>Easily losing possessions and being unable to locate them | Occupational therapist<br>O&M specialist<br>Psychologist/neuropsychologist<br>Teacher of students with visual impairments |

*(continued on next page)*

**TABLE 10.1** *(continued from previous page)*

| *Evaluation Areas* | *Sample Behavioral Indicators of a Potential Difficulty* | *Possible Evaluators* |
|---|---|---|
| **C. To Evaluate Functioning in Children with Profound Visual Impairment** | | |
| Evaluation of salient/preferred stimuli, responses, and environments over time | Attending to simple stimuli, which can become more complex over time<br>Responding through subtle movements or vocalizations, which can become more defined over time<br>Responding to slow-paced visual or auditory stimuli; pace can increase over time | Occupational therapist<br>O&M specialist<br>Psychologist/neuropsychologist<br>Teacher of students with visual impairments |
| Blindsight evaluation | Intermittently noticing stimuli brought in from the periphery<br>Responses can include smile, reaction to moving light, eye movement toward moving target, turning or reaching to a moving target, navigation around obstacles<br>Habituation to targets moved in repeatedly from same direction<br>Head rocks or moves back and forth when concentrating | Occupational therapist<br>O&M specialist<br>Psychologist<br>Teacher of students with visual impairments |
| Auditory processing assessment including knowledge of where sounds and speech are coming from and auditory search | Not knowing where voice is coming from; worse with background sound | Psychologist/neuropsychologist<br>Speech-language pathologist<br>Audiologist |
| **D. Additional Areas to Consider for All Children** | | |
| Auditory processing assessment including knowledge of where sounds and speech are coming from and auditory search | Not knowing where voice is coming from; worse with background sound | Psychologist/neuropsychologist<br>Speech-language pathologist<br>Audiologist |
| Additional neuropsychological testing | Problems associated with general attention, visual attention, visual information processing, executive functions | Psychologist/neuropsychologist |
| **Third-Tier Assessment: Evaluation within Functional Tasks or Situations (for visual processing issues)** | | |
| Reading | Reading is not fluent when text is matched to visual acuity<br>Reading is enhanced by occluding adjacent text (dorsal stream impaired)<br>Reading is not fluent. Cannot recognize letters (ventral stream impaired) | General education teacher<br>Reading specialist<br>Teacher of students with visual impairments |

*(continued on next page)*

**TABLE 10.1** *(continued from previous page)*

| *Evaluation Areas* | *Sample Behavioral Indicators of a Potential Difficulty* | *Possible Evaluators* |
|---|---|---|
| Mathematics | Inability to negotiate page of math problems<br>Needing graph paper (squared paper) of appropriate size and line thickness for all number work (numbers can't be aligned and jumble otherwise) | General education teacher<br>Teacher of students with visual impairments |
| Orientation and mobility skills | Getting lost in crowded environments only (dorsal stream problems)<br>Problems with route-finding based on intrinsic orientation skill and landmarks (ventral stream problems) | O&M specialist |
| Arts and crafts | Difficulty mentally rotating, invoking, and creating imagery from memory for artwork or to copy from images or real life | Art teacher<br>Teacher of students with visual impairments |
| Daily living skills | Varies with tasks to be performed | Occupational therapist<br>O&M specialist<br>Teacher of students with visual impairments |
| Social skills | Lacking eye contact (due to low acuity; inability to split attention when talking; or inability to recognize facial expressions)<br>Inability to see friends in a group (dorsal stream impaired) | Occupational therapist<br>O&M specialist<br>Psychologist/neuropsychologist<br>Teacher of students with visual impairments |
| Physical education and sports | Inability to jump off a bench (lower field impaired)<br>Inability to handle team sports (dorsal stream impaired) | O&M specialist<br>Physical education teacher<br>Teacher of students with visual impairments |
| Assistive technology | Can benefit from alternative means of access to curricula, materials, environment | Assistive technology specialist<br>Teacher of students with visual impairments |
| Other school subjects | Varies with tasks to be performed | Subject teacher specialists<br>Teacher of students with visual impairments |
| Environmental analysis of key environments | Environment has many elements that may be distracting or confusing<br>Environment contains elements that may not be within the perceptual range of the child | O&M specialist<br>Teacher of students with visual impairments |

*(continued on next page)*

**TABLE 10.1** *(continued from previous page)*

| *Evaluation Areas* | *Sample Behavioral Indicators of a Potential Difficulty* | *Possible Evaluators* |
|---|---|---|
| Understanding of CVI | Child does not understand that behaviors are different from peers<br>Caregivers bewildered with behaviors and not certain of ways to accommodate them to promote success in school and social situations | O&M specialist<br>Teacher of students with visual impairments |

2. What happens when a fast-moving object such as a cat, dog, or toy cart zooms toward or past your child unexpectedly? (Difficulty seeing things that are moving quickly, such as small animals)
3. When you point to something in the distance for your child to see, what happens? (Difficulty seeing something that is pointed out in the distance)
4. When presented with a pile of clothes, what does your child do to find a specific item in the pile? (Difficulty locating an item of clothing in a pile of clothes)
5. Can you describe how your child handles copying words or drawings? (Difficulty copying words or drawings)

These questions can be used as a screening tool for older children who do not have physical limitations in walking or copying words or drawings (for example, children who do not have cerebral palsy) and who do not have profound visual impairment. If a child has reported difficulty with activities identified in three or more of the five questions, it is an indication of possible CVI, and a subsequent in-depth history should be elicited as part of the first or second tier of assessment. In addition, use of open-ended questions to elicit the child's story and information about the child's performance is described in Chapter 11.

Information gathered from history taking can guide the assessment process and provide valuable insights into intervention needs for optimal habilitation or rehabilitation activities at home, school, and beyond. Chapter 11 contains detailed information about history taking for children with CVI. It describes how to conduct a visual history and a history-taking inventory, and includes an inventory of questions for caregivers of children with CVI. Chapter 20 presents history-taking guidelines specifically for infants with profound visual impairment. Lueck (2004b) provides a caregiver interview guide for the evaluation of functional vision in children. Some excellent sample interview questions are also offered by Roman-Lantzy (2007) for young children who have or may have *cortical* visual impairment (children with very limited functional vision as a result of brain damage). In addition, a preverbal assessment questionnaire (PreViAs) has been developed to investigate visual behaviors in children under 24 months of age in four domains: visual attention, visual communication, visual-motor coordination, and visual processing (Pueyo et al., 2014). Administered to primary caregivers, information derived from the questionnaire is designed to complement history-taking results in order to more fully understand the visual-cognitive needs of very young children who have CVI.

### *Observational Assessment*

Figure 10.2 provides an observation guide that can be used by school staff as an initial informal screening tool prior to more formal assessments such as formal testing by an eye care specialist, a functional vision evalua-

FIGURE 10.2

**Recording Form for Observational Assessment of Functional Vision**

## Observational Assessment of Functional Vision

**Child:** ______________________ **Date:** ________ **Evaluator:** ______________________________

**Reading Ability and Efficiency** (Describe reading characteristics noted such as print size, distance from page, lighting required, reading fluency, reading speed, ability to follow along a line of text, ability to locate next line of text, ability to locate material in different parts of a page as in a workbook.)

**Reading or Close-Viewing Behaviors** (Describe any head tilts, eccentric viewing, finger-pointing, keeping place, reading letter-by-letter, skipping words or letters.)

**Pictures** (Describe size of pictures viewed and seen, black/white vs. color, photographs, line drawings, pictures with complex backgrounds vs. single objects.)

**Preferred Viewing Distances for Near and Far Work** (Describe target including its size and distance.)

**Preferred and/or Optimal Positioning for Viewing** (Describe target and its position—held below, above, to one side or another.)

**Use of Writing Equipment** (Describe use of pens, pencils, markers, bold lined paper.)

**Writing** (Describe use of print and cursive letters, size, legibility. Reads own writing? What size?)

**Copying/Drawing/Cutting** (Describe time, legibility, omissions. For young children: coloring within lines, cutting along lines.)

*(continued on next page)*

**FIGURE 10.2** *(continued from previous page)*

**Artistic skills** (Describe limitations in creating artistic and diagrammatic representations.)

**Color Identification and Use** (Describe viewing of primary colors, pastels, and any color preferences.)

**Lighting Requirements, Performance in Different Lighting Conditions** (Describe performance variations in different lighting conditions, adaptation from light to dark or dark to light, effects of glare, lighting conditions of daily environments.)

**Contrast Needs** (Describe examples of performance with low-contrast and high-contrast materials.)

**Mobility and Distance Tasks** (Describe walking, running, large object location, any unusual behaviors such as tripping, bumping into objects below, above, or to the one side, hesitant gait, hesitant on going up or down stairs, slowing down in bright light or dim light.)

**Near Object Location and Reach** (Describe ability to locate desired small objects, their size, search techniques, direct or indirect reach for objects, over-reaching or under-reaching for objects.)

**Use of Eyeglasses** (Eyeglasses are kept clean, in good condition, and easy to locate. Describe use: worn regularly or for specific activities, takes off all the time, takes off to read or to see at distance, looks over the top regularly, pulls outward to look through when carefully examining objects.)

**Use of Optical Devices** (Devices are kept clean, in good condition, and easy to locate. Describe use: used for prescribed purposes, not used at all, used for other purposes, how held in relation to visual target and eyes.)

**Use of Special Equipment** (Describe specific type and use of computer, CCTV magnifier, electronic tablets, adaptive devices: such as reading stand, reading lamp, adaptive sports equipment.)

**Requests for Assistance** (appropriate, unusually demanding, not able to request.)

**Competing Sensory Stimuli in Environment that Affect Performance** (visual, tactile, kinesthetic, auditory, gustatory, olfactory)

**Other**

*Source:* Adapted from Lueck, A. H. (2004). Overview of functional evaluation. In A. H. Lueck (Ed.), *Functional vision: A practitioner's guide to evaluation and intervention* (pp. 96–97). New York: AFB Press.

tion by school personnel, or an assessment of appropriate learning media by school staff (see Chapters 12, 15, and 18). Teachers of students with visual impairments can assist with evaluations performed by school personnel. The tool can also be used for more in-depth observations once additional information about visual functions is available from an eye care specialist's examination and any new corrections for refractive error or accommodation are in place. The information gathered by this informal screening tool can help determine questions to ask the eye care specialist about a child's vision capabilities, and will also be helpful in providing information in response to his or her questions during formal clinical eye examinations. Observation protocols for young children and children who have severe cognitive and other impairments can be found in Chapter 14.

During the administration of formal tests in the first tier, the evaluator can observe a child's behaviors while conducting these evaluations, in addition to recording the test results. The ways in which a child approaches and reacts to the tasks can provide additional insights into the effects of the child's ocular or cerebral visual impairments and must be taken into account when reporting assessment results. An astute evaluator will note when a child displays behavioral manifestations of CVI that require further investigation and, moreover, will understand that the potential presence of CVI indicated by these behaviors may affect the child's performance of certain tasks. It is also possible that at this point a specific pattern of CVI can be detected for further examination during the second- or third-tier assessment phases. Some behaviors that might be noted by evaluators at this stage in the assessment process, and that might indicate the need for further evaluation, can be found in Table 10.2. The behaviors listed may also be observed during informal assessments, observational assessments, or tasks completed in curricular areas.

### *Identification of Behavioral Adaptations*

Children who have CVI may develop atypical ways of interacting with their environment, such as separating items from one another (for example, as a result of simultanagnostic difficulties). Behaviors with adaptive value need to be identified and encouraged, while non-adaptive behaviors are discouraged, and if possible, replaced with ones that are more beneficial. Figure 10.3 provides a form that can help in identifying and recording some behavioral adaptations for young children and children with visual and cognitive dysfunction, as well as understanding children's responses in test situations and during observation in usual environments. The information can also help in the design of appropriate interventions. (Additional behavioral adaptations for a wider range of children can be found in Tables 3.2–3.9 of Chapter 3.)

## Second-Tier Assessments

### *Assessment of Dorsal and Ventral Stream Dysfunction in Children with Functional Vision*

Assessments in the second tier provide further insights into higher-order visual processing concerns that may have been uncovered during the first tier. For children who have functional vision, the second-tier assessments are designed to examine in greater depth patterns of behavior associated with disorders of the dorsal and ventral

**TABLE 10.2**

## Behaviors That May Require Additional Evaluation of a Child

| *Behavior* | *Possible Indication* |
|---|---|
| **Effects of Ocular Visual Impairment Only** | |
| Narrows eyelids together when attempting to look at test material. | A need for higher refractive correction or sensitivity to glare. |
| Removes glasses or looks over them to view test material. | Glasses may be uncomfortable or may not be optimum prescription. |
| **Effects of Ocular and Cerebral Visual Impairments** | |
| Responds slowly or rapidly during testing. | Inability to discriminate details visually, unfamiliarity with materials, non-understanding of test demands, or other issues that need to be investigated. |
| Makes consistent errors on line acuity charts or other near or distance tasks. The nature of these errors should be noted. | Difficulty with crowded symbols, scanning, visual field, oculomotor concerns or other issues that need to be investigated. |
| Appears to be easily frustrated, giving up on visual tasks before visual limits are reached. | Difficulty focusing for extended time on visual task due to inability to decipher task related to reduced acuity, visual field, oculomotor issues, or processing issues. |
| Does not appear to understand task requirements. | Cognitive issues, cultural differences, instructions not given in primary language, auditory issues, or inability to see what is being referred to in the task. |
| Tires easily and needs rest time between tasks. | Difficulty focusing for extended time on visual tasks related to inability to decipher task due to reduced acuity, visual field, oculomotor issues, or processing issues. |
| Exhibits unusual head position or movement when responding to all or portions of the test material. | Null point nystagmus, eccentric viewing for central field impairments, location of target for optimum viewing to compensate for peripheral field impairment. |
| Attempts to move forward to see the test material. | Inability to decipher due to reduced visual acuity; may move forward to reduce amount of material in visual field to reduce visual clutter. |
| Requires additional cues to locate a visual target during test administration using vision (e.g., pointing to a test target, tapping on the test target, verbal description of where the test target is located, movement of the test target). | Inability to decipher task due to reduced acuity, visual field, oculomotor issues, or processing issues. |
| Shows better performance with familiar symbols, pictures, or objects. | Cognitive or visual processing issues or cultural differences. |
| Shows better performance when symbols, pictures, or words are isolated. | May be related to amblyopia, if diagnosed, or to visual processing issues. |
| Responds better when the test materials are moving. | May be related to visual processing issues. |
| Requires a long time to initiate a response to vision tasks, ultimately participating in them. | Inability to decipher task due to reduced acuity, visual field, oculomotor issues, or processing issues. |
| Appears to be easily distracted from a task by other stimuli in the environment. | Inability to decipher task due to reduced acuity, visual field, or sensory processing issues. |

*Source:* Adapted from Lueck, A. H. (2004). Overview of functional evaluation. In A. H. Lueck (Ed.), *Functional vision: A practitioner's guide to evaluation and intervention* (p. 105). New York: AFB Press.

FIGURE 10.3

## Observed Behaviors Recording Form

**Recording Form for Observed Behaviors for Young Children and Children with Visual and Cognitive Challenges**

**Child:** ______________________ **Date:** ________ **Evaluator:** ______________________________

The assessment team should determine which behaviors to encourage or discourage.

| *Behavior Observed* | *Conditions Under Which Observed* | *Description and Comments* |
|---|---|---|
| **Involuntary** | | |
| Nystagmus (indicate if null point observed)<br>Lack of eye contact<br>Verbal or motor response delay | | |
| **Habitual and Reactive** | | |
| Light gazing<br>Reactive behaviors (e.g., angry, distressed, disruptive in crowded, busy environments)<br>Hand waving<br>Eye pressing or poking (a maladaptive behavior) | | |
| **Habitual and Adaptive** | | |
| Head turn away when reaching<br>Photophobia (aversion to light)<br>Body movement such as rocking, head shaking (NOTE: This is adaptive for some children who need movement to engage vision but for others it may be a form of self-stimulation)<br>Eccentric viewing<br>Head movement to follow or scan, rather than eye movement<br>Close viewing distance adopted<br>Frequent breaks required<br>Use of voice, sound, scent, or compelling visual feature such as hair, glasses, bracelet, clothing to identify people<br>Objects stacked or lined up in order to look at them one by one rather than looking at them within a close-knit array of items | | |

stream. Patterns of behaviors associated with dorsal stream disorders are summarized in Figure 10.4. Behaviors associated with ventral stream disorders can be found in Figure 10.5. (See Chapter 3 for a more detailed discussion of dorsal and ventral stream dysfunction.)

Careful administration of tests for visual processing, visual attention, and general attention may be required during second-tier assessments. Use of commercially available tests of visual perception and other areas that look at brain function are discussed in Chapters 6, 12, 13, 17, and 25. Hyvärinen and Jacob (2011) also provide a discussion of these types of tests. Some additional methods to evaluate visual perceptual and visual cognitive disorders in children are discussed by Zihl and Dutton (2015). It is essential that any tests, along with any informal assessments, contain items that are above the visual acuity threshold of the child, within the child's motor-planning abilities (if this is an issue), and within the child's intellectual capabilities, in order to avoid misinterpretation of test results. During the administration of these tests, it is crucial to observe how a child approaches each task and to look at the types of errors that occur and whether they form patterns (for example, if the child consistently has difficulty picking out a figure embedded in other figures), rather than reporting overall scores that do not supply information about specific behaviors that need to be identified and addressed. The pattern of errors provides valuable information to the assessment team about intervention considerations. It is also important to examine a child's performance with three-dimensional objects as well as two-dimensional symbols to see if there is a difference in performance.

Teasing out information about dorsal and ventral stream functioning can require a degree of finesse. The following are some helpful suggestions:

- When seeking information about identification of faces, be sure that the student is not using other cues such as voice, familiar smell, location, clothing, or personal items (such as eyeglasses) to identify a specific person. Interview questions and the observation environment need to ensure that these factors are taken into account.
- Be sure to differentiate between difficulty with facial recognition—which manifests on a one-to-one basis—and issues with simultanagnosia, which causes inability to recognize multiple elements in a visual scene, and leads to inability in finding friends in a crowded environment. (See Chapters 3 and 6 for more information.)
- It is also important to distinguish between the inability to use visual cues for guidance in a particular direction (*topographic agnosia*, a ventral stream dysfunction), and getting lost when there is too much to see or do (*simultanagnosia*, a dorsal stream dysfunction). The management strategies for these two behaviors are very different (see Chapter 3). Impaired ability to pick out figures when there is foreground clutter or background pattern (simultanagnostic visual dysfunction) in the context of everyday living translates into problems with a "too busy" background pattern because of dorsal stream dysfunction. Children should therefore be observed for facial recognition capabilities with individual faces whose features are

FIGURE 10.4

## Patterns of Behavior Associated with Perceptual Visual Disorders Related to Dorsal Stream Dysfunction

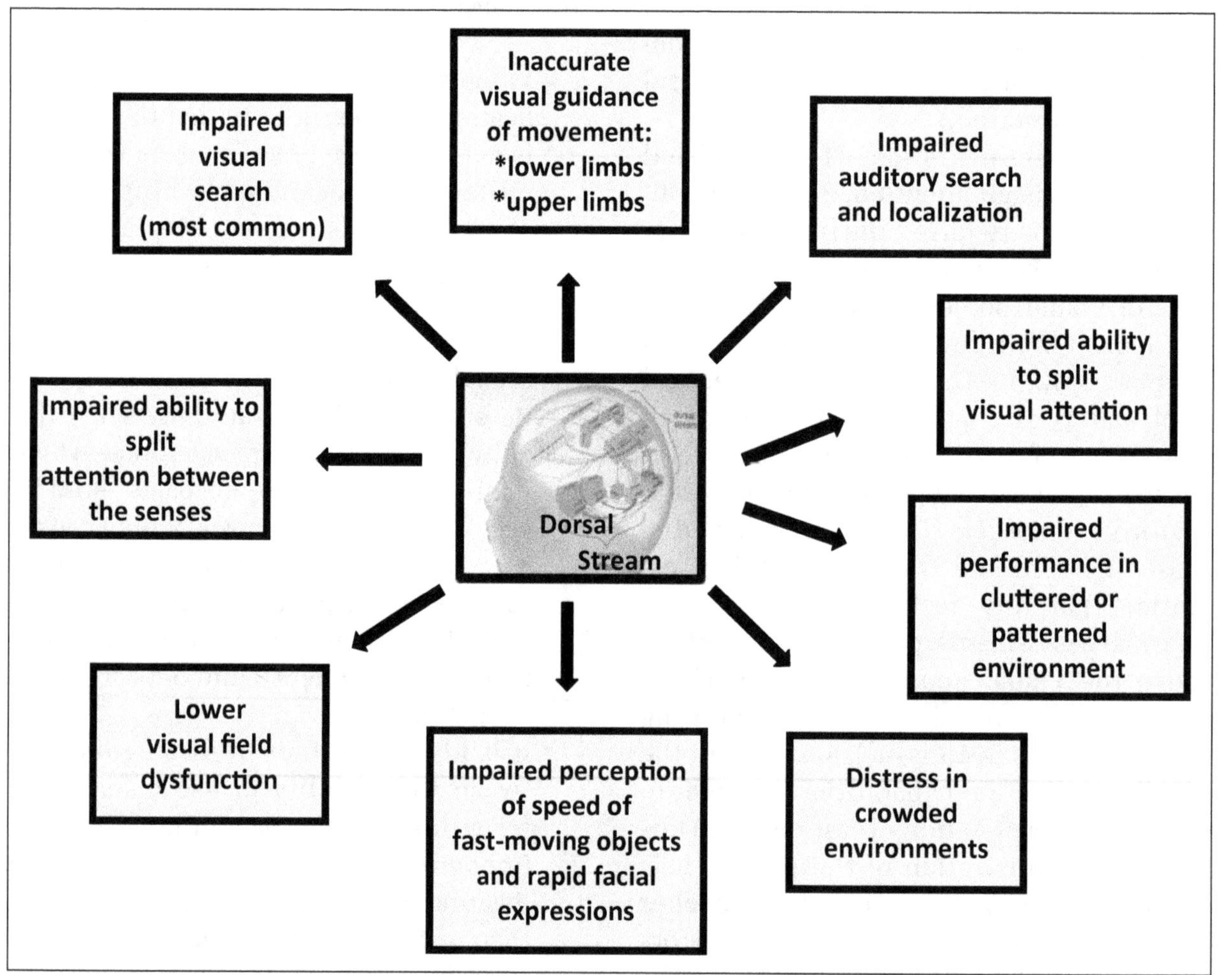


This figure refers to the effects of focal pathology, affecting elements of the dorsal stream and related areas serving speed of perception and the lower visual field. (Many children identified with CVI show some features of dorsal stream dysfunction, but other features may be masked by ones that are more severe.)

These features can occur in any number, combination, or degree, but when one is identified all the others need to be sought. Affected individuals tend to have no awareness of these dysfunctions, unless specifically taught about them. Since these disordered functions are unconscious ones, they cannot be aware of a lack or loss of what they never knew they had (*anosognosia*).

within their visual acuity range, rather than with faces in a crowd at a distance.

- Recognition and matching of colors is commonly normal, but many children with CVI have *color anomia* (inability to associate colors with their names). The strategy of associating colors to meaningful nouns (such as "lemon yellow") is rapidly effective in most cases. (See Chapter 3 for more information.)

FIGURE 10.5

## Patterns of Behavior Associated with Perceptual Visual Disorders Related to Ventral Stream Dysfunction

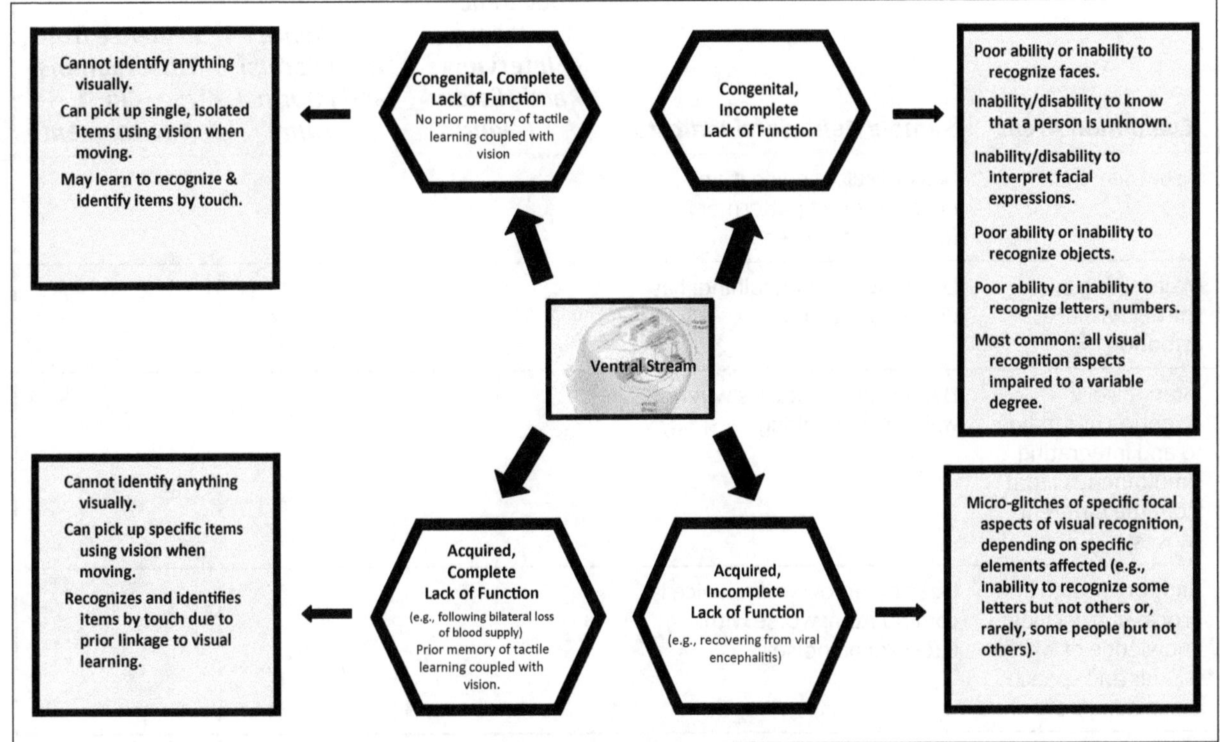


This figure refers to ostensibly isolated ventral stream damage due to focal pathology affecting ventral stream functions. Total ventral stream pathology is usually associated with low visual acuities due to concomitant damage to the occipital lobes. Innate orientation can be spared or impaired to a variable degree, leading to easily getting lost even in well-known environments. The features listed in the rectangular boxes highlight the nature of complete (or total lack of function) and incomplete or partial lack of function.

- Visual field impairments can result in subtle differences in performance where the visual field is reduced depending on the location and type of brain injury. (See Chapter 3 for more information.)

Figure 10.6 presents a summary form that can be used to record the results of a dorsal stream evaluation. Figure 10.7 presents a summary form for ventral stream evaluation. These forms may be completed individually by evaluators or collectively during team meetings. Another way to record assessment results is to use the Profile of Visual Functioning form found in Chapter 13 (see Figure 13.8; Hyvärinen & Jacob, 2011; Hyvärinen, Walthes, Freitag, & Petz, 2012).

### *Assessment of Children with Profound Visual Impairment*

For children with profound visual impairment in second-tier assessment, the evaluator must determine which, if any, visual stimuli evoke responses, the consistency of these responses, and how the environment can be optimized to encourage visual behaviors. The

FIGURE 10.6

## Summary Form for Evaluation of Dorsal Stream Disorders

| Summary of Evaluation for Dorsal Stream Disorders | | | | |
|---|---|---|---|---|
| ***Evaluation Areas*** | ***Sample Behavioral Indicators*** | ***Evidence from Interview and History Taking*** | ***Evidence from Formal and Informal Testing*** | ***Evidence from Observations in Environment*** |
| Visual search | Has difficulty finding items in background pattern or foreground clutter | | | |
| Maintaining and shifting visual attention | Looks away when talking; has difficulty copying | | | |
| Intersensory attention (attending to and integrating simultaneous input from the different senses) | Bumps into obstacles when walking and talking | | | |
| Auditory search and processing, including knowledge of where sounds and speech are coming from | Does not know where voice is coming from; worse with background noise | | | |
| Dysfunction of lower field of vision | Has difficulty going down steps and slopes | | | |
| Lower visual field impairment | Does not see nearest food, toys, and images | | | |
| Neglect of lower visual field | Walks over obstacles without being aware of them | | | |
| Visual guidance of movement of lower limbs | Looks at floor boundaries and probes with foot to identify if a step is present | | | |
| Visual guidance of movement of upper limbs and hands | Cannot accurately place items on table unless body is touching table<br>Reaches with wider than expected gap between fingers and thumb<br>Reaches with extended hand to touch item in order to identify its correct location | | | |
| Estimation of speed of moving targets | Perceives risk but walks out in front of traffic with incorrect timing | | | |

FIGURE 10.7

## Summary Form for Evaluation of Ventral Stream Disorders

| Summary of Evaluation for Ventral Stream Disorders | | | | |
|---|---|---|---|---|
| *Evaluation Areas* | *Sample Behavioral Indicators* | *Evidence from Interview and History Taking* | *Evidence from Formal and Informal Testing* | *Evidence from Observations in Environment* |
| Identification of people, facial expressions, objects, shapes, pictures, words | Does not recognize known people, incorrectly recognizes unknown people<br>Does not see language in facial expressions<br>Does not recognize objects, shapes, pictures, and words | | | |
| Orientation in surrounding environment (as related to topographic agnosia) | Gets lost easily in uncrowded places that should be known<br>Easily loses possessions and cannot locate them | | | |
| Orientation of lines; Creating, copying, and mentally rotating visual imagery | Has difficulty copying orientation of lines, copying or creating diagrams and pictures, and imagining visual imagery from different perspectives | | | |

manner in which a child responds can be documented (for example, vocalizations, gestures, change in activity level). Change in visual functioning over time can also be recorded. The CVI Range (Newcomb, 2010; Roman-Lantzy, 2007) can be used to monitor a variety of these behaviors over time as the child's vision improves. Other ways to observe, monitor, and record behaviors, such as level of visual attention, visual skills, dorsal and ventral stream function, and different types of visual stimuli, can be found in Chapter 14.

Evidence of blindsight can also be sought, such as an evident response to moving targets, lights, and colors in an impaired visual field (Boyle, Jones, Hamilton, Spowart, & Dutton, 2005). Children will use the small amount of vision they have when interacting with the world around them. Interventionists and families can use evidence of blindsight to encourage increased interaction and vision use.

Evaluation of auditory processing skills in children with profound visual impairment can be implemented in the second tier, if warranted by the first-tier auditory processing screening.

Furthermore, the vision of a child with profound visual impairment can improve over time. As this occurs, more emphasis can be placed on second-tier assessment practices relevant for children with functional vision (as described in the previous section) that matches their increase in vision.

### Third-Tier Assessments

The third assessment tier consists of evaluations of the child with regard to functional tasks or situations, including specific assessments related to school curricula. Third-tier assessments include observations of typical activities in a child's usual environments, as well as outcomes of assessments of reading, mathematics, daily living skills, O&M, and other significant activities for each child. It also includes an evaluation of the child's and family's understanding of the effects of CVI, plus an evaluation of elements in a child's typical environments that may affect performance. An example of a functional evaluation of reading performance for children with CVI was conducted by Ek, Fellenius, and Jacobson (2003), in which they investigated such elements as leisure reading behavior, word/letter perception, phoneme formation, the effects of crowding, as well as noting performance IQs and their change over time. More information on third-tier assessments in educational tasks can be found in Chapters 15, 16, 17, and 18.

#### *Effects of Competing Sensory Stimuli*

As mentioned earlier, environmental conditions can have a profound effect on performance outcomes for a child who has CVI. Simultaneous incoming stimuli from a variety of senses in addition to vision—auditory, olfactory, gustatory, tactile, or proprioceptive/kinesthetic input (movement of body)—as well as a sense of imbalance or discomfiture can interfere with the ability of children with CVI to accomplish visual tasks. Figure 10.8 provides an observation form that can be used to record the effects of competing sensory stimuli in critical tasks. This form has been completed for a hypothetical child who must find her food on a tray in the school cafeteria. The form also provides suggestions for environmental modifications to assist the child in completing her task more easily and efficiently. The observations can be used to generate recommendations for modifications or adaptations to the environment in order to help the child cope better with the effects of competing sensory stimuli.

## Considerations When Administering and Interpreting Assessments

The following are some additional issues and considerations that should be taken into account when administering and interpreting both formal and informal assessments:

- Be sure to give all students sufficient time to respond. Slowdowns among various information processing systems can lead to sluggish performance speeds for some evaluation procedures.
- Be sure to present the testing material and verbal directions and questions at a speed that the child can process.
- When administering visual tests, it is best to de-clutter the space before determining visual capabilities. Then the same visual skills should be examined under more cluttered conditions to determine if visual clutter affects performance.
- Be sure that a student's visual accommodation needs for near tasks have been

FIGURE 10.8

## Sample Observation of Competing Sensory Stimuli in Critical Tasks

### Observation Of Competing Sensory Stimuli In Critical Tasks

**Child:** Rebekah Huygens **Observation Date:** 4/15/15

**Evaluator:** C.Garcia **Task:** Finding food on lunch tray in cafeteria

**Auditory (sound)**
**Visual (sight)**
**Olfactory (smell)**
**Gustatory (taste)**
**Tactile (touch)**
**Proprioceptive/Kinesthetic (movement of body)**

| *Visual Task to be Performed* | *Location* | *Within What General Activity?* | *Competing Sensory Stimuli that Affect Successful Task Completion* | *Recommended Environmental Adjustments* |
|---|---|---|---|---|
| Finding food on tray | School cafeteria | Lunch | Movement of other children | Sit with class at a table along the wall at the edge of the cafeteria so there is less movement behind the table and no competing conversations beyond the table on one side |
| | | | Lunch tray and dishes are the same color (dark tan) | Be in the first class to arrive at the cafeteria so it is easier to get settled before most of the other children arrive |
| | | | Food is sometimes very close in color to dishes | Have a separate set of dark and light dishes available that can be selected based upon the food choice of the day so that the food can be readily located on the plate |
| | | | | Have a special tray that is high in contrast to the lunch dishes |

addressed by presenting these tasks at appropriate working distances and with the necessary spectacle correction worn for close viewing.

- Many children with CVI may have difficulty seeing fast-moving targets. It is best to determine this prior to administering any vision tests. See Chapter 3 for a discussion of a method for clinical observation of disordered perception of movement.
- Be sure to consider the child's physical and emotional status when analyzing behaviors. Was the student functioning at peak performance? If not, how was the child's performance affected? Consider illness, level of alertness, hunger, fatigue, medications, positioning, and discomfort

from pain, distress, seizure activity, or other influences. These factors will also likely affect a child's performance in the school setting and must be addressed in intervention programs.

- Evaluate a child's environment during testing to determine if the arrangement or amount of environmental stimuli is affecting performance. As already noted, surrounding stimuli (visual, auditory, olfactory, gustatory, and tactile/kinesthetic) can either support or detract from outcomes. This must be considered during assessment and addressed in the design of effective intervention programs.
- A very young child or a child with additional disabilities may have unique ways of responding to task demands. In addition, tasks may need to be presented in highly specific ways (for example, always presenting specific foods in a favorite bowl at snack time) in order for a child to understand them and be able to respond. It is important to acquire some knowledge of these behaviors from families and caregivers prior to testing. Evaluators need to be alert during testing for any unusual communicative methods used by the child.

## Assembling and Reporting Assessment Results

The assessment team works together to assemble information from the three tiers of assessment into a coordinated report or series of reports from different specialists that will provide guidance for intervention. Reports can be written in one of two ways. Checklists of key behaviors assessed can be provided along with a brief summary and list of recommendations for intervention and follow-up. Figure 14.5 in Chapter 14 provides a way to quickly record comprehensive assessment results for young children with CVI and for children with CVI and multiple disabilities. This type of approach is practical and often faster to produce, but more detailed information may be required to provide a full and accurate picture of a child. As an alternative, reports can be written in a continuous text format with a summary and recommendations at the end.

When reviewing reports, busy individuals often go directly to the summary at the end of the written report. Therefore, it is critical that a summary section be included in the final report that clearly and concisely recaps key elements in the assessment.

Reports need to include a list of evaluators involved in the process, assessment methods used, findings, and recommendations. They can match intervention goals to the challenges that need to be addressed and identify the child's areas of strength, which can be used to design effective strategies to achieve those goals. A background section with a brief history and summary of past assessment results should be included at the outset of the report. Any behavioral adaptations required during the assessment process (such as giving a student extra time to respond or simplifying the visual elements of a task presentation) should be mentioned, as these may need to be instituted in future assessments and in any subsequent intervention programs.

Reports need to paint a picture of the child, and for a child with CVI, this picture needs to present the ways in which the child views and experiences his or her world. Reports need to be factual and without judgment about the child and family. They also need to be free from professional jargon and written clearly so that the entire professional staff as well as the child's family can understand the results and their implications. Any technical terms should be followed by a brief description in parentheses (for example, myopia [inability to see clearly objects that are far away]). It is best that reports are organized in a way that allows readers to quickly locate items of interest to them (adapted from Lueck, 2004b).

Sidebar 10.2 provides an overall framework with some general headings that would be included in a comprehensive assessment report for children who have CVI. Within those headings, evaluators can include a checklist of items assessed or write continuous text explanations. Specific headings or items would be tailored for each child. For areas in which the child is having significant difficulty, recommendations for interventions that address each reported issue can be documented.

In general, recommendations included in the report are ones that will be considered for implementation by the child's educational team. Each recommendation needs to be carefully constructed so that it (a) addresses a primary concern identified for the child, (b) weaves the reason for the suggestion into the text, and (c) provides one or more suggested solutions. An example follows:

> **When attempting to locate items in his desk using** his vision, Marcel often gives up and seeks assistance from others. It is therefore suggested that visual clutter within Marcel's desk be kept to a minimum using a color-coded storage system. For example, his writing and cutting implements can be stored in a colored pencil case, and his papers can be kept in different-colored folders for different class assignments. Marcel should be encouraged to clean out and arrange items in his desk periodically as an organizational skill.

Sample assessment reports can be found in Appendix 10A and Appendix 10B. Reports will vary in content depending on the types of assessments carried out and the composition of evaluation teams. (For more information about the specific assessment tools and procedures mentioned in these reports, see Chapters 12 and 13.) A best practice among evaluators is to give the family and other team members a draft copy of the report to review prior to its discussion in a formal team meeting so that people have time to digest the material, suggest modifications, and prepare questions to ask at the assessment team meeting.

## Providing Feedback to the Family

Families expect to be told what conclusions have been reached based on the assessment process, what they mean, and what they can do to help their child. This information needs to be conveyed while it is fresh in everyone's mind. However, only a few key points can usually be remembered, so it is best to give the main findings in language that everyone can understand. If a technical term needs to be used, it is best used after the basic explanation. For example: "From the reports it appears that Martin has difficulty recognizing people's faces. If you want to look this up for more details, use the medical term *prosopagnosia,* which comes from the Greek *prosopos* (a face) and *agnosia* (not to know)." The second explanation is easier to understand because the listener is being led from the known into the unknown, rather than the other way round.

If the child and family require an interpreter, it is important to speak directly to the family rather than the interpreter. A pause

SIDEBAR 10.2

## Framework for a Team Assessment Report for Children Who Have CVI

The following is a general framework that can be used to prepare an assessment report for a child who has been assessed for CVI. Precise categories in a report will depend on a child's specific situation.

### Identification Information

- Name of child
- Date of birth
- Assessment date(s)
- Location(s)
- Name and title of evaluator(s)

### Purpose or Reason for Evaluation

### Background

- Diagnosis (visual diagnosis, other conditions)
- Relevant medical and educational history (including current medications)
- Summary and date of relevant eye reports
- Current educational placement information

### Current Assessment Results (list test or observation methods; address only those categories that are applicable)

- Functional vision (vision function results from eye doctors are listed in the Background section and mentioned here as needed)
- Auditory processing
- Visual processing
  - Visual attention
  - Visually guided movements
  - Perception of objects or faces/facial expressions
  - Simultaneous perception
  - Other
- Other attention issues
- Use of vision in typical tasks, situations, or curricular areas
- Adaptive behaviors
- Student's and family's understanding of vision capabilities and concerns
- Assistive technology
- Environmental analysis

### Summary

### Recommendation Areas (use only those categories that are applicable)

- Functional vision (including recommended object size or print size at recommended viewing distances for different tasks)
- Auditory processing
- Visual processing
  - Visually guided movements
  - Perception of objects or faces and facial expressions
  - Simultaneous perception
  - Other
- Other attention issues
- Use of vision in typical tasks, situations, or curricular areas
- Adaptive behaviors
- Student's and family's understanding of vision capabilities and concerns
- Assistive technology
- Environmental modifications
- List of adaptive equipment or assistive technology to be considered

at regular intervals allows time for the interpreter to convey the information clearly to the family.

It is critical that professionals be careful purveyors of information as well as good listeners, so they can respond to all questions the family might have and move the information forward at a pace the family can understand. When conveying assessment findings, evaluators should pause at regular intervals and invite questions, to be sure that information presented during the assessment process is understood, makes sense to all involved, and all questions and areas of concern have been addressed. The assessment team must also consider families' perceptions about which ideas or recommendations from the assessment process will be most helpful for their child. Finally, families benefit greatly when they know they can contact professionals on the team should any additional questions or concerns arise. It is important to let families know who they can contact and how to contact them in order to establish and maintain ongoing communication.

## Conclusion

Because of the wide range of behavioral manifestations of damage to the visual brain, as well as the various other conditions that accompany it, a coordinated multidisciplinary and multidimensional approach to assessment is crucial to understanding the behaviors of children with CVI and recommending strategies to address them. This chapter has presented an overview and model of this process, along with methods and forms to organize it, while Chapters 11–18, 20, and 24 present specific methods for the assessment of vision functions, functional vision, higher-order visual processing, and the use of vision within functional tasks as well as neuropsychological issues associated with CVI.

As teams focus on assessment methodology, it is important to remember that functional assessment is aimed at

- characterizing behaviors of children,
- understanding the reasons behind atypical behaviors whenever possible,
- determining behaviors that may be improved through direct training, and
- identifying behaviors that are strengths so they can be used to assist in areas where there are behavioral challenges.

In addition, methods to optimize learning environments to promote attention and successful task performance must also be identified during the assessment process. Finally, it is necessary to understand how children and their families view CVI and how a child operates in the world. This wealth of information leads to the design of programs that optimize the education of children who have CVI and also promotes increased understanding of the condition by the children and their families.

## References


Boyle, N. J., Jones, D. H., Hamilton, R., Spowart, K. M., & Dutton, G. N. (2005). Blindsight in children: Does it exist and can it be used to help the child? Observations on a case series. *Developmental Medicine & Child Neurology, 47*(10), 699–702.

Corn, A. L., & Erin, J. N. (Eds.). (2010). *Foundations of low vision: Clinical and functional perspectives* (2nd ed.). New York: AFB Press.

Duckman, R. H. (2006). *Visual development, diagnosis, and treatment of the pediatric patient.* Philadelphia: Lippincott Williams & Wilkins.

Dutton, G. N. (2003). Cognitive vision, its disorders and differential diagnosis in adults and children: Knowing where and what things are. *Eye, 17,* 289–304.

Dutton, G. N., Calvert, J., Ibrahim, H., Macdonald, E., McCulloch, D. L., Macintyre-Béon, C., et al. (2010). Impairment of cognitive vision: Its detection and measurement. In G. N. Dutton & M. Bax (Eds.), *Visual impairment in children due to damage to the brain* (pp. 117–128). London: Mac Keith Press.

Dutton, G. N., & Jacobson, L. K. (2001). Cerebral visual impairment in children. *Seminars in Neonatology, 6*(6), 477–485.

Ek, U., Fellenius, K., & Jacobson, L. (2003). Reading acquisition, cognitive and visual development, and self-esteem in four children with cerebral visual impairment. *Journal of Visual Impairment & Blindness, 97*(12), 741–754.

Fahsi, A. J., & McAndrews, S. L. (2012). Journal writing: Support for students with learning disabilities. *Intervention in School and Clinic, 47*(4), 234–244.

Gregory, G. H., & Kuzmich, L. (2004). *Data driven differentiation in the standards-based classroom.* Thousand Oaks, CA: Corwin Press.

Hatton, D. D., Schwietz, E., Boyer, B., & Rychwalski, P. (2007). Babies count: The national registry for children with visual impairments, birth to 3 years. *Journal of the American Association for Pediatric Ophthalmology and Strabismus, 11*(4), 351–355.

Henriksson, L., Raninen, A., Näsänen, R., Hyvärinen, L., & Vanni, S. (2007). Training-induced cortical representation of a hemianopic hemifield. *Journal of Neurology, Neurosurgery, & Psychiatry, 78*(1), 74–81.

Hyvärinen, L. (2003, November 15). *Assessment of vision in CVI.* Lectures presented at San Francisco State University. Retrieved October 7, 2011, from http://www.lea-test.fi/en/assessme/sfracvilect/index.html

Hyvärinen, L. & Jacob, N. (2011). *WHAT and HOW does this child see? Assessment of visual functioning for development and learning.* Helsinki, Finland: VISTEST, Ltd.

Hyvärinen, L., Walthes, R., Freitag, & Petz, V. (2012). Profile of visual functioning as a bridge between education and medicine in the assessment of impaired vision. *Strabismus, 20*(2), 63–68.

International Reading Association (2006). *Diagnostic teaching for primary level schooling: Facilitator's guide.* Paris: United Nations Educational, Scientific and Cultural Organization.

Lueck, A. H. (2004a). *Functional vision: A practitioner's guide to evaluation and intervention.* New York: AFB Press.

Lueck, A. H. (2004b). Overview of the evaluation process. In A. H. Lueck (Ed.), *Functional vision: A practitioner's guide to evaluation and intervention* (pp. 89–113). New York: AFB Press.

Macintyre-Béon, C., Ibrahim, H., Hay, I., Cockburn, D., Calvert, J., Dutton, N., et al. (2010). Dorsal stream dysfunction in children. A review and an approach to diagnosis and management. *Current Pediatric Reviews, 6*(3), 166–182.

Morse, M. T. (2012, October 1). Cerebral/cortical visual impairment. Paper presented at the Educational and Conference Center Series of the Southeastern Regional Education Service Center (SERESC). Retrieved December 15, 2012, from http://www.seresc.net/cerebral-cortical-visual-impairment

Newcomb, S. (2010). The reliability of the CVI Range: A functional vision assessment for children with cortical visual impairment. *Journal of Visual Impairment & Blindness, 104*(10), 637–647.

Pueyo, V., Garcia-Ormaechea, I., Gonzalez, I., Ferrer, C., de la Mata, G., Dupla, M., . . . Andes, E. (2014). Development of the Preverbal Visual Assessment (PreViAs) questionnaire. *Early Human Development, 90*(4), 165–168.

Rauschecker, J. P. (2011). An expanded role for the dorsal auditory pathway in sensorimotor control and integration. *Hearing Research, 271*(1–2), 16–25.

Roman-Lantzy, C. (2007). *Cortical visual impairment: An approach to assessment and intervention.* New York: AFB Press.

Salvia, J. E., Ysseldyke, J., & Bolt, S., (2013). *Assessment in special and inclusive education* (12th ed.). Belmont, CA: Wadsworth Publishing.

Walthes, R. C., Hyvärinen, L., & Petz, V. (2011, June). *Supporting children in achieving their potential—Communication as a key feature.* Paper presented at the 13th meeting of the Child Vision Research Society, Huizen, The Netherlands.

Ysseldyke, J., Salvia, J. E., & Bolt, S. (2009). *Assessment in special and inclusive education* (11th ed.). Belmont, CA: Wadsworth Publishing.

Zihl, J., & Dutton, G. N. (2015). *Cerebral visual impairment in children: Visuoperceptive and visuocognitive disorders.* Vienna: Springer-Verlag Wien.

# APPENDIX 10A
# Sample Vision Assessment Report: Emily

**Name:** Emily Granger
**Age:** 10
**Location:** Newtown Hospital Clinic; Newtown Elementary School
**Evaluators** Mary Reed, MD, Pediatric Ophthalmologist
Ivan Pulchowsky, M.A., Teacher of Visually Impaired Students

## Reason for Evaluation

Emily's vision was assessed for her school program in order to gain updated information about how she currently sees and uses her vision, as well as to recommend approaches and strategies that are likely to help her.

## Background

### Medical History

Emily was born prematurely and developed complications that led to a learning disability, cerebral palsy, and cerebral visual impairment (damage to the brain that affects vision). Emily's cerebral palsy affects her four limbs, but mainly her legs. She has spastic diplegia with a degree of upper limb involvement (muscle stiffness in her legs and arms). She is mobile when using her wheeled walker. Emily's receptive language is somewhat delayed according to a recent school report, but both her expressive and receptive language skills were more than adequate to complete tasks required during the assessment process. Emily does not have any auditory processing concerns according to school records. She currently receives services from an occupational therapist, physical therapist, teacher of students with visual impairments, and orientation and mobility (O&M) specialist.

An earlier vision report from her previous ophthalmologist two years ago, Dr. R. Tanaka, indicates that Emily's visual acuity (ability to see details) with both eyes viewing was slightly reduced (20/40 with single symbols). She was reported to have a reduced lower visual field, particularly on the left. She was previously found to have difficulty determining single elements in complex visual scenes as a result of visual crowding. At the time of her last assessment, it was questioned whether she had specific problems with recognition of objects and people. In the past she was found to lack focusing ability for near targets (poor accommodation).

### Current Educational Placement

Emily has an individual education program in a special class for children with moderate to severe disabilities. She goes to regular fifth-grade elementary school classes for art and music with the assistance of a paraprofessional. She receives services from a teacher of students with visual impairments, physical therapist, occupational therapist, and speech-language therapist.

Emily is able to recognize some, but not all, letters by sight and can name them. She has yet to link them with the sounds that the letters convey and remains at the pre-reading stage of education. At home and at school, the focus of her education is on life skills.

## Visual Assessment

### Need for Eyeglasses

Emily is slightly hyperopic with astigmatism. Her current spectacle prescription is +1.50/+0.50 at 90° in each eye. At present, spectacles do not measurably improve Emily's visual acuity, and this may be the reason she dislikes wearing them. However, the positive lenses in her prescription do provide limited magnification, allowing Emily to get closer to near tasks, and slightly reducing visual crowding for her, which may help in her schoolwork. Therefore, careful evaluation of Emily's performance with her current spectacles at school is suggested in order to determine whether they improve her performance on near tasks.

### Visual Acuity (Ability to See Details)

***Distance:*** Emily has an unchanged visual acuity for single symbols of 20/40 measured with the LEA Single Symbols Book with both eyes viewing, but with the crowded symbols on the LEA Line Distance Chart, it is 20/60.

***Near:*** Emily's near visual acuity for non-crowded symbols on the LEA Symbols Near Vision Card is 2.25M at 40 cm, but when the symbols are crowded, her visual acuity is 3.2M at 40 cm.

### Contrast Sensitivity (Ability to See Things against Different Background Shades)

This was tested with Cardiff Contrast Sensitivity Cards and was found to be 3 percent, which is slightly reduced.

### Eye Movements

Emily is able to move her eyes in all directions and follow a slowly moving target, but a fast-moving target (moving at a speed that other children of the same age would not find difficult) leads to loss of her ability to keep her eyes on the target. She also has difficulty moving her eyes quickly from one target to another. When asked to look from one item in a room to another, her ability to do so was very limited.

### Visual Fields (The Area Where Things Can Be Seen)

With the confrontation visual field test, using a penlight as a visual target in a dimly lit room, Emily was noted to have limited visual function in her lower visual field. Although she turned her head to look toward a slowly moving large target below the horizontal midline of her visual field when she looked straight ahead, she did not spontaneously look or reach for stationary items on the table in front of her unless she chose to look down to search the table.

In addition, her left visual attention is limited. Although she turns to look at an isolated moving target in the upper-left quadrant of her visual field, she is unable to do so if she is already looking at a central target. A moving target in the upper-right quadrant, however, is detected and responded to despite the presence of a distracting central target.

When Emily sits at a table with her chair turned about 15 degrees to her left, her ability to find items on the left side of the table is markedly improved. Her parents report that when she is eating at the table, they turn her plate around so she can see items that were previously on the left side of the plate, enabling Emily to finish her meal.

## Information from Observations and Structured History Taking with Emily's Parents

### *Color Vision (Ability to See and Distinguish Colors)*

According to Emily's parents, although Emily was previously unable to name colors, that is no longer the case. This may be a result of color identification training she received at school.

### *Facial Recognition Distance*

Emily can recognize people from across a room if there are plain walls with limited decoration and few people in the room. She cannot do this when there is a lot of pattern or clutter or a lot of people in the room. It is likely that she is unable to identify a person against a visually crowded background.

### *Significance of Facial Expressions*

In a quiet, plain room, with a one-to-one situation, Emily was able to discern the significance of facial expressions within a distance of 9 feet. She was able to recognize clear, static facial expressions, but when asked to interpret brief expressions, she was unable to do so. When her mother was placed among a group of school staff sitting against a visually complex background, 9 feet away in a brightly lit school entryway, Emily was unable to identify her mother or see her facial expressions. Emily's ability to see and recognize facial expressions appears to be intact, but is easily compromised when the expressions are rapid or when there are distracting elements present.

### *Simultaneous Perception*

Emily has been found to have difficulty processing multiple pieces of visual information at the one time. On the other hand, it was also found that she is able to complete a task with multiple visual elements when she focuses on the task without other visual distractions. She identified differently shaped beads in a box for a threading task, which she undertook successfully. Her parents reported this was not the case when her ability to do the task was assessed a year ago.

Although Emily does continue to have some difficulty when overloaded with visual information and distractions from the other senses, her capacity to deal with such situations appears to be improving.

### *Movement Perception*

Emily's parents report that she is unable to see things that move quickly. This accords with our observation that she cannot interpret rapid facial expressions. When asked to count fingers as they are extended from a stationary hand, she was able to do so accurately, but when asked to repeat this task for a vertically moving hand, she could only do so when the hand moved slowly in her central or right visual fields, but not in her left visual field.

### *Visual Guidance of Movement of the Hands and Arms*

Emily's parents report that she has difficulty coordinating her vision with her movement and will often miss items that she is reaching for. She compensates by reaching beyond what she wishes to pick up and then gathers the item up with a sweeping motion instead.

### *Visual Memory and Recognition*

Emily's mother reports that Emily is now able to identify shapes and colors, even though she was not able to a year ago. This was confirmed today by Emily's performance on both the near vision test and the bead-threading task that required shape and object identification. She did have some difficulty identifying and recognizing schematic drawings as representations of real objects.

*Fatigue and Visual Attention*

Emily's mother also reports that Emily has difficulty concentrating for more than 20 minutes, and this applies to her visual attention as well as other areas of attention. When asked to repetitively track an object across her field of vision, Emily developed nystagmus (jerky eye movements) and lost attention. After performing visual tasks for some time, Emily appeared to fatigue and her performance progressively declined, as did her motivation.

## Summary

Emily has an impairment of her vision resulting from difficulty processing information sent to her brain from her eyes. She has slightly reduced visual acuity and contrast sensitivity as well as limited function in her left visual field. She has limited visual attention on her left, and her vision fatigues easily. She processes information slowly. She is unable to count fingers that are displayed during rapid hand movement, and she cannot follow a fast-moving target. She has limited pursuit eye movements. Emily also has difficulty finding objects in a complex scene and cannot easily move her eyes from one item to another. This is combined with inaccuracy of visual guidance of movement. These features are consistent with the condition known as *dorsal stream dysfunction*. Emily is making very good progress; her clarity of vision and her ability to deal with visual crowding are both continuing to improve. However, Emily's visual impairment affects her ability to access educational materials using vision, and it is recommended that she continue to receive educational services from a teacher of students with visual impairments.

## Recommendations

1. Emily has eyeglasses, but they do not enhance her visual acuity. At the next assessment, it would be worthwhile to evaluate whether they improve her access to near material and her ability to read letters.
2. Emily reads 3.2M crowded symbols at 16 inches (40 cm). Since she prefers to hold her reading material at 8 inches (20 cm), the print should be 2 to 3 times her threshold size of 1.6M at 8 inches (20 cm). It is recommended that symbols be 3M to 4.8M font at 8 inches (20 cm) at the start of her next reading assessment.
3. Emily's limited eye movements make it difficult for her to scan across a page, so information presented to her needs to be limited to two or three items per page.
4. Emily has been supplied with a 1.5X dome magnifier that she likes to use to read smaller print. It also makes the reading material brighter and allows her to focus her attention on the important points in the text.
5. In an uncluttered and uncrowded environment with no distractions, Emily is able to see clearly both at near and at distance. However, people and objects need to be twice as close for her to see them with the same clarity of vision as a typically sighted person. This increases to fourfold when there is visual crowding, which also reduces Emily's ability to see things in the distance.

6. Although Emily can recognize people, she can only do this easily in a one-to-one situation, away from visual distractions. Having first gained her attention, anyone coming in to Emily's presence should therefore introduce themselves by name to ensure that Emily is aware of them and knows who they are.
7. When Emily is overwhelmed with information, as is often the case in school, she is unaware of feelings and emotions conveyed by others through facial expression. Such information therefore routinely needs to be conveyed through language, as it would be for someone who is unable to see.
8. Emily has inattention in her left visual field, as well as limited visual function in her lower visual field. Teachers and caregivers should be informed that Emily sees best straight ahead and to her right, and that a slight body rotation to her left or presentation of information off-center and to the right enhances her ability to see what is to her left. She needs to be reminded to "slow (down), look (down), check, and go" when using her wheeled walker. She already has an adjustable sloping workstation at school to enable her to see the lower part of a page better, and it will be worthwhile to consider arranging a similar workstation at home.
9. Emily does not see things that move quickly. She prefers to watch television programs and films with limited movement. This limitation in her vision, combined with her problems with visual crowding, needs to be recognized when walking with her in traffic, when showing her educational films, and when taking her to the theater and cinema, where productions need to be carefully chosen.
10. Emily has difficulty coordinating her vision with movement, and therefore misreaches at times. She finds it easier to look at an item, memorize its location, look away, and then reach for it. Anyone working with Emily needs to recognize that these strategies are adaptive for Emily, and they should not be discouraged.
11. Emily has problems with visual crowding and clutter but has shown improvement recently in her ability to find and work with objects in a cluttered array. Ideally, if an environment is plain and calm, with little decoration or noise, it will help Emily concentrate and accomplish what she wishes to see and do.
12. To reduce visual clutter, letters and pictures on a page need to be spaced out for Emily. An additional assessment of the size and degree of spacing of imagery and letters that meets her needs should be conducted by school staff.
13. Implementing a storage system where everything has its place and where search is focused in a single direction will enhance Emily's ability to find things herself. Approaches include using color to enhance specific storage locations or storing clothes in sets on single hangers.
14. Emily's inability to find friends in a crowd is causing social isolation, according to her mother. Her parents and school staff are therefore encouraged to find ways to ensure Emily's participation in social events at her school and in leisure time group activities.
15. In busy environments Emily has been reported to panic. This is probably because: (a) she does not know how far away people are from her and thinks they are going to crash into her; (b) noise can overwhelm her; (c) she becomes lost in crowded environments; and (d) she loses people easily and cannot find them again, giving her a sense of isolation, which can be frightening

for her. Emily can be introduced to busy locations at times when crowds and activity are reduced. It can help, for example, to go to parties early to allow the group of children to build up slowly. Shopping is best done when the stores are quiet. Emily can learn to answer a simple mobile phone that she can carry in case she gets lost, and she might be able to learn to call one or two telephone numbers programmed into the phone when she feels she requires help.

16. Emily's ability to use her vision, as well as her other skills, declines when she is tired, and she will benefit from short, well-timed rests between activities.

17. When starting on a new activity, it is important to gently but firmly draw Emily's attention to the task at hand.

18. When carrying out a task or activity, Emily tends to favor use of her right hand. She needs to continue to work with her occupational therapist to encourage the use of both hands.

19. Emily is gaining more independent living skills. At present, she manages with a standard plate and spoon. She is also learning how to use a microwave.

20. Emily should continue to receive evaluations and resultant services from an O&M specialist.

# APPENDIX 10B

# Sample Functional Vision Assessment Report for Education: Ranjit

**Name:** Ranjit Gupta
**Age:** 4.5 years
**Location:** Red Valley Elementary School
**Evaluator:** Lenora Schneider, Teacher of Visually Impaired Students

## Reason for Evaluation

Ranjit's functional vision was assessed to confirm that he would benefit for educational services for students with visual impairments and to determine appropriate instructional goals for his school program.

## Background

### Medical History

According to the report from his pediatric ophthalmologist from one year ago, Ranjit was born at 26 weeks' gestation and was diagnosed with both cerebral visual impairment (CVI) (compromised vision due to brain damage) and retinopathy of prematurity (ROP) (damage to the tissue lining the inner surface of the eye—the retina). His MRI scan report describes "periventricular white matter pathology (loss of white matter around the fluid-filled cavities in the brain), more marked on the left side of the brain." Ranjit had laser treatment for the ROP, experienced a partial retinal detachment (partial separation of a layer of tissue—the retina—from the inner surface of the eye) in the right eye, which now has minimal vision, and has retained some useful vision in the left eye. His lower visual field is reported to be limited in both eyes, and the visual field in his right eye is further limited nasally due to the detachment.

According to his latest ophthalmological report, Ranjit was unable to fixate and follow with his right eye, but he did respond to large targets presented in his upper-left and right fields of vision in the right eye. He was also able to respond to targets with his left eye. A previous eye report at 2 years of age indicated that Ranjit's vision was not testable with formal tests and that he had difficulty fixating and following with either eye. This suggests some improvement of vision over time. His latest reports also state that Ranjit has a reduced lower visual field in his left eye.

According to his ophthalmologist, Ranjit had 20/300 visual acuity in his left eye and does not need corrective lenses. There was no mention of any ocular motor dysfunction in previous reports.

Ranjit's medical history also indicates that he has impairment of movement on the right side (right hemiplegia due to cerebral palsy). He is able to walk independently and retains the use of both hands.

### Educational History

Previous educational records indicate that Ranjit has reduced vision and qualified for the services of a teacher of students with visual impairments. He has also received services from a physical therapist. This is his first year in the Anderson County School District. His full school records have not been received to date, but his Individual

Education Program from the previous district indicates that he received the services of a teacher of visually impaired students while he was there.

Ranjit is able to communicate well verbally and is enrolled in a daily preschool class that meets in the mornings only. His preschool teacher reports that Ranjit has difficulty following instructions in his class and often falls behind in his classroom activities. He does not play with peers unless it is in a structured playgroup with adult supervision. Ranjit knows basic shapes, primary colors, and some letters and recognizes his first name, according to his teacher, but he sometimes has trouble finding things during his art activities and around the classroom. He often plays alone on the periphery of the playground and appears to be reluctant to join in ball games outside.

## Functional Vision Evaluation

Ranjit's functional vision evaluation incorporated information from a parent interview, interviews with school staff, formal and informal assessment tools, and observations at school.

***Interviews:*** Ranjit's mother was interviewed prior to formal testing and observation. Questions were asked relating to Ranjit's visual functioning, and, since Ranjit had been diagnosed with CVI, a structured history-taking inventory was also used to prompt questioning. Ranjit's teacher was also interviewed about his use of vision in the classroom. Key results of these interviews have been incorporated below.

***Observations:*** Ranjit was observed in his classroom and on the playground during his preschool class.

### Distance Visual Acuity (Ability to See Details at a Distance)

Ranjit's classroom teacher reported that he makes a number of errors when reading letters and pre-primer words that he knows, so a symbol chart (house, heart, square, and circle) was used to evaluate functional visual acuity. Ranjit was asked to read the symbols on the LEA Symbol Chart 10-Line Pediatric Eye Chart at 5 feet with both eyes viewing, with and without a directional lamp for additional illumination.

With that test, he read down to the 100-foot symbol line, missing one letter on the right side of the line, and he was slow in identifying the letters. When each letter was touched with a black stick used as a pointer to assist Ranjit, he read along the line of letters more quickly. Ranjit's estimated Snellen equivalent functional acuity with this test was $5/80^{-1}$ which converts to $20/320^{-1}$ (or $6/95^{-1}$) with both eyes viewing.

Ranjit was then asked to identify single symbols on the LEA Symbols Low Vision Book at 5 feet with both eyes viewing, with and without a directional lamp for additional illumination. Ranjit read the single symbols more quickly and identified 63-foot symbols consistently at this distance. With single symbols, Ranjit's estimated Snellen equivalent functional acuity was 5/63. (This equates to 20/250 or 6/75.)

***Comments:*** The use of the directional lamp did not alter Ranjit's performance on either task. Ranjit appeared to tire more quickly when asked to read the line acuity chart, and he needed much encouragement to complete the task. Ranjit's performance improved when symbols were isolated or a "pointer" was used. He often missed letters at the right end of the line on the line acuity chart.

***Additional Observations/Reports:*** Ranjit's mother reports that he is not very interested in watching TV, but when there are slow-moving, large cartoon characters, he gets quite close to the screen to watch, moving his head to view individual elements. She feels that he listens to the TV more than he watches it. Ranjit also appeared to have difficulty naming children in his class when asked to locate them from 5 or more feet away. His mother says that he only can find his two brothers when they all go to the supermarket when they call out to him, and even then he can only locate them with difficulty. When in the supermarket, Ranjit does not recognize what is on the shelves until his mother tells him or he touches the food items or packages. His mother always lets him pick out his favorite cookies located on a lower shelf. He can find the shelf, but uses his hands to locate a single box to put in the shopping cart from the row of boxes of like items.

### Visual Acuity for Near Tasks (Ability to See Details at Near)

The Lea Near Vision Card (in both crowded and uncrowded symbol format) was presented to Ranjit. Ranjit was asked to read the smallest pictures on the card that he could see, and he was allowed to hold the card at his preferred distance. Ranjit chose to read the 1.6M uncrowded symbols (equivalent to 14-point Times New Roman font) at 6 inches (15 cm). From this, it was determined that Ranjit's best close viewing distance was 8 inches or 20 cm (using the formula 1.5 × closest viewing distance of 6 inches = 8 inches). Ranjit was then asked to read down the card held at 8 inches, from larger to smaller symbol sizes. Ranjit's reading was slow, even with large symbols. From the point at which Ranjit's reading was noted to slow down more significantly, it was determined that spaced symbols for Ranjit should be about 2.5M in height (equivalent to 22-point Times New Roman font) at 8 inches. This procedure was repeated for the more crowded symbols on the chart that are closer to a reading task. For these, Ranjit was most efficient with 3.2M symbols (equivalent to 29-point Times New Roman font). Copies of these symbols are attached to this report. Print sizes need to be adjusted to fit the demands of each reading task presented to Ranjit (depending on task difficulty, type of font used, and line spacing, for example), and provide a starting point for determining the best print size for a given task.

When given a typoscope (a reading window made from a black index card that isolates a line of symbols), Ranjit's speed and accuracy increased as he read across lines of both crowded and uncrowded symbols.

***Comments:*** Ranjit read uncrowded symbols more easily than crowded symbols, and his accuracy and speed increased with the aid of a typoscope (reading window) that isolated a line of symbols. A reading lamp did not affect Ranjit's performance.

***Additional Observations:*** To view material of interest, such as pictures in books or parts of toys, Ranjit positions his face about 6 inches away from the material.

### Contrast Sensitivity (Ability to Detect an Object from its Background)

Contrast sensitivity can affect the ability to see stairs, drop-offs, and faces. Using the Cambridge Low Contrast Gratings test held at 2.5 feet with both eyes viewing in typical classroom illumination, Ranjit was able to recognize the location of the plate with the stripes down to Plate 2, indicating a 2.7 percent Michelson contrast. This indicates a mild reduction in contrast sensitivity.

### Visual Field (Area of Vision)

The Confrontation Field Test, a gross test of functional visual fields, was administered with both eyes viewing in a dimly lit room using a penlight topped with a puppet cap as the target. Ranjit was asked to look straight ahead at the examiner's nose while the penlight was brought in from above, below, right, and left. Ranjit did not see the light from below until it reached the level of his lips and when brought in from the right in his upper field, he spotted it visually (his eyes moved quickly toward it) when it reached about 2 inches from his nose. Ranjit either pointed to the penlight when he first saw it or told the examiner when he first saw the light. Ranjit appeared to have full visual fields above and to the left, but his lower and right visual fields appeared to be quite reduced.

***Observations:*** When walking in the classroom and around his school, Ranjit was noted to bump into things on his right, and stumble over toys on the ground when he moved quickly around the classroom. Ranjit was noted to startle several times in his play outside when a bright soccer ball was coming toward him from various directions. On one occasion, for example, he didn't appear to notice the ball until it whizzed by him about 2 feet from his right side. He jumped away quickly. His mother reports that when crossing streets while holding her right hand and standing to her right, Ranjit will keep walking even when children in the neighborhood are moving quickly toward them from the right on bicycles or skateboards. He is not allowed to cross streets by himself. She also reports that Ranjit trips on curbs and cracks in the sidewalk. She says that she must always keep an eye on him when they are walking around the neighborhood. He has great difficulty walking down slopes and stairs if there is no handrail.

### Illumination Requirements

***Observations:*** Ranjit did not appear to perform differently on near or distance functional visual acuity tests when a reading lamp was focused on his visual task. He squinted, narrowing his eyelids, when outdoors in bright sunlight. When moving from outdoors to his classroom, he would stop for a few seconds before proceeding, appearing to need to take this time for his eyes to adjust to the changing light levels.

### Color Identification

Ranjit was able to name and match primary colors using colored blocks. His favorite color is green, the color of his family's pickup truck. His mother reports that Ranjit does not appear to have difficulty picking out his shirts or pants by color. She feels that color helps Ranjit find things in his piles of clothes and in his toy box. Ranjit was not able to complete a color vision screening test for young children; he could not see the shapes on the busy background in the Color Vision Made Easy test or understand the instructions for the subtle shades of color on the Quantitative Color Vision test. The latter test will be given when Ranjit is older and better able to understand task directions.

### Visual Processing

*Directions of Lines*

Ranjit showed no difficulty on the Mailbox Game when he had to align a "letter" with the orientation of a "mailbox" slot 1 foot away. He also showed no difficulty aligning the "letter" with the slot and inserting it as the slot was turned in various orientations.

### *Length of Lines and Objects*

On the Rectangles Games, Ranjit was able to match a series of rectangles of different dimensions when they were placed far apart from one another, but when placed against one another to make a larger pyramid shape, Ranjit hesitated throughout the task and made a number of matching errors. It is likely that Ranjit was able to decipher the length of lines of objects, but only when matching pairs were presented singly. Ranjit was able to match the length of straight lines constructed by the examiner out of colored blocks in the classroom.

### *Tracing, Copying, and Drawing*

Ranjit was asked to trace with his finger the stripes (or gratings) on the Lea Gratings test held at 11.5 inches (29 cm); he used his left hand. He was able to do this accurately with the wider gratings that measured 2.0 cm wide, 1.0 cm wide, and 0.5 cm wide at the 11.5-inch distance. (If lines are presented at twice the distance, for example, the width of the lines must be doubled for the same performance; if the lines are presented at half the distance, the width of the lines can be reduced by one half.) Samples of the size gratings that Ranjit could trace are attached to this report. (Although the gratings Ranjit could trace are listed in cycles per centimeter, their actual width in centimeters is reported here for ease of interpretation.)

***Observations:*** During his class's art lesson with crayons, it was clear that Ranjit chooses to use his left hand. Ranjit drew a picture about a field trip to the local zoo. His drawing was primarily on the left side of the page, and components on the right side were distorted. His face was about 4 inches from the paper as he drew. When asked to copy shapes right after the examiner drew them—a horizontal line, a vertical line, a circle, and a square—Ranjit's vertical line was about the same length as the examiner's line, but his horizontal line was very short, because he took his pencil off the paper just after it had crossed his midline from left to right. When Ranjit was shown how to rotate the paper to view his work and finish a figure, he became very excited and lengthened several horizontal lines to better match the models. His circle was a good approximation of the shape; his square looked very similar to the circle. Ranjit's teacher reports that Ranjit is having difficulty copying letters as he learns to write his first name although he can point to them and does recognize his first name when it is written for him.

### *Perception of Faces*

Ranjit had no difficulty identifying the expressions on the faces in the Heidi Expressions Test Game when he looked at the cards from a distance of 6 inches.

***Observations/Interviews:*** Ranjit's mother and teacher indicate that he can identify them by their faces when they approach him silently from about 5 feet away. He was also able to tell a smiling face from an angry face from this distance for static expressions, but not when the expressions were maintained for only a brief time. From within 5 feet, Ranjit was noted during the classroom observation to identify his teacher, a classroom aide, and some students, using what appeared to be his vision alone, rather than from voice or other cues. His teacher and classroom aide both have short brown hair.

## Eye-Hand Coordination

Ranjit threaded large colored beads on a bright orange cord without difficulty. When threading beads of different highly contrasting colors, Ranjit picked out each bead by color visually as it was named before placing it on the cord. Ranjit also stacked colored plastic rings onto a ring stand without difficulty.

## Visual Perceptual Skills

### *Visual Perceptual Skills with Drawings*

Ranjit was shown selected items to determine if further testing was warranted to evaluate his performance on visual perceptual tasks. Ranjit showed consistent errors on tasks locating a picture amidst a busy background and identifying a known figure when parts were missing.

***Observations/Interview:*** Ranjit was not able to locate a favorite interactive toy among a pile of toys during playtime in his classroom. When the toy was placed on a shelf of contrasting color, Ranjit walked directly to it to pick it up. Ranjit's mother reports that he often leaves food on the near and right sides of his plate and can be surprised to find he has missed some. He is learning to rotate his plate to compensate. She also has to help him identify his shirts from a pile of shirts of similar colors that she is sorting for Ranjit and his brothers.

### *Movement Perception*

***Figure in Motion:*** The Pepi Test that assesses the perception of slow motion was attempted with Ranjit, but he did not decipher the picture of the Dalmation as a picture of a dog from dots in the busy background. The examiner was not certain that Ranjit had sufficient near vision to discern the elements of the picture of the slowly moving dog on the background dots.

***Interview:*** Ranjit's mother reports that Ranjit startles when they are in their front yard and their neighbor's small dog runs up to greet them. Ranjit does not appear to see the dog running up and only notices it when the animal finally reaches them. This could relate to the dog's not being seen in Ranjit's lower visual field, to an inability to see fast movement, or a combination of both. Ranjit participates in ball games with his two brothers by running to get a bright, large ball after his brothers hit it or pitch it and it stops moving. His mother reports that he loves doing this rather than throwing or hitting the ball because he can do this with much success. Hitting the ball and throwing it to someone else to hit are hard for him.

***Observation*:** Out on the schoolyard, Ranjit did not play ball games with the other children. He stayed on the side of the play area, and when a ball went out of bounds, the children told him where it was. He then ran to fetch it back for play. He tended to stay at the side of the play yard when there was a lot of activity and joined in only when one of his many friends came to get him. When the activity in the playground became calmer, Ranjit walked more in the central part of the yard independently to be with the other children. His friends often called out to him, but also had to come up close, so that he knew where they were. Ranjit did not appear to be able to locate the direction of his friends when they called to him. When sitting at a table at the front of the class, Ranjit did not appear to look directly at his teacher as she walked animatedly back and forth during a review of what happened on a field trip to the zoo with the class.

## Summary

Ranjit has decreased visual acuity due to retinopathy of prematurity and cerebral visual impairment. He does not need to wear eyeglasses according to his ophthalmologist. Ranjit can read 1.6M (equivalent to 14-point Times New Roman font) when symbols are presented singly at 6 inches. When presented with a line of symbols, Ranjit slows down and makes more errors. For groups of symbols as found in print reading, Ranjit requires at least 3.2M symbols (equivalent to 29-point Times New Roman font) when held at his best close viewing distance of 8 inches. Copies of the 1.6M and 3.2M equivalent symbols have been attached to this report so that teachers can use these as a guide for symbol or print size to use at 8 inches for Ranjit.

Ranjit has reduced areas of vision in his right and lower visual fields. He does not appear to always detect things on his right or in his lower visual field according to interview reports and observations. Further investigation is required to determine if visual inattention to the right visual field is operating. Ranjit also has mildly reduced ability to see contrast differences between two adjacent surfaces, and this can affect his ability to see faces, stairs, drop-offs, and low-contrast educational materials.

Ranjit did not appear to have problems with color perception. Typical classroom illumination did not pose difficulties for Ranjit. Ranjit appeared to have difficulty noticing and following fast-moving visual targets, based on interview reports and observations. Some visual perceptual tasks appear to be difficult for Ranjit when they involve locating similar shapes that differ in size or orientation, locating a form against a busy background, and filling in missing parts of a known figure. Finally, Ranjit has difficulty selecting objects from a group or pile of objects, according to interview reports and observations.

## Recommendations

1. Ranjit has difficulty accessing educational materials using his vision and would benefit from the services of a teacher of students who are visually impaired.
2. Ranjit had some difficulties identifying items in a group or pile of items and matching a group of rectangles, finding items amidst visual clutter, and completing incomplete figures. He also has difficulty copying the letters in his name and tracing stripes as their widths decrease in size. Appropriate adaptations need to be made to accommodate Ranjit's visual perceptual needs. These include spacing out material so that he can see individual items, providing materials that are large enough for Ranjit to copy, considering early keyboarding skills to assist with writing, and special attention to copying, tracing, and cutting tasks using materials that are clearly visible to Ranjit.
3. Ranjit does not appear to be able to locate the direction of his friends when they call out to him. If auditory processing is established as a concern for Ranjit, then this must be taken into account in Ranjit's educational programming. (An auditory processing assessment is recommended as a follow-up to this report.)
4. Ranjit would benefit from his teacher moving more slowly when presenting lessons since Ranjit cannot follow her fast walking motions and fast hand gestures. Fast-moving TV shows and movies and classroom activities may be difficult for Ranjit to process.
5. Ranjit does not need special lighting for his near and distance tasks. However, he does squint (narrow his eyes) in bright light and appears to require additional time to adapt to significant changes in lighting (for example, going from bright sunlight outdoors to his classroom). It is recommended that Ranjit be evaluated for sunshades

during his next clinical eye examination or low vision evaluation and, until that time, some generic sunshades be tried with Ranjit along with a cap with a visor when Ranjit is outdoors in bright sunlight to see if these items help him.

6. Ranjit has reduced ability to see things at a distance. For distance viewing, objects and people need to be 16 times larger (or he needs to be 16 times closer) than for people with typical vision for Ranjit to see them when they are crowded together or against a busy background. When an object stands out from the background, it only needs to be 12 times larger than for those with typical vision.
7. Ranjit read slowly along lines of symbols regardless of symbol size. It is recommended that, at present, Ranjit learn to read using a typoscope to isolate single words with a print size of 3.2M (equivalent to 29-point Times New Roman font) at 8 inches as a starting point. Teachers will need to determine if a sans serif font such as Arial would be better for Ranjit. Arial, for example, is a larger font than Times New Roman. (That is, "words in Arial" and "words in Times New Roman" appear to be different sizes even though they are in the same font size.) Therefore, the point size of the sans serif font selected might require adjustment. In addition, it may be that after some experimentation, a different print size or viewing distance is determined to be more comfortable and efficient for Ranjit, and the size of print used may differ with the visual and cognitive demands of different reading tasks. Ranjit can use a typoscope to isolate single words or a short line of words that are spaced apart. Words can also be outlined with Ranjit's favorite color, green, to attract and maintain his attention. Teachers can experiment to see if another color may be more efficient for the word outlines (such as red or orange). Letters in words should be spaced a little bit apart.
8. Ranjit has reduced vision on his right side. It is therefore recommended that Ranjit sit on the right side of his classroom so that most activities occur in his left field of vision. (The psychological assessment and orientation and mobility assessment can help determine if Ranjit has visual inattention to his right.) In addition teachers and other staff members should ensure that items that Ranjit needs to see are placed in his available field of vision. Ranjit may also require training in ways to scan with his head or body, depending on the nature of the field impairment. Ranjit tends to sit rotated with his left side closer to the table, both at home and at school. This could well be an adaptive behavior for lack of attention to the right and does not need to be corrected.
9. Ranjit also has a constricted and inefficient lower visual field. He can be taught to move his work pages upward so that he can take in the entire page, or he can use a reading stand or tilted workstation to elevate and orient his work material in order to see the lower part more readily. Care should be taken to ensure that Ranjit travels safely in areas with stairs, curbs, uneven ground, and where items may be unexpectedly on the floor in his path of travel.
10. At 1 foot, objects and pictures should be at least 0.5 inches (1.25 cm) high for Ranjit to see them easily. At 2 feet they should be at least 1 inch high (2.5 cm), and at 3 feet they should be at least 1.5 inches (3.75 cm) high. School staff will need to experiment to determine if Ranjit actually needs slightly larger ob-

jects, especially when against a busy background or when presented close together in groups.

11. It is recommended that the teacher of students with visual impairments discuss the use of magnifiers with Ranjit's eye care specialist as a way to assist in providing larger print for Ranjit, as well as isolating words so that he can read more fluently. The use of a typoscope to isolate words or lines of words can also be tried with Ranjit, as mentioned in an earlier recommendation.
12. Ranjit's educational materials should be in high contrast so that Ranjit can see them easily.
13. Workbooks or work pages should be simplified for Ranjit by removing extraneous visual content or masking it so that Ranjit can more easily locate material on each page.
14. Ranjit appears to have difficulty with visual clutter. Efforts should be made to provide an uncluttered environment for him. This includes his workspace, his work tasks, his classroom environment, and his play environments. Teachers and other staff members need to be aware that Ranjit does not function well when materials, objects, or people are close together, as he cannot sort them out visually. Noise, movement, and visual distractions should be kept to a minimum. Ranjit's play areas need to be carefully organized so that he can readily find his way around objects in them and locate items of interest. Materials that he uses in class activities should be stored in different colored containers for each type of item, for example. There should be ample space between items on shelves where his leisure time toys and storybooks are located. Using linear storage systems, in which Ranjit places his possessions himself, will mean that he only needs to search in one dimension and can use memory and color as aids to promptly locate his possessions.
15. Ranjit does not always have friends to play with in his classroom, where activities are fast-paced and active. Efforts should be made to design activities in which Ranjit can participate independently with a group, and when this is not possible, activities should be monitored in ways that encourage his participation, such as working with an assigned "buddy" or partner, encouraging Ranjit to lead an activity, or having the children take turns.

## Recommendations for Further Assessment

The following referrals are suggested to complement the recommendations made in this report.

1. Since Ranjit has mildly reduced contrast sensitivity as well as difficulty tripping over materials in the classroom and identifying fast-moving objects, it is recommended that he be evaluated for orientation and mobility (O&M) services. Ranjit's ability to walk independently in areas where children are playing can be evaluated during this assessment. The O&M evaluation can determine if special techniques are needed to accommodate his lower and right visual field impairment while traveling or playing. Until additional recommendations are available from the O&M assessment, Ranjit should continue to be allowed to play on the periphery of the outside play area where he feels secure away from the fast-moving objects and crowds of children. Teachers should be made aware that he may need some assistance in negotiating the area when it is crowded with children or when the

activity around him is fast moving. For example, Ranjit could have a friend assigned to him at these times.

2. Referral for further neuropsychological evaluation by a school psychologist is recommended to determine Ranjit's visual and other processing abilities so that appropriate interventions can be implemented to assist in any areas of need that may be found.
3. Ranjit's auditory processing skills require further assessment, and he should therefore be referred to the school psychologist or speech-language therapist for this purpose.
4. Ranjit may benefit from low vision optical and electronic devices for reading. It is therefore recommended that he receive a clinical low vision evaluation to determine his potential to use these devices.
5. A thorough learning media assessment is recommended for Ranjit once results from the recommended clinical low vision evaluation have been received. The learning media assessment should include an evaluation for the use of braille for reading as well as the use of assistive technology for his schoolwork, such as optical and electronic devices, including touch tablets. When the learning media assessment has been completed, the most effective reading medium or media can be determined for Ranjit.

# 11

# Assessment of Functional Vision: History Taking for Children with CVI

*Gordon N. Dutton*

Taking a detailed history from parents or caregivers is the first step in assessing a child with cerebral visual impairment (CVI). The information obtained not only allows professionals to understand the nature of the child's vision, but also provides them with information needed to plan the assessment of vision. Carefully crafted questions presented to family members within a welcoming environment can lead to an accurate and revealing account of the visual difficulties and behaviors exhibited by a child with CVI and the ways in which his or her family has coped with and adapted to them. History taking contributes to effective and comprehensive assessment (see Chapter 10), and provides information crucial to guiding intervention and future educational programs.

Parents and caregivers may not be fully aware of how much they know, having lived with and adapted to their child's behaviors (particularly in the case of an only child with no siblings for comparison). The first meeting with the child and caregivers gives the professional a chance to seek a comprehensive account of any visual difficulties and their impact, any associated behaviors, and the feelings the parents or caregivers may have about the child's condition. It also offers an opportunity to probe the family's wishes and hopes for the child's future. From the information gathered in the course of taking the history, a cohesive story or picture begins to emerge of the child's vision, his or her behaviors, and the effects on the child and the family, including coping methods and adaptations. This story, in turn, can point the way to planning appropriate assessment and intervention that is tailored to the individual child.

A child's key medical history from the caregiver's perspective can also be sought if necessary, by specifically asking for a summary of important medical information during the interview. However, the interviewer should have reviewed the child's previous medical history from available records, prior to the start of the interview. A pathological label or diagnosis provides the origin of the problem, and an anatomical label derived from scans of the brain offers information about the site and extent of any damage to the brain. Functional and behavioral descriptors of the child's condition also need to be obtained and recorded, and some of this information will be supplemented by the interview process.

## The Skill of Eliciting the History

It takes some skill and preparation for an interviewer to make people comfortable, gain their trust, and deliver key questions that follow a respondent's lead. This requires setting the stage for the interview and being familiar with the types of questions that facilitate a free flow of information. The environment in which the interview is conducted, the demeanor of the interviewer, and the nature of the questions are prepared ahead of time. The remainder of this chapter describes in detail the different components of history taking. An audio recording of an actual history-taking session between the author and the mother of a child with CVI (Emerald Education Systems, n.d.) is available to illustrate the real-life interchange between interviewer and family member in attempting to seek out the details of the child's story.

### Location

- Use a clean, tidy, uncluttered room with plenty of space and a suitable play environment for the child.
- Allow for a drink or a snack for the child.

### Demeanor

- Use a calm voice.
- Be welcoming, kind, engaging, and friendly.
- Involve the child in the process whenever possible by asking about his or her experiences.
- Make the child feel important and the focus of events, particularly at the beginning and the end of the meeting. At the beginning, provide a friendly welcome and invite the child to come and play with the toys if he or she wishes, and at the end, make sure to thank the child for all he or she has contributed.
- Remember to pay sufficient attention to siblings if they are present. (Brothers and sisters can often take part in the interview and can provide useful information.)

### Structuring the Questions

The way a question is asked can significantly influence the answer. *Open questions* are neutral in tone and invite interviewees to share information of any kind. In contrast, *leading questions* subtly prompt people to give an answer that may be anticipated by the interviewer. *Closed questions* are narrower in scope, and are often specific to the point of allowing only certain answers to the question posed; they therefore limit the interviewee's response. The question, "What are your concerns about David's vision?" is open and does not lead. The question, "What happens when you take David into a supermarket?" is a closed but non-leading question, whereas the question "Does David become upset when you take him into a supermarket?" is both a closed and a leading question, as the expected answer is implied; such a question may act as a prompt to the person being interviewed.

Each type of question has its place. Open, non-leading questions are needed to elicit the child's and the family's story for the first time. Closed, non-leading questions are used to develop topics being discussed and find out more about the issues that have been raised. Closed, leading questions can be helpful later on in the interview to determine possible effects of CVI on the child, and how best to help the child once the overall picture has been elicited using an initial open, non-leading approach.

Closed, leading questions do have a role in an interview. These types of questions can help parents recognize the behavioral features being sought out by the interviewer as possible indicators of the presence of CVI in their child. It may never have occurred to them that the behaviors they see every day are in any way unusual, so such information may not be volunteered; therefore, leading questions can become key in eliciting this information.

For example, a large proportion of children with low visual acuity or perceptual visual impairment prefer to sit very close to a television, to compensate for their low acuity and to diminish visual crowding. Many parents discourage this behavior. So if an interviewer asks the open, leading question, "Where does your child sit while watching TV?" the response given by the parents reflects their instruction to the child, rather than the child's natural behavior. The closed, leading questions, "Does your child try to get close to the TV? If so, how close?" elicit information that might otherwise be missed.

Often such questions lead to moments of realization that behaviors that families thought were normal (and therefore would not think of identifying or reporting) are in fact the results of reactions or strategies the child uses to circumvent or compensate for visual disorders. However, leading questions must be used advisedly, and the responses interpreted carefully because a minority of families can absorb this information and use it in the future to change or enhance their reports of the child's behavior. Such an outcome is counterproductive for the child.

## Stages of the Interview

Finding out about impairment of vision resulting from damage to the brain in children is carried out in a number of stages:

1. Seeking the history
2. Clarifying the history
3. Expanding the history
4. Asking informed questions to seek out patterns of visual behavior
5. Using a question inventory, if required, to characterize the visual difficulties in order to provide help and advice for each issue
6. Finding out the impact the visual difficulties have on the child and the child's family
7. Determining the previous history and what the family has been told by other professionals
8. Understanding the wishes and agenda of the child and the family
9. Making sense of the information and seeking cross-correlation of reported behaviors to validate their presence and features
10. Assembling the history and drawing conclusions
11. Documenting the history obtained
12. Using the information gathered from history taking to guide further assessment

### Seeking the History

When finding out information for the first time, it is important to ask open questions along the lines of "What have you noticed about David's vision?" Then it is important to sit and listen without interrupting. Parents and caregivers often come to a first meeting with a particular agenda based on their concerns about their child. If they are interrupted, this can break their train of thought and useful information will be lost. It can be helpful to suggest to parents in advance of the meeting that it is worth coming with a list of questions because important material can be left out of a family's account when there is a lot to communicate.

At this stage, the interviewer should take note of all the key issues. They can be recorded as a list, or it can prove helpful to note them down in the form of a diagram to visually organize the information about the child's visual behavior—sometimes referred to as a "mind map"—or a chart or similar graphic (see Figure 11.1 for one possible template). This kind of organized diagram can represent the child's vision in the center, with the issues that are raised during the interview noted in an array radiating outward from this central concept. Space is left to make additional notes as the interview proceeds and themes are developed. In the author's experience, this type of recording can be particularly helpful when a large number

FIGURE 11.1
**Mind Map Diagram**

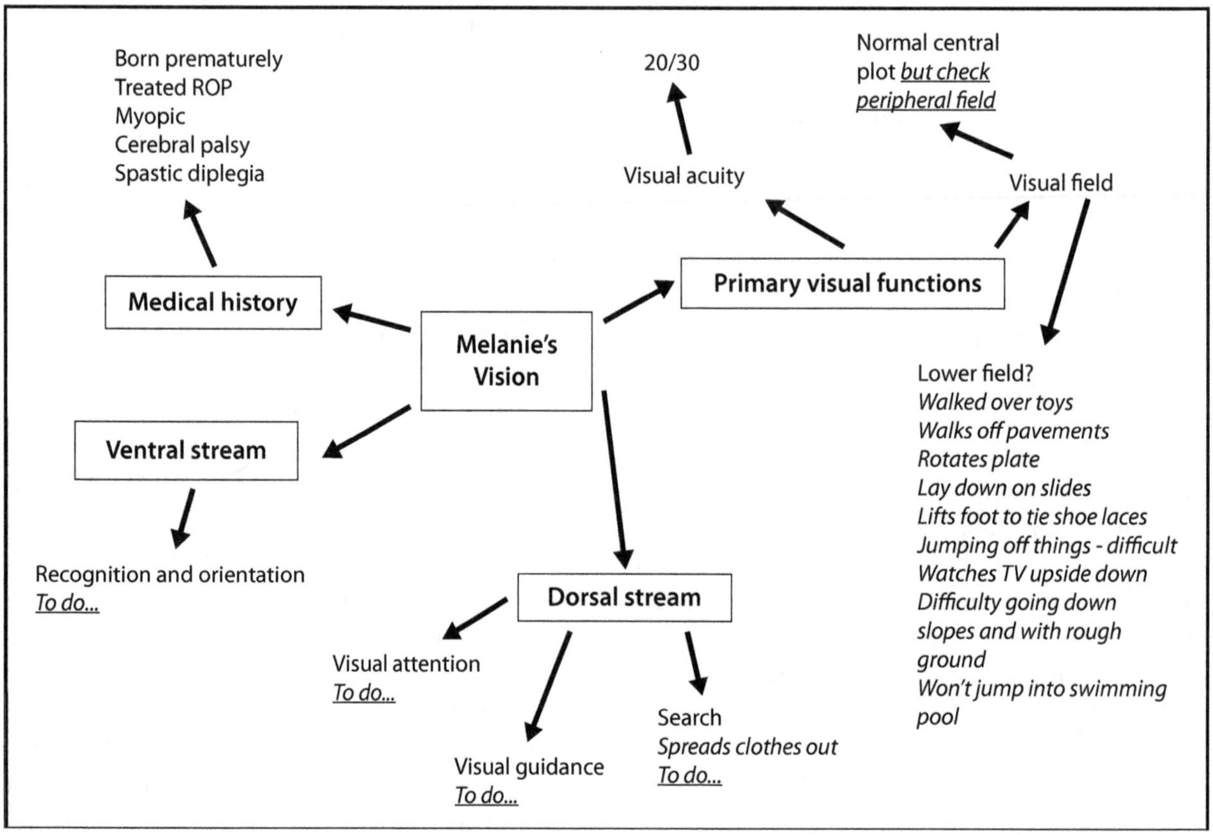

Born prematurely
Treated ROP
Myopic
Cerebral palsy
Spastic diplegia
20/30
Normal central plot *but check peripheral field*
Visual acuity
Visual field
**Medical history**
**Primary visual functions**
**Melanie's Vision**
**Ventral stream**
Lower field?
*Walked over toys*
*Walks off pavements*
*Rotates plate*
*Lay down on slides*
*Lifts foot to tie shoe laces*
*Jumping off things - difficult*
*Watches TV upside down*
*Difficulty going down slopes and with rough ground*
*Won't jump into swimming pool*
Recognition and orientation
*To do...*
**Dorsal stream**
Visual attention
*To do...*
Search
*Spreads clothes out*
*To do...*
Visual guidance
*To do...*

A mind map diagram providing a template for seeking and recording information about behaviors related to CVI. This diagram illustrates notes taken for a child named Melanie.

of visual difficulties are reported. A story concerning the child's visual behaviors can emerge somewhat randomly, but the diagram can be filled in like the details of a painting. The mind map portrayed in Figure 11.1 depicts notes recording information emerging about a girl named Melanie during an interview that is presented later in this chapter.

## Clarifying the Story

Once the family has finished recounting what they wish to say, clarify any incomplete or unclear issues. Then explore each issue in terms of "time, place, and person," as appropriate, to further develop the information provided. For example, if a parent states, "David gets distressed when we go somewhere that's busy," the interviewer can inquire about the details as follows:

### *Time*

Q: When did you first see this behavior?
A: When he was a toddler.
Q: How often does it happen?
A: Whenever we go to the supermarket. We don't take him anymore.
Q: How long does it last when it happens?
A: For the whole time he is in the shop, and for a while afterward as he calms down.
Q: Has it happened recently? If so, what were the circumstances?
A: Yes, last month during Christmas shopping. He had to go back and sit quietly in the car with his dad.

### *Place*

Q: Where does this happen? Can you give any examples?
A: Yes. He went to a party. We took him early when it was quiet, but as soon as the games began and the boys ran around, he hid in a corner and wouldn't come out.

### *Person*

The word "person" in this context refers to the nature of the child's experiences and behaviors.

Q: What is his behavior like?
A: It varies. Sometimes he becomes withdrawn like at the party; other times he can get distressed and angry.
Q: Is there anything that makes it better?
A: He's great when he is out walking in the countryside. We never see this behavior then.
Q: Is there anything that makes it worse?
A: Additional noise. He will stand in the corner crying with his fingers in his ears.
Q: Does it upset David when it happens?
A: Oh yes. He's 7 years old, and he doesn't want to be different, but he is beginning to understand that he is.

The behavior described in this account could stem from a range of reasons, but for a child with CVI, the story is typical of a child who is unable to process a lot of information as a result of dorsal stream dysfunction. This realization would lead the interviewer to ask questions concerning behaviors related to both dorsal stream and ventral stream dysfunction, as well as behaviors consistent with lower visual field impairment, which is a common accompaniment.

## Expanding the Story (Thinking in Threes)

The primary challenge in gathering information is to detect whether manifestations of CVI are present, and if so, the various ways in which they may be affecting a child,

SIDEBAR 11.1

### Structure–Function–Outcome: Triplets of Ideas to Keep in Mind during CVI History-Taking Interviews

***Think:***

1. Structure
2. Function
3. Outcome

***Structure:*** *Structures in the brain that may be involved*

1. Visual pathways and occipital lobes
2. Dorsal stream and posterior parietal lobes
3. Ventral stream and temporal lobes

***Function:*** *Functions that can be directly affected*

1. Occipital lobes
   - **A.** Image clarity
   - **B.** Visual fields
   - **C.** Seeing motion
2. Dorsal stream
   - **A.** Visual guidance
   - **B.** Visual search
   - **C.** Visual attention
3. Ventral stream
   - **A.** Face recognition
   - **B.** Shape recognition
   - **C.** Orientation

*Functions depending on vision that can be affected*

- **A.** Visual memory
- **B.** Visual imagination
- **C.** Visual representation (art)

***Outcome:***

1. Visual dysfunctions can affect:
   - **A.** Access to information (both distant and near)
   - **B.** Social interaction
   - **C.** Visual guidance of movement of arms, legs, and body
2. The adaptations the child makes include:
   - **A.** How to make best use of intact vision
   - **B.** Avoidance of difficult situations
   - **C.** Unusual social behaviors
3. Psychological impacts include:
   - **A.** Emotional: behaviors and feelings
   - **B.** Interpersonal: interactions with other children
   - **C.** Physical: fatigue, because of the effort needed to cope

keeping in mind the wide range of issues that need to be considered. To fully understand a child's profile and condition, an evaluator needs a way of remembering the key issues. Most people can effectively consider things in sets of three, so if one thinks in sets of three, it is often possible to consider a wide range of issues without overlooking key elements. One possible working model is to remember the following set of three factors: structure, function, and outcome (see Sidebar 11.1). For example, the anatomical *structure*—the posterior parietal lobe—serves the *functions* of visual guidance of movement, visual search, and visual attention. The *outcome* of the damage impairs these functions, leading to typically observed behaviors. This framework for thinking can be effective in making sure key issues are covered and important items are not overlooked.

## Asking Informed Questions to Seek Patterns of Visual Behavior

As described in previous chapters, visual behaviors resulting from CVI tend to occur in recognizable patterns (see, for example, Figures 10.4 and 10.5 in Chapter 10), which can be effectively detected, traced, and described by applying the "structure, function, outcome" model. When one element is not easily identifiable in a given instance, evidence of dysfunction of the other two elements needs to be sought by asking pertinent and focused questions. Specific questions are needed because past observers may already have incorrectly attributed these behaviors to inappropriate behavior or lack of intelligence on the part of the child, and they may not be thought of as being related to problems with vision.

### *Sample Interview: Melanie*

The following condensed interview shows how the approach and principles just presented can be applied. The interview takes place with Melanie, an 11-year-old who has recently moved to a new school, and her mother. Melanie and her parents have requested an assessment on account of her vision to make sure she receives appropriate instruction and consideration at school. (A sample mind map illustrating notes taken during this interview appears in Figure 11.1.)

Melanie has had visual difficulties for years, but she feels that no one has ever really listened to her. She was born prematurely at 28 weeks instead of the normal 40 and was in an incubator for a long time. She had to have laser treatment to her eyes for retinopathy of prematurity, and is now myopic (short-sighted or nearsighted). Her legs are weak and stiff, and her walking is ungainly because she has the type of cerebral palsy called spastic diplegia. She is pursuing a mainstream curriculum at school and is particularly good at language, but her arithmetic and math skills are below what is typical for her school level. All her visual difficulties have, in the past, been attributed to her eyes.

Melanie's visual acuity is 20/30 in each eye. Her contrast sensitivity is slightly reduced. Her plotted visual fields were said to be normal, but only the central visual fields were recorded. She is wearing contact lenses for her myopia. There is scarring at the periphery of the retina of both eyes due to her laser treatment.

INTERVIEWER: What concerns do you have about Melanie's vision?

MOTHER: Where to begin? We have had concerns about Melanie's vision since she was a toddler. She learned to walk when she was 2 years old, which we thought was a bit late. She had weak legs, of course, but there was something else. She walked over her toys as if they were not there. She would walk off the edge of pavements and still does, don't you? *[Mother addresses Melanie, who nods]*

*[The interviewer starts to draw a mind map and thinks: "I need to ask questions about the lower visual field and check whether Melanie can see her feet as she walks. And because lower visual field impairment is commonly associated with dorsal stream dysfunction, as the lower visual field pathway and dorsal stream pathway are close to each other, I'll need to ask my dorsal stream questions as well, then move on to the ventral stream questions."]*

MOTHER: She could never find her toys in her toy box, and always asked me to find them for her.

*[Interviewer thinks: "Yes, impaired visual search of dorsal stream dysfunction."]*

MOTHER: Now she is much older, but she still has similar difficulties. You tell him, Melanie.

MELANIE: I still step off pavements if I'm not careful, and Mom is always telling me off for spreading my clothes over the bed, but if I don't, I can't find them!

*[Interviewer thinks: I'll ask the lower visual field questions first, then the dorsal stream, then the ventral stream questions, and follow up with a few other questions about the current situation.]*

INTERVIEWER: Are there any places where it is difficult to walk? *[Closed, non-leading question to further investigate walking.]*

MELANIE: Yes. I can't walk down steep slopes, and it's really difficult on rough and uneven ground.

INTERVIEWER: Do you ever leave food on the side of the plate nearest to you? *[Closed, leading question]*

MOTHER: *[Interrupts]* She always used to but doesn't do it any more, do you? *[She addresses Melanie]*

MELANIE: No I don't, I've learned to turn the plate around when no one is looking.

INTERVIEWER: Do you watch television in an unusual way?

MOTHER: What do you mean?

INTERVIEWER: Some children lie on the floor or on the sofa in a way that others don't.

MOTHER: Ah yes. You used to lie on your back on the floor and watch the TV upside down, Melanie, and now you have a TV in your bedroom and you do the same thing from your bed.

*[Interviewer thinks: "Yes, that's typical of lower visual field impairment. We'll have to check this out."]*

INTERVIEWER: How did Melanie go down slides when she was little? [*Closed, non-leading question]*

MOTHER: She always lay on her tummy. If you sat her upright at the top of the slide she used to cry and try to climb off.

MELANIE: That was because I felt as if I was sliding down into a cloud of nothingness.

*[Interviewer thinks: "I'll ask about other adaptations."]*

INTERVIEWER: How do you tie your shoelaces?

MELANIE: What do you mean?

INTERVIEWER: Do you lift your foot up?

MOTHER: Yes, she stands at the bottom of the stairs and leans slightly against the wall for balance as she puts her foot on the third step to tie her shoe.

MELANIE: But I have to do it that way, because if I don't, I can't see my foot properly.

INTERVIEWER: What happens if you jump off something like a chair, a bench, or a low wall?

MELANIE: I used to avoid jumping off walls. But my dad was in the army, and he taught me to jump off, and then do a commando roll if I feel I am going to fall over so that I don't hurt myself. It works well.

[*Interviewer thinks: "That's unusual, but a good idea." (The author has heard this description on two occasions.)]*

INTERVIEWER: How about jumping into swimming pools?

MOTHER: Melanie panics when she is standing at the edge of a pool, and will only go down the ladder.

MELANIE: You would freak out too if you didn't know where the edge was and didn't know the height of the water in the pool. Do you remember the time I jumped on top of that little boy?

INTERVIEWER: Does Melanie walk slowly or quickly?

MOTHER: She tends to move quickly.

*[Interviewer thinks: "That's typical of lower visual field impairment too. I'll move on to asking my dorsal stream dysfunction questions."]*

This section of the interview proceeded with the family being given "free rein" to tell their story through the use of closed, nonleading questions as well as judicious use of closed, leading questions to clarify details of behaviors known to be a problem. This part of the interview, which seeks evidence of lower visual field impairment, has helped reveal a range of adaptive behaviors, all of which the author has often heard from other patients. The interviewer needs to be able to visualize common behaviors for the range of possible difficulties, for both younger and older children, and to formulate appropriate questions as the interview unfolds. Families whose experiences are sought in this way become progressively more relaxed during the interview as they realize they have met someone who is taking a sustained personal interest in their child, and they may at last have found someone who understands their child's visual difficulties and adaptive behaviors and can do something to deal with these difficulties.

## Using a Question Inventory to Characterize Visual Difficulties

Figure 11.2 presents an inventory of closed questions that can be used for a wide range of children with CVI, to identify visual processing problems in order to provide specific advice matched to the needs of each child. (A question inventory is a checklist of questions to ask, but unlike a questionnaire, an inventory seeks clarification of salient responses; a questionnaire does not typically allow further information to be sought.) This inventory should be used only after history taking has been carried out, as outlined in this chapter. This is because the questions are leading in nature, and it is essential to ensure that descriptions of any behavioral features typical of CVI have been volunteered first. Significant responses from this inventory are discussed, clarified, and incorporated into the overall descriptive profile of the child that is emerging. A set of history-taking questions for infants with profound visual impairment can be found in Chapter 20.

## Ascertaining the Impact of Visual Difficulties

When a child has a profound visual impairment, its effects are usually well understood by the family, and appropriate actions are usually taken. When visual difficulties are less severe, and the child has adopted strategies to cope with them (see Chapter 7), such difficulties can be easily missed and the child's behaviors attributed instead to specific behavioral disorders. The impact of less severe visual impairment can, therefore, be wide-ranging and profound without it being recognized. The questioning strategy therefore needs to seek information about the following issues:

- The impact of the visual impairment on the child with regard to:
  - Social interactions and relationships
  - The context of education concerning:
    - Near vision tasks (reading and writing)
    - Middle distance tasks (reading music and seeing information conveyed by facial expressions)
    - Distance vision tasks (accessing information from the whiteboard and TV)
- The impact of the visual impairment on the family, when appropriate, with regard to:
  - Social interactions and relationships
  - Work
  - Income

## Determining Previous History

For families of some children, the interview will be their first, and the parents will want explanations for how their child behaves. For

FIGURE 11.2

## Questions to Ask Parents and Caregivers of Children with CVI

This question inventory is designed for children with visual acuities of 20/200 (6/60) or better (Macintyre-Béon, Young, Calvert, et al., 2012; Macintyre-Béon, Young, Dutton, et al., 2013). For children with poorer visual acuities, the question inventory can serve as a useful reminder of difficulties to ask about, but responses to the questions may also relate to ocular causes.

For each of the questions, check the box that best accords with the child's behavior. Children with typical vision tend to have responses of "never" with two or three responses of "rarely," except for questions 37 and 38, for which clarification needs to be sought for positive answers.

| ***Questions seeking evidence of visual field impairment or impaired visual attention on one or both sides*** | ***Never*** | ***Rarely*** | ***Sometimes*** | ***Often*** | ***Always*** | ***N/A*** |
|---|---|---|---|---|---|---|
| **Does your child . . .** | | | | | | |
| 1. trip over toys and obstacles on the floor? | | | | | | |
| 2. have difficulty walking down stairs? | | | | | | |
| 3. trip at the edges of pavements going up? | | | | | | |
| 4. trip at the edges of pavements going down? | | | | | | |
| 5. appear to "get stuck" at the top of a slide or hill? | | | | | | |
| 6. look down when crossing floor boundaries (e.g., where linoleum meets carpet)? | | | | | | |
| 7. leave food on the near or far side of his or her plate? | | | | | | |
| If so, on which side? | near ☐ | | far ☐ | | | |
| 8. leave food on the right or left side of his or her plate? | | | | | | |
| If so, on which side? | right ☐ | | left ☐ | | | |
| 9. have difficulty finding the beginning of a line when reading? | | | | | | |

*(continued on next page)*

**FIGURE 11.2** *(continued from previous page)*

| | | | | | | |
|---|---|---|---|---|---|---|
| 10. have difficulty finding the next word when reading? | | | | | | |
| 11. walk out in front of traffic? | | | | | | |
| If so, which side? | right ☐ | left ☐ | both ☐ | | | |
| 12. bump into doorframes or partly open doors? | | | | | | |
| If so, which side? | right ☐ | left ☐ | both ☐ | | | |
| 13. miss pictures or words on one side of a page? | | | | | | |
| If so, which side? | right ☐ | left ☐ | both ☐ | | | |

| ***Questions seeking evidence of impaired perception of movement*** | ***Never*** | ***Rarely*** | ***Sometimes*** | ***Often*** | ***Always*** | ***N/A*** |
|---|---|---|---|---|---|---|
| **Does your child . . .** | | | | | | |
| 14. have difficulty seeing passing vehicles when he or she is in a moving car? | | | | | | |
| 15. have difficulty seeing things which are moving quickly, such as small animals? | | | | | | |
| 16. avoid watching fast-moving TV? | | | | | | |
| 17. choose to watch slow-moving TV? | | | | | | |
| 18. have difficulty catching a ball? | | | | | | |

| ***Questions seeking evidence of difficulty handling the complexity of a visual scene*** | ***Never*** | ***Rarely*** | ***Sometimes*** | ***Often*** | ***Always*** | ***N/A*** |
|---|---|---|---|---|---|---|
| **Does your child . . .** | | | | | | |
| 19. have difficulty seeing something that is pointed out in the distance? | | | | | | |
| 20. have difficulty finding a close friend or relative who is standing in a group? | | | | | | |
| 21. have difficulty finding an item in a supermarket (e.g., finding the breakfast cereal he or she wants)? | | | | | | |



*(continued on next page)*

**FIGURE 11.2** *(continued from previous page)*

| | | | | | | |
|---|---|---|---|---|---|---|
| 22. get lost in places where there is a lot to see (e.g., a crowded shop)? | | | | | | |
| 23. get lost in places that are well known to him or her? | | | | | | |
| 24. have difficulty locating an item of clothing in a pile of clothes? | | | | | | |
| 25. have difficulty selecting a toy from a toy box? | | | | | | |
| 26. sit closer than about 1 foot (30 cm) from the television? | | | | | | |
| 27. find copying words or drawings time-consuming and difficult? | | | | | | |
| ***Questions seeking evidence of impairment of visually guided movement of the body and further evidence of visual field impairment*** | ***Never*** | ***Rarely*** | ***Sometimes*** | ***Often*** | ***Always*** | ***N/A*** |
| 28. When walking, does your child hold onto your clothes, tugging down? | | | | | | |
| 29. Does your child find uneven ground difficult to walk over? | | | | | | |
| 30. Does your child bump into low furniture such as a coffee table? | | | | | | |
| 31. Is low furniture bumped into if it is moved? | | | | | | |
| 32. Does your child get angry if furniture is moved? | | | | | | |
| 33. Does your child explore floor boundaries (e.g., between linoleum and carpet) with his or her foot before crossing the boundary? | | | | | | |
| 34. Does your child find inside floor boundaries difficult to cross? | | | | | | |
| a. If so, boundaries that are new to him or her? | | | | | | |
| b. Or boundaries that are well known to him or her? | | | | | | |

*(continued on next page)*

**FIGURE 11.2** *(continued from previous page)*

| ***Questions seeking evidence of impairment of visually guided movement of the upper limbs*** | ***Never*** | ***Rarely*** | ***Sometimes*** | ***Often*** | ***Always*** | ***N/A*** |
|---|---|---|---|---|---|---|
| 35. Does your child reach incorrectly for objects, reaching beyond or around the object? | | | | | | |
| 36. When picking up an object, does your child grasp incorrectly, missing or knocking over the object? | | | | | | |
| ***Questions seeking evidence of impaired visual attention*** | ***Never*** | ***Rarely*** | ***Sometimes*** | ***Often*** | ***Always*** | ***N/A*** |
| 37. Does your child find it difficult to keep on task for more than 5 minutes? | | | | | | |
| 38. After being distracted, does your child find it difficult to get back to what he or she was doing? | | | | | | |
| 39. Does your child bump into things when walking and having a conversation? | | | | | | |
| 40. Does your child miss objects that are obvious to you because they are different from their background and seem to "pop out" (e.g., a brightly colored ball against the grass)? | | | | | | |
| ***Questions seeking evidence of behavioral difficulties associated with crowded environments*** | ***Never*** | ***Rarely*** | ***Sometimes*** | ***Often*** | ***Always*** | ***N/A*** |
| 41. Do rooms with a lot of clutter cause difficult behavior? | | | | | | |
| 42. Do quiet places or the open countryside cause difficult behavior? | | | | | | |
| 43. Is behavior more difficult in a busy supermarket or shopping center? | | | | | | |
| 44. Does your child react angrily when other restless children cause a distraction? | | | | | | |

*(continued on next page)*

**FIGURE 11.2** *(continued from previous page)*

| ***Questions evaluating the ability to recognize what is being looked at and to navigate*** | ***Never*** | ***Rarely*** | ***Sometimes*** | ***Often*** | ***Always*** | ***N/A*** |
|---|---|---|---|---|---|---|
| **Does your child . . .** | | | | | | |
| 45. have difficulty recognizing close relatives in real life? | | | | | | |
| 46. have difficulty recognizing close relatives from photographs? | | | | | | |
| 47. mistakenly identify strangers as people known to him or her? | | | | | | |
| 48. have difficulty understanding the meaning of facial expressions? | | | | | | |
| 49. have difficulty naming common colors? | | | | | | |
| 50. have difficulty naming basic shapes such as squares, triangles, and circles? | | | | | | |
| 51. have difficulty recognizing familiar objects such as the family car? | | | | | | |

*Source:* Adapted with permission from Dutton, G. N., Calvert, J., Ibrahim, H., Macdonald, E., McCulloch, D. L., Macintyre-Béon, C., & Spowart K. (2010). Impairment of cognitive vision: Its detection and measurement. In G. N. Dutton & M. Bax (Eds.), *Visual impairment in children due to damage to the brain* (pp. 117–128). London: Mac Keith Press.

others, there may have been a number of previous encounters with a range of professionals who may have given different explanations of the findings, and who may have provided a range of interpretations. Before giving any explanations, or making any plans, it is wise to ask the question, "What have you been told already?" followed by "What do you understand about your child's vision?" The answers to these questions are crucial to knowing how to explain what has been identified and what needs to be done. If an explanation is given that is contrary to the parent's beliefs or previous explanations they've been provided, it has the potential to cause difficulties. If the child had previously attended a different school, it is important to find out as much as possible from the parents about what was done and how they were involved.

## Understanding the Wishes and Agenda of the Child and the Family

In the United States, special education services received by a child are determined through a mandated assessment process and implemented by an educational team that carries out an Individualized Family Service Plan for very young children, an Individualized Educational Program for school-aged children, or an Individual Transition Plan (related to long-term adult outcomes) in later school years. Both the child and the family are part of this team, and the family's wishes need to be reflected in the child's educational program. It is essential that team members work together to determine what the professionals, the child, and the family understand about the child's situation, and what the child's and family's preferences, goals, and expectations may be, so that educational, medical, and related arrangements, planning, as well as the advice and guidance that is given, address the family's and child's expectations and needs.

### Correlating the Information with Features of CVI

The framework and approach described in Chapter 3 allows the interviewer to determine whether the family's account of their experiences is consistent with features of CVI or not. Very rarely is a history inconsistent, but if the expected patterns of visual behavior typical of CVI do not cluster in a consistent way, then alternative explanations for what the family is describing need to be sought. In this author's experience, when taking a history about CVI for the first time, the story given is nearly always consistent with the model described in Chapter 3, and explanations may be found for each element.

### Assembling the History and Drawing Conclusions

The exact pattern of visual behavior for each child is unique, but the model described in Chapter 3 allows a coherent history to be assembled from the behaviors the parents describe and the descriptions provided by the child.

### Documenting the History

Once the interview is complete, it can be helpful to take a break to write down all the key elements.

### Using the Information to Guide Further Assessment

There is a wide range of assessment methods available for the evaluation of vision (see Chapter 12; Corn & Erin, 2010; Lueck, 2004). The knowledge gained from the assessment of basic visual functions and the history can be used to decide what, if any, further tests are required. Tests that would neither add to what is already known nor contribute to future care do not need to be carried out.

## Conclusion

Taking a history about a child with CVI can be very informative. A large amount of salient information can be elicited in a short time. Parents, caregivers, and teachers have observed the behaviors of the children under their care over long periods of time and have a wealth of information available that can be used to understand the characteristics and impact of CVI on the individual child and to design targeted strategies to address identified needs. The knowledge gained from history taking is fundamental to providing optimal educational approaches. Explaining the reasons underlying a child's behaviors to their parents, caregivers, and teachers also gives them a greater understanding of what they can do to change their own behavior to benefit the child.

## References

Corn, A. L., & Erin, J. N. (2010). *Foundations of low vision: Clinical and functional perspectives* (2nd ed.). New York: AFB Press.

Dutton, G. N., Calvert, J., Ibrahim, H., Macdonald, E., McCulloch, D. L., Macintyre-Béon, C., et al. (2010). Impairment of cognitive vision: Its detection and measurement. In G. N. Dutton & M. Bax (Eds.), *Visual impairment in children due to damage to the brain* (pp. 117–128). London: Mac Keith Press.

Emerald Education Systems. (Producer). (n.d.). Dr. Dutton interviews the mother of a child with CVI [Audio recording]. Available at http://www.pplvr.com/news/1948.

Lueck, A. H. (Ed.). (2004). *Functional vision: A practitioner's guide to evaluation and intervention.* New York: AFB Press.

Macintyre-Béon, C., Young, D., Calvert, J., Ibrahim, H., Dutton, G. N., & Bowman, R. (2012). Reliability of a question inventory for structured history taking in children with cerebral visual impairment. *Eye, 26*, 1393.

Macintyre-Béon, C., Young, D., Dutton, G. N., Mitchell, K., Simpson, J., Loffler, G., . . . Hamilton, R. (2013). Cerebral visual dysfunction in prematurely born children attending mainstream school. *Documenta Ophthalmologica, 127*(2), 89–102.

# 12

# Assessment of Visual Function and Functional Vision: Clinical Assessment and Suggested Methods for Educators

*Barry S. Kran and D. Luisa Mayer*

As emphasized in previous chapters, visual difficulties resulting from cerebral visual impairment (CVI) in children range from profound visual impairment to disorders of higher-order visual functions such as visual recognition, visual search, and visual guidance of movement (Colenbrander, 2010). This chapter outlines an approach to evaluating the vision of children with CVI and how they use their vision for various tasks and activities. *Vision* is a broad term, encompassing all that goes into producing an individual's visual world, including central visual acuity, peripheral visual field, higher-order visual processing, and interaction with other senses, as well as previous experience.

Increasing numbers of children with CVI are being referred to pediatric low vision clinics for guidance concerning their low vision care, habilitation, and advocacy for additional services. As discussed in more detail at the end of this chapter, appropriate assessment can lead to interventions that address a child's needs from birth throughout his or her school years, and beyond.

The procedures for assessing vision presented in this chapter are based on the practices of the New England Eye Low Vision Clinic at the Perkins School for the Blind. The clinic's clientele are mainly from New England, with one-third also attending the school. They range in age from birth to 22 years, with the majority over 5 years of age. Referrals come from pediatric ophthalmologists, teachers of students with visual impairments, and parents, and often include cases with suspected, but as yet undiagnosed, visual disabilities. Whether they have been diagnosed or not, all children who come to the clinic are assessed in order to characterize their visual abilities. This, in turn, provides guidance for the development of appropriate habilitation strategies by school staff and families.

The clinical assessment team at the Perkins New England Eye Low Vision Clinic comprises an orientation and mobility (O&M) specialist, a vision scientist, and an optometrist. All members of this team specialize in low vision and work closely together. This team approach has significantly enhanced patient care, and while this professional grouping may be relatively unique, it can be adapted by clinical practitioners, educators, and therapists to align with local resources and needs (Kran & Wright, 2008). Working independently, neither educators nor clinicians can address all of the needs of children with CVI, but shared reporting and good communication among all involved will help bring out an individual's full potential.

This chapter discusses the types and range of visual impairments that may accompany CVI, as well as the child-centered assessment process that can effectively address children's needs. The process comprises pre-assessment (discussed in detail later in this chapter), observation, optical and eye examination, assessment of visual functions and functional vision, and resulting recommendations.

Tests of central vision are considered in this chapter before tests of peripheral vision or visual field. In general, the testing that is least intrusive to the child is carried out first. However, the sequence of testing in an actual examination session may well differ. For example, initial assessment of the visual field can help guide how best to evaluate central vision. If lack of attention to the right side is observed in a child then it may be best to carry out central visual function assessment from the child's left side.

## Categories of Visual Impairment

The anatomical classification of the visual system employed by vision professionals comprises the following:

- Ocular visual impairment (OVI) (involving the eye, optic nerve, and optic chiasm)
- Cerebral visual impairment (CVI) (involving damage or disorder of the visual pathways behind the optic chiasm)
- Visual difficulties related to ocular-motor dysfunction (visual fixation or tracking problems, ocular misalignment, and impairment of accommodation)

It is not uncommon for children with CVI to have elements of all three (Colenbrander, 2010; Huo, Burden, Hoyt, & Good, 1999).

## Visual Function and Functional Vision

Thorough assessment of vision involves estimation of both visual function and functional vision. Measuring *visual function* involves quantitative measurement of the limits of vision for each eye, where thresholds of visual acuity, contrast sensitivity, and visual field are determined in a clinical setting (Colenbrander, 2010; see Chapter 1). In such cases, visual stimuli that become progressively less visible are shown until the limit at which they can only just be seen is measured. This limit, or threshold, such as the lowest line of letters that can be read on an acuity chart or the lowest level of dark-light contrast between a letter and its background, is the measure of visual function. *Functional vision* refers to real-life evaluation of visual functions, with both eyes open, within the performance of tasks, activities, or skills, and often involves qualitative judgment of how vision is used and the limits it imposes on daily living. Parents, teachers, and caregivers, as well as clinicians can all report on a child's functional vision.

Both measures of visual function and assessments of functional vision help professionals understand how a child with CVI sees. The eye care provider uses this information clinically to support diagnosis and to contribute information that can be used to optimize the plan for a child's education and care at home. Since many eye care providers do not assess both visual function and functional vision, teachers of students with visual impairments, O&M specialists, and other professionals trained to assess functional vision can provide important observations and supporting documentation to the family and the rest of the educational team, as well as to the low vision specialist.

The following case study shows how insufficient information on both visual function and functional vision can lead to limited understanding of the child's behaviors and inadequate service delivery.

**A 5½-YEAR-OLD BOY, MIKHAIL, WAS SEEN IN THE CLINIC** for a third opinion. Two other eye care clinics had given different opinions. One had identified profound visual impairment, while the other found that he did not meet the criteria for legal blindness.

Mikhail had been born prematurely. Diagnostic head scans had shown clefts with brain tissue lacking in both cerebral hemispheres (schizencephaly). He had developmental delays, hearing impairment in both ears, seizure disorder, and cerebral palsy, but was mobile. He tended to bump into objects (with or without wearing eyeglasses) and to panic in crowded or unfamiliar places, such as the playground or grocery store. Mikhail was nearsighted (short-sighted or myopic) with astigmatism. He had horizontal nystagmus, and strabismus. He received numerous services including those of a teacher of students with visual impairments.

Mikhail had difficulty finding the examiner's hand for a handshake and used touch rather than vision to do so. He walked with assistance. He was very cautious and used his free hand to explore ahead and to explore his surroundings, which he investigated with both hand and mouth.

Mikhail's motor impairments did not explain his behavior. He had difficulty reaching accurately for salient objects and looked away as he did so. His unaided grating acuity (discussed later in this chapter) with both eyes open, obtained three months after the last measure, was 20/94, below normal for his age (Johnson, Kran, Deng, & Mayer, 2009). He had constricted visual fields, but not sufficiently so to explain his behavior. It was clear, after a detailed assessment, that he had significant CVI with impaired acuities and visual fields. His motor behavior was consistent with impaired visual guidance of movement or optic ataxia, and his distress in crowded places was suggestive of difficulties resulting from visual crowding, both consistent with dorsal stream dysfunction, a previously unsuspected diagnosis. Considerable time was needed to explain the different opinions, and to present new approaches to his management.

## Clinical Examination and Functional Vision Assessment

This section reviews the stages of a clinical low vision examination, which includes assessment of both visual function and functional vision. It is important for education professionals to understand how findings from a clinical examination have been determined and how to interpret these findings in order to implement effective functional vision assessments for educational purposes. Suggested methods for educational professionals to conduct functional vision assessments of the various visual functions discussed have also been included.

A clinical low vision examination follows a general eye examination, in which diagnosis, measures of basic visual function, and medical and optometric recommendations are determined. The information from a clinical low vision examination expands on that information in order to provide guidance for habilitation by school staff and families. (For more information about the content of general eye exams, clinical low vision evaluations, and educational functional vision assessments, see Corn & Erin, 2010; Lueck, 2004.)

## Pre-Assessment

Before seeing the child, the available information is reviewed to determine:

- The circumstances that led to visual and other possible impairments
- Any medical, educational, and other interventions and how effective they have been
- History-taking issues to address (see Chapter 11)
- The choice of environment in the exam room and the best approach for the child
- The initial selection of assessment methods and their sequence
- Whether the known visual impairments explain the difficulties described
- Issues to consider and assess that could enhance quality of life and education

The following case study illustrates the incorporation of these considerations when planning the assessment.

**Teresa, a 2½-year-old girl who was born at 28** weeks gestation, is under treatment for epilepsy. She receives therapy for low muscle tone and global developmental and speech delays. Periventricular white matter pathology is evident on a brain MRI. She had previously undergone laser treatment on both eyes for retinopathy of prematurity (ROP). She has low visual acuities, with a variable convergent strabismus (eye turn). Her ophthalmologist has attributed her low vision to her ROP. She is not registered with the state blindness agency, and was referred to the low vision clinic by her teacher of students with visual impairments to seek advice on preschool vision services.

Teresa was not tolerating her spectacle correction for high myopia and patching for right amblyopia. Her visual attention, even with eyeglasses, is described as fleeting and variable. She pays attention when there are a few familiar surrounding objects, but she becomes inattentive with too many surrounding objects or with background noise. She looks away from a toy when reaching to grasp it. Teresa is beginning to make intermittent eye contact when spoken to.

These features lead to the suspicion of dual ocular and cerebral visual disabilities commonly seen in prematurely born children (Dutton, 2013). A goal of the current clinical low vision evaluation is to find out if the behaviors described relate to the retinal findings, to CVI, or to both. Teresa's seizures and overall developmental delay indicate possible CVI and impaired attention related to her developmental status.

The approach will be to ensure a simplified environment for examination, with conversation kept to a minimum during assessment. The impact of visual crowding and auditory distraction on Teresa's use of vision will be explored. Her visual functions and functional vision will be assessed. Postural instability can impair visual attention, and this will be explored. For example, will her use of vision be more engaged when she is supine (lying on her back)? Her interaction and attention with familiar versus novel objects, as well as her coordination of vision during reaching and playing, will be evaluated. Her spectacles and their fit will be checked, and her refraction and focusing (accommodation) will be tested. Would an undercorrection of her distance spectacles be better tolerated (helped by thinner, lighter lenses), and would this improve her near and intermediate visual attention?

Visual behaviors suggestive of CVI to look out for include poor visual searching and scanning; poor visually guided movements of hands and arms; lack of visual attention for faces, objects, complex pictures, or scenes; and impaired recognition of objects and pictures. Careful history taking will elicit information about recognition of familiar people and places, the ability to find a parent in a group, visual guidance of movement of the limbs through surrounding space, and distress in crowded places. The structured history-taking inventory described in Chapter 11 will be applied, with recognition of its limitations at this child's young age.

Vision impairment secondary to ROP can range from a minimal to a profound visual acuity deficit. This child's expressive language difficulties suggest that tests that do not require language or reading skills such as preferential looking grating cards or Cardiff cards will be needed initially; icon-based tests such as LEA Symbols or the Patti Pics [discussed later in this chapter] will be used, presented singly with matching or naming responses, depending on Teresa's cognitive level and communication abilities. Visual acuities with both eyes open will be tested first, before trying to cover each eye for monocular testing. If Teresa is found to have very poor visual acuity, light gazing, or visual inattentiveness, these behaviors could be related to ROP, CVI, or both.

Visual field assessment will seek evidence of constriction (associated with Teresa's prior ROP laser treatment), lower visual field impairment (associated with periventricular white matter pathology), and evidence of visual neglect (for further discussion of this topic, see the section later in this chapter and Chapter 3). An eye movement examination will focus on the ability to look from one target to another and the pattern, quality, and maintenance of the fixation and looking.

The outcome of the assessment will be communicated in clear, easy-to-understand language, verbally and in writing.

## Approach to Assessing the Child

Suggestions provided in the sections that follow outline practices developed in a clinical setting, but many elements of this approach can be readily incorporated into educational settings as well.

### *Preparing the Assessment Environment*

In order to obtain as much information as possible, the child needs to be treated as a unique individual; staff members need to become acquainted with each child, his or her health, education, and family situation, and any indicators of ocular and cerebral visual impairment. In a sense, the clinic is a proxy for a home, with the doctor being the host. The examiner's job is to make sure that the guest (the child) has his or her needs met. If the examiner is an attentive "host" then the data collection and visit should be successful. If the examiner is not attentive to the needs of the child, or is too rigid in approach, then it will be frustrating for everyone. No child with CVI is "typical," so a predetermined or standard approach cannot be applied. Being a good host involves setting aside enough time (typically an hour) to ensure the child's comfort as well as sufficient data collection. Appropriate attire should be worn—no ties, large earrings, loose long hair, or necklaces that can be pulled or grasped by the child. Constant observation, inviting input from those accompanying the patient, and monitoring feedback from the patient all aid in directing the course and approach to the examination.

A range of toys that appeal to the visual, auditory, and tactile senses and multisensory combinations are used to engage the child and to assess visual and visual-motor responses, as well as the impact of auditory or tactile stimulation on visual responses. For children who respond to visual materials displayed at a distance, having a computer-based acuity system with speakers and an Internet connection allows the assessors to use cartoons, games, or music to encourage distance fixation. (They can also be used for breaks during testing.) However, for some children, video or auditory stimuli can be distracting or can cause agitation, so obtaining information from parents and teachers accompanying the child will be important.

Busy backgrounds and cluttered environments such as wall posters and a jumble of objects that may distract or agitate a child need to be minimized with the use of white walls and storage cabinets with low contrast knobs. Overhead lighting and adjustable spotlights can fine-tune illumination in the room and control the amount of visual clutter.

### *Greeting the Child, Taking a History, and Observing During Assessment*

The child should be greeted warmly and made to feel important. Hypotheses gained from reviewing letters and reports are put to the test by closely observing the child's behavior throughout the visit. For example, does the child make eye contact when first introduced? If so, at what distance? Is he or she sitting in a stroller with eyes closed, hand in mouth, but listening, as evidenced by sometimes opening the eyes and turning to a familiar voice? How does the child interact with caregivers? Does the child engage with the surroundings and watch as people pass by? Does the examiner need to get close before the child is aware of the examiner's presence?

Some children startle when they hear new voices or sounds. Others are wary in new environments. Care is needed in the directness of one's approach. Does the child see a hand extended for a handshake? If both hands can be used, is the correct one extended? Does an independently mobile child hesitate on entering the room? If so, is this related to vision, motor issues, wariness, shyness, or a combination of issues? As the child enters the room (independently or escorted), does the child look around? What items, of what size, and at what distance attract attention? As the child sits down and becomes comfortable, does visual attention improve? Is eye contact made after the child settles down? Is there a head turn while looking at the examiner, perhaps to minimize nystagmus? Is there a variable or constant eye turn?

The caregiver's concerns are sought, salient medical and educational information is garnered, and examination commences. A team of examiners can "divide and conquer," with one quietly taking the history, while others measure the child's vision as they play and interact with him or her. In other settings, clinical data can be collected first, while the child is still engaged and cooperative, and the history can be elicited during a later break to select and prioritize further tests.

## Observing for Features of CVI

Using open questioning, information is obtained from those accompanying the child about the child's visually guided movements, ability to search, and recognition of familiar people and places. In the authors' experience, formalized CVI surveys using inventories are not commonly used in medical settings in North America. Reasons for this include the lack of large-scale validation studies of such instruments and lack of time to administer and integrate results with other information, such as the neuropsychological assessment of higher-order functions, cognitive abilities, and learning disabilities, as well as occupational therapy reports. (See Chapter 13 for discussion of neuropsychological assessment.) In North America, vision educators tend to use the Roman-Lantzy (2007) CVI Range survey for very young children and those who are clearly developmentally impaired with profound visual impairment.

For developmentally impaired children with profound visual impairment, evidence of basic CVI-associated behaviors is sought from family members or caregivers. These behaviors include light gazing or aversion, avoidance of new faces or novel toys, difficulty attending visually when there is sound, difficulty looking while reaching and touching, greater attention to attractive stimuli such as reflective materials than to ordinary toys and visual materials, or greater attention to moving rather than static objects (Roman-Lantzy, 2007). These functional visual responses can also be observed and documented by personnel familiar with these techniques on the clinical assessment team or within the child's education program.

The inventory presented in Chapter 11 (Dutton et al., 2010; Macintyre-Béon et al., 2012) is designed for use with children whose acuity and function are indicative of perceptual visual impairment.

## Measuring and Interpreting Visual Functions

The following sections describe the various tests used during an evaluation of visual functions and functional vision. Most tests of visual functions are performed under standardized conditions. Vision educators, including teachers of students with visual impairments and orientation and mobility specialists, as well as other vision professionals, may use some of the vision tests described with adequate training. However, if standardized tests such as those for visual acuity are performed in a different environment (such as in a school by the vision educator), the results may not be consistent with the formal tests conducted by an eye care specialist. For this reason, some eye and vision professionals feel that the actual size of test objects (such as icons or letters), and the test distance should be reported on functional vision assessments, rather than the visual acuity notation. (However, see discussion of assessment of functional near reading acuity and Sidebar 12.1 later in this chapter.) With any test, the conditions of the test (such as lighting; the child's comfort in the testing situation; use of the testing task; and extra assistance, such as more time to respond or pointing letter by letter, or letting the child respond by pointing rather than verbally) and whether the child is wearing eyeglasses should be reported. With regard to tests of eye movements and eye alignment as well as external ocular health assessment, it is most appropriate for vision educators and others in the community to report and functionally interpret their observations rather than make a diagnosis. Table 12.1 summarizes the types of assessments, including the visual functions assessed in an eye examination, low vision assessment, and functional vision evaluation.

The tests and procedures discussed in this chapter are those that are most valuable when assessing individuals with visual impairments and other disabilities. Careful, accurate assessment of visual functions (such as acuity, contrast sensitivity, and visual field) is essential for optimal diagnosis and management of visual disorders. All assessments of vision are carried out with the child wearing the appropriate spectacle correction whenever possible. Measurement is done as reliably as possible using methods that match the age, developmental level, cognitive abilities, motor skills, attention levels, positioning requirements, and the temperament of the child. Tests that encroach least upon the child's space and need the least cooperation are done first to gain confidence and trust.

The visual functions of each eye are measured separately because one eye may be

TABLE 12.1

## Common Assessment Activities in Different Types of Vision Evaluations

| | *The Eye* | | *Visual Functions* | | |
|---|---|---|---|---|---|
| | **Ocular Health** | **Refractive Error** | **Visual Acuities** | **Visual Field** | **Contrast Sensitivity** |
| **Basic Eye Examination** | Usually | Usually | Usually | Usually | Sometimes |
| **Low Vision Examination** | Only if indicated for eye health check or to check for recent vision change | Often modified techniques; alternative instrumentation | Often modified techniques; alternative instrumentation | Often modified techniques; alternative instrumentation | Often modified techniques; alternative instrumentation |
| **Functional Vision Evaluation** | | | Observation of behavior during replication of tests done within basic or low vision examination | Observation of behavior during replication of tests done within basic or low vision examination | Observation of behavior during replication of tests done within basic or low vision examination |

[a]Response to light: (a) variation of visual function at different lighting levels; (b) glare discomfort; (c) glare disability (or veiling glare)—an adverse consequence of extraneous light within the visual environment; (d) light adaptation: the gradual change in the ability to see when going from one light level to another.

*Source:* Reprinted from Lueck, A. H. (2004). Comprehensive low vision care. In A. H. Lueck (Ed.), *Functional vision: A practitioner's guide to evaluation and intervention* (p. 12). New York: AFB Press.

more severely affected by refractive error, eye disorder, or eye movement difficulties. Knowledge of the visual functions of each eye can help explain visual behaviors in children with asymmetrical eye disorders or impaired eye movements. For example, a child with an eye turn (strabismus) may have lower visual acuity resulting from an abnormal optic nerve, or a high refractive error in the eye that turns. In these cases, the eye turns because it does not see well. Without this information, it might be assumed that the child's eye turn is a result of an eye movement disorder only (see Chapter 8). Head and eye postures in such children need to be interpreted in relation to the visual function of each eye. For children with measurable and useful vision in only one eye, the implications for daily life skills (mobility, reading, orientation, and viewing at distance) need to be conveyed to vision service providers and parents.

In contrast, functional vision is assessed with both eyes viewing to understand the child's use of vision in everyday activities. This information is used to optimize the child's experiences in the home, school, and community by ensuring optimal visibility of all elements that the child interacts with. Observations of functional vision can be done

| *Visual Functions* | | | | *Functional Vision* |
|---|---|---|---|---|
| **Response to Light**[a] | **Color Vision** | **Oculo-Motor Function** | **Accommodation** | **Use of Vision in Functional Tasks** |
| Sometimes | Sometimes | Usually | Usually | Infrequently |
| Special procedures | Often modified techniques; alternative instrumentation | Usually | Often modified techniques | Frequently |
| Observation of changes in behavior and performance in different lighting conditions | Observation of behavior during replication of tests done within basic or low vision examination | | | Observation of behavior and performance while completing various functional tasks |

during the clinical low vision assessment and in educational and home settings by qualified personnel. These observations are discussed later in this chapter and throughout the assessment portion of this book.

## Assessment of Visual Functions

The following sections discuss visual testing in children with CVI, focusing on three specific visual functions: visual acuity, contrast sensitivity, and visual fields. Table 12.2 summarizes the tests that are used to measure these visual functions for a range of ages and developmental levels. Many of the methods discussed can be applied by qualified education personnel as they conduct functional vision assessments.

### Visual Acuity

Visual acuity refers to the ability of an individual to see, or resolve, fine detail. Technically speaking, it is measured by the ability to distinguish each component of the black-and-white parts of an image as being separate from one another. More specifically, it is the measure of the thinnest black lines and white gaps, presented as letters, images, or

TABLE 12.2

## Tests of Visual Functions, Indications, and Functional Concerns

| *Visual Function* | *Tests and Stimuli* | *Indications, Requirements, Comments* | *Functional Concerns* |
|---|---|---|---|
| **Visual Acuity** | **Test Types (printed or digital)** | | |
| Visual acuity measures detail vision in all types of visual impairments.<br>Monocular visual acuity is used to diagnose and manage ocular and oculomotor disorders. Binocular visual acuity provides information on *functional* visual acuity. | **Recognition Acuity Tests**<br>**A. Chart** (entire range of acuity levels) Multiple lines of five optotypes (letters, numbers, symbols) 20/200 to 20/20 (6/60 to 6/6 - typical) | A. Chart best for functional visual acuity; requires good fixation and scanning (but one can isolate a line); EDTRS is standard chart format - 0.1 logMAR difference in optotype size between levels. | Compare full chart with line or isolated optotype to elicit behaviors showing difficulties with crowding and complexity, for example, decreased ability to sustain performance along with possible lethargy and lack of physical tone.<br>Note unusual head-eye positions (as a result of nystagmus, strabismus, monocular acuity deficit, or other oculomotor causes). |
| | **B. "Crowded" isolated optotypes** with surrounding bars/box | B. "Crowding" with surrounding bars provides equal or slightly lower visual acuity as the line acuity; good scanning is not required but good fixation is. | |
| | **C. Isolated optotypes** | C. Isolated optotypes are best for 2- to 4-year-olds, and for those with attention and visual crowding problems. | |
| | **Test Stimuli** | | |
| | **Optotypes** | *Choice depends on cognitive abilities:* | |
| | **A. Letters**—Sloan, Bailey-Lovie, HOTV, Keeler LogMAR Crowded Test | A. Child must know the alphabet; naming or matching response must be possible. HOTV is easiest but overestimates letter acuity. | |
| | **B. "E" (game) or Landolt C** | B. Tests require orientation discrimination (the opening of E, or gap in C) and directional response (pointing) or matching. Good for non-readers, and those from other cultures or who speak different languages. | |
| | **C. Symbol pictures** (LEA, Patti Pics) | C. Naming, signing, or matching; generally successful with cognitively normal 2- to 3-year-olds and multiply impaired children; however, shapes may not be equally discriminable. | |
| | **D. Object pictures** (Kay Pictures, Lighthouse, Allen Pictures) | D. Images may not be equally discriminated; Kay Pictures have age norms for age 3–4 years and good test reliability. | |

*(continued on next page)*

**TABLE 12.2** *(continued from previous page)*

| *Visual Function* | *Tests and Stimuli* | *Indications, Requirements, Comments* | *Functional Concerns* |
|---|---|---|---|
| | **Reading Acuity** | | |
| | Words or sentences in lines on chart; tested at near | Child must know alphabet; threshold acuity is the line above the line where reading is slowed or labored.<br>No tests are available for the early reader; young children can point to letters in words on first- to third-grade-level reading test. | *Functional* reading is assessed binocularly.<br>Note difficulties during testing.<br>Recommend 2–5 times larger print than threshold acuity level for reading. |
| | **Preferential Looking Acuity** | | |
| | **A. Acuity cards**—preferential looking methods<br>1. Teller Acuity Cards, Keeler Acuity Cards—large grating patch on right or left on wide rectangular cards; cards have central viewing hole; acuity is the finest grating examiner judges the child can see.<br>2. Cardiff Acuity Test—the target images consist of dark and light lines outlining the pictures on the upper or lower half of a gray card; line thickness is the measure of acuity. Picture disappears when the limit of acuity is reached.<br>3. Pacific Acuity Test—test stimuli are two ovals, one a schematic face and the other a non-face, composed of dark and light lines as in Cardiff, on the upper or lower half of gray cards. Recognition acuity (preference for face vs. non-face) is testable in children older than 18 months, while only resolution acuity (either or both stimuli detected) is successful at younger ages (Lowery et al., 2014). | *For individuals who cannot be tested with recognition acuity tests:*<br>A.1. Teller and Keeler Acuity Card tests measure visual acuity over wide range (Teller 20/11 [57 cpd] to 20/4700 [0.13cpd]). Therefore, these tests can assess a range of visual impairment ages and diverse disorders. Horizontal or vertical card positions provide flexibility for testing ocular motor disorders and field defects.<br>A.2. Cardiff tests only to 20/640 (1.0 cpd), thus limited in very low vision; useful with toddlers and children who are interested in pictures; naming picture may represent recognition acuity.<br>• Inflexible card position because of orientation of picture.<br>• Less useful in children with CVI with low acuity than large-grating tests, perhaps as a result of sparse elements.<br>A.3. Whether the Pacific Acuity Test will have advantages for clinical testing of acuity in children with visual impairments remains to be determined. | Grating acuity is tested at near (38-55 cm); therefore, visual acuity deficit resulting from myopia may not be detected.<br>Child may have reduced attention for intermediate and far distances than grating acuity suggests.<br>The time to test and whether and how much the environment needs to be altered is important for therapeutic intervention.<br>Grating acuities may overestimate recognition acuity, and should not be used for legal purposes. |

*(continued on next page)*

**TABLE 12.2** *(continued from previous page)*

| *Visual Function* | *Tests and Stimuli* | *Indications, Requirements, Comments* | *Functional Concerns* |
|---|---|---|---|
| | **B.** LEA Paddles<br>1. Large gratings and matching gray on paddles; acuity is taken as finest grating child prefers over gray. | B.1. Measures acuity in narrow range of widths, in large steps.<br>Potential for examiner bias because of examiner's knowledge of location of grating during testing.<br>Potential distractions by surroundings and examiner's face. | |
| **Contrast Sensitivity (CS)** | **Stimuli & Test Formats** | | |
| Contrast sensitivity measures the ability to see objects that have low contrast with background.<br>Contrast sensitivity is used to monitor ocular disorders (e.g., macular lesions, cataracts) and to assess reduced vision not shown or under-estimated by visual acuity.<br>It provides a guide to ensuring optimum visibility of educational material. | **A. Optotypes (letter or symbol)**<br>1. Large, same size Sloan letters of varying contrast on chart (Pelli-Robson and Mars tests). | A.1. Measures contrast sensitivity for low spatial frequency letters. | Poor contrast sensitivity impairs visually guided mobility, face recognition, reading, and activities of daily living.<br>Contrast sensitivity may be more reduced than predicted by visual acuity. |
| | 2. Letter size varies with contrast level on separate charts (e.g., Bailey-Lovie, Rabin). | A.2. Measures letter acuity for different low contrasts. | |
| | 3. Sloan letter acuity; high contrast and low (10%) contrast on same chart (Colenbrander Mixed Contrast Test). | A.3. Measures high contrast letter acuity and 10% contrast letter acuity with same chart; good for quick check of high and low contrast visual acuity. | |
| | 4. Card test booklets—same size, large letters or symbols in a line surrounded by a box, different contrast on each card (Sloan letters, Patti Pics, LEA Symbols). | A.4. Measures contrast sensitivity for letters or symbols; large interval between contrasts, easy to test; lowest contrasts too high for assessing mild to moderate contrast sensitivity deficits. | |
| | **B. Gratings**<br>1. Spatial frequency and contrast of small circular gratings that vary on the same chart (e.g., FACT); grating orientation is discriminated. | B.1. Measures grating contrast sensitivity for a range of spatial frequencies; requires discrimination of 3 grating orientations. | |
| | 2. Large field grating paired with gray, contrast varies across pages; gratings are detected vs. gray (Cambridge Low Contrast Gratings). | B.2. Measures contrast sensitivity for one low spatial frequency grating; simple responses: point to grating or observe looking; the highest contrast is low for severe CVI. | |

*(continued on next page)*

**TABLE 12.2** *(continued from previous page)*

| *Visual Function* | *Tests and Stimuli* | *Indications, Requirements, Comments* | *Functional Concerns* |
|---|---|---|---|
| | **C. Edges**<br>1. Circular areas bisected by contrast differences (edges); four orientations of edges are discriminated (Melbourne Edge Test).<br><br>2. Schematic Faces—large image on paddles or sheets varying in contrast; detection of lowest contrast face (Hiding Heidi, Peek-A-Boo Patti). | C.1. Measures contrast sensitivity for very low spatial frequency stimulus; orientation discrimination required.<br><br>C.2. Easy and fast to use; examiner bias and distractability are problems as with grating paddle tests; contrast intervals are large; 1- to 2-year-olds see lowest contrast. | |
| **Visual Field** | **Perimeters, Stimuli, and Methods** | | |
| Visual field, peripheral or side vision, is measured to monitor and treat retinal and optic nerve disorders and cerebral damage. Binocular visual field provides information on functional visual field. | **A. Hemispheric perimeters**—clinical standard; light spot projected on inner surface.<br><br>**B. Automated static perimetry**—spot brightness is varied to measure light sensitivity in different areas of visual field; brief light stimuli.<br><br>**C. Kinetic perimetry (e.g., Goldmann)**—spot is moved by examiner from non-seeing to seeing; spot size and brightness variations provide visual fields of different size.<br><br>**D. Double-arc perimeter**<br>1. White sphere kinetic perimetry—white sphere on thin wand moved by examiner along one of four arcs. | A. Measures field quantitatively; patient's response: beep when detect light.<br><br>B. Efficient test strategies; specific stimuli to test different ocular disorders; requires good central fixation, vigilant attention, and good motor reaction time.<br><br>C. Kinetic test requires less strict control over fixation than static test; examiner can vary the stimulus and rate of kinetic scan for young or less attentive children; examiner can monitor orienting response to peripheral light.<br><br>D.1. Measures field extents in four quadrants; observer monitors child's orienting response; large-scale age norms; studies of pediatric clinical conditions at risk of field disorders, including CVI (Quinn et al., 1996; Quinn et al., 2011; Scher, Dobson, Carpenter, & Guthrie, 1989; Van Hof-van Duin et al., 1998). | CVI is often associated with lower field defects, hemianopia (right or left), and general constriction of visual fields. |

*(continued on next page)*

**TABLE 12.2** *(continued from previous page)*

| *Visual Function* | *Tests and Stimuli* | *Indications, Requirements, Comments* | *Functional Concerns* |
|---|---|---|---|
| | **E. Hemispheric perimeters–** experimental | | |
| | 1. LEDs embedded in inner surface, flickering, in fixed positions (Mayer, Fulton, & Cummings, 1988). | E.1. Examiner monitors child's central fixation and orienting to peripheral LEDs by video camera; limited age norms; clinical test to screen major field defects. | |
| | 2. Projected light spot, kinetic scan (Werth & Schadler, 2006). | E.2. Two observers independently judge child's orienting; norms and clinical cases. | |
| | **F. Confrontation testing**–various peripheral stimuli and central fixation targets; optimal testing with small toy for fixation and toy or light on long wand. | F. To detect major field defects–dense and complete or partial and constriction; not quantitative.<br>• Most useful for young and multiply impaired children when formal perimetry cannot be used.<br>• Strategies for CVI–test in four quadrants and careful testing of inferior field; if vision is low, use flickering light stimulus in darkened room. | |

gratings that can be seen by the individual as separate (discriminated) under correct lighting conditions (standards for which vary internationally; see Visual Functions Committee, 1984, for details). Visual acuity is calculated from the smallest optotype (or line of optotypes, the standard symbols for testing vision) that the individual can read at a specified distance. This is equivalent to the resolution *threshold* for image detail.

Visual acuity is commonly recognized by professionals as the single most useful visual function test and is measured early in the examination of a child, starting first with both eyes open to ensure the most reliable results. Visual acuity can be impaired by disorders in any part of the visual pathway.

The choice of test is dictated by the child's age and developmental level (see Table 12.2.). Clinically, the most complex level of visual acuity testing is known as *recognition acuity,* but when the child is not able to identify a letter, number, or symbol by naming, pointing, matching, or other means, then grating acuity (ability to distinguish patterns of alternating black and white lines) is tested, as described later.

### Recognition Acuity

Letters and symbols used to test visual acuity are called *optotypes.* This term refers to the fact that not only must the child see the parts of the letter or symbol as separate to "discriminate" the image, he or she must also recognize it to be able to report that he or she has seen it.

Letter acuity—that is, recognition of letters—is the clinical standard for measuring visual acuity, and is the most widely used test. Young, nonreading and nonverbal patients can be tested using symbols. The most widely used in the United States are Patti Pics and LEA Symbols. Picture drawings, such as Kay Pictures, are more commonly used in the UK and have age norms for young children. (See the Resources section at the end of this chapter for more information.) Although these tests are very useful for measuring acuity in young patients, there may be differences in the discriminability of symbols and pictures in a given test (Charman, 2006) that can affect test reliability. Testing visual acuity with symbols can be done at 2½ to 3 years of age in typical children and in children with developmental delays of a similar mental age. Young children can respond by naming, signing, or matching the test optotypes to those on a sample card.

Various formats of optotypes are used to test recognition acuity. These include a complete letter chart with lines of progressively smaller size (such as the well-known Snellen chart), a single line of letters presented at a time, a line of letters surrounded by a box, or an isolated optotype (letter or symbol) with or without crowding bars—that is, isolating the optotype by placing a bar on four sides.

A complete letter chart is easily read down to the acuity level by older children who read fluently. The standard used today is the ETDRS chart (so-called because it was originally developed as part of the Early Treatment for Diabetic Retinopathy Study). Younger and visually impaired children may need a single line of optotypes or an isolated optotype to be tested successfully (see Table 12.2 for some examples). The crowding—or the inability to recognize objects in the presence of other nearby objects—produced by presentation of an entire chart full of letters or even a single line of letters may reduce visual acuity in an eye with amblyopia or "lazy eye." This may also be seen in the child with simultanagnostic dysfunction caused by dorsal stream dysfunction (see Chapter 3). Disordered visual scanning resulting from apraxia of gaze or abnormal eye movements may also cause reduced visual acuity for crowded optotypes.

Computer-based visual acuity testing systems provide flexibility of choice in optotypes, test formats, and test procedures, but these are primarily for testing distance acuity. Near vision reading acuity charts are needed to test reading of whole words and sentences, and to assess functional visual acuity for reading, as discussed in the next section.

Observations of the following should be made during recognition acuity testing:

- ***Reading from left to right*** (or right to left in some scripts, and vertically down in others) is a learned skill that needs to be taught. The younger child may not start from the correct side, as they may not have learned that skill yet. Missing optotypes on the right can result from a right-sided visual field defect, and those missed on the left from a left field defect. For children who read in a language from left to right, reading performance can be severely affected by a right-sided visual field defect, especially if it is acquired; the same is true for children who read from right to left and have a left-sided visual field defect. (See the Visual Field section later in this chapter.)

- ***Lack of ability to read the letters in the middle of a line*** (unless these letters are pointed out) may indicate amblyopia (usually for one eye). When both eyes are equally affected, the cause may be the simultanagnostic vision of dorsal stream dysfunction (see Chapter 3).
- ***Low lighting conditions*** may impair visual acuity, especially in children with cataracts and disorders of the retina or optic nerve. If a child appears not to see well in dim lighting, visual acuity needs to be measured in standard as well as dim lighting.
- ***Discomfort in normal room lighting*** requires testing with some reduction in background illumination, while the vision of children with profound CVI should be re-evaluated under dim lighting, as it may be better than in normal lighting (Good & Hou, 2006).
- ***An unusual head and eye position*** may be seen during acuity testing. This may be the position used by a child to minimize "camera shake" of his or her visual image resulting from involuntary to-and-fro eye movements (nystagmus) in order to improve vision. (See the discussion on nystagmus later in this chapter.) The child who lacks central vision in both eyes may shift the eyes and head to the position that gives best clarity of vision, by looking slightly to the side of the optotypes on the chart.

### Testing Recognition Visual Acuity at Near

Near visual acuity is tested for different purposes. In a clinical examination, near acuity is tested for each eye separately in order to gain information about the child's visual status and eye health, as well as to assess the effect of optical correction on near vision. Information regarding the child's functional near vision is measured with both eyes open. Near acuity tests usually measure recognition acuity using optotypes as the visual target. The smallest line of optotypes or single optotype that the child can read at a standard distance measures the child's near visual acuity.

However, people do not read or do other close work for extended periods of time using the smallest optotypes they can see. For example, if all the print in a textbook were the size of footnotes, students would not be able to read for prolonged periods. People typically read and work with material above their visual acuity threshold. This can be measured using a functional near visual acuity assessment that determines the best size of optotypes for near tasks at a given distance (that is, how large these must be above threshold visual acuity), using both eyes for comfortable viewing. Functional visual reading acuity is defined by the font size, style, spacing, and viewing distance that allows the child to read comfortably and effectively without fatigue. It can be different for different reading tasks.

Functional near acuity is also tested for people who have low vision to find the best level of enlargement and optical magnification devices for close work. This is often assessed using word reading cards and sometimes with sentence reading cards. Sentence reading cards provide a measure of *reading acuity.* That is, they can be used to determine the threshold for reading and can be used in a systematic way to provide initial information about the optimal size of print for reading. Measurement of threshold is useful in order to understand the smallest elements in a near visual display (reading, pictures, real objects) that a child can see at a specified distance—for example, whether the child can see footnotes in a textbook. But for reading and other extended visual tasks, it is essential to provide the child with material that is *above* threshold. It has been estimated that the size above threshold acuity that promotes the most efficient reading of text can range from two to five times the threshold level, depending on the reading material and the capabilities of the student (Bailey et al., 2003).

For children with CVI, additional aspects of text presentation—such as spacing of symbols and between lines of symbols, letter contrast, the format of the text on the page—and the child's visual capabilities—including visual field, eye movement capabilities, accommodation capabilities, illumination needs, and ability to discriminate color—must be considered when assessing vision for reading.

Methods that estimate reading acuity and optimal print size must systematically take into account accommodation needs (how close the child can hold the reading material before the image begins to blur), as well as print size and viewing distance. Sidebar 12.1 presents one method for determining the best print size and viewing distance for print reading and other reading tasks. M (meter) notation, a measure of print size, is a useful way to present reading acuity measures since it provides an actual symbol size from which to work. For instance, 1M print is 1.45 mm in height. (Appendix 12A

SIDEBAR 12.1

## Determining Appropriate Print Size

***Amanda Hall Lueck, Gordon N. Dutton, and Ian L. Bailey***

A system to determine appropriate print size developed by Lueck and Bailey (in press) is presented here as an initial step in determining appropriate print size for print reading and other reading tasks.

Use a chart with a sequence of text in different print sizes such as the MNRead Acuity Chart (Legge, Ross, Luebker, & LaMay, 1989) which has sentences at the third-grade reading level, with specific differences in size between successive lines. (For details of how this and other LogMAR charts are constructed, see Greer, 2004, p. 185.) It is available in many languages (Virgili et al., 2004), and assesses reading acuity using sentences. The LEA near reading card (spaced and unspaced symbols; see the Resources section) can be used for children who cannot read words. (Note that point-size equivalents used in the examples given here are for New Times Roman font, the font used on most reading acuity cards.) The following are some points to consider in carrying out this procedure:

- Allow the chart to be held with both hands. Avoid leaning the arms against the tabletop when possible.
- The reader should be wearing eyeglasses if they have been prescribed for reading tasks.
- Testing should be done in optimal lighting conditions for reading. If testing is done in less than optimal lighting conditions, this should be noted as lighting may affect test results for some children.

### A. Determining Best Close Viewing Distance

- Ask the reader to read the smallest print possible on the chart. The chart can be held at any distance.

*(continued on next page)*

- Measure the viewing distance used to read the smallest print the child can read. This is the *closest viewing distance.* (As children read smaller and smaller print sizes, they will hold the reading chart closer and closer. When they reach the smallest print size they can read, it means that print will begin to blur if they hold the material any closer.) Reading speed is slowed when struggling to read the smallest print.
- Since readers cannot sustain reading at the closest viewing distance, it is best to estimate the *best close viewing distance* by multiplying closest viewing distance by 1.5.

### B. Determining Critical Angular Size at the Best Close Viewing Distance

- Ask the reader to hold the chart at the best close viewing distance. (Note: The chart can be held at a longer distance, but not at a shorter distance than the best close viewing distance; however, the best close viewing distance is recommended.)
- Be sure the print is as clearly visible to the child as possible by having the child wear any prescribed eyeglasses for refractive error (myopia, hyperopia, astigmatism) or to correct for accommodation needs (reading glasses).
- Begin with the largest print on the chart at this distance and have the child read down the chart from larger to smaller print sizes. Be sure to maintain the same reading distance as the child reads smaller and smaller print sizes even though the child may want to bring the card closer as print gets smaller. (Note: It is not always necessary to begin with the largest print on the card, but it is important that the initial print size to be read is well above the size the child is expected to read.)
- Identify when reading first slows down noticeably. (This slowdown is usually quite obvious.)
- Record the print size that is one step larger (one line larger) on the reading chart than the size for the first slowdown. This is the smallest print size that was read with best speed.
- The *critical angular size* is the print size that is one step larger than the size causing the first slowdown at the viewing distance at which the chart was held. (For example: If the slowdown occurs at 1.0M [9-point] print held at 12 inches [30 cm], the critical angular size is one step up on the chart, or 1.25M [11-point] print at 12 inches [30.5 cm].)
- Remember that if the viewing distance is changed, an adjustment must be made to the print size so that it stays in the same proportion to the viewing distance. For example, if the viewing distance is reduced by half, then the print size must be decreased by half. If the reading distance is increased by two, then the print size must be increased by two.

### C. Additional Steps to Determine Optimal Print Size and Presentation of Print for Specific Reading Tasks

- Optimal print size can vary by reading task and also by font style. Once the initial assessment process (Parts A and B) has been completed, the child's teacher of students with visual impairments can determine the appropriate size print and font for different reading tasks by monitoring the child's accuracy, reading style, and speed of reading, using this information on print size and viewing distance as a starting point.
- Print fonts have different features and different spacing between letters that affect vision differently. Care should be taken regarding the specific font used with children with CVI who have difficulties with crowding. Simple, sans-serif fonts with generous gaps between letters, words, and lines may be best.
- To recommend the width of a pen point or nib for a child to use in writing and drawing,

*(continued on next page)*

SIDEBAR 12.1 *(continued from previous page)*

start with the width of the stroke of the letters in the print size on the near vision chart at the child's threshold near acuity measurement enlarged by two to five times. (Note that letter stroke width is 1/5 the overall width of the letter.) Examples can be provided by lines drawn by different exact pen widths. Remember that the stroke width should not be so large that the gaps between the lines become so small as to render the figure illegible. These gaps between lines need to be the same size as the width of the stroke (Arditi, 2004).

- The optimum size may need adjustment depending on the child's fixation ability (nystagmus); ability or inability to read all optotypes (or words) in sequence on a line; ability to read down the chart; and speed and accuracy of reading in "real world" tasks. Be sure, however, that the print size selected is not so large as to actually slow down children's reading because fewer letters can be deciphered at any one time (Bailey et al., 2003).
- Observe any difficulty naming optotypes or reading words in order along the line, such as missing an optotype or a word in the middle or at the end of the line. Note any difficulty finding the next line down or skipping of lines. If the child has any such difficulties, this can be a result of visual crowding.
- Determine whether a line guide above the line to be read enhances reading (by diminishing crowding, but not interfering with access to the next line).
- Near acuity tests with wider spacing between optotypes may be needed for the child with difficulties reading crowded material.

provides additional information about these and other notation systems and presents a table of print size equivalents for Times New Roman font.)

Print features that have been found to promote ease of reading (Arditi, 2004) include the following:

- Increased point size (or vertical letter size); font styles with the same point sizes differ in size. For example, the letter *h* depicted in Arial font is larger than an *h* depicted in the same point size in Times New Roman font.
- Large letter aspect (width to height) ratio, giving fewer characters per line.
- Fonts with extra space between letters.
- Fixed-width fonts where all letters occupy the same space.
- Dark colors against light colors give greatest contrast, or vice versa.
- Bold stroke widths with sufficient spacing.
- Filled fonts, in which the entire letter is a solid color (as opposed to outlined fonts).
- Serif and sans-serif fonts can both be highly legible, but serifs can render reading more difficult for children with CVI, possibly due to the greater visual crowding.
- Absence of special effects (such as shadowing and three-dimensional shading).

Charts to measure reading acuity should match the reading level of the child. Some children who cannot read well can be tested by asking them to name the letters that they see rather than read the words on a sentence chart. This changes the validity of the test, but it still enables teachers to make an estimate of the print size that the child can work with most efficiently. When impaired reading means that letter, word, and sentence reading cards cannot be used, the LEA Near Acuity Test system, with symbols that approximate the size and spacing of letters in word reading tasks, provides an alternative (Hyvärinen, Näsänen, & Laurinen, 1980). Performance using these closely spaced symbols (non-spaced symbols) can be compared with performance using symbols with more space in between (spaced symbols), also available in the LEA Near Acuity Test. Again, when selecting the size of objects and pictures for non-readers, they need to be 2 to 5 times larger than near acuity at threshold (Bailey et al., 2003). Teachers can fine-tune this estimate for each individual child.

### *Recognition Acuity in Children with Ventral Stream Dysfunction*

Bilateral damage to the ventral stream in the temporal lobes of the brain is rare in children, but when it occurs, the affected child is unable to recognize people, shapes, and forms (see Chapter 3). Yet acuity may be relatively spared, as may the dorsal stream, leading to the paradox that the child can move freely through a world that cannot be seen very well. Measurement of acuity can be carried out with gratings, Cardiff cards, and even picture-based tests, described here, which can be pointed to, even if they cannot be recognized or named. Although the child does not know what the pictures represent, the ability to use the finger to trace the line of picture on a Cardiff card, for example, allows the visual acuity to be estimated.

### *Preferential Looking Acuity*

Visual acuity can be tested using patterns of alternating black-and-white lines (called *gratings*) and preferential looking techniques. These patterns are used for children who cannot identify symbols by naming, matching, or touching them with their hands or feet, and they have a long history in the study of visual functions and visual perception in infants (Dobson, Mayer, & Candy, 2009; Fulton, Hansen, Moskowitz, & Mayer, 2013; McDonald et al., 1985; Teller, 1997). Preferential looking techniques are based on the observation that very young infants and severely visually impaired children will look at large, high-contrast patterns in preference to a plain image with no pattern when the line thicknesses are wide enough to be seen by the child. Toddlers may lose interest in simple gratings, and show more interest in a picture test such as the Cardiff Acuity Test (Adoh & Woodhouse, 1994; Woodhouse et al., 1992), which pairs simple pictures such as a house, car, or duck with a plain, gray area on the same card. The ideal design of grating-based acuity tests involves printing the black-and-white images on a gray background so that the image disappears and blends into the gray background if it cannot be differentiated or detected.

Commercially available tests of grating acuity are available: Teller Acuity Cards II, Keeler Cards, and Cardiff Acuity Test (see the Resources section at the end of this chapter). In these tests, the stimuli are printed on rectangular cards, which helps minimize visual distraction. The stimulus is printed on one side of each card, usually held horizontally for Teller Acuity Cards and Keeler Cards and vertically for the Cardiff Acuity Test. When the stimulus is visible, the child will typically look to the side of the card with the stimulus, but not the blank side. This test design allows the tester to remain unaware of the stimulus location until he or she judges whether the child detects it, thus minimizing potential tester bias. Age norms are available for the Teller and Cardiff tests, and considerable research has been published on Teller grating acuity in diverse ocular and cerebral disorders (Dobson et al., 2009).

Behaviors during preferential looking testing indicating that the child detects the stimulus include turning the eyes toward the grating, pointing to the grating, or naming the Cardiff Acuity Test pictures. Such responses are robust and obvious when larger grating widths are shown. Finer grating and line widths engender subtler visual behaviors, including scanning both sides and briefly holding gaze on one side. (Judging these visual responses is challenging for the novice tester and is less accurate than for experienced testers.) The finest stimulus pattern (smallest black-and-white lines) that the child sees, as judged by the examiner, is taken as the child's threshold or visual acuity.

For all preferential looking–based grating or line acuity measures, test-retest differences in acuity may be greater than expected when compared with recognition acuity testing (Mash & Dobson, 2005; Mayer et al., 1995) unless testers are well trained in a strict protocol (Harvey, Dobson, Tung, Quinn, & Hardy, 1999). The differences may also be larger for visually impaired and multiply impaired persons.

The new Pacific Acuity Test, conceived as a "recognition" acuity test, uses images created by dark and light lines, as with Cardiff Acuity Test pictures (Lowery, Hayes, Sis, Griffith, & Taylor, 2014). Two large oval stimuli matched in size—one a schematic face and the other not a face—are printed on upper and lower portions of gray cards. The finest line width of the face that the child reliably prefers, as judged by the examiner, is the measure of recognition acuity. Detection of the stimuli without preference for the face is the measure of resolution acuity. Pacific Acuity Test recognition acuity is testable in most typical children older than 18 months, while success is much lower under age 18 months. Although the Pacific Acuity Test is a promising new acuity test, how children with ocular visual impairment, CVI, or other developmental disabilities will perform remains to be determined.

Paddle and disc-grating tests are more portable and easier to administer. They are also less expensive. Gratings are printed on both sides of hand-held paddles (in the LEA Gratings or the Patti Stripes Square Wave Grating paddles) or small discs (see the Resources section), with one paddle or disc side containing a blank gray stimulus. The blank paddle is paired with the grating paddle, and preferential looking responses are observed, as with Teller Acuity Cards and the Cardiff Acuity Test. However, the potential for examiner bias because of knowledge of the location of the grating during testing and the potential distractions for the child (because the test images are on two different paddles with other objects, such as examiner's face, between the paddles) may render these tests less accurate. Paddle grating tests do not have the research background and clinical history as do Teller Acuity Cards and Cardiff grating acuity tests. It is unknown whether grating acuity measured with paddles and discs are comparable to those measured with Teller Acuity Cards stimuli. However, if the teacher of students with visual impairments or other vision educator wishes to measure acuity with a paddle or disc-grating test, the following guidelines are recommended:

- Present gratings paired with the matching gray paddle multiple times to be sure the child is detecting the grating.
- Keep a consistent distance between the child and the paddles, and measure this several times during testing.
- Be as objective as possible in judging shifts in the child's gaze. Children with CVI and severe visual impairment often make random shifts in gaze to the right and left that may not be related to the test stimulus.
- Movement of an object can cause a gaze shift, so we recommend presenting the grating and the gray paddle next to each other simultaneously and without movement. Acuity for a moving grating pattern can be better than for a non-moving grating. However, there are no norms for this mode of testing.
- Test the child at different distances to confirm the grating acuity by detection of different cards. Note that some children lose attention to these stimuli held farther than 30–40 cm (12–16 inches) away.

### *Grating Acuity Testing in Children with CVI*

Most children with severe to profound CVI can only respond reliably to a grating acuity test because they cannot match or name symbols on a recognition acuity test. The way the grating stimuli are presented is important. The orientation of the cards and the distance at which they are presented need to be considered. Elimination of distractions and the way the child is held or positioned during testing are also important. The way in which the cards are presented needs to match the child's responses, capabilities, and reactions, and this requires training. Some tips about testing:

- It is common for children with CVI to respond to a grating stimulus with a brief glance, without the sustained fixation of the typical child.
- Some children with CVI withdraw and turn away from the grating card, perhaps due to a startle reaction when the card is presented, or to difficulty attending to the new visual stimulus.
- Attention to grating stimuli may be obtained in a dimly lit room if a light source is projected from behind the child onto the acuity cards.
- Children with severe to profound CVI may respond to acuity gratings presented directly in front of the face, since here the target fills the child's field of view. The examiner then needs to compare the child's responses to the grating with their response to the blank side of the card when each side is presented directly in front of the face. Detection of the grating may be indicated by eye widening, cessation of roving eye movements, stilling of extraneous movements, or small back-and-forth eye movements. Paddle and small card grating tests (discussed later in this chapter) also lend themselves to this method of testing.
- Children with CVI who are not interested or attentive to gratings of any size, except perhaps very coarse ones, may prefer to gaze at lights or reflective surfaces. Very high contrast translucent patterns on a light box may be needed to elicit a looking response.
- Some less attentive or highly distractible children with or without CVI may not attend to finer gratings after having given fairly typical responses to coarser ones. These children do not actively look for finer gratings, as do typical toddlers and older children, even those with a vi-

sual impairment. This may indicate that threshold has not been obtained and that other factors that reduce looking behaviors are at play. Such results need to be qualified by a statement of how likely it was that threshold was measured.

- Experience suggests that children with more severe CVI may not be engaged by the Cardiff Acuity Test picture stimuli, perhaps because of the limited amount of line elements or lack of interest in schematic images. These children typically make more robust and reliable responses to the large field Teller Acuity Card gratings.
- When presenting Teller Acuity Card gratings in the standard mode, with the grating on one side and blank on the other, a consistent lack of response to one side provides evidence of possible hemianopia or neglect on that side. The cards can be rotated vertically to test acuity in these cases. For the Cardiff Acuity Test, lack of response to the lower half of the grating stimulus when presented vertically suggests a possible lower visual field deficit.

An important use for grating visual acuities is in the creation of communication systems for children who are nonverbal, as is the case for many children with CVI. Vision service providers can use this information, in collaboration with the communication specialist and parents, as explained in Sidebar 12.2.

SIDEBAR 12.2

## Using Grating Visual Acuities to Select Pictures for Use with Communication Systems

### Designing Communication Systems

Many children with CVI who are nonverbal require augmentative communication systems, such as photographs and schematic pictures representing objects, events, and activities. Making recommendations for the design of such communication systems is a very important area of assessment by both the vision educator and the eye care provider. It also relies on input from parents and teachers and a review of materials (such as books, an iPad, or handouts) they bring or report. The nature of the visual stimuli, how they are presented, the ways the child responds, and how reliable these responses are need to be understood. When asked by parents and speech-language specialists to provide recommendations regarding communication (see the discussion on selecting optimum optotype and object size in the earlier section on Visual Acuity), it is strongly recommended that the child's teacher of students with visual impairments participate in assessing and discussing, with speech-language therapists and teachers, aspects of the child's visual communication system.

### Using Grating Acuity to Guide Communication Picture Size

For those who have low visual acuities, details in photographs and picture symbols need to be made visible by ensuring that all salient elements and features can be seen. In addition, spacing between features must be wide enough for the picture to be identifiable. Other important considerations include the number of images presented, how they are arranged and spaced, and whether they are colored or not. Picture communication apps are available for new digital devices using photographic images or commercial symbols. Ultimately, determining

*(continued on next page)*

**SIDEBAR 12.2** *(continued from previous page)*

optimal size, number, and spacing requires collaboration between the communication specialist, parents, and vision service providers.

The following is an initial method based on preferential looking grating acuities to calculate dimensions for picture icons that are widely available (such as Mayer-Johnson symbols with Boardmaker or "Symbol Stix," an iPad app; see Resources section), or to make picture drawings by hand. Grating visual acuity measured using preferential looking can guide the width of lines of "critical features" in schematic pictures or self-made drawings used for communication systems (see Appendix 12B). This can be done by the vision educator or speech-language therapist.

- First, decide on the likely critical communication features. For example, the smile and eyes on the Mayer-Johnson smiley face are probably the key identifying features.
- Second, using the grating at the child's acuity level, measure the width of one black or white bar (on Teller Acuity Cards or Keeler Cards) or the width of the central white line outline of the Cardiff picture.
- Third, enlarge the printed smiley face so that the smile line and eyes are equal to between 2 and 5 times the measured width of the grating bar. The overall picture will be enlarged by the same factor. The choice of this enlargement factor will depend on the child's acuity and cognitive abilities, as well as previous trial-and-error experiences. (There is a line width that is impracticably large to enable recognition of all but the most basic details. For example, the width of a grating of 0.4 cpd [20/1400, 6/420] is 0.8 cm [7/32 inch], and this would make very large pictures.)
- When commercial picture icons are not available, too crowded, or too expensive, self-created drawings are a good alternative using a pen point or nib matched to the required line thickness. This technique can also be used to enhance pictures. For example, in many books, the eyes may be so small that they are invisible and need to be enlarged appropriately.

### *Interpretation of Grating Acuity*

Grating acuities of children under 4 years of age must be compared with normal values based on age, since visual acuity continues to improve over a long period of time after birth for typically developing children. For example, at age 1, a binocular Teller Acuity Card grating acuity of about 20/200 (6/60) is within normal limits for age, while at 2 years of age, the acuity is below age norms. By 5 to 8 years of age, grating acuities have reached near adult values. (Recording forms and norms with which to compare a child's measured grating acuity accompany the Teller Acuity Card and Cardiff Acuity tests.) Some clinicians and vision scientists advocate against interpreting grating acuities in terms of Snellen fractions (the commonly used description of visual acuity in which the top number represents the testing distance and the bottom number represents the letter size). Instead they apply the more appropriate metric for gratings, cycles per degree (cpd) (Hyvärinen & Jacob, 2011).[1] However, clinicians, patients, and vision specialists are accustomed to thinking in

[1] One cycle includes one dark and one light stripe. Gratings are specified in cycles per centimeter (cpcm). Acuity in cycles per degree is derived from the cycles per centimeter using the testing distance. Gratings are converted to Snellen notation by calculating the minutes of arc of one-half cycle (dark or light stripe), which equate to the stroke of an optotype.

terms of the Snellen fraction and find the measure "cycles per degree" difficult to conceptualize, so this value is often converted into Snellen notation to aid understanding. Appendix 12C shows the equivalents of acuities in cycles per degree with Snellen fractions as well as with other measures of visual acuity.

However, in countries where entitlement to certain vision services (such as eligibility for the services of a teacher of students with visual impairments in the United States) is contingent on a child's measured visual acuity, use of grating acuities poses a dilemma. Grating acuity measures may not qualify a child for services for those with "legal blindness" because grating acuities can be better than those obtained by recognition acuity tests, and they can overestimate recognition acuity in children with macular lesions and optic nerve disorders (Mayer, Fulton, & Hansen, 1985; Mayer, Fulton, & Rodier, 1984; White & Loshin, 1989). Amblyopia severity may also be underestimated by grating acuity in some (Geer & Westall, 1996; Mayer et al., 1984; McKee, Levi, & Movshon, 2003), but not all cases (Drover, Wyatt, Stager, & Birch, 2009; Sharma et al., 2003).

Despite these caveats, for a preschool child with evident CVI, grating acuity may be the only feasible acuity test. Appropriate vision services should always be advocated if the eye care provider judges the need. If grating acuity is better than 20/200 (6/60), or 3 cpd, but the child manifests vision consistent with legal blindness, instead of reporting a grating acuity that is not a comparable measure to Snellen, it is appropriate for the optometrist or ophthalmologist to report that the child as "functioning at the level of legal blindness." If appropriate, the diagnosis of "cortical or cerebral blindness" is reported by the eye care specialist. ("Cortical blindness" is the accepted term for medical and legal purposes in the United States, in concert with the federal reporting mechanism of the American Printing House for the Blind [2012].)

### *Visual Evoked Potentials to Objectively Estimate Visual Acuity*

Another method of estimating visual acuity is by measuring electrical signals created in the child's visual brain in response to viewing changes in black-and-white patterns generated on a computer screen. These electrical signals are called visual evoked potentials (VEP) (Hamilton et al., 2013). As the pattern shown gets progressively smaller, the VEP signals become smaller too, until they can no longer be detected. The dimensions of the pattern at which this happens lead to an estimate of visual acuity; however, the VEP estimate may not reflect the quality of the child's vision. VEP grating acuities are not equivalent to behavioral grating acuities but have a parallel course of development in children with CVI (Lim et al., 2005). VEP testing is available only in a medical setting, such as some pediatric ophthalmology departments, other specialized clinics, and in research laboratories. It is particularly useful for children who are unable to cooperate with other methods of testing, and may have value as a predictor of later visual status in children with CVI (Watson, Orel-Bixler, & Haegerstrom-Portnoy, 2010).

## Contrast Sensitivity

Contrast refers to differences in brightness of adjacent surfaces or of objects against a background. Contrast sensitivity is a measure of the ability to see these differences. *High contrast* is seen between white and black, whereas *low contrast* is seen between white and very light gray. Contrast sensitivity is measured by determining the smallest difference in contrast (expressed as a percentage) that a person can detect between objects, or elements of objects, and the background. This limit or threshold for contrast detection is specified in percent contrast, or, as contrast sensitivity, as the inverse of the contrast proportion. In this chapter, the terms *contrast threshold* as well as *contrast sensitivity* are used.

Note that when reading or reporting results, it is important to know if they have been measured using the Weber or Michelson methods to avoid misinterpreting them.[2] Contrast for optotypes is measured using the Weber method and contrast for gratings is measured by the Michelson method. As a rule of thumb, up to about 20 percent Weber contrast, the Weber value is about double the Michelson value.

The perception of contrast between object and background depends on the size of the object. Large objects that contrast little with the background may be seen, while small objects with the same contrast may not be seen and may need a greater contrast to render them visible. Under bright lighting, contrasts as low as 0.5 to 1 percent Michelson (1–2 percent Weber) can typically be seen by those with normal contrast sensitivity (perceptually, this is a very light gray against a slightly grayer background, or vice versa). On the other hand, those with reduced contrast sensitivity resulting from visual impairment may need 10 or more times this degree of contrast to perceive an image or object that normally sighted viewers can see. Contrast sensitivity is reduced when visual acuity is reduced, but the degree of reduction in contrast sensitivity is not always predictable from the measure of visual acuity. For some individuals, contrast sensitivity gives a better understanding of functional vision than other visual function measures. Vision educators may choose to use simple, affordable tests of contrast sensitivity (such as face contrast tests, grating detection tests, and symbol flip book tests discussed later in this chapter) with many of their clients or ask a low vision specialist to perform this assessment. Interpretation of contrast sensitivity results is also discussed later in this chapter.

In adults, a reduction in contrast sensitivity impairs visually guided mobility, reduces reading speed, impairs face recognition, and interferes with daily life skills (Leat & Woo, 1997; Owsley, 2003; West et al., 2002). For young children there is little published research concerning the effects of a poor ability to discern contrast. Parents and teachers often describe that their visually impaired child pays less attention to people's faces and has poorer fine motor and mobility skills than would be expected from their measured visual acuities. Measurement of contrast sensitivity in children with visual impairments is therefore warranted, but the results need to be interpreted qualitatively (see Table 12.2). Children with CVI may have problems in attending to and perceiving in complex environments, and difficulty integrating visual and motor skills that contribute to their deficits in contrast sensitivity. It is important to understand a child's contrast vision in order to determine if visual behaviors are specifically related to contrast sensitivity impair-

---

[2] Percent contrast is calculated in the Weber method as

[Luminance Maximum minus Luminance Minimum / Background Luminance] [ × 100]

and in the Michelson method as

[Luminance Maximum minus Luminance Minimum / Luminance Maximum plus Luminance Minimum] [× 100] ment, or some other visual function or visual perception issue.

### *Contrast Sensitivity Tests for Older Children*

The most useful and valid tests currently available measure contrast sensitivity for large letters with a size that maximizes their visibility (Woods & Wood, 1995). Two such tests are the Pelli-Robson Low Contrast Test (Pelli, Robson, & Wilkins, 1988) and the Mars Letter Contrast Sensitivity Test (Arditi, 2005) (see the Resources section at the end of this chapter). The stimuli in these two tests are letters of the same size printed on a chart in rows that decrease in contrast in regular progression down the chart, from 100 percent to below visibility. These two tests provide comparable results and have good test-retest properties (Dougherty, Flom, & Bullimore, 2005; Elliott, Bullimore, & Bailey, 1991). Both are efficient, requiring only a few minutes to administer. However, the ability to identify letters of the alphabet is required. Norms for the Pelli-Robson test for 6-year-olds show the average contrast threshold to be 2.4 percent Weber (Hargadon, Wood, Twelker, Harvey, & Dobson, 2010) versus 1.6 percent Weber for adults (Leat & Wegmann, 2004).

Other tests of contrast sensitivity require the child to identify the orientation of small patches of gratings (e.g., Functional Acuity Contrast Test [FACT]; see Ginsburg, 1984, 1996, and Resources section) or the orientation of the edge between halves of small circles (Melbourne Edge Test; see Verbaken, 1989, and Resources section) over a range of contrasts (see Table 12.2). Although considerable research has been done on grating orientation contrast sensitivity tests in adults, there are concerns about their reliability and clinical validity (see Owsley, 2003; Pesudovs, Hazel, Doran, & Elliott, 2004; Woods & Wood, 1995). More recent research suggests that the Melbourne Edge Test has good reliability and sensitivity to visual impairments (Haymes & Chen, 2004). However, because these tests require discrimination of the orientation of grating or edge, they may not be applicable to young children, especially those with CVI.

## Contrast Sensitivity Tests for Young Children

Contrast sensitivity tests using *symbols* are available for young children (e.g., Patti Pics and LEA Symbols; see Table 12.2 and Resources section). A convenient and efficient format for these tests is a booklet with successive pages each containing a rectangular box of five symbols printed in different contrasts (Variable Contrast Patti Pics Flip Book and LEA Symbols Low Contrast Test [see Resources section]). The same symbols can be used to test acuity, making it possible to interpret a child's contrast deficit in relation to acuity. The symbols of 9.5M or 10M size at 30 cm distance are nearly the same size as the Pelli-Robson test (Leat & Wegmann, 2004). Limitations of these tests are that the lowest available contrast level (1.25 percent Michelson) is not low enough to reach threshold even in the youngest typical children who can be tested (1- to 2-year-olds) (Leat & Wegmann, 2004), and the intervals between the levels are relatively large (1.25, 2.5, 5, 10 percent), precluding small changes in contrast sensitivity from being measured.

*Preferential looking contrast sensitivity* with the Cardiff Contrast Sensitivity Test employs the same images and card format as the Cardiff Acuity Test. The contrast of successive cards is progressively reduced, from 46 to 1 percent. Age norms are provided; the lower limit of the normal range for 2- to 4-year-olds is 3 percent contrast (Michelson), while for 1- to 2-year-olds it is 16 percent contrast. Thus there is a broader range for younger children, 1 to 16 percent, versus 1 to 3 percent for older children. This test works well with high-functioning children with CVI, but those with more severe CVI are not so easily engaged, perhaps because of the sparse elements in the pictures or the lack of higher contrast stimuli.

The *Cambridge Low Contrast Grating Test* (Verbaken, 1989; Wilkins, Della Sala, Somazzi, & Nimmo-Smith, 1988) consists of a ring binder with pages of successively reduced contrast gratings with wide stripes (low spatial frequency), paired with a matching blank page. Children can either point to the grating stimulus, or the examiner judges the child's preferential looking responses. At a 2.5-foot distance the grating covers a large area (16 × 16 degrees) and is a good stimulus for the child with low vision. It is rapid and simple to administer. Contrasts range from below 1 to a maximum of 13 percent. Lack of higher contrast stimuli is a limitation, especially for those with marked CVI. Norms for children have yet to be published, although a qualitative severity classification ascribes contrast threshold of 1 percent or less to be near normal, 2 percent mildly reduced, 3–4 percent moderately reduced, and 5–13 percent severely reduced (Haegerstrom-Portnoy, 2004).

*Large schematic faces* of diminishing contrast printed on boards or "paddles" are designed for young, visually impaired children using preferential looking techniques similar to the paddle grating tests (Hiding Heidi Low Contrast Face Test, Peek-a-Boo Patti Low Contrast Vision Test; see Resources section). A blank white card is the "control" and is paired with a "face" stimulus. The control paddle can be placed over the face paddle and then slid to one side to reveal the face. Fixation on the face indicates its detection. The tests are portable and easy to administer. As with the grating paddles, however, examiner bias has to be guarded against. These tests have faces of 100 percent contrast, although the next lowest available contrast is at 25 percent; this prevents measurements between 100 and 25 percent contrast. The lowest contrast is 1.25 percent. The intervals between contrasts are relatively large (doubling of contrast, e.g., 1.25, 2.5 percent), which means that small changes in contrast sensitivity cannot be detected. The complexity of the faces produced by features of different widths (different spatial frequencies) may make them more interesting to children than repetitive grating patterns; however, this complexity could limit their diagnostic value (Charman, 2006). Although contrast sensitivity measured with the Hiding Heidi faces does not closely correspond to Pelli-Robson contrast sensitivity in adults with low vision (Leat & Wegmann, 2004), they serve a useful function in helping parents who watch the test being carried out understand how faces and expressions may not be recognized by their child and what to do to enhance contrast levels of objects in everyday tasks to rectify this (see Chapter 13).

## Interpreting Contrast Sensitivity Test Results in Children

Testing the child's contrast sensitivity in front of parents and teachers allows them to discern and understand the visual disability. However, the question is, what is the impact of poor contrast sensitivity? We can extrapolate from studies of letter contrast sensitivity in adults with low vision (e.g.,

Leat & Woo, 1997; West et al., 2002) to children tested with symbol or grating tests (converting from Weber contrast to Michelson contrast):

- The ability to see symbols of 1.5 percent Weber contrast or gratings of 1–2 percent Michelson contrast facilitates early reading skills without the need for increased contrast.
- Mobility problems tend to arise at contrasts lower than 12 percent Weber (6 percent Michelson), even with intact visual fields.
- Activities and skills of daily living are impaired but possible if contrast thresholds are between 4 and 10 percent Weber (2–5 percent Michelson).

For children whose contrast sensitivity can only be tested with face stimuli, it seems acceptable to consider that if a young patient can detect the lowest contrast levels available in Hiding Heidi and Patti Pics tests (1.25 percent Michelson), there should be no significant effect on visually guided behavior. However, the specific adverse impact of reduced contrast sensitivity in young children is not known.

## Contrast Sensitivity in Children with CVI

Contrast sensitivity in children with CVI has been found to be reduced compared to controls in a study using visual evoked potential testing (Good, Hou, & Norcia, 2012). Clinical experience shows that children with CVI have more variable and less visual attention for low-contrast visual stimuli than those children with comparable visual acuity deficits as a result of ocular or ocular-motor visual impairment. This implies that in children with CVI, contrast sensitivity may be lower than what would be anticipated from the visual acuity. In the authors' experience, children with CVI who have grating visual acuities between 20/130 (6/39) (4.6 cpd) and 20/270 (6/81) (2.2 cpd) may detect only Weber contrasts of 16 to 25 percent, while normative data from the Cardiff Acuity Tests suggest that they should detect contrasts of at least 5 percent Michelson, or 10 percent Weber.

### *Recommendations for Children with Low Contrast Sensitivity*

Children with visual impairments need to have high-contrast materials for visual learning and fine motor tasks. Stair edges and other features in the child's environment need to be enhanced for safe mobility. Although studies into the difficulties caused by low contrast sensitivity in children with CVI are needed, based on studies in adults with low vision (Leat & Woo, 1997; West et al., 2002), the authors tentatively suggest the following as starting points for making practical assessments:

- Enlargement of high-contrast print in individuals with visual acuity of 20/60 or better is likely to be needed if contrast threshold is 4–5 percent Weber (2–2.5 percent Michelson) or higher (poorer contrast sensitivity).
- A contrast threshold higher than 4–10 percent Weber (2–5 percent Michelson) may require provision of high-contrast materials for skilled activities.
- Contrast threshold for letters, symbols, or gratings higher than 12 percent Weber (6 percent Michelson) warrants referral to an O&M instructor, even if the child has no visual field defect.
- For children with poor contrast sensitivity, increase the color contrast and/or

size of details more than would be predicted to be needed from visual acuity.

- For children with severe CVI and diminished contrast sensitivity, try light box stimuli (Roman-Lantzy, 2007), but only if it has been determined that high-level background lighting does not overwhelm the child and interfere with the child's ability to use his or her vision.
- If color vision is impaired, create a high degree of contrast with variations of the same color hues (e.g., dark red versus light red).

## Visual Field

The visual field is the area of a person's surrounding environment that they can see at any one time. Areas of reduced or absent perception in any part of the visual field are called visual field defects. They result from an abnormality (disorder, disease, or damage) anywhere along the visual pathway, from the eye to the visual brain. Figure 2.4 shows the types of visual field defects that result from damage along the visual pathway. The location of the damage predicts the type of visual field defect and its severity predicts the extent and degree of loss. Although the location of damage revealed by a head scan can be used to predict the condition of the visual field, recovery from very early onset damage can make the prediction inaccurate in some cases.

The visual field is arguably the second most important visual function measured in clinical practice after visual acuity. Visual field defects can occur without impairment of visual acuity. Visual field defects resulting from retinal or optic nerve disease or disorder are often different in each eye, whereas when there is damage to visual pathways behind the optic chiasm, visual field defects for each eye have similar distributions (see Chapters 2 and 3). As a result, testing the visual field with both eyes open when there is damage to the visual pathway behind the optic chiasm effectively measures the same field defect for each eye.

Defects of an individual's visual fields may not correspond to their *functional visual field*, which is revealed by how the individual performs and acts in daily life using peripheral vision with both eyes open. The starting point for evaluating the individual's functional visual field is to measure the field with both eyes viewing. The measured functional visual field may be different from the field predicted from testing each eye. For example, in patients with strabismus, functional field extent may be smaller on the side of the eye that turns in (esotropia) and expanded in individuals with outward eye turn (exotropia).

### *Visual Field Defects Suggested by the Child's Medical History*

The medical history helps to identify risk factors for visual field impairment, guide testing for it, and assist in interpretation of test responses. Examples include the following:

- ***Injury, malformation, or surgery for epilepsy in one brain hemisphere*** can cause a visual field defect (such as hemianopia or quadrant field defect) on the opposite side.
- ***Children born very prematurely*** may have had injury to developing white matter. This typically affects parieto-occipital brain areas, causing inferior visual field defects.
- ***Severe hypoxic ischemic brain injury*** can cause marked generalized visual field constriction.
- ***Severe diffuse brain injury*** may appear to cause a lack of central vision, but with

retained ability to respond to peripheral objects.

- ***Optic nerve hypoplasia or atrophy*** can lead to lateral and inferior field defects and scotomas (blind spots) that are different for each eye.
- ***Vigabatrin medication for epilepsy*** can cause generalized visual field constriction resulting from toxicity to the retina.
- ***Metabolic or mitochrondrial brain disorders and epilepsy*** can lead to poor attention to peripheral objects, resembling generalized visual field constriction.
- ***Moderate to severe CVI*** may cause constriction of the entire visual field, hemianopia, or bilateral lower visual field defect.

### Visual Field Defects and Functional Consequences

A literature search does not reveal any published information on how visual field defects affect developmental milestones and activities of daily life of young children. In adults, visual field defects can affect safety in relation to driving (Rubin et al., 2007), cause falls (Ramrattan et al., 2001), impair mobility (Lovie-Kitchin, Mainstone, Robinson, & Brown, 1990; Turano et al., 2004), and impair skills of daily living (see Owsley, 2003). Hemianopia can impair reading (Pouget et al., 2012), while central visual field defects reduce reading speed and efficiency independent of visual acuity or contrast sensitivity deficits (Legge, Ross, Isenberg, & LaMay, 1992) and limit pleasure in reading (Ramrattan et al., 2001). Adults with visual field defects can benefit from rehabilitation services (Rubin et al., 2007).

Clinical experience suggests that visual field defects in infants and young children can interfere with accurate, visually guided reach and fine motor skills. They may also delay crawling and walking, impair attention at distance, and disturb visual scanning and search behaviors essential later on in life for developing reading skills. Visual-motor skills for children of all ages can be impaired by field defects. Mobility is particularly impaired by lower field defects, and orientation is impaired by hemianopia. In these instances, it is important to have a comprehensive O&M evaluation for environmental modifications and visually guided mobility.

### Clinical Measures of the Visual Field

Visual fields are measured by eye care specialists using a device called a bowl perimeter, a hemisphere with peripheral stimulus targets of spots of light projected onto or embedded into its inner surface. Some specialists test with a flat screen (tangent screen) using a small object on the end of a thin wand as the peripheral stimulus. Arc perimeters are also used with similar stimuli. A variety of perimetry methods may be used. *Static* perimetry presents spots of light in fixed locations that are progressively brightened until visible. In *kinetic* perimetry (with a hemisphere, tangent screen, or arc) the stimulus is moved from a peripheral to a more central location until it is seen. Kinetic perimetry is much easier for young children, while the sustained attention required for static perimetry is too demanding, even for typical children under age 8 and for many disabled older children. In testing with a hemispheric perimeter, the child sits with his or her chin on a chin-brow rest, looking at a small target in the center of the bowl. The child lets the examiner know when a second light is seen in his or her peripheral vision by pressing a beeper. The test can be introduced as a game for the child to "shoot the stars." Typical children can perform kinetic perimetry at 4 years of age (Mayer & Fulton, 2005), and some older children with multiple impairments can also be tested with this technique.

Hemispheric and arc perimeters have been used with preferential looking procedures to measure visual fields in normal infants and young patients in specialized clinical and research settings (see examples in Table 12.2: kinetic arc perimetry, LED hemispheric kinetic perimetry, projection kinetic perimetry) (Mayer & Fulton, 1993; Mayer, Fulton, & Cummings, 1988; Quinn et al., 1996; Quinn et al., 2011; Werth & Schadler, 2006). Normal maturation of the visual field and disorders affecting the visual field have been studied in young patients with these techniques (see Fulton et al., 2013). However, despite their value for research and for clinical trials, these methods have limited use in many clinical settings because specialized equipment and trained and experienced staff are needed.

### *Confrontation Visual Field Testing*

The most practical way of estimating visual fields in a young child or child with severe cognitive impairment is to present a target in the child's peripheral visual field and observe the child's orienting eye and head movements. Known as *confrontation visual field testing*, this method does not require a perimeter or other instrumentation but takes advantage of the young child's natural orienting responses. This orienting movement occurs in the newborn and throughout life. The child's visual fixation is attracted to a target while another target is presented in the peripheral visual field. Orienting eye and head movements and verbal responses are carefully observed. Each practitioner has his or her own favorite confrontation methods and test objects, including wiggling fingers, small toys, or examination hand lights. There are no standard methods or test objects for confrontation testing, especially with disabled children (although there are well-described methods for cooperative adults; see Anderson, 1987; Kerr, Chew, Eady, Gamble, & Danesh-Meyer, 2010; Shahinfar, Johnson, & Madsen, 1995).

For vision educators and others working with children in the community, confrontation testing can be useful in assessing the child's functional visual field, with both eyes viewing, with some caveats. Responses to peripheral objects can be affected by the area in front and to the side of the child if there are distractors, by the relative size and interest value of the central fixation stimulus and the peripheral stimulus, and by the capability of the child to make eye-head orienting movements. If an area of the child's visual field appears to be constricted, consider the impact of distractors, the ability to shift gaze between central and peripheral targets, the latency of the response, the presence of an eye turn, and the potential effect of eyeglasses. Observations and results from confrontation testing by a vision educator or other nonspecialist should be reported without interpreting the possible cause of the visual field abnormality.

For suggestions and procedures in confrontation field testing, see Sidebar 12.3.

### *Limitations of Confrontation Visual Field Testing in Young Patients*

Only major and dense field defects (large areas of the field in which no object of any size or brightness can be seen) can be reliably detected by confrontation testing (Kerr et al., 2010; Shahinfar et al., 1995). Such field

## SIDEBAR 12.3

# Suggestions for Confrontation Visual Field Testing

### *Suggestions for Stimuli and Procedures in Confrontation Testing*

The features of the central fixation stimulus and the peripheral target need to be appropriate for the child's visual difficulties, age, attention, and cognitive abilities. The key to effective and accurate testing is maintaining the child's central fixation when the peripheral target is being presented to ensure that the child does not anticipate the peripheral target position and search for it.

The following are suggestions and guidelines for confrontation testing that may be helpful for vision educators and others, as well as indications regarding possible visual field defects.

#### *Central Fixation Target*

- The examiner's face is an effective central stimulus for many children. When feasible, children can be asked to look at the examiner's nose. The examiner can talk to the distractible child to elicit gaze to his or her face. However, talking by the examiner may cause the child with marked CVI to become visually inattentive.
- Although the examiner's face can be an effective central target, it is large, so it can be preferable to use a visible toy (or light) held in one hand.
- The central target should be interesting but not so interesting that it prevents or delays looking at the peripheral target.
  - Difficulty disengaging attention, or "sticky fixation," occurs in some children with CVI whose visual field may be functionally constricted (Harvey, Dobson, & Narter, 1997; Mayer & Fulton, 1993).
  - For children with sticky fixation it can be best to use only a peripheral target without a central target.
  - Sticky fixation is an indicator of the apraxia of gaze that is characteristic of Balint's syndrome, with its associated simultanagnosia, impaired visual guidance of movement, difficulty attending to more than one element at once (see Chapter 3), and sometimes associated with lower visual field impairment that needs to be looked for.

#### *Peripheral Target*

- The peripheral target needs to be salient enough to bring about a quick shift in fixation to it. Some children will respond more rapidly to a peripheral target when it is moved or wiggled than when it is held steadily.
- Placing the peripheral target (toy or light) on the end of a stick or wand has advantages for the child who anticipates target location from the examiner's arm movement.
- Shifting attention to the peripheral target can be gained by verbal prompts, such as "Where's '[toy name]'?" or "Where's the white ball?" (for children who know the names of objects).
- Severely visually and multiply impaired children may not attend or orient to central or peripheral objects in normal room lighting. A salient light stimulus, such as a flickering light in a dimly lit or dark room, may be most effective.
- An LED stimulus, with different settings of luminance and flicker, mounted on a flexible wand, is commercially available (see the Resources section of this chapter). This target is most useful to test cooperative young children with good fixation.

The following are some methods of presentation in confrontation testing:

- The peripheral target must be moved at a speed that is appropriate to the attention of the child. Too fast and it may not be spotted, and the field may appear constricted when it

*(continued on next page)*

is not. Too slow and the child may lose fixation and look around for the target.

- Detection of the peripheral target is seen as a rapid shift in gaze from the central target to the peripheral target.
- In severely visually impaired children and those with CVI, the orienting response may be a slow head movement toward the peripheral light; and localization of the light may be inaccurate.
- The child's head is kept straight (helped by a parent or assistant), not turned to the right or left, or tilted down when testing, which may be compensatory for a visual field defect. Other examiners may choose to orient their own positions during testing to compensate for the child's head turn.
- Alternative methods for children who can anticipate and look for the peripheral lights include:
    - Present two light wands at once, one in the child's right hemifield and the other in the left (or in two adjacent quadrants). Illuminate only one target sequentially in each hemifield, and compare the child's responses. Central fixation must be well maintained for this to be effective.
    - One examiner holds the child's attention and fixation on the central target, and another examiner presents the peripheral target from behind the child. The child's head movement toward the target observed by the examiner presenting the central target confirms the judgment of the child's eye-head orientation.
    - The peripheral target is made to "pop out" from behind an occluder large enough to cover the examiner's head and upper torso, with a small hole to look through to see the child. The target is mounted on a wand and is rapidly protruded from behind the occluder. A game is played where the child has to spot the target the moment it appears.

### *Testing for Specific Visual Field Defects Using Confrontation*

Testing the lower field quadrants carefully is critical, as lower field defects are common in children with perinatal brain damage and CVI. Hemianopic field defects occur in children with early brain damage, in those with cerebral malformations, and as a consequence of childhood stroke. Upper field defects are less common but are also important to seek out, for example, in children with chorioretinal colobomas (as with CHARGE syndrome).

- The examiner tests each field quadrant, conceptualized by dividing the field "pie" into four pieces, with horizontal and vertical divisions intersecting at fixation.
- The peripheral target is moved along an imaginary line bisecting each quadrant.
- Orienting eye-head movements in the oblique directions are easily detected by the examiner who can ignore right-left eye-head movements from distractions.
- If the child does not appear to detect the peripheral target in a quadrant, this can be confirmed by moving the target horizontally and then vertically from within the area thought to have no vision. The boundaries of the quadrant with no vision are confirmed by fixation head or eye movements at the right locations.
- A complete right or left hemianopia (half-field defect) can also be probed in this way using horizontal movement of the target from the blind area to the sighted one.

defects include hemianopia, the inability to see from the visual midline to the extreme periphery in one half-field, and quadrantanopia, the inability to see in a quarter section of the visual field, conceptualized, for example, as the pie-shaped segment on a clock face between 3 and 6 or 6 and 9. Testing field defects in adult patients can be improved by testing with two different confrontation methods (Kerr et al., 2010). Sometimes the results are suspected but not certain when, for example, a possible right hemifield defect or possible inferior left field defect is recorded. To confirm the results, testing with different objects (Kerr et al., 2010) or repeated testing at a later stage is advised.

Apparent overall constriction of the visual field may result from an impaired ability to shift visual attention, as occurs in Balint's syndrome ("sticky fixation"), as mentioned previously. This result reflects the child's *field of visual attention*, or the area within which the child is able to attend and, therefore, to see, and is arguably as significant as an anatomically based visual field constriction. The field of visual attention represents a nonanatomical constriction that can exist in the field of each eye as well as with both eyes open. Children with CVI often show marked overall field constriction, which may result from extensive damage to visual areas of the brain or to an impaired field of visual attention. A visual field constriction secondary to anatomical, attentional, or functional causes needs to be understood and addressed.

### Testing for Lower Visual Field Defects

A lower visual field impairment may be suspected by parents and vision educators, but may not be identified by the methods of testing previously described. Reported concerns typically include:

- Falling over things while walking
- Bumping into obstacles on the floor
- Difficulty going down stairs or slopes
- Difficulty walking over uneven ground
- Walking off curbs when going down, or missing or tripping on them when going up
- Keeping the head tilted down when moving around or when in unfamiliar surroundings
- Exhibiting great caution when moving around, and staying close to parents when outside
- Missing objects that are near to the child's body on the table surface
- Missing material on the bottom of pages

If a field defect has not been detected by careful confrontation testing, one can ask the independently mobile child without motor impairment who understands instructions to look straight ahead and raise one leg straight up until the foot is seen. The foot is often lifted much higher before it is seen than in children with typical vision. This suggests that lower visual field impairment can be so peripheral that it is not detectable by traditional testing, yet is disabling. For the child seated at a table who is looking straight ahead at a target, a toy can be surreptitiously placed just in front of the child, where it cannot be seen, and progressively moved away until the child reacts to it. This can graphically illustrate the very same peripheral lower visual field deficit.

Other possible reasons for the difficulties described above are:

- Lower motor impairment (such as spastic diplegia) without lower field defect may cause difficulties when moving.

- The child may be very goal-oriented when moving and may pay no attention to what is around or below him or her while moving toward something of interest. This child may bump into obstacles to the side as well as below.
- Impaired attention or impaired visual guidance of movement of the lower limbs, despite intact visual fields, is seen in some children (Dutton et al., 2004).
- Impaired movement perception may be identified. When affected children move fast, visual clarity is presumably lost.
- In children with nystagmus, the need to keep the eyes steady using the head and eye position in which the nystagmus is least (the null position; see Chapter 8) may make them reluctant to look down, probably because the increased eye movement when looking down blurs vision. A child whose eyes are misaligned when looking down may also keep the head erect or even tilted up to avoid double vision when looking down.

## Central Visual Field Defects

A different problem occurs when interpreting behaviors of a child with a central visual field defect. The authors have observed several children reported to have CVI who each had a long history of poor eye contact, with difficulty recognizing people and difficulties in visual perceptual and motor skills. The cause, however, was not CVI, but a central scotoma in each eye resulting from disordered retinal or optic nerve function or bilateral occipital lobe damage. To measure a central scotoma requires careful quantitative perimetry, and the fixation behaviors of a child must be observed along with visual acuity to infer central scotoma. Looking off-center or eccentric fixation (using the peripheral retina) is a hallmark of a central scotoma.

### *Common Misconceptions about Visual Field Defects in Children*

Parents often misunderstand their children's vision because of misconceptions about visual field defects, for example, thinking that a visual field defect must be in the far periphery ("out there"), while not realizing that the defect might involve the whole half-field from the vertical midline to the periphery, as in a hemianopia, or the whole inferior field up to the child's visual horizon. They may also fail to recognize that homonymous visual field defects affect both eyes symmetrically, believing that only one eye (the eye on the side of the hemianopia) is affected. Such misconceptions can be avoided by clear explanation and simulation of the specific field defect measured. For simulation, safety goggles can be placed on the parent's face, with portions of the lens area corresponding to the area of the visual field defect blocked off for both eyes. Parents are often shocked or surprised by the perceptual effect of a complete visual field defect. They must be reassured that while the simulated hemianopia is experienced as blackness, the field defect actually experienced by the child is *absence* of vision akin to not seeing behind oneself.

### *'Functional' Visual Field in the Child with a Visual Field Defect*

Some children with major visual field defects do not appear impaired in the way one would predict. A child with a hemifield defect may not show difficulties avoiding obstacles when mobile and may not bump into things on the affected side; there may be no demonstrable or reported difficulties in school performance or in daily life activities. The apparent lack of impairment may be a result of the child's use of compensatory scanning toward the hemifield defect. A head turn toward the hemifield defect and even head thrusting toward the side of the defect may be compensatory and aid the child's scanning into the non-seeing field area. Typically, the history of such a child indicates early postnatal or prenatal brain injury. Children with later-onset brain damage causing visual field defects are less likely to develop compensatory head turns and good scanning skills. Another explanation is that the child may have intact reflex vision (or blindsight [see Chapter 3]) that brings about reflex looking into the non-seeing area (Boyle, Jones, Hamilton, Spowart, & Dutton, 2005; Tinelli et al., 2013).

Thus, the functional visual field of a child (or older person) with a field defect depends in part on their compensatory abilities and skills. Yet, when parents are questioned, they may remark that when routine behaviors are challenged by an unusual situation or unique demand, such as walking through an unfamiliar room with a lot of furniture, the effects of the field defect become evident. This is especially concerning with regard to the safety of the child when mobile. This emphasizes the importance of intervention by an O&M specialist for children with a visual field defect, regardless of how well they appear to compensate.

### Visual Neglect

*Visual neglect* can closely resemble lack of vision on one side due to hemianopia, and can accompany hemianopia. It refers to lack of attention to visual space on one side (spatial neglect) or to one side of the body (body neglect). (See Chapter 3 for a more detailed discussion of visual neglect.) The neglected side is opposite to the brain hemisphere that is damaged, which is usually of the temporal-occipital area but also the parietal area (see review by Milner & McIntosh, 2005). The cause of neglect is usually stroke or hypoxic ischaemic encephalopathy (insufficient supply of oxygen and blood supply to the brain), and it can occur in adults and children. If there is spatial neglect and a field defect, they occur on the same side. Left spatial neglect is more common than right spatial neglect (see Chapter 3).

Visual neglect relates to the body and is not compensated for by head and eye movement, and a turn of the body to compensate is often seen, both when seated at a table and when walking (see Chapter 3, Figure 3.5). Spatial neglect in children is rarer than in adults, possibly because of brain plasticity and recovery of damaged connections. However, subtle signs of contralateral neglect may persist into preschool years in children with early-onset unilateral brain damage (Trauner, 2003).

*Spatial neglect* can be elicited by presenting the child with two similar objects in mirror image positions on both sides of the child. The child with neglect will attend only to the object in the non-neglected hemifield. However, when only one object is presented to the neglected side, it may be detected if the child is alert and engaged. *Hemispatial neglect* should be distinguished from *body neglect* (in which there is lack of awareness of the neglected side of the body), although it is unclear how frequently they occur together. Spatial neglect is difficult to differentiate from lack of visual field on one side in infants and young children who have yet to develop the cognitive skills required for the tests that are most diagnostic in adults. In one type of "cancellation" test, able children at age 4–5 years are asked to cross out small items covering a page; affected children omit items on the affected side. Another test indicative of neglect is line bisection, where the patient is asked to exactly bisect horizontal straight lines with a mark (Ting et al., 2011). A bias in making the mark to one side indicates hemispatial neglect on that side. This test is difficult for young children. Nevertheless, both tests are used where possible as neither is diagnostic of neglect in all affected children. Such tests should be administered by qualified professionals trained in their use.

Other indications of hemispatial neglect in adults are drawing only one-half of an image (for example, a clock face), biasing a drawing to the non-neglected side, missing pictures or letters on one side of a page, missing familiar objects on one side of a table, leaving food on one side of the plate, poor auditory attention to stimuli on one side, collisions with objects on one side, and a bias in navigating familiar places. Parent interviews and Dutton's CVI inventory (Dutton et al., 2010; see Chapter 11) can provide information on possible neglect in children. It is possible to observe behaviors suggesting neglect such as biased drawing and writing, or biased pointing at pictures during an assessment. A child's performance on a test involving removal of objects from a large array may show a bias away from the neglected hemifield (Trauner, 2003). However, caution is warranted as a visual field defect on one side can cause these difficulties with or without neglect.

In young children following a stroke, hemiplegia (paralysis) of the side of the body opposite the stroke is common. These children may have body neglect of the hemiplegic side as well. This means they are unaware of their arm and leg on that side. Therapy to treat hemiplegia also treats the neglect. A number of children seen in New England Eye Low Vision Clinic at Perkins have been treated with "constraint" neuroplastic therapy whereby the non-paretic (not paralyzed) arm is constrained to force use of the paretic arm. Not only does the child show improved use of the paretic arm and hand, but he or she also shows improved awareness of that side of the body and the field on the paretic side. Thus, the motor therapy may improve the spatial neglect. As further evidence for the possibility that motor therapy may improve sensory awareness in spatial neglect, some orientation and mobility specialists encourage children with hemiplegia who are able to walk to use a cane that is held in the hemiplegic hand if possible, and have the child use it to explore space on the side of the hemiplegia (in addition to intensive physical therapy).

### *Recommendations Regarding Visual Field Defects in Young Children*

If, after careful testing, it is strongly suspected that the child has a major hemifield defect, or a complete lower visual field defect, or a quadrantic field defect, the New England Eye Low Vision Clinic at Perkins provides a set of recommendations for family members, one for young infants, and one for school-age children. Some recommendations are provided in Sidebar 12.4. (For the complete fact sheets and recommendations, see Mayer, n.d.a and b.)

If a defect of the upper visual field is identified that is affecting both eyes—which is rare in children with CVI—there is a concern about the child bumping into things that protrude at eye or head level (into the affected field). In young, small children,

SIDEBAR 12.4

## Recommendations for Young Children with Visual Field Defects

The following suggestions for teachers of students with visual impairments, orientation and mobility specialists, physical therapists, occupational therapists, speech-language pathologists, and parents are helpful when working with children who have visual field defects:

- When a child is learning a new visual skill, such as a visual-motor task, position the visual materials toward the child's seeing field (in a child with left hemianopia materials should be placed in the child's right visual field, for a child with right hemianopia materials should be placed in the left visual field, and in a child with lower field loss, materials should be placed in her or his upper visual field).
- For learned visual tasks or when transferring learned skills to other favorite or meaningful activities, shift materials more toward the non-seeing field to encourage its use.
- Encourage reaching, grasping, and manipulating of objects in the non-seeing field.
- Teach the child to visually scan or gaze into their non-seeing field for single and multiple objects by causing the objects to produce sounds, pointing to them, and talking about them.
- Systematic scanning should be practiced early, following the sequence of reading in the child's cultural language (for example, left to right for English).
- For the child with a visual field defect on the weak side of body (for example, in hemiplegic cerebral palsy), when stimulating use of the weak hand, ensure that the hand is seen (for example, by presenting objects for reaching biased to the seeing field, or in the central visual field). A large object, such as a face, placed in the child's near space may be seen only partially; to ensure the whole face is seen, come toward the child from the seeing field.
- Help the child explore his or her whole spatial environment, especially in unfamiliar spaces.
- For the child with a generally constricted visual field and reduced visual acuity, as in CVI, visual materials to advance perception and learning should be placed in the child's central visual field; stimulating scanning into the peripheral field may require using salient stimuli such as lighted and musical objects.
- For mobility, safety is always an important consideration and modifications of the environment should be made to ensure safe movement.
- When teaching orientation and visual efficiency skills for moving in the environment, the location and severity of the child's visual field defect should be taken into consideration.

As a general principle, when a child is searching for something he or she wants, that item should be placed in the area of the impaired visual field to encourage and bring about successful search, but when the child needs to learn from visually presented information that is not motivating in the same way, it should be placed in the sighted area.

family members are cautioned regarding table edges, leaving drawers open, and so forth. If the upper field defect is large, the small child may not see or attend to an adult's face. Classroom materials positioned higher on the wall may not be seen.

Constricted visual fields are usually accompanied by significant visual acuity and contrast sensitivity deficits (less often in children with hemifield or quarter field defects). First, we think about types of visual materials that the child can see and respond to.

Then, we consider optimal placement of the visual materials. For children with cerebral palsy, the head may need to be turned or tilted. For those who have communication displays or computer tablets attached to their wheelchairs by an armature, the display or tablet needs to be adjusted for their principal gaze direction.

Methods of rehabilitation of visual function for major visual field defects that have been proven effective in some studies of adults (Pouget et al., 2012; Trauzettel-Klosinski, 2011a, 2011b) can also be applied to children with visual field defects, although there is little information regarding their efficacy in children. These include training hemianopic patients to use compensatory eye movements; training in the use of eccentric fixation for central field loss; magnification of text for reading; using optical devices such as telescopes for distance viewing, and prisms for hemianopias and hemispatial neglect (Milner & McIntosh, 2005); and training in cane use and tactile guidance. Training compensatory eye movements in children with hemianopia and lower field defects can be incorporated into interventions by the child's teacher of students with visual impairments and occupational therapist, while teaching cane use and tactile guidance are essential components of O&M instruction. Optical and digital magnification devices are also crucial visual aids for children as well as adults.

## Color Vision

Little is known about color vision in children with CVI. In those affected children who have the ability to perform tests of color vision, no abnormality tends to be found. In the authors' experience, in some children who are unable to perform the tests, their ability to see colors turns out to be a visual strength. Children with CVI may respond better to colored pictures than to black-and-white pictures in picture communication systems. Although anecdotally children with CVI are said to prefer red or yellow objects to other colored objects, the only research study on this topic found that children with CVI had no greater preference for blue, green, yellow, or red stimuli (Cohen-Maitre & Haerich, 2005).

There are, however, situations in which it is useful to assess the ability to see and tell the difference between colors. Between 4 and 8 percent of men and 0.4 percent of women worldwide have difficulty telling the difference between red and green (Birch, 2012), and those affected by CVI are no exception. The best-known tests for this disability are the Ishihara color plates (see the Resources section) and those with similar formats (Dain, 2004). Numbers or patterns made up of specifically colored spots of varying size have to be identified from among other spots with colors chosen to test for impaired red-green discrimination, and the rarer blue-yellow color vision deficit. For patients with acuity no worse than 20/200 and who can accurately identify a circle, the preferred color vision screening tool for young children is Color Vision Testing Made Easy (see the Resources section). To pass, the patient needs to identify a circle (which is present on each of the cards) on at least seven of the nine plates (Cotter, Lee, & French, 1999). False positive results can be obtained as a result of low acuity or simultanagnosia, sometimes making it difficult for the child with CVI to identify the overall picture from among the spots (Brazis, Graff-Radford, Newman, & Lee, 1998). This is when it can be helpful to use the Panel 16 test (see the Resources section) or similar tests that do not have this problem. Panel 16 and similar tests entail matching two sets of paired round colored discs with each other. The results can help determine if the child with CVI has a color vision disorder in the process of assessing his or her functional vision. While children with simultanagnosia may succeed in this type of test, it does require sustained visual attention; poor attention may result in poor performance and inaccurate results. Quantitative, diagnostic color vision tests require specific lighting for accuracy of diagnosis and screening. Thus, if a color vision difficulty is strongly suspected, consider referring the child to an eye care provider for formal testing.

Inability to name colors is the most common scenario in children with CVI and others with developmental delays, and this can be misinterpreted as poor color vision. The Panel 16 test provides a way of showing parents and caregivers that it is color naming rather than disordered color vision that is the cause of the problem. A child who does not yet name colors may be able to match colors of different objects, or different items of clothing, thus demonstrating the difficulty is a result of a language or cognitive difficulty rather than a color vision deficit. Parents and vision educators can make this observation.

## Eye Movements

Our eyes need to be able to move in all directions to search for an object of interest and to lock onto a target (fixate) in order to give attention to a static or moving object. Children with CVI commonly have impaired ability to move the eyes or control them. (This is discussed in detail in Chapter 8.) During an assessment, eye movements and alignment are examined carefully, watched, and interpreted from the start of the initial observation and throughout the evaluation process. (See For Further Reading at the end of this chapter for additional information on eye movements.) Vision educators and others working with this population, such as occupational therapists, to the extent of their training, should observe a student's ability to fixate, track, change fixation, and align his or her eyes.

### Assessment of Eye Movements, Focusing, and Binocular Visual Functions

Formal assessment of eye movements requires a range of illuminated and non-illuminated objects and toys. In a child with CVI, better attention may be given to a familiar rather than a novel toy.

Assessment of eye movements using a moving toy is a good starting procedure because it can be made into a game, performed at what the child feels to be a safe distance, and it can help establish rapport. It addresses the following questions:

- Can each eye fixate and follow an object of interest?
- Can an object be followed by moving the eyes without moving the head?
- Do the eyes work together as a team?
- Do the eyes turn in to focus appropriately?
- How do the findings relate to how the child uses his or her vision?

#### *Fixation*

Fixation is the ability to keep the eyes steady on a target. Give a big smile to the child as the child enters the room. Does the child look at your eyes? Is this maintained as you move your head? This simple, informal procedure not only helps to establish rapport, it gives preliminary information about the child's ability to see and fixate.

Lack of fixation is a serious concern for parents, although the capability may not be identified by that name. "Why does my child not make eye contact with me?" is a common question. Lack of vision in both eyes resulting from refractive error, eye disorders, or CVI is one reason; disordered control of eye movements is another.

Fixation can be assessed as part of the clinical low vision examination and during the functional vision assessment. A penlight, finger puppet, or small toy is held in front of the child, and the evaluator judges the ability of the eyes to move to look at it, as well as the accuracy of the eye movements. Normally the eyes turn and look directly at the target in a single, accurate movement. If the movement is inaccurate, the eyes may have undershot or overshot the toy, with a second move being made to get the eyes on target. If the eyes do not turn and look, there may be impaired eye movement, or vision may be poor or absent. Some children adopt an atypical head or head and eye position, and fixation is assessed with the child's habitual posture, as well as with the head held straight.

If fixation on a simple penlight is poor, the examiner must determine if this is improved by turning the background light down and by cutting out background sound to diminish visual and auditory distractions. Is there a delay in taking up fixation? If so, how long is this, and is the delay diminished by eliminating distractions? If a small fixation target does not bring about fixation, how big does a toy need to be to gain fixation? (Knowing this can provide a guide to the starting point for assessing visual acuity.)

Teachers of students with visual impairments and others working with this population should report what they are using to assess fixation as well as its saliency to the environment. For example, did the child respond better to a novel or a familiar stimulus, or was a dim room with an illuminated target needed? Also, did the child locate or fixate on an object (or person) and was an auditory prompt required for the child to do this?

### *Eye Alignment and Strabismus*

Assessment of ocular alignment requires sufficient vision in each eye for the two pictures sent to the brain to be joined in the mind. (See the discussion of sensory fusion later in this section.) If a patient has such poor vision that he or she cannot locate a penlight or significant object, then precise assessment of eye alignment cannot be made.

If there is an eye turn (strabismus) present, it is important to note whether the eye is turned inward (esotropia) or outward (exotropia), upward (hypertropia) or downward (hypotropia) (see Chapter 8). If the vision educator observes an apparent eye turn that has not been documented by the child's eye doctor, the vision educator should describe the observations, but avoid labeling them with a diagnosis. A complete examination by the eye care provider will be able to diagnose the educator's important observations. (See Sidebar 12.5 for a description of the Hirschberg test to evaluate degree of strabismus.)

The following assessments for strabismus are performed by an eye care provider:

- Is the strabismus constant or intermittent? (For example, strabismus that is present only when tired may be a result of an uncorrected refractive error and indicates that a test for eyeglasses is needed.)

SIDEBAR 12.5

## Hirschberg Test to Evaluate Degree of Strabismus

The Hirschberg test to evaluate degree of strabismus is typically performed by trained eye care personnel, and is based on the following principles:

- When a discrete light source is shown into the eyes, a bright glint is seen reflecting off the front (corneal) surface of each eye.
- The position of the glint is the same in both eyes if they are grossly aligned, but not when there is an obvious strabismus (see Chapter 8).
- The greater the difference in position of the glint in each eye, the greater the degree of strabismus. This Hirschberg test provides a way of seeing and estimating the degree of strabismus without the need for the child to cooperate.

An eye care specialist can perform additional tests to determine a more precise categorization of the type of eye deviation and to explore possible reasons for the eye deviation. If those working with a child in the community observe an asymmetry in the position of the light reflexes in the child's eyes, it should be communicated to the family and eye care provider.

---

- Is the strabismus stable or variable in degree?
- Is the strabismus present when looking at near visual targets as well as when looking into the distance?
- If the viewing eye is covered, does the squinting eye (the eye with the eye turn) move to look at the target? (If not, it is likely to have very poor vision.) When the cover is removed, does the originally squinting eye turn in again, or has the strabismus reversed so the other eye is now squinting? (If it does reverse, the vision in both eyes is nearly equal and the strabismus is said to be alternating.)
- If the eyes are turned inward, does wearing eyeglasses for farsightedness (longsightedness or hyperopia) help straighten the eyes, and if so by how much? (In such children, the eyeglasses improve eye alignment and visual development and need to be worn full time.)

In addition, eye care providers use prisms to measure the angle of the strabismus. A prism bends light. When a prism is placed appropriately in front of a squinting eye, the squint is apparently reduced. The measure (in prism diopters) of the size of the squint is determined by the strength of the prism that makes a squinting eye look straight.

### *Near Point of Convergence*

When one looks at something up close, the eyes turn in so that they both receive the same picture. This is called convergence (see Chapter 8). The ability to converge can be poor in children with CVI. Poor convergence may be an indicator of poor focusing ability and each can cause difficulties when reading.

Convergence is assessed in children whose eyes are aligned normally. To assess convergence, a small object of interest or a penlight is used. The child is asked to look at the target or light that is held approximately 50 cm (20 inches) away. The child is asked what he or she sees. The child should report seeing one light, and the assessor should observe good eye alignment (symmetrical glints or light reflexes in each pupil). The child is told that the light will move toward his or her nose and is asked to say if the light appears double at any point. The light is then slowly brought toward the child while the examiner observes the eyes. The eyes should continuously converge as the light is brought toward the child's nose. Alignment to the light is normally maintained up to 6 cm (about 2.4 inches) from the nose. If alignment is not maintained, then the distance at which the child reports double vision (known as the *break point*) is noted, while the evaluator continues to move the light closer. The light is then slowly moved away until the child reports seeing only one light again (this is called the *recovery*). Both distances are noted. If, as the light is brought toward the child, an eye turn is observed but double vision is not reported, this is because one eye is not seeing at this point; this is called *suppression*. A break at more than 8 cm (or about 3 inches) from the child and a recovery greater than 10 cm (or about 4 inches) away suggests that convergence is deficient, and further investigation is required. (More information can be found in Scheiman & Wick, 2008.) If vision educators and others in the school community find new or abnormal results, referral to the eye care provider is warranted to evaluate and confirm the findings.

### *Sensory Fusion and Stereopsis*

The ability of the mind to join the incoming, slightly disparate images from the two eyes into a single perceived image is called sensory fusion. This ability is impaired when information from one eye cannot reach the brain (such as with a congenital cataract), if a constant unilateral deviation is present, or if a significant difference in refractive status exists. In such instances, the brain learns to suppress information from one eye to ignore discordant information.

If a person looks at a few items on a table in front of him or her and covers one eye, he or she will notice that the scene appears flat. Upon uncovering the eye, the picture regains its three-dimensional appearance. This three-dimensional appearance is called *stereopsis* (see Chapter 8). (A small proportion of typically sighted people do not have stereopsis and are not able to experience this phenomenon.)

Stereopsis is a form of fusion and is apparent when three-dimensional depth is perceived by the brain by combining the images from the two eyes. The further away something is from an individual, the less important stereopsis becomes for judging depth. Thus, stereopsis is typically measured at near; grosser degrees of stereopsis are obtained with farther measurement distances. The poorer the visual acuity, the poorer the degree of stereopsis. With acuity below 20/200, stereopsis is minimal. (For a more detailed discussion of stereopsis, see Steinman, Steinman, & Garzia, 2000.) Sensory fusion is best assessed by the eye care provider.

Stereopsis is measured by the individual looking at images designed to appear three dimensional with both eyes viewing. The difference between the image components seen by each eye is progressively reduced until it is insufficient for the target to be seen three dimensionally. A range of tests is available on the market. The most appropriate tests of stereopsis for the range of children with CVI that are seen in the New England Eye Low Vision Clinic include the following:

- Random Dot E test
- LEA Symbols Stereoacuity Test

- PASS test
- Frisby test
- The Lang stereotest

(See the Resources section at the end of this chapter for more information.)

### Implications of Eye Turns for Functional Vision in Children with CVI

*A constant turn of one eye* results in the eye that is not turned being the preferred eye for detailed vision. It is common in children with CVI. If the eye turn is associated with low vision in the affected eye, the cause is most likely to be "lazy eye," or amblyopia. Treatment, prescribed by the eye care provider, might include daily part-time patching of the preferred (better seeing) eye, or atropine drops in the preferred eye to blur vision. Both are used to increase use and function of the amblyopic eye with poorer vision by increasing input from the non-preferred eye to the visual brain. During the time the preferred eye is being treated, the child's acuity and contrast sensitivity are reduced to the level of the non-preferred eye. For those working with the child in school or in the community, this typically means the child's activities may need to be changed, necessitating the need for a community-based evaluation of function by the vision educator. Some accommodations that might be considered include enlarged materials and preferential seating so that the child can see when the better functioning eye is being covered or blurred using eye drops. The vision educator may also provide input about how to most effectively engage the student with visual-based activities during the periods when the patch is on. (For more information about implications of eye turns for functional vision, see Chapter 8.)

### Nystagmus

Nystagmus is a rhythmic, involuntary oscillation of one or both eyes (Hertle, 2006). The most common association with nystagmus in children with CVI is periventricular leukomalacia (Jacobson & Dutton, 2000). Each of the aspects described below needs to be borne in mind when assessing a child with nystagmus associated with CVI.

When measuring visual acuity with both eyes open, an evaluator may observe the child using a combination of head and eye postures to adopt the "null position" (a position of the eyes, which may be accompanied by a head turn, in which the oscillations of a person's nystagmus are least; see Chapter 8) to minimize the nystagmus. The child's posture when viewing at distance can, for example, be a head turn to the right with the eyes looking left; while at near, the eyes may turn in excessively (esotropia), resulting from overconvergence of the eyes that also reduces the nystagmus and lends clarity to the near vision.

Individuals with nystagmus typically choose their null positions, especially when looking at something that is small and difficult to see at distance or near, or when maintaining focused vision for an extended period of time. It is not unusual for the child with a null position to maintain it while following an object of interest; to do so, the child moves his or her head rather than the eyes. Scanning the scene while moving around tends to involve moving the head more than the eyes. Other functional concerns include variability in the ability to sustain a visually demanding task; this may explain difficulty maintaining comprehension when reading.

Magnification aids, line guides, and audio-based options may be useful to relieve the visual demands of academic work for children with nystagmus. At near, some children overconverge their eyes to reduce the nystagmus. If the child is using this approach at near, and this results in near acuity that is significantly better than acuity at distance, then viewing a distant scene by means of the screen of a digital camera and zooming in may provide a clearer view into the distance. This is worth evaluating.

Providing a sharp image for individuals with nystagmus with an appropriate, full-time spectacle correction is of critical importance to maximize visual acuity, visual attention, and the ability to sustain the use of vision. Individuals with nystagmus will probably read best by holding their eyes in the null position and moving either the page, or their head, to read across the page. Some small amount of refixating and fast eye movements (saccades) may be noted as well. It does not make sense for eye care specialists or vision teachers to train scanning and tracking in the same manner as they would for someone without nystagmus; as the eyes move away from the null point, the frequency and amplitude of the nystagmus increases and the acuity decreases. Prismatic spectacles with special lenses that shift the images in both eyes to help move the null point to the center can aid management of the child with nystagmus, but can also disorient children with CVI. A tentative prescription is always tested and modified as necessary for the best balance of maximum improvement in head, body, and eye position with movement through space, as well as hand-eye coordination. Horizontal nystagmus tends to cause more blur horizontally than vertically, and vertical control of eye movement may be better. For this reason a minority of children choose to read vertically (rotating the page 90 degrees sideways so that the lines of text go up and down the page; see Chapter 3 and Figure 3.2), and testing the speed of vertical reading in comparison with horizontal—bearing in mind that the child has not done this before—warrants consideration in high-functioning children.

Practitioners can work on improving the efficiency and accuracy of the child's use of his or her eyes in combination with either the head or hands. For example, a child might prefer to move the book in free space or on an X-Y table under the video magnifier. Or a child may hold the reading material still and move the head to move the eyes across the page or screen. Moving both the head and text is typically too difficult to sustain without loss of place or fatigue. The clinic team at New England Eye Low Vision Clinic at Perkins prefers a uniform approach to the training of scanning, which can be reinforced by the mobility instructor, vision teacher, classroom teacher, and parents. As we read English print from left to right and from the top down, this strategy is advised for both classroom tasks as well as for orienting at distance. The direction of scanning is adapted for children who read in other language formats. Scanning and moving the finger along lines of small images and numbers may be a useful exercise that can be set up as a "game." This approach is a starting point from which modifications may be necessary for individuals with field loss or other issues.

### *Pursuit Eye Movements and Saccades*

The ability to continuously watch and follow a moving target is known as *pursuit eye movement.* A target, such as the one used to assess fixation, is smoothly moved away from the point of central fixation to left, right, up, and down, and obliquely in all directions of gaze. Jerking eye movements and lack of eye movement, compensated for by head movements instead, are the features to look for. As already noted, children with nystagmus who have a preferred head and eye position may not follow objects without using the head. (In young children, movement of the head normally accompanies pursuit eye movements, but this diminishes to become minimal by age 7 (Maples & Ficklin, 1988). Whether the child is assessed in the clinic or in the community, the type of target, speed of movement, and surrounding illumination may affect the child's ability to fix and follow and is important to note as it has functional consequences for the child. *Saccades,* or fast eye movements (see Chapter 8), are initially assessed simply by watching the child as he or she looks from one item to another around the room. What the child looks at, and how small the items are, as well as the frequency and accuracy of the eye movements, gives useful information about how well the child can see and whether or not the movements are within normal parameters. The target is then held centrally and a second target is introduced in succession to the right, left, above, and below the central target, and the child is asked to look from the central target to each eccentric location. Saccades can be delayed, inappropriate, or inaccurate, with the eye movements overshooting or undershooting the target, followed by a second movement to target. In the assessment, note not only the targets and environment and how they affect performance, but also the approximate distance between the targets.

### The Natural Eye Movements of Balance (Doll's Eye or Labyrinthine Eye Movements)

Eye movements of balance—the doll's eye reflex or labyrinthine eye movements—are completely automatic. When a person tips his or her head in total darkness, the balance system automatically rotates the eyes to look to the horizon (if it were visible). This automatic righting system of the eyes works in tandem with the automatic righting system of the body and allows us to remain erect, but can be deficient in children with the type of cerebral palsy that is dyskinetic, with poor control of body movement.

Normally, as the head moves, the eyes are stabilized, but in some children with CVI and cerebral palsy, this stabilization is likely impaired, probably with associated blurring of vision (G. N. Dutton, personal communication, April 2013). Testing for dysfunction of these eye movements is best left for those with specialized training (such as neuro-ophthalmologists and other health care providers).

## Refractive Errors

Refractive errors and accommodation, discussed in detail in Chapter 9, are best assessed by a qualified eye care provider, as are tests to determine whether a child needs eyeglasses. (See also the section on Visual Acuity in this chapter.)

## Learning Media Assessment

In addition to assessment of visual functions and functional vision, a learning media assessment is appropriate for any individual with a visual impairment. A learning media assessment evaluates optimal access to auditory, tactile, as well as visual information and can be worthwhile to determine the potential productive use of additional senses for learning (Koenig & Holbrook, 1995).

Functional vision assessments, as well as the results of the clinical evaluation, provide important basic information that can be used as part of this process to determine the most appropriate learning media for students who have visual impairments. See Chapter 15 for detailed consideration of how functional vision and learning media assessments are used to determine the selection of appropriate literacy media.

## Observations of Visual-Motor, Visual Perceptual, and Social Skills

Some children with CVI have a range of additional sensory, physical, and cognitive difficulties. Visual-motor and visual perceptual skills may be compromised, and CVI can also interfere with a child's developing social skills. During the clinical low vision examination and functional vision assessment by educators, observations of visual-motor, visual perceptual, and social skills can be noted and reported. Referrals to additional specialists can be made for more in-depth evaluation as needed. Further information about visual processing skills related to higher order visual functions can be found in Chapters 6, 7, and 13.

### Visual-Motor Skills

The visual-motor skills of greatest concern in relation to CVI in young children include those that can be observed when reaching and pointing, shape fitting (as in puzzles), stacking blocks, and stringing beads. Although accuracy of reaching and pointing is important, the focus of interest is on the child's coordination of gaze while reaching/pointing and interacting with objects. Does the child look at the object as he or she reaches for it, or look away before reaching, or glance at the object and then look away? Lack of coordination between visual gaze and motor actions is almost a hallmark of CVI in the young child. Some children with CVI will feel things presented to them before looking at them.

Also observed is the child's ability to effectively use the hand and fingers; whether they are able to grasp and hold an object, how they fit shapes into a puzzle, how accurately they reach for and stack objects, and how they use their vision for hand-eye coordination tasks such as stringing large beads on a thick string.

Children with severe developmental delays and poor neuromuscular control (cerebral palsy) may not have the motor control to point or even reach, although many can touch objects or images with the whole hand, with assistance if needed. Objects placed low in the child's visual field may not be seen because of a lower field defect or the child's head control may be too poor to shift head and eyes down. Placement of material on a raised, slanted surface may be tried if head control is poor. The child is closely observed for gaze direction: is it toward the object or image as their hand touches? Do they keep their gaze away from the hand and object?

With the recent advances in digital devices, tablet apps are particularly helpful for informal assessment of young patients' functional vision (see Appendix 18A to Chapter 18 regarding use of technology devices). Cause-effect apps (in which a child receives immediate feedback for an action, such as on-screen "fireworks" that appear immediately after a child taps the touch screen) are very useful for children who have severe cognitive delays. Questions to be asked include: How accurate is the child's touch on the screen? Does the child make a connection between touch and action? Do sounds distract or enhance responses? Do children visually attend as they touch the screen? Writing and drawing apps on a tablet are also used as they are very appealing to children, have multiple colored options, and allow for multiple attempts and saved images of writing or drawing attempts.

### Visual Perceptual Abilities

The visual perceptual abilities of young children and children who have major cognitive challenges are screened by observing the child's gaze at single objects, shifts of gaze between objects, and whether preferences are shown among several alternating presentations (also an indicator of short-term memory). Two-dimensional pictures are presented, usually from simple, colorful picture books, and the examiner can observe whether and how the child scans the images, whether the child fixates on them, and whether he or she attends to the most salient components (such as a baby's face). Children who are capable are asked to show or point to named pictures of features (such as the eyes or mouth on a baby's face). Children who can name things are asked "What is the baby doing?" in a photo book showing various baby activities.

Regarding the tablet apps, the images the child attends to, both simple and complex, are noted, as well as whether the child maintains gaze on the images while touching them. Shape and color matching and identification can be assessed during motor tasks. However, there are now apps that informally allow assessment of these more complex visual functions.

The more subtle disorders of visual perception tend not to be immediately evident unless structured history taking leads to a direct search for more details about the specific disabilities uncovered and further assessments take place (see Chapters 6, 10, 11, and 13). Over time and through interprofessional collaboration and report sharing, more subtle but important perceptual issues tend to emerge.

### Social Attention

Social attention for young children and children with major cognitive challenges can be examined by observing whether, when, and how the child makes eye contact with the examiner. Children with the more severe forms of CVI often avoid eye contact or social interaction with the examiner until well into the session. Young children may be shown a large mirror, and whether they look at their own image and the image of the person holding them is noted (for example, if they ask, "Where's Mommy?" as they look in the mirror).

## Examination Results and Recommendations

This chapter has focused on the clinical low vision evaluation of visual function and functional vision for children who have CVI, as well as features that can be incorporated into a functional vision assessment by educators. This section covers the delivery of results and recommendations following a clinical low vision assessment for children who have CVI. Educators need to know what to expect as a result of a clinical low vision evaluation and how to effectively incorporate these results into programs for children and families. (Information about ways to report assessment results conducted by educators to families and other professionals can be found in Chapter 10.)

After a clinical low vision assessment, observations and findings need to be discussed with the family and others attending the examination, such as the child's teacher of students with visual impairments. Many parents are anxious and ultimately want to hear good news but may be steeling themselves for more bad news. The discussion with the parents should initially try to focus on concrete things that were accomplished and things that the child handled well or did well. Noting the child's improvement from the previous exam is a positive start. Then, discussion regarding the key findings and observations should ensue. In both speaking with the family and in the written notes, it is very important not to blame the child when certain measures could not be obtained. The examiner might note, for example, "The examiners were unable to successfully engage the child" rather than "the child was uncooperative or untestable." Using the host/guest analogy again, it is the host's job to make sure that the guests have a good time, not the other way around. Shifting the responsibility for success to the care team rather than to the child or parents will likely be greatly appreciated by the family and others present for the examination.

Recommendations are based on the initial concerns, the results of the examination (both the functional vision components, as well as the actual clinical vision function data such as, but not limited to, visual acuity, contrast sensitivity, and visual field test results), and the evaluators' understanding of some of the issues facing the child at his or her age and developmental level with respect to any motor and cognitive impairments. Recommendations are often made relating to computer access for writing as well as learning to read and reading tasks. Eyeglasses to correct a refractive error or to compensate for an eye turn or null point, low vision devices, possible treatment of amblyopia, and other general ocular health issues are discussed and prescribed, if appropriate, and accepted by the child and parents. The need for community-based assessments of functional vision (by the teacher of students with visual impairments) and evaluation of the environment and mobility (by an O&M specialist), along with some suggestions regarding accommodations prior to these assessments are also provided.

For children with reduced best-corrected acuity or reduced field, the data and observations made during the evaluation and information gleaned from the other reports is used to discuss a treatment plan that requires action or follow-up (such as follow-up on a device or spectacles, review of a CVI screening tool, or additional testing), or to request or advocate for other services. The latter often include the need for the vision educator or other specialist to conduct further evaluations, or the possibility of direct service to aid with the training and utilization of a magnifier or a monocular telescope. Referrals, as needed, for other services such as occupational or physical therapy or augmented communication services are made. Referrals to other eye care or medical specialists may also be recommended.

It can be emotionally difficult for the eye care specialist and family members to discuss issues concerning the visual impairment-to-blindness continuum. Many parents who are relatively new to the world of visual impairment are not sure what "blindness" means. Some think it means a complete lack of vision. If the family members state that the chief reason for the appointment is to understand their child's vision and possibly register with a blindness agency, it is imperative that the professional gently probe what the family understands regarding how their child uses vision as well as their understanding of the term "blindness," both in the social and the legal context. This information, and a sense of where the family is in their understanding and emotional readiness with regard to the child's condition, are obtained throughout the assessment of the child so that the ultimate discussion at the end of the exam can be positive, practical, and coherent, with the hope of minimizing the emotional elements.

After describing positive attributes of the exam and findings, there should be a discussion of the visual continuum (20/20 vision through light perception and visual field information, as needed) directed to the legal definition of blindness (see Chapter 1) and their child's status in relation to that definition. In spite of all of these efforts and the apparent education and acceptance by parents of their child's use of and level of vision, hearing the eye care specialist use the term *blindness* as a descriptor for their child, even if it is modified as "*legal* blindness," can be quite emotional for some families. Other parents may have already reconciled themselves to this diagnosis and are ready to take full advantage of the label and use it to maximize receipt of needed services. Referral, as needed, to various parent vision groups, agencies, or local affiliates of organizations is provided. Given the underlying diagnosis (such as cerebral visual impairment) and the age of the patient, it may be relevant to discuss the need and benefits of registering the child sooner rather than later to obtain government or educational services. Should findings change over time such that the child no longer meets the definition of legal blindness or visual impairment required to obtain services, then a discussion regarding removal of that label can be included, as well as the role of the clinic in the ongoing care of the child.

How frequently a child needs to be seen for follow-up care is also discussed with the family. Factors to consider include the level of information obtained at the initial examination, the need for additional testing by others (medical or educational professionals), the medical stability of the child, proximity in time to key transition points (such as the transition from early intervention to preschool), the ability of the local eye care physician to obtain information from the child, and the need for follow-up on devices dispensed. An attempt to find common ground for the timing of future meaningful and constructive visits is pursued.

## Conclusion

Individuals with visual impairment need care and services as soon as the suspicion of visual impairment is confirmed. The teacher of students with visual impairments or early intervention vision specialist may need support to document observations and to help prioritize the approach to engaging vision both at a basic level and for the performance of more complex visual tasks as time passes. Early identification and prescription of spectacles for refractive error, compensation of an eye turn, or for null point are substantial interventions that can have a dramatic impact on function. Further, issues regarding contrast and complexity can be addressed among the eye care specialist, vision educator, and family. Knowledge of how the child is operating in space can aid in determining the need for a bifocal versus a single-vision lens. Later on, as gross and fine motor skills are developed, consideration can be given to providing bifocals or multiple pairs of eyeglasses. Special prism glasses may also be considered for individuals with visual field impairment or neglect.

As children approach school age and have the requisite visual-motor skills, optical or electronic magnification devices can be considered for both academic and nonacademic tasks. It is important for children to feel comfortable using devices for activities of daily life rather than just in the classroom. They also need support in using these devices, both at home and in school. In lower grade levels, use of a video magnifier as a learning center in the classroom is often suggested, so that the child's classmates can benefit and appreciate the device. Use of computers and tablets is also discussed when relevant.

As the child's needs change, academic or otherwise, advocacy for these new tasks and school and life goals, and the eye care provider's role in reaching these goals are explored. It is also critically important to respect the decisions of the child. Children are told that there are many devices and approaches ("toys in the toy box," so to speak), and if they appreciate what a device is doing but think that it is ugly or that there is no way they want to be seen in public with it, then alternative ways to accomplish the specific task as independently as possible are explored.

Finally, as students begin to plan for life after high school, it is important that their potential needs are considered proactively. This may include demonstration of various devices that might be beneficial for them in the community. In this process, ongoing communication with the family, vision educators, and most importantly with the students themselves, are necessary to best prepare for and meet their needs in a timely and appropriate fashion.

## For Further Reading

### General Information about Functional Vision Assessment for Educators


Chen, D. (Ed.). (2014). *Essential elements in early intervention: Visual and multiple disabilities* (2nd ed.). New York: AFB Press.

Corn, A. L., & Erin, J. N. (Eds.). (2010). *Foundations of low vision: Clinical and functional perspectives* (2nd ed.). New York: AFB Press.

Lueck, A. H. (Ed.). (2004). *Functional vision: A practitioner's guide to evaluation and intervention.* New York: AFB Press.


## Technical Reference Texts


Anderson, D. R. (1987). *Perimetry: With and without automation* (2nd ed.). St. Louis, MO: C.V. Mosby.

Ciuffreda, K. J., & Tannen, B. (1995). *Eye movement basics for the clinician.* St. Louis, MO: Mosby-Yearbook.

Hoyt, C. S., & Taylor, D. (2013). *Pediatric ophthalmology and strabismus* (4th ed.). Philadelphia: Elsevier Saunders.

Leigh, R. J., & Zee, D. S. (2006). *The neurology of eye movements* (4th ed.). New York: Oxford University Press.

Scheiman, M., & Wick, B. (2008). *Clinical management of binocular vision: Heterophoric, accommodative and eye movement disorders* (3rd ed.). Philadelphia: Lippincott.

Steinman, S. B., Steinman, B. A., & Garzia, R. P. (2000). *Foundations of binocular vision: A clinical perspective.* New York: McGraw-Hill Medical.

Weissberg, E. (2004). *Essentials of clinical binocular vision.* St. Louis, MO: Elsevier Science.

Wong, A. M. F. (2008). *Eye movement disorders.* New York: Oxford University Press.

Wright, K. W., Spiegel, P. H, & Thompson, L. S. (Eds.). (2006). *Handbook of pediatric neuro-*

*ophthalmology.* New York, NY: Springer Science+Business Media, Inc.

## References


Adoh, T. O., & Woodhouse, J. M. (1994). The Cardiff Acuity Test used for measuring visual acuity development in toddlers. *Vision Research, 34*(4), 555–560.

American Printing House for the Blind. (2012). *New APH federal quota census facilitates the inclusion of students with cortical visual impairment (CVI).* Louisville, KY: Author. Retrieved September 13, 2014, from http://www.aph.org/cvi/quota.html

Anderson, D. R. (1987). *Perimetry: With and without automation* (2nd ed.). St. Louis, MO: C.V. Mosby.

Arditi, A. (2004). Selecting fonts for readers with low vision. In A. H. Lueck (Ed.), *Functional vision: A practitioner's guide to evaluation and intervention* (pp. 419–421). New York: AFB Press.

Arditi, A. (2005). Improving the design of the letter contrast sensitivity test. *Investigative Ophthalmology & Visual Science, 46*(6), 2225–2229.

Bailey, I. L., Lueck, A. H., Greer, R., Tuan, K. M., Bailey, V. M., & Dornbusch, H. G. (2003). Understanding the relationships between print size and reading in low vision. *Journal of Visual Impairment & Blindness, 97*(6), 325–334.

Birch, J. (2012). Worldwide prevalence of red-green color deficiency. *Journal of the Optical Society of America A: Optics, Image Science, and Vision, 29*(3), 313–320.

Boyle, N. J., Jones, D. H., Hamilton, R., Spowart, K. M., & Dutton, G. N. (2005). Blindsight in children: Does it exist and can it be used to help the child? Observations on a case series. *Developmental Medicine & Child Neurology, 47*(10), 699–702.

Brazis, P. W., Graff-Radford, N. R., Newman, N. J., & Lee, A. G. (1998). Ishihara color plates as a test for simultanagnosia. *American Journal of Ophthalmology, 126*(6), 850–851.

Charman, W. N. (2006). Spatial frequency content of the Cardiff and related acuity tests. *Ophthalmic and Physiological Optics, 26*(1), 5–12.

Cohen-Maitre, S. A., & Haerich, P. (2005). Visual attention to movement and color in children with cortical visual impairment. *Journal of Visual Impairment & Blindness, 99*(7), 389–402.

Colenbrander, A. (2010). Towards the development of a classification of vision-related functioning—A potential framework. In G. N. Dutton & M. Bax (Eds.), *Visual impairment in children due to damage to the brain* (pp. 282–294). London: Mac Keith Press.

Corn, A. L., & Erin, J. N. (Eds.). (2010). *Foundations of low vision: Clinical and functional perspectives* (2nd ed.). New York: AFB Press.

Cotter, S. A., Lee, D. Y., & French, A. L. (1999). Evaluation of a new color vision test: "Color vision testing made easy." *Optometry and Vision Science, 76*(9), 631–639.

Dain, S. J. (2004). Clinical colour vision tests. *Clinical and Experimental Optometry, 87*(4–5), 276–293.

Dobson, V., Mayer, D. L., & Candy, T. R. (2009). *Teller Acuity Cards II (TAC II).* Chicago: Stereo Optical Company, Inc.

Dougherty, B. E., Flom, R. E., & Bullimore, M. A. (2005). An evaluation of the Mars Letter Contrast Sensitivity Test. *Optometry and Vision Science, 82*(11), 970–975.

Drover, J. R., Wyatt, L. M., Stager, D. R., & Birch, E. E. (2009). The Teller Acuity Cards are effective in detecting amblyopia. *Optometry and Vision Science, 86*(6), 755–759.

Dutton, G. N. (2013). The spectrum of cerebral visual impairment as a sequel to premature birth: An overview. *Documenta Ophthalmologica, 127*(1), 69–78.

Dutton, G. N., Calvert, J., Ibrahim, H., MacDonald, E., McCulloch, D. L., Macintyre-Béon, C., et al. (2010). Structured clinical history-taking for cognitive and perceptual visual dysfunction and for profound visual disabilities due to damage to the brain in children. In G. N. Dutton & M. Bax (Eds.), *Visual impairment in children due to damage to the brain* (pp. 117–128). London: Mac Keith Press.

Dutton, G. N., Saeed, A., Fahad, B., Fraser, R., McDaid, G., McDade, J., . . . Spowart, K. (2004).

Association of binocular lower visual field impairment, impaired simultaneous perception, disordered visually guided motion and inaccurate saccades in children with cerebral visual dysfunction—A retrospective observational study. *Eye, 18*(1), 27–34.

Elliott, D. B., Bullimore, M. A., & Bailey, I. L. (1991). Improving the reliability of the Pelli-Robson contrast sensitivity test. *Clinical Vision Sciences, 6*(6), 471–475.

Fulton, A. B., Hansen, R. M., Moskowitz, A., & Mayer, D. L. (2013). Normal and abnormal visual development. In C. S. Hoyt & D. Taylor (Eds.), *Pediatric ophthalmology and strabismus* (4th ed., pp. 23–30). Philadelphia: Elsevier Saunders.

Geer, I., & Westall, C. A. (1996). A comparison of tests to determine acuity deficits in children with amblyopia. *Ophthalmic and Physiological Optics, 16*(5), 367–374.

Ginsburg, A. P. (1984). A new contrast sensitivity vision test chart. *American Journal of Optometry and Physiological Optics, 61*(6), 403–407.

Ginsburg, A. P. (1996). Next generation contrast sensitivity testing. In B. Rosenthal & R. Cole (Eds.), *Functional assessment of low vision* (pp. 77–88). St. Louis, MO: Mosby Year Book, Inc.

Good, W. V., & Hou, C. (2006). Sweep visual evoked potential grating acuity thresholds paradoxically improve in low-luminance conditions in children with cortical visual impairment. *Investigative Ophthalmology & Visual Science, 47*(7), 3220–3224.

Good, W. V., Hou, C., & Norcia, A. M. (2012). Spatial contrast sensitivity vision loss in children with cortical visual impairment. *Investigative Ophthalmology & Visual Science, 53*(12), 7730–7734.

Greer, R. (2004). Evaluation methods and functional implications: Children and adults with visual impairments. In A. H. Lueck (Ed.), *Functional vision: A practitioner's guide to evaluation and intervention* (pp. 177–253). New York: AFB Press.

Haegerstrom-Portnoy, G. (2004). Evaluation of young children. In A. H. Lueck (Ed.), *Functional vision: A practitioner's guide to evaluation and intervention* (pp. 115–154). New York: AFB Press.

Hamilton, R., Bradnam, M. S., Dutton, G. N., Lai Chooi Yan, A. L., Lavy, T. E., Livingstone, I., . . . Mackinnon, J. R. (2013). Sensitivity and specificity of the step VEP in suspected functional visual acuity loss. *Documenta Ophthalmologica, 126*(2), 99–104.

Hargadon, D. D., Wood, J., Twelker, J. D., Harvey, E. M., & Dobson, V. (2010). Recognition acuity, grating acuity, contrast sensitivity, and visual fields in 6-year-old children. *Archives of Ophthalmology, 128*(1), 70–74.

Harvey, E. M., Dobson, V., & Narter, D. B. (1997). The influence of a central stimulus on visual field measurements in children from 3.5 to 30 months of age. *Optometry and Vision Science, 74*(9), 768–774.

Harvey, E. M., Dobson, V., Tung, B., Quinn, G. E., & Hardy, R. E. (1999). Interobserver agreement for grating acuity and letter acuity assessment in 1- to 5.5-year-olds with severe retinopathy of prematurity. *Investigative Ophthalmology & Visual Science, 40*(7), 1565–1576.

Haymes, S. A., & Chen, J. (2004). Reliability and validity of the Melbourne Edge Test and High/Low Contrast Visual Acuity chart. *Optometry and Vision Science, 81*(5), 308–316.

Hertle, R. W. (2006). Nystagmus and ocular oscillations in infancy and childhood. In K. W. Wright, P. H. Spiegel, & L. Thompson (Eds.), *Handbook of pediatric neuro-ophthalmology* (pp. 289–323). New York: Springer Science+Business Media, Inc.

Hoyt, C. S., & Taylor, D. (2013). *Pediatric ophthalmology and strabismus* (4th ed.). Philadelphia: Elsevier Saunders.

Huo, R., Burden, S. K., Hoyt, C. S., & Good, W. V. (1999). Chronic cortical visual impairment in children: Aetiology, prognosis, and associated neurological deficits. *British Journal of Ophthalmology, 83*(6), 670–675.

Hyvärinen, L., & Jacob, N. (2011). *WHAT and HOW does this child see?* Helsinki, Finland: VISTEST Ltd.

Hyvärinen, L., Näsänen, R., & Laurinen, P. (1980). New visual acuity test for pre-school children. *Acta Ophthalmologica (Copenhagen), 58*(4), 507–511.

Jacobson, L. K., & Dutton, G. N. (2000). Periventricular leukomalacia: An important cause of visual and ocular motility dysfunction in children. *Survey of Ophthalmology, 45*(1), 1–13.

Johnson, C., Kran, B. S., Deng, L., & Mayer, D. L. (2009). Teller II and Cardiff acuity testing in a school-age deaf blind population. *Optometry and Vision Science, 86*(3), 188–195.

Kerr, N. M., Chew, S. S., Eady, E. K., Gamble, G. D., & Danesh-Meyer, H. V. (2010). Diagnostic accuracy of confrontation visual field tests. *Neurology, 74*(15), 1184–1190.

Koenig, A. J., & Holbrook, M. C. (1995). *Learning media assessment of students with visual impairments: A resource guide for teachers.* Austin: Texas School for the Blind and Visually Impaired.

Kran, B. S., & Wright, D. W. (2008). A telephone survey of low vision services in U.S. schools for the blind and visually impaired. *Optometry—Journal of the American Optometric Association, 79*(7), 378–390.

Leat, S. J., & Wegmann, D. (2004). Clinical testing of contrast sensitivity in children: Age-related norms and validity. *Optometry and Vision Science, 81*(4), 245–254.

Leat, S. J., & Woo, G. C. (1997). The validity of current clinical tests of contrast sensitivity and their ability to predict reading speed in low vision. *Eye, 11*(Pt 6), 893–899.

Legge, G. E., Ross, J. A., Isenberg, L. M., & LaMay, J. M. (1992). Psychophysics of reading: Clinical predictors of low-vision reading speed. *Investigative Ophthalmology & Vision Science, 33*(3), 677–687.

Legge, G. E., Ross, J. A., Luebker, A., & LaMay, J. (1989). Psychophysics of reading: VIII, the Minnesota low-vision reading test. *Optometry and Vision Science, 66*, 843–853.

Lim, M., Soul, J. S., Hansen, R. M., Mayer, D. L., Moskowitz, A., & Fulton, A. B. (2005). Development of visual acuity in children with cerebral visual impairment. *Archives of Ophthalmology, 123*(9), 1215–1220.

Lovie-Kitchin, J. E., Mainstone, J. C., Robinson, J., & Brown, B. (1990). What areas of the visual field are important for mobility in low vision patients? *Clinical Vision Sciences, 5*(3), 249–263.

Lowery, J. P., Hayes, J. R., Sis, M., Griffith, A., & Taylor, D. (2014). Pacific Acuity Test: Testability, validity, and interobserver reliability. *Optometry and Vision Science, 91*(1), 76–85.

Lueck, A. H. (2004). Comprehensive low vision care. In A. H. Lueck (Ed.), *Functional vision: A practitioner's guide to evaluation and intervention* (pp. 3–24). New York: AFB Press.

Lueck, A. H. & Bailey, I. L. (in press). *Decision-making: A guide to print size selection.* Louisville, KY: American Printing House for the Blind.

Macintyre-Béon, C., Young, D., Calvert, J., Ibrahim, H., Dutton, G. N., & Bowman, R. (2012). Reliability of a question inventory for structured history taking in children with cerebral visual impairment. *Eye, 26*(10), 1393.

Maples, W. C., & Ficklin, T. W. (1988). Interrater and test-retest reliability of pursuits and saccades. *Optometry—Journal of the American Optometric Association, 59*(7), 549–552.

Mash, C., & Dobson, V. (2005). Intraobserver reliability of the Teller Acuity Card procedure in infants with perinatal complications. *Optometry and Vision Science, 82*(9), 817–822.

Mayer, D. L. (n.d.a). *Visual field loss in children.* Watertown, MA: New England Eye Low Vision Clinic at Perkins. Retrieved from http://www.perkins.org/assets/downloads/low-vision-clinic/handout-visual-field-loss-child-rev1-31-11.pdf

Mayer, D. L. (n.d.b). *Visual field loss in infants.* Watertown: MA: New England Eye Low Vision Clinic at Perkins. Retrieved from http://www.perkins.org/assets/downloads/low-vision-clinic/handout-visual-field-loss-in-infants-rev-1-31-11.pdf

Mayer, D. L., Beiser, A. S., Warner, A. F., Pratt, E. M., Raye, K. N., & Lang, J. M. (1995). Monocular acuity norms for the Teller Acuity Cards between ages one month and four years. *Investigative Ophthalmology & Visual Science, 36*(3), 671–685.

Mayer, D. L., & Fulton, A. B. (1993). Development of the human visual field. In K. Simons (Ed.), *Early visual development: Normal and abnormal* (pp. 117–129). New York: Oxford University Press.

Mayer, D. L., & Fulton, A. B. (2005). Visual fields. In C. S. Hoyt & D. Taylor (Eds.), *Pediatric ophthalmology and strabismus* (3rd ed., pp. 78–86). London: Elsevier Science Ltd.

Mayer, D. L., Fulton, A. B., & Cummings, M. F. (1988). Visual fields of infants assessed with a new perimetric technique. *Investigative Ophthalmology & Visual Science, 29*(3), 452–459.

Mayer, D. L., Fulton, A. B., & Hansen, R. M. (1985). Visual acuity of infants and children with retinal degenerations. *Ophthalmic Pediatrics and Genetics, 5*(1–2), 51–56.

Mayer, D. L., Fulton, A. B., & Rodier, D. (1984). Grating and recognition acuities of pediatric patients. *Ophthalmology, 91*(8), 947–953.

McDonald, M. A., Dobson, V., Sebris, S. L., Baitch, L., Varner, D., & Teller, D. Y. (1985). The acuity card procedure: A rapid test of infant acuity. *Investigative Ophthalmology & Visual Science, 26*(8), 1158–1162.

McKee, S. P., Levi, D. M., & Movshon, J. A. (2003). The pattern of visual deficits in amblyopia. *Journal of Vision, 3*(5), 380–405.

Milner, A. D., & McIntosh, R. D. (2005). The neurological basis of visual neglect. *Current Opinion in Neurology, 18*(6), 748–753.

Owsley, C. (2003). Contrast sensitivity. *Ophthalmology Clinics of North America, 16*(2), 171–177.

Pelli, D. G., Robson, J. G., & Wilkins, A. J. (1988). The design of a new letter chart for measuring contrast sensitivity. *Clinical Vision Sciences, 2*(3), 187–199.

Pesudovs, K., Hazel, C. A., Doran, R. M. L., & Elliott, D. B. (2004). The usefulness of Vistech and FACT contrast sensitivity charts for cataract and refractive surgery outcomes research. *British Journal of Ophthalmology, 88*(1), 11–16.

Pouget, M.-C., Levy-Bencheton, D., Prost, M., Tilikete, C., Husain, M., & Jacquin-Courtois, S. (2012). Acquired visual field defects rehabilitation: Critical review and perspectives. *Annals of Physical and Rehabilitation Medicine, 55*(1), 53–74.

Quinn, G. E., Dobson, V., Hardy, R. J., Tung, B., Palmer, E. A., Good, W. V., et al. (2011). Visual field extent at 6 years of age in children who had high-risk prethreshold retinopathy of prematurity. *Archives of Ophthalmology, 129*(2), 127–132.

Quinn, G. E., Dobson, V., Hardy, R. J., Tung, B., Phelps, D. L., & Palmer, E. A. (1996). Visual fields measured with double-arc perimetry in eyes with threshold retinopathy of prematurity from the cryotherapy for retinopathy of prematurity trial. *Ophthalmology, 103*(9), 1432–1437.

Ramrattan, R. S., Wolfs, R. C., Panda-Jonas, S., Jonas, J. B., Bakker, D., Pols, H. A., . . . de Jong, P. T. (2001). Prevalence and causes of visual field loss in the elderly and associations with impairment in daily functioning: The Rotterdam study. *Archives of Ophthalmology, 119*(12), 1788–1794.

Roman-Lantzy, C. (2007). *Cortical visual impairment: An approach to assessment and intervention.* New York: AFB Press.

Rubin, G. S., Ng, E. S. W., Bandeen-Roche, K., Keyl, P. M., Freeman, E. E., & West, S. K. (2007). A prospective, population-based study of the role of visual Impairment in motor vehicle crashes among older drivers: The SEE study. *Investigative Ophthalmology & Visual Science, 48*(4), 1483–1491.

Scheiman, M., & Wick, B. (2008). *Clinical management of binocular vision: Heterophoric, accommodative, and eye movement disorders* (3rd ed.). Philadelphia: Lippincott.

Scher, M. S., Dobson, V., Carpenter, N. A., & Guthrie, R. D. (1989). Visual and neurological outcome of infants with periventricular leukomalacia. *Developmental Medicine & Child Neurology, 31*(3), 353–365.

Shahinfar, S., Johnson, L. N., & Madsen, R. W. (1995). Confrontation visual field loss as a function of decibel sensitivity loss on automated static perimetry. Implications on the accuracy of confrontation visual field testing. *Ophthalmology, 102*(6), 872–877.

Sharma, P., Bairagi, D., Sachdeva, M. M., Kaur, K., Khokhar, S., & Saxena, R. (2003). Comparative evaluation of Teller and Cardiff acuity tests in normals and unilateral amblyopes in under-two-years-olds. *Indian Journal of Ophthalmology, 51*(4), 341–345.

Steinman, S. B., Steinman, B. A., & Garzia, R. P. (2000). *Foundations of binocular vision: A clinical perspective.* New York: McGraw-Hill Medical.

Teller, D. Y. (1997). First glances: The vision of infants. The Friedenwald lecture. *Investigative Ophthalmology & Visual Science, 38*(11), 2183–2203.

Tinelli, F., Cicchini, G. M., Arrighi, R., Tosetti, M., Cioni, G., & Morrone, C. (2013). Blindsight in children with congenital and acquired cerebral lesions. *Cortex, 49*(6), 1636–1647.

Ting, D. S., Pollock, A., Dutton, G. N., Doubal, F. N., Ting, D. S., Thompson, M., et al. (2011). Visual neglect following stroke: Current concepts and future focus. *Survey of Ophthalmology, 56*(2), 114–134.

Trauner, D. A. (2003). Hemispatial neglect in young children with early unilateral brain damage. *Developmental Medicine & Child Neurology, 45*(3), 160–166.

Trauzettel-Klosinski, S. (2011a). Current methods of visual rehabilitation. *Deutsches Ärzteblatt International, 108*(51–52), 871–878.

Trauzettel-Klosinski, S. (2011b). Rehabilitative techniques. *Handbook of Clinical Neurology, 102*, 263–278.

Turano, K. A., Broman, A. T., Bandeen-Roche, K., Munoz, B., Rubin, G. S., & West, S. K. (2004). Association of visual field loss and mobility performance in older adults: Salisbury eye evaluation study. *Optometry and Vision Science, 81*(5), 298–307.

Van Hof-van Duin, J., Cioni, G., Bertuccelli, B., Fazzi, B., Romano, C., & Boldrini, A. (1998). Visual outcome at 5 years of newborn infants at risk of cerebral visual impairment. *Developmental Medicine & Child Neurology, 40*(5), 302–309.

Verbaken, J. H. (1989). *Contrast sensitivity testing with low contrast acuity charts: Manufacturer's guide*. Melbourne: Australian Vision Charts.

Virgili, G., Cordaro, C., Bigoni, A., Crovato, S., Cecchini, P., & Menchini, U. (2004). Reading acuity in children: Evaluation and reliability using MNREAD charts. *Investigative Opthalmology & Visual Science, 45*(9), 3349–3354.

Visual Functions Committtee. (1984, October). *Visual acuity measurement standard*. Presented to the Consilium Ophthalmologicum Universale, International Council of Ophthalmology, Kos, Greece. Retrieved from http://www.icoph.org/dynamic/attachments/resources/icovisualacuity1984.pdf

Watson, T., Orel-Bixler, D., & Haegerstrom-Portnoy, G. (2010). Early visual-evoked potential acuity and future behavioral acuity in cortical visual impairment. *Optometry and Vision Science, 87*(2), 80–86.

Werth, R., & Schadler, G. (2006). Visual field loss in young children and mentally handicapped adolescents receiving vigabatrin. *Investigative Ophthalmology & Visual Science, 47*(7), 3028–3035.

West, S. K., Rubin, G. S., Broman, A. T., Munoz, B., Bardeen-Roche, K., & Turano, K. (2002) How does visual impairment affect performance on tasks of everyday life? The SEE project. *Archives of Ophthalmology, 120*(6), 774–780.

White, J. M., & Loshin, D. S. (1989). Grating acuity overestimates Snellen acuity in patients with age-related maculopathy. *Optometry and Vision Science, 66*(11), 751–755.

Wilkins, A. J., Della Sala, S., Somazzi, L., & Nimmo-Smith, I. (1988). Age-related norms for the Cambridge low contrast gratings, including details concerning their design and use. *Clinical Vision Science, 2*(3), 202–212.

Woodhouse, J. M., Adoh, T. O., Oduwaiye, K. A., Batchelor, B. G., Megii, S., Unwin, N., et al. (1992). New acuity test for toddlers. *Ophthalmic and Physiological Optics, 12*(2), 249–251.

Woods, R. L., & Wood, J. M. (1995). The role of contrast sensitivity charts and letter contrast tests in clinical practice. *Clinical and Experimental Optometry, 78*(2), 43–57.

# APPENDIX 12A

# Table of Print Size Equivalents for Times New Roman Font

*Ian L. Bailey*

| *M-Units* | *x-height (mm)* | *Points (N)* | *Jaeger (J values)* |
|---|---|---|---|
| 0.20 | 0.29 | 2.0 | |
| 0.25 | 0.36 | 2.5 | |
| 0.32 | 0.47 | 3.0 | |
| 0.40 | 0.58 | 3.5 | J1 |
| 0.50 | 0.72 | 4.5 | J1/J3 |
| 0.63 | 0.92 | 5.5 | J1/J5 |
| 0.80 | 1.16 | 7.0 | J1/J6 |
| 1.00 | 1.45 | 9.0 | J2/J8 |
| 1.25 | 1.8 | 11 | J3/J10 |
| 1.6 | 2.3 | 14 | J4/J12 |
| 2.0 | 2.9 | 18 | J4/J13 |
| 2.5 | 3.6 | 22 | J6/J14 |
| 3.2 | 4.7 | 28 | J7/J16 |
| 4.0 | 5.8 | 36 | J14/J16 |
| 5.0 | 7.3 | 45 | |
| 6.3 | 9.2 | 56 | |
| 8.0 | 11.6 | 72 | |

***Technical Notes***

This table shows the correspondence between point size and M-units when using the Times New Roman font. For reading charts, it is usual to use print in Times New Roman typeface or similar fonts. Height alone is not sufficient to give a measure of visual acuity. The viewing distance must also be specified.

***M Notation***

- Low vision clinicians and vision scientists consider the best indicator of the visibility of print to be the height of the smallest letters.
- Low vision clinicians and vision scientists express the size of the print in M-units, which indicate the distance in meters at which the height of the smallest letters forms an angle of 5 minutes or arc (or 1/12 degree).
- 1.0 M print has a height of 1.45 mm. That is, letters that are 1.45 mm high subtend an angle of 5 minutes of arc when at a distance of 1.0 meter.

- The M-unit rating of a sample of print can be determined by measuring the height of the smallest letters and dividing by 1.45. (For example, letters that are 2.9 mm tall are 2.0 M units.)
- Measurements of reading acuity (visual acuity for reading material) typically specify both the testing distance and the size of the smallest letters that can be read. (For example, 2.0 M print at 40 cm, which may be written as 0.40/2.0M.)

***Point Notation***

- For typeset material, the best indicator of the visibility is the height of the smaller lowercase letters (those without ascending or descending limbs).
- The height of the letter x (the "x-height") is usually taken to be the representative lowercase letter.
- Printers indicate the size of print in points, with 1 point equal to 1/72 inches (or 0.35 mm).
- For 12-point print, the total height is 12/72 inches (4.2 mm). This total height includes the numbers, the capitals, and the ascenders of the tall lowercase letters as well as the lowercase letters with descending limbs (*g, j, p, q,* and *y*).
- Most charts used for the clinical testing of reading use the Times or Times New Roman serif fonts.
- For Times, Times New Roman, and similar fonts, dividing the point size by 9 gives a good estimate of the M-unit size of the small letters. (18-point Times = 2.0 M)
- Helvetica and Arial are common non-serif (or sans-serif) fonts.
- Their lowercase letters are a relatively larger proportion of the total height, and their ascenders and descenders are relatively stubby.
- For Helvetica, Arial, and similar fonts, dividing the point size by 8 gives a good estimate of the M-unit size of the small letters. (16-point Arial = 2.0 M)
- Capital letters and numbers are taller than the small lowercase letters.
- If the reading material is "all-caps" or all numbers, then dividing the point size by 6 provides a good estimate of the M-unit size. (18-point all-caps = 3.0 M)
- Times, Times New Roman, Helvetica, and Arial all have very similar heights for their numbers and capital letters, and the factor of 6 can be applied to all.

***N Notation***

- Some reading test charts have print sizes labeled with an "N" followed by a number.
- The "N" indicates that the font is Times New Roman and the number gives the size in points.

***Jaeger Notation***

- Some reading charts have print sizes labeled with a "J" followed by a number.
- The "J" stands for "Jaeger," named after the ophthalmologist who introduced new reading charts in 1854.
- However, the system is not standardized for size. Within any "Jaeger chart," smaller numbers mean smaller print.
- From one "Jaeger chart" to another, however, there can be wide variations in the relationship between print size and the J numbers. For example, on one chart J1 might be 0.4M in size, but on another, J1 might be 0.5M.

# APPENDIX 12B

# Line Thickness and Spacing Guide for Children with Visual Impairments

*Iain Livingstone*

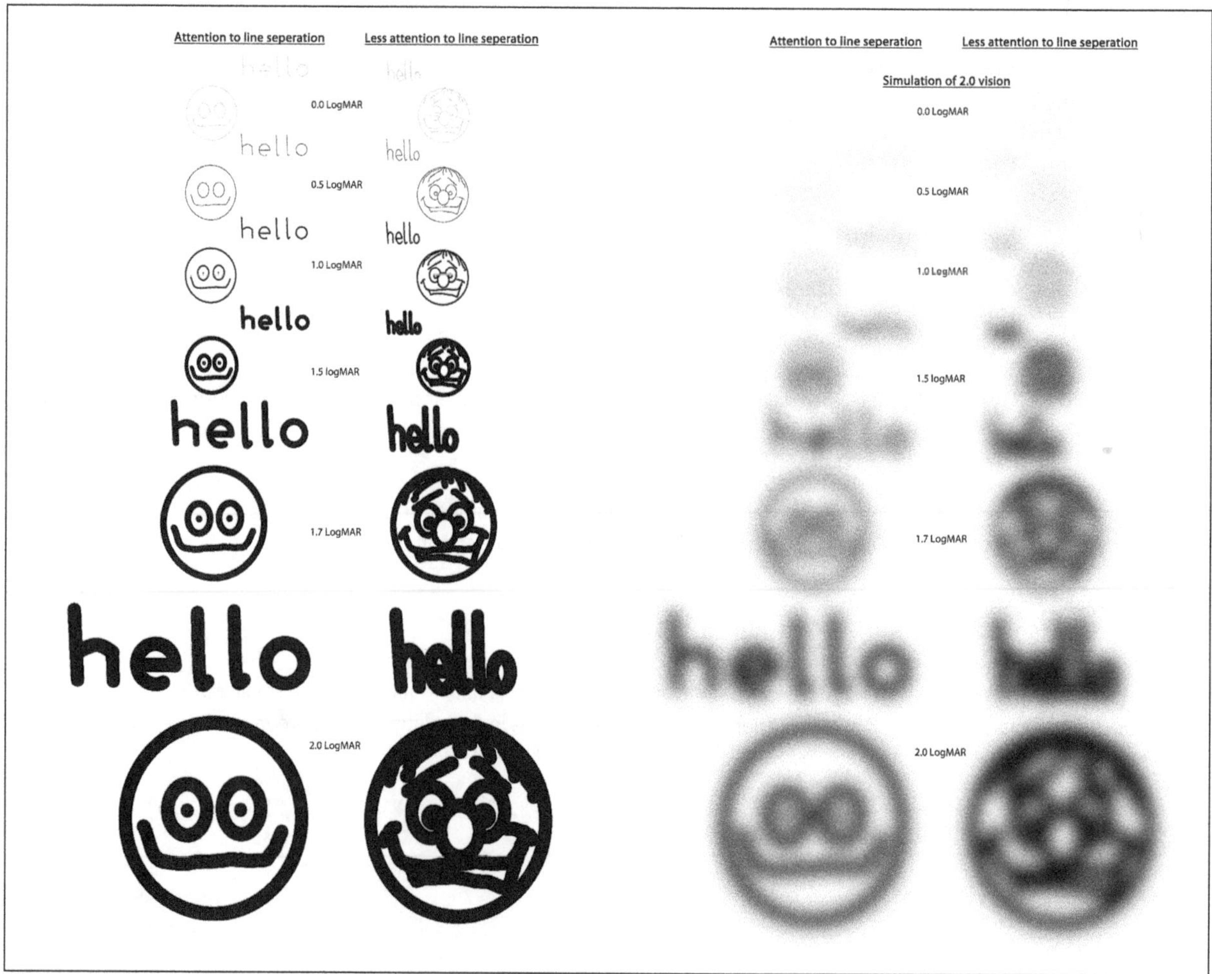


These graded images of a face are related here to logMAR visual acuity (see Appendix 12C). The images on the right have been degraded with Sight-Sim software (www.sight-sim.co.uk) to simulate a visual acuity of 2.0. Images have been constructed with two amounts of separation between the lines used. It can be seen that appropriate line thickness and line separation are equally important in the construction of educational materials.

# APPENDIX 12C

# Conversion Table for Notations of Visual Acuity

*Ian L. Bailey*

| *Alternative Specifications of Visual Acuity* These do not require the specification of distance | | | | | *Specification of Visual Acuity as "Snellen Fractions"* These include specification of the testing distance | | | | |
|---|---|---|---|---|---|---|---|---|---|
| **Log MAR** | **MAR** | **VAR** | **Decimal** | **Cycles** | **6 meters** | **5 meters** | **4 meters** | **1 meter** | **20 feet** |
| −0.3 | 0.50 | 115 | 2.0 | 60 | 6/3.0 | 5/2.5 | 4/2.0 | 1/0.5 | 20/10 |
| −0.2 | 0.63 | 110 | 1.6 | 48 | 6/3.8 | 5/3.2 | 4/2.5 | 1/0.63 | 20/12.5 |
| −0.1 | 0.80 | 105 | 1.3 | 38 | 6/4.8 | 5/4 | 4/3.2 | 1/0.8 | 20/16 |
| 0.0 | 1.00 | 100 | 1.0 | 30 | 6/6 | 5/5 | 4/4.0 | 1/1.0 | 20/20 |
| 0.1 | 1.25 | 95 | 0.8 | 24 | 6/7.5 | 5/6.3 | 4/5.0 | 1/1.25 | 20/25 |
| 0.2 | 1.6 | 90 | 0.63 | 19 | 6/9.5 | 5/8 | 4/6.3 | 1/1.6 | 20/32 |
| 0.3 | 2.0 | 85 | 0.5 | 15 | 6/12 | 5/10 | 4/8.0 | 1/2.0 | 20/40 |
| 0.4 | 2.5 | 80 | 0.4 | 12 | 6/15 | 5/12.5 | 4/10 | 1/2.5 | 20/50 |
| 0.5 | 3.2 | 75 | 0.32 | 9.5 | 6/19 | 5/16 | 4/12.5 | 1/3.2 | 20/63 |
| 0.6 | 4 | 70 | 0.25 | 7.5 | 6/24 | 5/20 | 4/16 | 1/4 | 20/80 |
| 0.7 | 5 | 65 | 0.20 | 6.0 | 6/30 | 5/25 | 4/20 | 1/5 | 20/100 |
| 0.8 | 6.3 | 60 | 0.16 | 4.8 | 6/38 | 5/32 | 4/25 | 1/6.3 | 20/125 |
| 0.9 | 8 | 55 | 0.125 | 3.8 | 6/48 | 5/40 | 4/32 | 1/8 | 20/160 |
| 1.0 | 10 | 50 | 0.10 | 3.0 | 6/60 | 5/50 | 4/40 | 1/10 | 20/200 |
| 1.1 | 12.5 | 45 | 0.08 | 2.4 | 6/75 | 5/63 | 4/50 | 1/12.5 | 20/250 |
| 1.2 | 16 | 40 | 0.063 | 1.9 | 6/95 | 5/80 | 4/63 | 1/16 | 20/320 |
| 1.3 | 20 | 35 | 0.05 | 1.5 | 6/120 | 5/100 | 4/80 | 1/20 | 20/400 |

***Technical Notes:***

1. The primary scale is LogMAR, which is the common logarithm of the Minimum Angle of Resolution.
2. Minimum Angle of Resolution (MAR) is the angular size of the smallest detail that can just be resolved.
3. When MAR = 1.0, logMAR = 0 .0 and the component parts of the test target are separated by an angle of 1 minute of arc (1/60 degree).
4. VAR = Visual Acuity Rating is an arbitrary scale which gives convenient units. VAR = 100-50 × logMAR.
5. Decimal acuity values are the reciprocal of the MAR (minarc) Decimal = 1/MAR.
6. Cycles per degree may be used when the test targets are gratings. One cycle includes one dark and one light stripe.
7. Snellen fractions specify both the viewing distance and the height of the optotype (letter, number, or symbol).
8. The number representing the height of the letter is the distance at which the component parts of the letters subtend an angle of 1 minute of arc (1/60 degree).

# Resources for Clinical Vision Assessment

The following listing includes some sources for obtaining the tests and assessment tools referred to in this chapter. Contact information for the companies listed appears at the end of the section. This information was current at the time of publication. For more information about these assessments, see the references listed in the chapter.

## ASSESSMENT TESTS

### *Color Vision*

**Color Vision Testing Made Easy**
Source: Konan Medical USA
www.konanmedical.com/colordx

**Ishihara's Test for Colour Deficiency**
Sources: Color Blindness
www.colour-blindness.com/colour-blindness-tests/ishihara-colour-test-plates/

Stereo Optical
www.stereooptical.com/shop/vision-testing-products/orignal-ishihara-color-test/

**Panel 16 Quantitative Color Vision Test**
Source: Good-Lite
www.good-lite.com/Details.cfm?ProdID=101

### *Contrast Sensitivity*

**Bailey-Lovie Chart Set**
Precision Vision
precision-vision.com/all-products/contrast-eye-charts/low-contrast-single-contrast-level-variable-size/variable-distance/baileyloviechartset.html

**Cambridge Low Contrast Grating Test**
Source: Haag-Streit USA
http://store.haag-streit-usa.com/productcart/pc/Cambridge-low-contrast-gratings-p81.htm

**Cardiff Contrast Sensitivity Test**
Source: Richmond Products
www.richmondproducts.com/shop/index.php?route=product/product&product_id=340

**Colenbrander Mixed Contrast Test**
Source: Precision Vision
http://precision-vision.com/products/contrast-eye-charts/mixed-threshold-contrast-charts/mixed-contrast.html

**FACT (Functional Acuity Contrast Test)**
Source: Stereo Optical
http://www.stereooptical.com/shop/vision-screeners/functional-vison-analyzer/

**Hiding Heidi Low Contrast Face Test**
Sources: Bernell
www.bernell.com/product/GF3500/383

Good-Lite
www.good-lite.com/Details.cfm?ProdID=44

**LEA Symbols Low Contrast Test**
Source: Good-Lite
www.good-lite.com/Details.cfm?ProdID=56

**Mars Letter Contrast Sensitivity Test**
Source: Precision Vision
http://precision-vision.com/all-products/contrast-eye-charts/mixed-threshold-contrast-charts/threshold-contrast/marslettercontrastsensitivitytest.html

**Melbourne Edge Test**
Source: National Vision Research Institute of Australia
http://www.nvri.org.au/pages/-products-logmar-charts-and-more-.html

**Patti Pics Low Contrast Flip Book**
Source: Precision Vision
http://precision-vision.com/products/contrast-eye-charts/low-contrast-single-contrast-level-variable-size/variable-distance/pattipicslowcontrastflipbook.html

**Peek-a-Boo Patti Low Contrast Vision Test**
Sources: Bernell
www.bernell.com/product/2795/376

Precision Vision
http://precision-vision.com/all-products/testing-aids/fixation/peek-a-boopattilowcontrasttest.html

**Pelli-Robson Contrast Sensitivity Chart**
Source: Precision Vision
http://precision-vision.com/all-products/contrast-eye-charts/mixed-threshold-contrast-charts/threshold-contrast/pelli-robsonsloanlettercontrastchart.html

**Rabin Test for Contrast Sensitivity**
Source: Precision Vision
http://precision-vision.com/all-products/contrast-eye-charts/mixed-threshold-contrast-charts/threshold-contrast/completerabincontrastsensitivityset.html

**Sloan Letters Low Contrast Chart**
Source: Good-Lite
https://www.good-lite.com/Details.cfm?ProdID=350

### *Eye Movements (Stereopsis)*

**Frisby Stereotests**
Sources: Bernell
www.bernell.com/category/952

Stereotests Ltd.
www.frisbystereotest.co.uk/

**The Lang Stereotest**
Source: The Fresnel Prism and Lens Co.
www.fresnel-prism.com/products/lang-stereotest-1-or-2/

**PASS (Preschool Assessment of Stereopsis with a Smile) Test 1, 2, & 3**
Source: Vision Assessment Corporation
http://visionassessment.com/1011.shtml

**Random Dot E**
Sources: Precision Vision
http://precision-vision.com/products/stereo-vision-tests/random-dot-e.html

Stereo Optical
http://stereo-optical-2.myshopify.com/collections/schools-public-health/products/random-dot-e

**Stereopsis Butterfly with LEA Symbols**
Source: Good-Lite
www.good-lite.com/Details.cfm?ProdID=314&category=19&Secondary=60

### *Visual Acuity*

**Allen Acuity Test Cards**
Western Ophthalmics
www.west-op.com/presalactesc.html

**Bailey-Lovie Chart Set**
Source: Precision Vision
http://precision-vision.com/all-products/contrast-eye-charts/low-contrast-single-contrast-level-variable-size/variable-distance/baileyloviechartset.html

**Cardiff Acuity Test**
Sources: Good-Lite
www.good-lite.com/Details.cfm?ProdID=341

Richmond Products
www.richmondproducts.com/shop/index.php?route=product/product&path=1_18_121_554&product_id=1401

**The "E Game"**
Source: Richmond Eye Associates
www.richmondeye.com/vision-tests/#distance

**HOTV Eye Chart**
Sources: Good-Lite
www.good-lite.com/results.cfm?category=9

Precision Vision
http://precision-vision.com/products/illuminator-cabinets/small-914-original-cabinet-and-charts/3-meter-10ft-acuity-charts/hotveyechart10ft.html

**Kay Picture Test**
Source: Kay Pictures
www.kaypictures.co.uk/lowvision.html

**Keeler Acuity Cards for Infants**
Source: Keeler Eye Shop
www.keeler.co.uk/Keeler-Acuity-Cards-for-Infants-753.htm

**Keeler LogMAR Crowded Test**
Source: Keeler Eye Shop
http://www.keeler.co.uk/LogMAR-Crowded-Test-200.htm

**Landolt C Eye Chart**
Source: Precision Vision
http://precision-vision.com/products/acuity-charts-high-contrast/3-meters/landoltcfoldingchart.html

**LEA Gratings Paddles**
Sources: Good-Lite
www.good-lite.com/Details.cfm?ProdID=41

Vision Associates
http://visionkits.com/lea-grating-paddles.html

**LEA Symbols and LEA Numbers Near Vision Card**
Sources: School Health
https://www.schoolhealth.com/vision-hearing/eye-charts-cards/lea-symbols-numbers/lea-symbols-pocket-near-vision-card

Vision Associates
http://visionkits.com/products/tests/acuity/near/lea-symbols-lea-numbers-near-vision-card.html

**Lighthouse Near Acuity Test Chart**
Source: Good-Lite
https://www.good-lite.com/Details.cfm?ProdID=760&category=3&Secondary=71

**LogMAR Charts**
Source: Carleton Optical
www.carletonltd.com/catalogue/logmar-charts

**MNRead Acuity Chart**
Source: Precision Vision
http://precision-vision.com/request-quote/mnreadchart1-w-detail

**Pacific Acuity Test (PAT)**
Sources: Bernell
www.bernell.com/product/GL360000/376

Good-Lite
www.good-lite.com/Details.cfm?ProdID=731

**Patti Pics Vision Testing System**
Source: Precision Vision
http://precision-vision.com/all-products/low-vision/low-vision-test-materials/pattipicscolenbranderlowvisionchart.html

**Patti Stripes Square Wave Grating Paddles**
Source: Precision Vision
http://precision-vision.com/all-products/testing-aids/fixation/pattistripessquarewavegratingpaddles.html

**Sloan Striped Visual Acuity Chart**
Source: Precision Vision
http://precision-vision.com/products/illuminator-cabinets/small-914-original-cabinet-and-charts/6-meter-20ft-acuity-charts/sloanstripedvisualacuitychart.html

**Teller Acuity Cards II (TAC)**
Sources: Bernell
www.bernell.com/product/TAC/1268

Precision Vision
http://precision-vision.com/

Stereo Optical
www.stereooptical.com/shop/vision-testing-products/teller-acuity-cards-ii-half-set/

### *Visual Field*

**LEA Flicker Wand**
Source: Good-Lite
www.good-lite.com/Details.cfm?ProdID=457

## SOURCES OF OTHER MATERIALS

**Boardmaker**
Source: Mayer-Johnson
www.mayer-johnson.com/what-is-boardmaker

**Symbol Stix**
Source: n2Y
www.n2y.com/products/symbolstix

## CONTACT INFORMATION FOR SOURCES OF PRODUCTS

**Bernell**
4016 N. Home Street
Mishawaka, IN 46545
(800) 348-2225 or (574) 259-2070
www.bernell.com/

**Carleton Optical**
Pattisson House
Addison Road, Chesham
Buckinghamshire HP5 2BD

United Kingdom
www.carletonltd.com/
carleton@carletonltd.com

**Color Blindness**
www.colour-blindness.com

**Good-Lite Company**
1155 Jansen Farm Drive
Elgin, IL 60123
(800) 362-3860
Fax: (888) 362-2576
www.good-lite.com

**Haag Streit USA**
3535 Kings Mills Road
Mason, OH 45040
http://store.haag-streit-usa.com

**Kay Pictures Ltd.**
55 Grove Road
Tring, Hertfordshire HP23 5PB
United Kingdom
+44 (0)1442 823507
Fax:+44 (0)8701 236191
www.kaypictures.co.uk/
contact@kaypictures.co.uk

**Keeler Ltd.**
Clewer Hill Road
Windsor SL4 4AA UK
+44 (0)1753 857177
Fax:+44 (0)1753 827145
www.keeler.co.uk
info@keeler.co.uk

**Konan Medical**
15 Marconi
Suite A
Irvine, CA 92618
(949) 521-7730
www.konanmedical.com

**Mayer-Johnson**
2100 Wharton Street
Suite 400
Pittsburgh, PA 15203
(800) 588-4548 or (412) 381-4883
Fax: (866) 585-6260
www.mayer-johnson.com/

**n2Y**
P.O. Box 550
Huron, OH 44839
(419) 433-9800 or (800) 697-6575
Fax: (419) 433-9810
www.n2y.com/

**National Vision Research Institute**
Australian College of Optometry
Corner Keppel and Cardigan Streets
Carlton VIC 3053
Australia
+61 3 9349 7484
http://www.nvri.org.au/pages/contact-us.html
info@nvri.org.au

**Precision Vision**
944 First Street
La Salle, IL 61301
(815) 223-2022
http://precision-vision.com
info@precision-vision.com

**Premier Ophthalmic Services**
22773 Citation Road
Frankfort, IL 60423
(800) 597-7152 or (815) 464 3331
Fax: (815) 464-3343
http://premierop.com

**Richmond Eye Associates**
4600 Cox Road
Innsbrook Corporate Center
Markel Plaza, Suite 120
Glen Allen, VA 23060
(804) 270-0330
Fax: (804) 270-1003
www.richmondeye.com

**Richmond Products Inc.**
4400 Silver Avenue SE
Albuquerque, NM 87108
(505) 275-2406
Fax: (810) 885-8319
www.richmondproducts.com/

**Stereo Optical**
8623 W. Bryn Mawr Avenue
Suite 502
Chicago, IL 60631
(773) 867-0380 or (800) 344-9500
www.stereooptical.com/contact/
sales@stereooptical.com

**Stereotest Ltd.**
137 Brookhouse Hill

Fulwood, Sheffield S10 3TE
United Kingdom
44 (0) 114 230 7819
www.frisbystereotest.co.uk/
sales@frisbystereotest.co.uk

**Vision Assessment Corporation**
2675 Coyle Avenue
Elk Grove Village, IL 60007
(847) 239-5889 or (866) 887-9692
Fax: (847) 440-9017
http://visionassessment.com/
info@visionassessment.com

**Vision Associates**
295 N.W. Commons Loop
Suite 115-312
Lake City, FL 32055
(407) 352-1200
Fax: (815) 363-7919
www.visionkits.com

**Western Ophthalmics**
Colony Park Business Center
19019 36th Avenue West,
Ste. G
Lynnwood, WA 98036
(425) 672-9332
Fax: (425) 672-3528
www.west-op.com
info@west-op.com

# 13

# Assessment of Functional Vision: Assessment of Visual Processing in Children with CVI

*Sander Zuidhoek, Lea Hyvärinen, Namita Jacob, and Anne Henriksen*

When cerebral visual impairment (CVI) is suspected, and a child's visual functions and functional vision have been assessed (as discussed in Chapter 12), the child's abilities in the area of visual processing are investigated. The goal of this chapter is to address the evaluation of visual processing of children with CVI—that is, how visual information from the eyes and visual pathways is recognized and interpreted by the brain to make sense of what is seen—and to suggest currently available methods and strategies of doing so.

As earlier chapters have already indicated, the assessment of children with CVI aims to discover their visual capabilities and requires the collation of information from a variety of sources to best understand how a child functions. Two approaches with different emphases to assessment are considered in this chapter. One is a multidisciplinary approach with a neuropsychological core. Neuropsychology is the science that connects behaviors to brain structures and functioning. Damage to or atypical development of brain structures results in disorders in brain functions. In CVI, visual impairment is caused by disorders in one or more functions that allow us to see, resulting from damage to or atypical development of one or more brain structures. Therefore, neuropsychological knowledge about particular brain structures and their functional role in allowing visual awareness and behavior is the cornerstone for determining the exact nature of a child's visual impairment; assessment of these functions using neuropsychological tools forms the basis for determining which of the functions causes the impairment. This provides insight into how a particular child experiences the world, and as such forms the basis for treatment to reduce the problems the child encounters in daily life.

The second approach considers higher-order visual functions and their disorders (visual selective attentional functions, visual perceptual functions, visual memory functions, visual working memory functions, guidance of movement [visual-motor functions], and the capacity to choose to give and maintain visual attention; see Chapters 1 and 6) within the context of performance of meaningful "real world" tasks over time, to guide interventions, without placing an emphasis on diagnosis.

As has been highlighted throughout this book, assessment of children with CVI requires expertise from a multidisciplinary team. The two approaches mentioned are complementary and can be implemented by different team members to afford a broad perspective of the child's vision. Testing in real-world situations is encouraged since even subtle differences in task demands can lead to differences in task performance. Suggested ways to implement and organize assessments from multiple perspectives can be found in Chapter 10.

The selection of methods to evaluate visual processing in children with CVI depends on the severity of the visual condition and the presence and severity of additional impairments. As noted previously in this book, children who have CVI can be grouped into three overlapping categories:

- Those with profound visual impairment (due to lower and/or higher visual dysfunctions), many of whom have additional cognitive and motor disabilities.
- Those with functionally useful vision (with impairment due to lower and/or higher dysfunctions) who have additional cognitive and/or motor disabilities.
- Children who have functionally useful vision who work at or near the expected academic level for their age group; they may or may not have additional disabilities. These children have normal or near normal lower visual functions, but primarily have disorders in higher visual functions (see Chapters 1 and 10).

Children in each of these categories tend to be managed by different groups of professionals, and it is important to consider evaluation techniques that address the needs of all three groups. Issues in the assessment of children with multiple disabilities are indicated in this chapter so that readers can see how material can be applied to children with severe cognitive or physical impairments.

The chapter begins with Part A, an introduction to the evaluation of higher-order visual functions in general, followed by some guidelines for the assessment of children who are able to participate in neuropsychological testing situations. Part B presents specific information about testing protocols and includes suggestions for test modifications to provide practitioners with applicable screening procedures. Profiles of vision functions and/or visual functioning have been suggested to better illustrate the vision needs of people with visual impairments (e.g., Hyvärinen, Walthes, Freitag, & Petz, 2012; Flom, 2004; Looijestijn, 2008). In part Part C, one such profile of day-to-day visual functioning for children with CVI as well as case studies are presented.

## PART A: Identification of Visual Functions and Neuropsychological Testing Considerations

*Sander Zuidhoek*

Neuropsychological assessment aims to determine the quality of brain functions in order to identify the cause of distortions or deviations in a person's behavior or experience of the world. The brain houses many visual functions. *Visual functions* can be defined as the essential basic building blocks provided by brain processing that give rise to and determine the quality of visual experience and behavior. Disorders in any of these functions result in distortions in visual experience or visual behavior. The nature of the distortions depends on the functions in question.

To be able to help reduce a child's visual problems in daily life, we need an understanding of how the child experiences the world visually. In order to understand this, we need to know the nature and quality of the visual functions, especially those that alter visual experience, and neuropsychological tests can be used to determine the quality of higher-order visual functions. There are a multitude of real-world tasks that may be difficult for a child with CVI to perform and can be targeted for assessment; the list is endless. Neuropsychological assessment of the quality of higher-order visual functions aims to identify the *causes* of the child's difficulty with those particular tasks. Thus, the information gained from neuropsychological assessment can be used to understand some of the reasons, related to higher-order visual functions, underlying a child's difficulties in the performance of a variety of typical tasks in the school, home, and community.

The approach to assessment of visual processing presented in this section requires an understanding of the integrated neuropsychological model of visual processing—or how visual information from the eyes and visual pathways is processed throughout various sectors of the brain to make sense of or to act on what is seen—as presented in Chapters 2 and 6. Briefly:

- Processing in the brain's visual systems, and thus seeing, depends on attention.
- Attention is controlled according to prioritizing top-down processes performed by the executive system and bottom-up processes initiated by salient events and stimuli in the outside world.
- These prioritizing processes are driven by the inside world (urges, emotions, and motivations), but take into account possible environmental threats and social factors.

When an individual needs to attend to visual information:

1. *Initial processing* occurs in the occipital lobes, in which a representation of the outside world is present (the visual field).
2. *A selection of a part of the visual field* is made. The first selection takes place by the direction of the gaze, which can be driven either by stimuli in the outside world (via the superior colliculi) or by free will (by prefrontal cortex and the frontal eye fields).
3. *The size of the selected area* is made by a network containing the occipital lobes, temporo-parietal areas and parts of the thalamus. Selected elements are processed further, resulting in their perception.
4. *Recognition functions* are performed in the networks of the temporal lobes and adjacent structures (connected to the occipital lobes via the ventral stream) serving the functions of object and face recognition, route-based orientation, and recognition of landmarks.
5. *Visual-spatial functions* in the brain's parietal lobes are employed to understand visual-spatial information.
6. Functions associated with *"vision for doing"* are served in the parietal lobes of

the brain (connected to the occipital lobes via the dorsal stream), which can affect awareness of directions and distances (which in orientation and mobility [O&M] are called spatial awareness, body awareness and orientation, attention, and eye-hand coordination).

7. The *mirror neuron system (MNS)* is networked in various parts of the brain. This high-level system affords rapid awareness of the significance of other people's hand movements, expressions, gestures, and moods that we experience as mirroring our own feelings and motor functions. MNS functions are evident from early infancy.

This is a simplified model of thinking related to common sites of damage when these functions are impaired. However, in the brain with atypical development of pathways and connections, some functions and connections may not be present or may have alternative locations.

## How Brain Damage Can Affect Assessment of Vision

Due to the interconnection of networks, brain damage can also cause changes in measures obtained of standard visual functions for a child. For example, there can be variations in measured visual acuity levels for children with CVI related to the ways in which it is measured due to the nature and severity of damage in the different parts of the cortical area responsible for the recognition of abstract forms. The standard *visual* functions, measured in a thorough ophthalmological or optometric examination, are the foundation for the assessment of visual functioning, but need to be further assessed as specific *brain* functions if a child shows evidence of using vision in atypical ways in some cognitive functions.

For instance, visual acuity that is measured with optotypes as recognition visual acuity (see Chapter 12) may be normal in someone with normal eyes and visual pathways but who has damage to areas of the visual brain serving recognition if measured with the LEA Symbols line test chart, but low if measured with the LEA Numbers chart, and not measurable at all with a line acuity letter chart such as the ETDRS (Ferris, Kassoff, Bresnick, & Bailey, 1982). This is discussed further later in this chapter.

Visual processing disorders often coexist with damage to other brain functions that cause motor problems, intellectual disability, central auditory processing disorders, and losses in executive functions and attention. The assessment of visual processing functions therefore often requires adaptations in the observations and measurements of standard visual functions as well as visual processing functions (see also Chapters 6 and 12).

The executive system, as presented in Chapter 6, also has considerable impact on the manifestations of dysfunction in higher as well as lower visual functions. Without an evaluation of the executive system, general attention functions, and visual selective attention functions, as well as emotional characteristics of the child, the impact of visual functions cannot be adequately interpreted. Acknowledging and accepting this implies that in order to assess higher visual functions, broad neuropsychological examination, as well as behavioral and personality assessment are desirable, if not necessary, across the spectrum of children who are suspected as having a form of CVI. The availability of resources to conduct this type of assessment varies by country or region.

Since many children with CVI may not have access to this type of evaluation due to limited resources or limitations in the application of available tests to children with severe additional disabilities, a variety of methods to examine visual processing are reviewed and clarified in this chapter.

## The Hierarchy of Functions

Our ideas of what it means to be visually impaired are based on our ideas of what it means to see well. In order to identify the visual functions, we need to have intersubjective agreement on what seeing well means. This section takes into account the hierarchical relationship of groups of functions within the visual system in addition to the hierarchical position of the visual system from the neuropsychological viewpoint described in Chapter 6.

The following is a list of functions that constitute seeing well—that is, what would be the most desirable capabilities for each visual function. Note that any function arises from multiple components that contribute to that function. For example, the function of acuity depends on several eye and brain structures, which perform different subfunctions that make up the fundamental visual function of acuity. The first set of items, numbered 1–6, comprise the lower visual functions. Items 7–12 include the higher visual functions, covering visual selective attentional functions, perceptual understanding and consciousness, and visual-motor processing (or how visual perception and movement are coordinated by the brain); these higher visual functions are related to a physical outside world of here and now. The last group, items 13–15, includes higher visual functions that require memory and working memory, and make up the visual world we create with our minds.

- **I.** Groups of lower visual functions
  - **A.** Visual sensory functions
    - **1.** Having a large, binocular visual field.
    - **2.** Having good visual acuity in both good and poor lighting conditions and for near and distant tasks (with eyeglasses if needed).
    - **3.** Being able to perceive subtle contrasts.
    - **4.** Adapting quickly to dark and/or richly illuminated spaces.
    - **5.** Being able to discern the full range of colors (sensory functions).
  - **B.** Oculomotor functions
    - **6.** Being able to move the eyes in harmony in all directions (oculomotor functions).
- **II.** Groups of higher visual functions
  - **C.** Visual selective attentional functions
    - **7.** Being able to select both big portions as well as small details from a large amount of visual information, at will, as brought about by salient stimuli in the environment—that is, global and local visual attention, in a top-down fashion (driven by executive functions) as well as a bottom-up fashion (driven by external events).
  - **D.** Visual perceptual functions
    - **8.** Being able to consciously see and identify whatever has been selected (visual consciousness and visual identification—the

"what" pathway [see Chapters 2 and 6]).

9. To understand the spatial characteristics of what is seen, understanding the intrinsic spatial characteristics of a visual scene, understanding where the perceived object(s) are in relation to oneself and other objects, and how they are oriented (visuospatial perception—the "where" pathway [see Chapters 2 and 6]).
10. Knowing (a) whether the perceived object is moving, and if so (b) how fast, (c) in what direction (a special form of visuospatial perception—the "where" pathway), and (d) whether the movement characteristics are recognizable.

E. Visual-motor functions

11. Being able to perform fast and accurate actions to a visually selected object or part of an object (visual-motor processing—the "how" pathway [see Chapters 2 and 6]) and being able to move freely through the environment by means of visual guidance.

F. Visual emotional functions

12. Having an emotion or feeling about significant images, without cognitively interpreting them—for example, patients with impairments in the identification of faces may experience warm feelings when confronted with a picture of their children, without actually identifying them. (This visual function is not addressed in more detail in this chapter, since its impairment is very rare among children.)

III. Higher visual functions that require memory and working memory

G. Visual memory functions

13. Being able to recognize and/or recall the identity and spatial properties of a perceived object or objects (in short-term, longer-term, and long-term memory)—functions that are needed for recognition and recall (e.g., drawing) of visual objects and visuospatial figures, memory of visuospatial (environmental) information and routes (used for navigation).

H. Visual working memory functions

14. Being able to generate and manipulate a mental visual image working memory).

I. Visual processing speed

15. Being able to react to and perceive visual stimuli quickly. (Some people respond slowly to visual stimuli without showing a dysfunction in any of the aforementioned visual functions or the attentional or executive functions.)

All these groups of functions implicitly or more explicitly refer to qualitative notions: good, fast, rather quickly. In determining how well or poorly a child is doing at one of the functions, one always needs to make a comparison of how well a child at the same developmental age would do or what is set as a performance level for a particular age group. For this, normative data on valid and reliable tests are required. (It should also be mentioned that many standardized tests cannot be administered to children with CVI due to their sensory, cognitive, or physical limitations, and the normative data from such tests often cannot be applied to such children.)

## Considerations in the Assessment of Higher Visual Functions

### *Obtaining a Complete Picture of the Child*

To be able to interpret a child's visual behavior and unusual visual strategies or behaviors relating to impairments in the processing of visual information, we need to have a complete, comprehensive picture of the child. We need to know the child's salient medical and developmental history, the quality of all of the child's sensory (including lower visual), cognitive, sensorimotor, and body functions, the child's former and present environments and the child's interactions with these, his or her personal history, and the child's personality characteristics. Integration and understanding of these pieces of information and their interrelationships are required to explain the child's behavior in any situation and results on any test or observation protocol. In addition, to focus diagnostic assessment and to be able to actually help a child in daily life, one needs to know a particular child's limitations in daily life activities and problems in participating in society as precisely as possible, as well as the child's abilities and strengths.

For example, knowing that "the child has difficulty reading" and his or her lower visual functions appear to be in order, is an insufficient basis to commence intervention, treatment, or educational programming. It is necessary to know the exact cause or causes. The gathering of information should be aimed at specifying and explaining the nature of the reading difficulty; it makes a big difference knowing whether the child has difficulty reading because he or she finds the letters too small, because of difficulty learning the form of the letters, or difficulty remembering and linking the sound to letter groups or phonemes. The child's optics and focusing must be checked and appropriate eyeglasses provided if needed. It is important to know if reading problems occur primarily at school or at home, the type of material the child is reading (books, sheet music, etc.), and the lighting conditions under which the limitations occur. In addition, the child's developmental age is an important factor, since he or she may just not be ready for some components of reading yet.

Furthermore, there may be problems and limitations in domains other than those spontaneously mentioned by the child, caretakers, or teachers. Thus, an active stance is required to uncover all possible problems and limitations. Looijestijn (2002, 2007) has devised a semi-structured interview, the Visual Activities and Participation (VAP) Scales, for the purpose of uncovering many of the problems and limitations in daily life. It has the parents, child, or both estimate independently of one another the extent to which the specific difficulties are caused by visual or other factors. In order not to miss anything, it contains 40 questions.

Additional disabilities need to be known so that the ways they affect use of vision and task demands can be considered in planning details of the assessment, in interpreting results, and in treatment of the problems in daily life. For example, demands on vision and cognitive functions are different for a child with CVI who can walk compared to a child who must use a wheelchair in route orientation. For the child in the wheelchair, the planning of routes is a more complex task because uneven surfaces and thresholds require attention to a different constellation of details along the route, and the path ahead needs to be rendered visible for a longer distance than for a walking child.

Finally, the individual's emotional state is a crucial element in every part of the assessment process, particularly in children. In comparison with adults, children bend relatively easily to their own emotions, urges, and wishes. This may be even more evident in children who are emotionally damaged, for example as a result of repeated failing on visual tasks. Consider a child who is used to failing visual tasks. He or she is likely to be afraid of failing again when confronted with an unknown visual task. The child's emotions may even lead to a child's executive decision to feign disinterest or promote other fake needs to avoid doing the task. To *hypothesize* socio-emotional problems of this sort, the examiner "just" needs experience and a keen eye. In order to *determine* whether, indeed, they are part of the child's problems, however, and if so, to what extent, the examiner needs to gather a lot of information. In fact, to interpret a child's emotions and psychological health, one should know about the child's personality, history, role in the family, the nature of the child's friendships, the way schoolteachers see and respond to the child, the child's physical health, and how all these important factors relate and interact, since they all can have a detrimental effect on the child's self-confidence.

### Taking Developmental Age into Account

Developmental age is an important factor in the interpretation of test or task performances. The emotional, executive, and attentional prerequisites for neuropsychological testing are such that children under the developmental age of 6 have yet to master the required executive control and attentional capacities to provide reliable data. As a consequence, most neuropsychological instruments are constructed for children who are 6 years of age and older. Despite these limitations there are good behavioral questionnaires (CBCL [Achenbach, 1991], BRIEF [Gioia, Isquith, Guy, & Kenworthy, 2000]), instruments (BSID II [Van der Meulen, Ruiter, Lutje Spelberg, & Smrkovsky, 2002]), and intelligence tests (WPPSI IV [Wechsler, 2012]), which can be used to map the younger child's developmental age, as well as their weaknesses and compensatory abilities.

However, it is important to note that there is no such thing as "intelligence" as a single entity. Intelligence tests are sets of rather arbitrary subtests that trigger their own random combinations of different cognitive, visual, and motor functions; their respective qualities determine the subtest scores that together form a total IQ score. Since different intelligence tests ask very different things of children, they do not measure the same thing. For example, some intelligence tests place the emphasis on verbal abilities and active manipulation of the materials used; some emphasize executive functions; some require fine motor and drawing skills or mental and motor speed. As a result, the performances (and scores) of children with atypical development of cognitive or motor functions in particular can vary substantially, depending heavily on which intelligence test has been used. Thus, information gained from these tests must be interpreted with caution and requires an understanding of the effects of atypical functioning on performance variables and outcomes.

Use of the concept of developmental age must be managed with caution. Children with visual impairment, including those with CVI, may have different developmental trajectories than typical children, depending on their degree of vision and additional impairments; developmental ages cannot be directly compared as a result (Warren, 1994). While it may help in the selection of tests and the interpretation of test results, children with visual impairments may have alternative developmental milestones in a variety of developmental domains (see Chapter 4). Furthermore, the performance of children with limited sensory or motor input cannot be fairly compared with the performance of nondisabled children on the same task because, in reality, the task presents different perceptual, cognitive, and motor demands for children with sensory and motor disabilities.

When administration of items from available neuropsychological tests is not possible, for example in children with severe cognitive and other disabilities, then the multidisciplinary evaluation team will need to rely on collaborative information collected about the child's performance through observation. Knowledge of the cognitive and emotional prerequisites of seeing, as well as of the lower and higher visual functions, as described previously in this chapter and in Chapter 6, helps in structuring the observations into hypotheses in terms of impairments of specific functions. In such instances, hypotheses may guide treatment, as a definitive diagnosis about which higher-order visual functions are impaired may not be possible.

To be able to specifically diagnose a dysfunction in higher visual functioning, however, the child needs to have broad neuropsychological testing to rule out attentional and/or executive dysfunctions. For example, without neuropsychological examination, one can never be sure that a child does *not* have a disorder in sustaining attention. For example, when a child is eyeing the testing material intently, this is no guarantee that the child is actually looking at it. Perhaps the child is listening to whatever is going on, paying attention to thoughts, or, for all we know, may be having an epileptic absence.

### *Using Simple, Singular Tasks*

Ideally, the key to choosing a valid task is to ensure that it will prompt, stimulate, or trigger just one function. However, no such task exists; any task requires many brain functions. So it is important to make sure that the demand on the executive and attention functions is as low as possible by

- using simple, short instructions,
- avoiding having the child choose from multiple pictures if possible,
- not presenting more than one test item on one page, and
- acknowledging that picture-naming tasks depend on active vocabulary.

A trained and skilled psychologist can apply tests that do not follow these principles, but one has to be aware that they do not measure what one would hope they measure; they involve a lot more, especially attentional and executive functions, and (more implicitly) motivation and emotions. In addition to contaminating the test outcome by requiring other than visual functions, the constructs many of these tests propose (such as "visual form constancy" or "visual figure-ground") evaluate more than one dominant visual cognitive function. (This is discussed in more detail later in this chapter.) As a consequence, they may help one *hypothesize* which functions may be impaired, but more tests or tasks are needed to identify the actual dysfunctions. Therefore, when trying to assess visual functions, ideally, tasks that target the intended function as cleanly as possible should be used; that is, tasks that make minimal demands on executive and attentional functions, as well as on other visual functions.

To successfully generate hypotheses about or diagnose dysfunctions in higher visual functions, it is necessary to have a good understanding of how visual selection, visual perception, and visual behavior come about. An effective model is needed that acknowledges that visual task performance involves the whole person. As discussed in Chapter 6, the model also needs to consider:

- emotions, needs, motivations, and the direct environment, which need to be interpreted and suppressed by . . .
  - executive functions, which control . . .
    - general attentional functions, with which the visual sensory modality is or is not selected, and
    - visual selective attentional functions, the first group of higher visual functions.

Only after these elements have exerted their influence do the cerebral visual pathways come into play—the perceptual and visual-motor functions that lead to identification ("what" pathway), visuospatial processing ("where" pathway), and visual-motor action ("how" pathway). As a consequence, we need to assess, or at least have a good idea of, all the elements just specified before one can finally get to draw conclusions about the actual perceptual and visual-motor functions.

A schematic summary of Zuidhoek's hierarchical neuropsychological model of visual perception is presented in Chapter 6, Figure 6.6. As discussed in detail in Chapter 6, the model incorporates both top-down and bottom-up processing: it shows both the "inside world" and the "outside world" and their connections with executive and attentional processes that in turn affect the "outside" and "inside worlds" through visual-motor and perceptual processing, respectively, creating an ongoing conceptual loop.

## Selecting which Visual Processing and Visual-Motor Functions to Assess

Another crucial question when it comes to understanding, seeing, and, therefore, diagnosing disorders in higher visual functions is, What functions do we find inside the "what," "where," and "how" pathways? In other words, what visual perceptual and visual-motor functions are there? It is possible that there may be hundreds of higher visual perceptual and visual-motor subfunctions that, in principle, can all be impaired independently of one another or any other functions. To assess them all is impossible. To perform meaningful clinical assessment, we need to identify those functions that matter in daily life, those that, if impaired, hamper task performance in a way that is meaningful and isolate those functional units that cause the specific problems and limitations in any particular child. For example, problems with spatial and recognition functions make it especially difficult to teach mathematics and reading to many children with brain damage who do not have the same virtual space as their peers, have several weak recognition functions and poor or no visual imagination, and who sometimes also have poor function in some parts of visual memory.

## PART B: Procedures for the Evaluation of Visual Processing

*Sander Zuidhoek, Lea Hyvärinen, Namita Jacob, and Anne Henriksen*

As indicated at the beginning of this chapter, an important approach to the assessment of visual processing is the consideration of higher-order visual functions in the context of the performance of everyday tasks. Observations and conclusions gathered from this approach can be combined with neuropsychological findings, as just described in the foregoing section, to obtain insights and information about a child's visual abilities and challenges. The following discussion considers a variety of assessment procedures that can be used to evaluate the performance of higher-order visual functions. The assessment suggestions listed here are intended in particular for those for whom neuropsychological assessment is not possible. This may occur when a neuropsychologist is not available, or when children cannot access current neuropsychological test batteries due to their visual or cognitive constraints.

### The Importance of Tests of Vision Functions

As mentioned earlier, lower visual functions need to be assessed before it can be determined how impairments in higher visual functions may potentially affect visual performance. Many of these tests are discussed in Chapter 12 and include line visual acuity charts with letters or numbers, single letter or number visual acuity charts, grating acuity tests, tests of contrast sensitivity, tests of stereopsis, tests of color perception, and tests of visual field. Standard vision tests targeting sensory functions assess more than the quality of the eyes, however. They actually require both oculomotor and higher visual functions, as well; good performance on tests that assess lower visual functions require accurate saccades, visual selective attentional functions, visual consciousness, and visual perceptual functions, which are all functions performed by the brain. It is, therefore, not possible to treat the measurement of higher visual functions as if they are separate from the findings of these other measures.

For example, recognition visual acuity of normally sighted *adults* is practically the same when measured with any of the following three sets of optotypes—Sloan letters, LEA Numbers, or LEA Symbols—because each of these three sets of optotypes has been calibrated with the same test, the Landolt C test, and they follow the same internationally recommended layout. If a person with CVI is assessed for recognition of abstract forms, all three tests should be used. The differences in the results depict differences in the function of the specific neural areas responsible for each individual set of optotypes. When testing young children, the LEA Symbols, being close in appearance to geometric forms that are well known by young children, may give a line better visual acuity than LEA Numbers and more than a line better with a test based on 4 Sloan letters. This is an easy way to become aware of the developmental level of a child's recognition of abstract forms, or changes in recognition functions in a child or adult with a progressive brain disorder. These three tests and the Landolt C test are printed on a test card called Visual Perception Card 4-1 (available from www.Good-Lite.com; see the Resources section in Chapter 12). Each test seeks responses by matching—that is, has a purely visual test situation.

## Evaluating the Quality of the Visual Image as the Child Sees it

Grating acuity tests, discussed in Chapter 12, can be used in an adapted way as tests of early visual processing. Figure 13.1 shows a drawing by an engineer who had amblyopia in one eye. He looked at the gratings with his amblyopic (lazy) eye, then while viewing with his normally sighted eye, he drew what he saw. The broad straight lines appeared straight, but the fine straight lines did not, and the finer they were, the more distorted they appeared.

Young children are not able to give a verbal description of grating line distortion, but they can show what they see by moving their finger along the lines. If a child sees the broad lines as straight, the child's finger glides smoothly along while tracing the broad line, but when presented with the finer lines, the finger may show varying irregular movements. When looking at the finest lines, the child often says that there are "no lines." This means that in the primary visual cortex, where the incoming visual information is sorted and coded (or encoded), the capacity is too limited to define the many fine lines, even though the child's measured optotype visual acuity value suggests that finer lines should be visible.

FIGURE 13.1
**Grating Line Distortion**

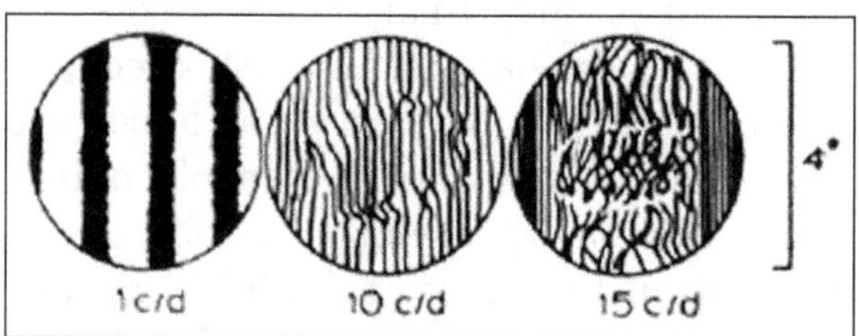


These drawings of straight lines of differing widths from a grating acuity test were made by an adult with amblyopia in one eye who drew what his amblyopic eye perceived. The finer the lines were, the more distorted they appeared to the amblyopic eye.

*Source:* Hyvärinen, L., & Jacob, N. (2011). *WHAT and HOW does this child see?* (p. 36). Helsinki, Finland: VISTEST Ltd.

Thus the quality of encoding of fine grating lines should be suspect if grating acuity is lower than expected, based on the optotype acuity value. This observation takes little time, so it is worth including it in routine test batteries. Its importance is shown by the following case history:

**A CHILD WITH CVI SELDOM HAS ONLY ONE TYPICAL SYMPTOM.** In an exceptional case, a teenager had a rare specific difficulty in interpreting the body language of others. She was known to have had an epileptic focus in the right temporal lobe, identified by electroencephalography (EEG) as a child. She had been seizure-free for several years without medication. During her visual assessment, all measured values were normal, except that grating lines were not perceived as straight, while the 8 cpcm (cycles per centimeter) lines were not perceived at all, despite the requisite optotype visual acuity. This additional phenomenon helped explain why the girl had not been able to cut materials in alignment with the weave of the cloth during her sewing class; she simply could not see them. This symptom had been misinterpreted and dealt with negatively, which had made the girl's favorite subject so unpleasant that she had refused to participate further.

This case shows that thorough assessment of vision of children with mild epileptic activity can reveal involvement of unsuspected brain areas where no findings are found in the EEG.

## Determining Methods to Evaluate Higher Visual Functions

The choice of which specific tests to administer must take into account information that has been gathered from earlier observations, available reports, and history taking (see Chapters 10 and 11). It is also necessary to determine the kind of visual, auditory, and tactile communication required in the administration of each test. Questions to ask when determining tests to administer include the following:

- What further observations might be needed before starting testing in order to understand the functional level of the child?
- Does the child need training in matching or in feeling the size and surface structures and qualities with his or her hands?
- Are there features of the visual field that can interfere with test situations? If the visual field has not been carefully evaluated, it should be one of the first tests. During visual field testing, the assessors can also learn more about the child's communication style, visual sphere (the area around the child within which he or she can most easily attend to visual information), the speed of responding, and ways of responding. Thus, further adaptation of the test situations is possible to meet the child's communication and conceptual needs.
- Does the child's specific medical condition or behavioral style lead one to suspect certain patterns of visual processing that need to be addressed by specific tests? (See Chapter 3.)
- What communication methods are best used with the child, and who should communicate with the child during evaluation sessions?
- How can the visual and auditory environment best be set up for the child?
- How should the child be prepared for testing in terms of level of alertness and body position?

## Specific Procedures for the Evaluation of Visual Processing

The tests and procedures described in the following sections provide methods for initial evaluation of higher visual functions, including perception of orientation, perception of location, disorders of perception of motion, disorders of visual identification, fundamental visuospatial functions and navigation, disorders in visual-motor ability, disorders in visuospatial cognition, and difficulties in copying figures. The methods for these fundamental visuospatial functions described in this section are particularly appropriate for those for whom standardized, formal neuropsychological assessment tools are not available. The methods to assess the first class of higher visual functions, the visual selective attentional functions, are not described in the following sections; these functions and the ways to assess them are discussed in detail in Chapter 6, as well as in Table 13.1, presented later in this chapter.

### *Orientation Perception*

The tests and procedures listed in this section measure perception of orientation—that is, the relative direction of an object. For all tests of perception of orientation, it is important that the child understands the meaning of the questions and can carry out the tasks set by giving a prior demonstration and seeking understanding.

It is important to note that there is a difference between *relative* orientation perception and *absolute* orientation perception. If a child is able to see subtle differences between orientations (relative orientation perception), it does not necessarily mean that the child is able to understand the orientations with respect to the surrounding space (more absolute orientation perception). For example, a child who has no difficulty noting the difference between two lines that differ by only 3 degrees may easily misinterpret the hands of an analog clock without numbering by as much as 5 minutes, which amounts to 30 degrees. This also stresses the need to relate orientation perception tasks with orientation in real-world activities for children with CVI, since task-specific findings can be directly applied to intervention plans.

***The Rectangles Game.*** The Rectangles Game (Hyvärinen, 2014) consists of five dark-colored and five light-colored rectangular shapes of various matching lengths and widths (see Figure 13.2). It evaluates recognition of the length of objects and lines (in part a temporal lobe recognition function) and eye-hand visual guidance and configuration in grasping (a parietal lobe motor function). The normal grasping functions should be accurate and with normal speed. In one variation of this game, placing a rectangle on its correct counterpart is guided by visual comparison of the length of the rectangle given to the child and those on the table. If a child's grasping function is poor, the purely visual task can be modified by asking the child to point to the rectangle among the five rectangles on the table that has the same length as the one held by the tester. Before using this test it is wise to identify whether the child can understand and recognize the differences in length and understands the words "shorter" and "longer."

***The Mailbox Game.*** In the Mailbox Game, children are asked to orient a card to a slot representing a mailbox (a visual orientation task) and also to post the card through the slot (a visual-motor task). Figure 13.3 shows two children being assessed and trained in the concept of the direction needed for eye-hand coordination (a parietal function) as they are directed to "post" a card through the mailbox slot. Figure 13.3A shows the child posting the card through the slot. In the test

FIGURE 13.2
**Rectangles Game**

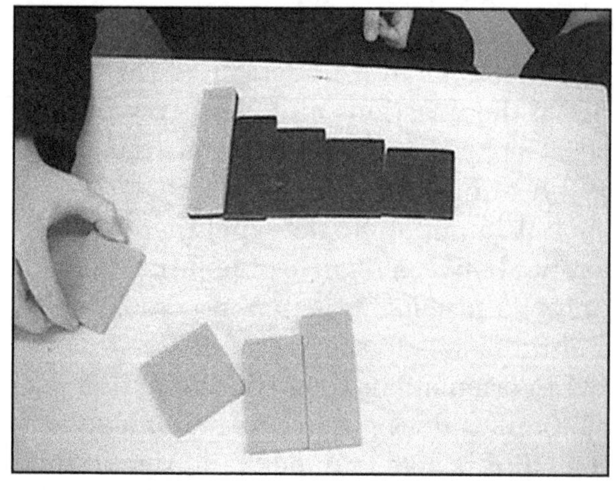

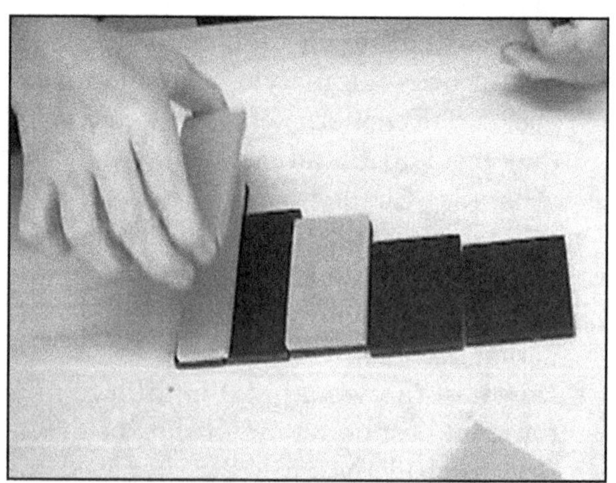

*Source:* Reprinted with permission from Hyvärinen, L., & Jacob, N. (2011). *WHAT and HOW does this child see?* (p. 125). Helsinki, Finland: VISTEST Ltd.

FIGURE 13.3
**Direction of Lines: Mailbox Game**

A
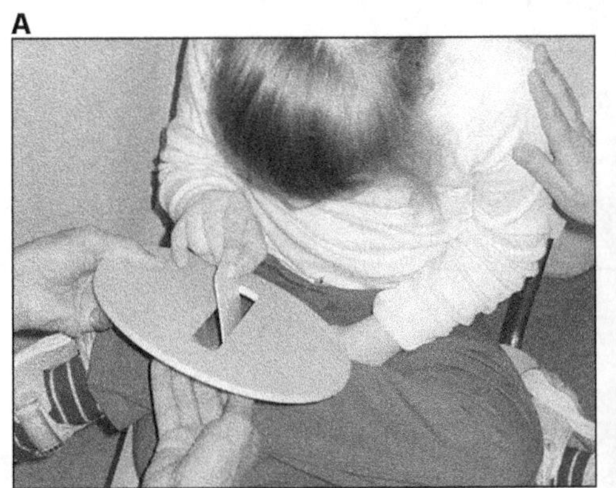
B
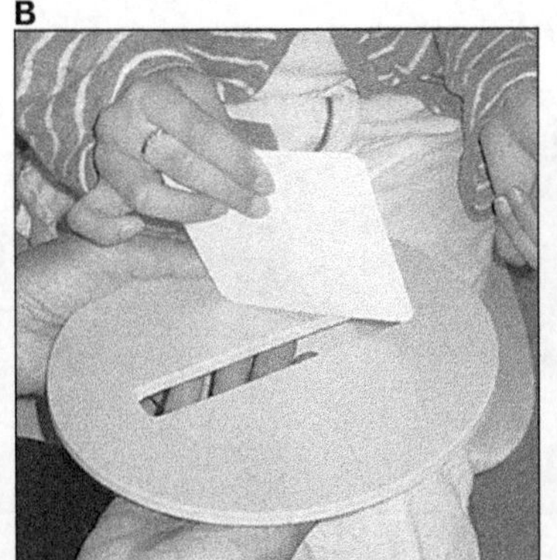
C
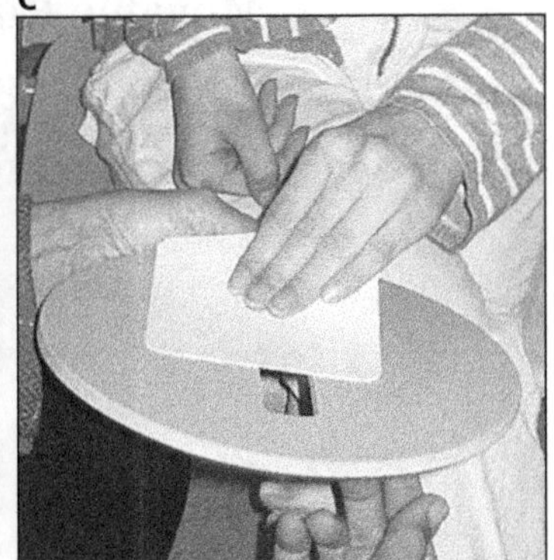

*Source:* Reprinted with permission from Hyvärinen, L., & Jacob, N. (2011). *WHAT and HOW does this child see?* (p. 126). Helsinki, Finland: VISTEST Ltd.

situation (Figure 13.3B), the card is handed to the child in an orientation at right angles to the direction of the slot. Figure 13.3C shows that the child's concept of visual-motor orientation has yet to develop, as the child unsuccessfully attempts to deliver the card through the slot in the same orientation as it was given

***The Movable Rod Method.*** The movable rod method of line orientation comparison is a purely visual test that requires demonstrating the ability to recognize when given lines are oriented in the same direction. It is based on the pure recognition function in which the orientation of a movable rod (which rotates around one fixed end) is matched to a fixed rod (see Figure 13.4). In this test variant, the tester shifts the movable rod, using small movements, until the child says that the moving rod is in the same direction as the fixed rod. The child is asked to compare the orientation of one line to the orientation of the other by answering the simple yes-or-no question, "Are these lines in the same direction?" Similar visual tasks can be arranged using magnetic rods or other narrow objects to create angles or parallel lines, making sure that the line thickness and separation between lines are within the child's functional visual acuity limit.

***Benton's Judgment of Line Orientation Test.*** Benton's Judgment of Line Orientation Test (Benton, Sivan, Hamsher, Varney, & Spreen, 1994) is more complex and can be used for the more able child. The orientation of two lines has to be judged against 11 others and requires a lot of attentional orchestration by the child. In addition, the lines are rather crowded, which poses a problem for those who have trouble adopting a small visually attended area (local visual selective attention). Moreover, the two test lines differ in length, and in some cases are so short that they require mental imagery to help compare them to the other lines.

A modification of this procedure for children with CVI is to present a child with two lines of the same length in different orientations and then to ask if the lines have the same orientation or not. This is a clear and practical method to examine a perceptual task involving the judgment of line orientation.

FIGURE 13.4
**Direction of Lines: Using a Movable Rod**

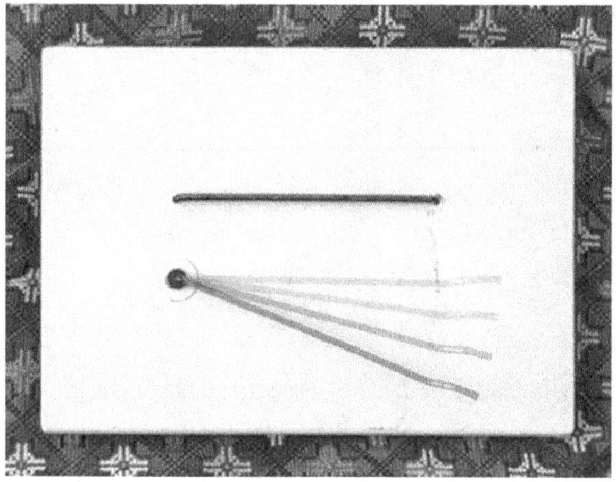

*Source:* Courtesy of Lea Hyvärinen.

FIGURE 13.5
**Perception of Location Task**

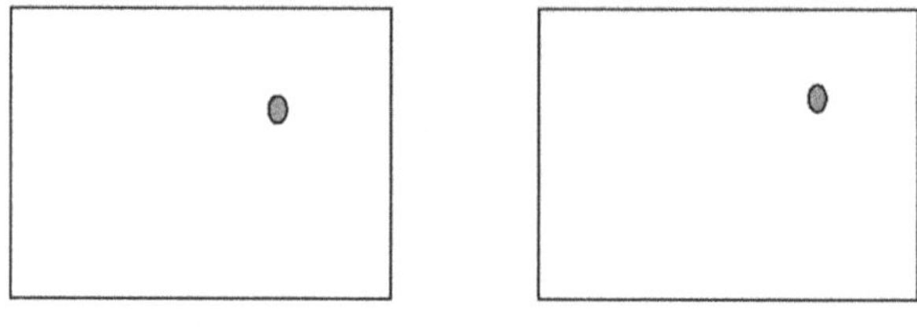

### *Perception of Location*

One may argue that knowing where an object is located is the most basic function or functional unit of all visuospatial understanding; the name "where" pathway for the dorsal stream pathway also suggests this is so. There is no test that specifically addresses the ability to judge an object's location. Two subtests of the Visual Object and Space Perception Battery (VOSP; Warrington & James, 1991) come close, but do not meet the criteria of good location perception tests.

One subtest involves the perception of the exact middle of squares (which covers only a very limited conception of location); the other requires matching the location of a dot in one square to the location of multiple, rather crowded numbers in another. This again depends on the ability to zoom in to details using local visual selective attention. In addition to these limitations and validity issues, this test is designed for people of 15 years of age and older.

Learning from the weaknesses of these subtests, it is suggested that if one wants to know how well a child understands spatial location, one would want to use a task in which the child compares the location of a dot in a square or circle with the location of a dot in a similar square or circle, and is asked to provide a simple yes-or-no response to the question, "Are these dots [they might be called ladybugs] in the same place on the window?" (see Figure 13.5).

Goal-directed visual-motor tasks are processed subconsciously by the "how" pathway and require accurate internally mapped representations of the surroundings that are used to perform fast and precise body and limb movement. Conscious appreciation of where things are located in relation to each other, how they are oriented, whether they move or not, and, if so, in which direction and how fast, are processed separately (see Chapter 3). To understand visual spatial figures like the ones presented in the Test of Visual Perceptual Skills (TVPS; Martin, 2006) (such as location and orientation of parts of a figure) or of objects in space (location with respect to other objects and self, orientation, static or moving, direction and speed of movement), one needs four higher visual functions: the ability to

- select the figure as a whole by using global visual selective attention,

- zoom in to details using local visual selective attention,
- judge the locations of the parts of the visuospatial figure using the location perception function, and
- judge the orientation of the parts of the figure.

In addition to these higher visual functions (and lower visual functions), one needs to be motivated, have an intact executive system, and have intact general attentional functions.

## *Identifying Disorders of Perception of Motion*

Motion perception is integral to moving through the visual world. It is important in negotiating traffic, and playing sports, and is required to identify the fleeting elements of facial expression and gesture that enhance communication. The capacity to see movement can be observed through children's behaviors in moving environments such as traffic and by discussing how moving cars or balls are perceived. It can also be observed by asking the child to count fingers on a fast, to-and-fro, horizontally moving hand as it gradually slows down in front of the child. This provides a useful indicator of whether motion perception may be impaired (see Chapter 3). Some tests have been developed to evaluate the detection of movement—that is, Is there something moving? Standardized tests to assess a child's ability to judge the speed and/or direction of the movement have yet to be developed. This gap needs to be filled urgently.

### FIGURE IN MOTION

***The Pepi Test.*** The Pepi Test (Hyvärinen & Jacob, 2011) investigates the ability to assemble the component parts of an image that does not have a specific profile, but only becomes evident and recognizable through the character of its movement. This is known as *figure-in-motion processing.* This test helps to reveal whether an infant from the age of 4 months or a young child can perceive—and when older, describe—the moving picture on a computer screen. This test facilitates observation of pursuit eye movements and the quality of motion perception, as well as whether the figure in motion can be recognized.

At the start of the Pepi Test, a small, red-and-white grating, designed to entice the infant or child to look at it, is presented in the center of the screen. When it disappears, the image of a Dalmatian appears in one of the corners of the screen and slowly moves diagonally to the opposite corner. The assessor can observe when the child notices the picture—(1) immediately, when it first appears in the corner of the screen, (2) as the figure moves closer to the center, or (3) at different distances, as the dog moves diagonally across the screen from each of the four corners.

Both children and infants typically look at the central target then make fast eye movements to look at, then follow, the target. Children with CVI may see only something moving but fail to identify it. They tend to look at the screen briefly two or three times but then lose interest. They can indicate the direction of the movement, but are unable to appreciate that a dog is present and identify it. Some children only look at the fixation target, and then their eyes wander around the screen as if looking for something to see. If they can talk, they may mention only "the small red picture in the middle." They may not have even perceived the moving picture, which has no discrete outline, and can be seen only if the visual and attentional systems can detect and process the figure in motion. The child's eye movements and behavior are observed closely throughout the test as the image is observed.

If the child detects the figure only when it is close to the middle of the screen, when it has come from one side but not the other, this suggests that the ability to give attention on the affected side is limited, or that the child has a visual field impairment.

By using the information from this test, one can find out whether a child's attention is pulled exogenously to the location of the onset of the stimulus and whether the child is capable of following the movement. If the child is observed to be capable of tracking the direction of movement with his or her eyes, this does not necessarily mean that what has been seen has been understood.

#### IDENTIFICATION OF BIOLOGICAL MOVEMENT

***Johansson's Walking Man.*** Johansson's Walking Man (Hyvärinen & Jacob, 2011; Johansson, 1976) involves a slowly walking figure depicted by a few moving dots. Biological movement such as walking can typically be recognized at distances at which a person cannot be recognized by facial features but can be recognized by clothing or by the nature of the movement itself. Children who have disorders of periventricular white matter, for example, may be unable to identify this form of biological movement (Pavlova, Staudt, Sokolov, Birbaumer, & Krägeloh-Mann, 2003). Variants of this test are available on the Internet.

### *Identifying Disorders of Visual Recognition and Identification*

With respect to the question "What is it?" seeing well means recognizing and identifying not only objects, faces, geometric shapes, and colors, but also pictures of objects, shapes, and faces. The assessor needs to find out which objects or pictures a child understands and which he or she does not. Different levels of identification that we may want to assess can be distinguished.

In assessing identification of pictures, faces, shapes, and color, the following considerations need to be taken into account:

- Is the child capable of visually identifying (matching, naming, accurately using, or pointing to) single real objects that should be known according to developmental age?
- If so, is the child capable of visually identifying smaller or larger but realistic versions of objects in three dimensions?
- The next step is to find out if the child is able to identify photographs in two dimensions, realistic color and black-and-white pictures, and abstract color and black-and-white pictures.
- In addition, if a child is suspected of having problems in face recognition, given the requisite functional visual acuity and appropriate viewing distance, this should be assessed as well. Disorders of face recognition (prosopagnosia) are considered distinct from disorders in object recognition (object agnosia), since a specific part of the "what" pathway is dedicated to face identification and recognition, and disorders in face recognition often occur independently of those of object recognition.
- The visual identification of geometric shapes is a tricky subject, since this depends on a child's understanding of spatial relationships and, as such, depends heavily on the development of the dorsal ("where") pathway, which in itself depends on the development of global visual selective attention.
- With respect to colors, there are big functional differences between experiencing

colors (a sensory function), being able to match them (sensory and understanding), and being able to name them (understanding). If there seem to be problems in the understanding of colors, one would want to find out at which of these three levels the child experiences difficulties.

There are many subtests that can be used to find out how well a child is able to identify pictures of objects or animals, and some not very good ones to assess whether children are able to learn new faces. To the authors' knowledge there is none to identify well-known faces or to identify them as unknown.

In testing visual recognition, the following considerations must be taken into account:

- The test image details need to be visible to the child.
- Global visual selective attention plays an important role in object and face recognition and identification.
- Naming may pose a problem in children with word-finding disorders.
- Tasks that have children pick one out of multiple pictures require a lot of attentional control; the assessor needs to make sure they look carefully at every picture before choosing.

In addition, it is important to know the extent to which the child understands *visual scenes*, which have more ecological value since they can include daily life situations, the understanding of which is crucial for day-to-day functioning. Understanding visual scenes entails identification of the parts of the scene, but also depends on many more functions. The ability to attend to large areas with each fixation (global visual selective attention) plays an important role in uncovering the relationships between the parts, the actors and objects, in the scene. The ability to attentionally "zoom in" (local visual selective attention) to examine the key components of the scene plays a substantial part in visual scene understanding. In addition, reasoning and knowledge about the world (an executive function) play important roles in understanding the scene.

Identification of *incomplete pictures and pictures from an unnatural viewpoint* can also be investigated. Identifying this kind of special stimulus requires additional high visual functions and some executive problem-solving skills, which in turn depend on attentional functions.

- Understanding pictures that are incomplete (such as the examples in Figures 6.3 and 6.4 in Chapter 6) predominantly requires the ability to use large visually attended areas per fixation and to decrease the attended area size (by executive functions) in order to select and recognize details (if available). In addition, it requires executive visual imaging ability to mentally complete the picture in working memory.
- Identifying pictures from an unnatural vantage point—for example, a familiar face presented upside down or a bicycle seen from above—may also require mental manipulation (mental rotation) in visual working memory and thus involves executive functioning in the form of mental image rotation.

Several tests can be used to screen for visual recognition of faces and expressions, which are specific to ventral stream functions and can be impaired independently of other, more general object identification. The perception of expressions depends on processing the face as a whole, using global visual selective attention, which is required for mirror neuron function. Perception of detail by serial selection of elements requires effort, while selecting single elements can lead to incorrect interpretation of the expression.

***Heidi Expressions Test Game.*** The Heidi Expressions Test Game (Hyvärinen, 2012), which consists of a set of cards containing six different basic expressions, can be used to evaluate the perception of faces with young children to see which details the child can perceive and recognize. There can be great variation in the nature and degree of atypical visual capabilities in face perception, depending on how damage to a specific higher cortical area affects the amount of visual information received. For example, some children with face blindness can perceive faces well, or at least vaguely, but cannot connect the information to memory and therefore cannot recognize people. There are also children with sufficient visual acuity who appear not to perceive facial structures at all and describe seeing "only skin," perceiving a light-colored oval without any structure. If a child has a poorly functioning cortical area for perception and recognition of faces, it is possible that information related to the parts of a face has been conveyed through tactile and haptic information only, and the child does not know, for example, that a curved line in the lower part of the picture depicts a mouth, despite the ability to point to parts of the face.

***The Hiding Heidi Test.*** The Hiding Heidi Test (Hyvärinen, 2013) can be used to find out at what distance an infant or young child can respond to visual communication (see Figure 13.6). In some cases, this can also be measured by observing the child's behavior when the mother or father approaches the child.

Since the contrast of faces can vary considerably, the test uses a "standard face" designed based on the work of Fantz (1970). The resulting smiling face, which is presented at different contrast levels, is close to the dimensions of the human face, and can be used to help elicit the child's optimum communication distance. The test is presented in a typical preferential-looking situation (see Chapter 12). If an infant smiles in response to the presented face, like the 3-month-old infant shown in Figure 13.6, the child must be able to see, interpret, and respond with a normal social smile. The test is sometimes used to estimate contrast sensitivity, although it was not designed for that purpose, nor does it define the width of the normal communication range at certain ages. It is useful in assessing vision when an infant's vision seems to be subnormal. If, at the usual communication distance of the child's family, the infant responds only to

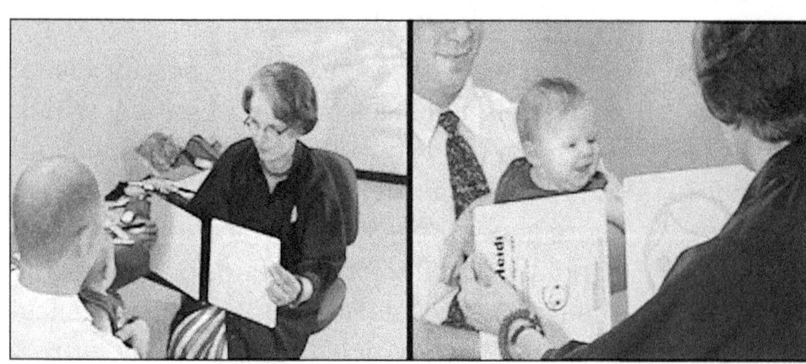

FIGURE 13.6
**Hiding Heidi Test**

*Source:* Reprinted with permission from Hyvärinen, L., & Jacob, N. (2011). *WHAT and HOW does this child see?* (p. 62). Helsinki, Finland: VISTEST Ltd.

the full-contrast picture, the 25 percent, and the 10 percent contrast picture, but not to lower-contrast images, it means that adults need to be closer and wear high-contrast makeup to render their faces visible.

The Hiding Heidi test has played an important role when teachers have found it hard to believe that a visually impaired student cannot see the teacher's face in the classroom and therefore has difficulty in following what he or she says. When it is demonstrated in the classroom that the child with atypical visual functioning cannot see 2.5 percent contrast picture from the first row, while the other children see it from the back of the classroom, the teacher can understand the importance of staying near the visually impaired student so that the child will receive the same visual communication as the other students.

### *Estimating Facial Recognition Distance and Speed*

The distance at which facial expressions can be recognized and the speed at which they can be seen can both be estimated. The examiner initially adopts a smile, a frown, or a sad look while close to the child, explaining that he or she is happy, angry, or sad, to prepare the child for the task at greater distances. The examiner then adopts these expressions at progressively greater distances until they can no longer be identified by the child. This procedure helps to determine the child's facial expression recognition distance, which everyone who interacts with the child should be aware of.

For estimating speed of recognition, the expressions can be displayed, at a close distance, either fleetingly or for intermediate or long durations. Many children with CVI are unable to capture the meaning of the fleeting expressions that typical children have no trouble perceiving. These approaches to estimating distance and speed for recognizing facial expressions are subjective, but with practice can prove very helpful.

## Issues in Assessing Fundamental Visuospatial Functions

The tasks used to assess the functions that form the basis of visuospatial understanding—location perception, orientation perception, movement perception, perception of movement speed, and perception of direction of movement—are all table tasks. Although these tasks involve the use of visual-spatial patterns, figures, and shapes and make sense with respect to understanding of visuospatial information presented on a table, the performance cannot be construed as an indicator of the capacity to handle larger scale visuospatial tasks in daily life, such as navigating, which involve a lot more than visual selective attentional functions and visuospatial perception functions. In addition to general attentional functions and extensive executive coordination, they can involve the use of visual imagery and mental rotation, as well as many other complex multimodal integration processes in which visual, vestibular, and even auditory information is integrated into map or route information. In addition, navigation often requires selection and perception of memory for landmarks and their sequence.

Many visuospatial functions are hard to evaluate, primarily due to lack of good assessment instruments as well as the nature of the processing required. Visual working memory functions—for example, the ability to form mental visual images—are hard to test. One could ask a child to draw something from memory or fantasy, which requires the creation of a mental image, but the drawings of children reflect much more than just the quality of the mental image, and may be hampered by motor disability. Mental image manipulation—for example, the ability to rotate a mental image—can be assessed by the Standardized Roadmap Test of Direction Sense (Money, 1976), which requires the ability to imagine oneself making turns using a simplified map that requires mental viewer-centered rotation and knowledge of the difference between right and left. In contrast, there are no standardized tests that assess mental object rotation capability, in which the mental rotation of an object (object-centered rotation) requires functions other than imagining mental *viewer*-centered rotation (Wraga, Creem, & Proffitt, 1999).

### *Identifying Disorders in Visual-Motor Ability*

Validated clinical tests that allow motor and visual-motor ability to be distinguished have yet to be developed. The difference between visual-motor and motor functions can be explained as follows: After the executive system selects a part of an object using visual selective attention, the *visual-motor system* instantly translates the coordinates produced in the internal mental map of the surroundings into finger, hand, foot, head, or trunk coordinates to facilitate fast and accurate goal-directed visual-motor action, such as pointing, grasping, kicking, catching, or walking through a doorway. The *motor system* performs the actions. A visual-motor disorder can be distinguished from a motor disorder by the individual's ability to perform a particular movement flawlessly without visual information, but lack of speed and accuracy when visual input is required to guide the movement.

Although some tests, like the Beery-Buktenica Developmental Test of Visual-Motor Integration (Beery VMI; Beery, Buktenica, & Beery, 2010) and the eye-hand coordination subtest of Developmental Test of Visual Perception (DTVP–3; Hammill, Pearson, & Voress, 2013), may appear to assess visual-motor functions (or visual-motor integration), they actually do not. They predominantly assess visual attentional and visuospatial perceptual functions (VMI), or do not distinguish between motor and visual-motor dysfunctions (DTVP–3) and do not take into account performance speed. As a consequence, children who score well on both these tasks may still have considerable visual-motor disorders, resulting, for example, in slow or badly aimed grasping, kicking, or catching a ball.

### *Identifying Disorders in Visuospatial Cognition*

Although many tests aim to assess visuospatial perception ("Where is it?"), it is hard to find one that identifies which impaired higher visual *function* or *functions* are responsible for a child's impaired performance. For one, tasks that appear to be primarily visuospatial in nature, like spatial construction tasks, often require a range of executive functions and abilities, to a greater extent than identification tasks. Sustained attention, orchestration of attentional processing, planning, working systematically, flexibility of strategy, envisioning the visual imagery of the end result, mental image rotation, and active mental imagery all contribute. The ability to change the size of the attended visual area (with visual selective attention preceding processing in the "where" pathway) determines what is perceived. A large visual area needs to be adopted to appreciate the spatial configuration of multiple elements (global visual selective attention), but to estimate the spatial characteristics of the elements, the capacity to attentionally "zoom in" (local visual attention) is also needed. As a consequence, knowledge about a child's executive functions, as well as the general and visual attentional functions is needed to be able to interpret a child's visuospatial functions or abilities and has a greater role than in identification tasks.

Another problem in assessing visuospatial functions is that the many available tests do not cover *functions*, but employ constructs or stimulus characteristics that can be broken down into more than one visual function or functional unit. For example, visual-spatial discrimination is a construct; it takes many functions to discriminate between visual-spatial figures. Global visual selective attention, however, is a function: it is a fundamental functional action the brain performs that allows us to select a large area of the visual field. This function—and the other visual-selective attentional and visual-spatial perceptual functions—is required to be able to discriminate visual-spatial figures. The use of constructs in available tests is not very helpful and may even be misleading when trying to find out which functions or functional units are not working well.

Consider, for example, some of the constructs TVPS uses to assess visuospatial functions. In addition to leaning heavily on sustained attention and flexibility in assigning local and global visual selective attention, plus not including time scores, the test presents constructs like visual discrimination, visual figure-ground, visual form constancy, and visual closure as if they are functions or functional units.

But we do not have a visual discrimination function. Nor do we have a visual figure-ground function, a form-constancy function, or a visual closure function. These are simply constructs used to describe the tasks at hand. To have diagnostic value, it is important to break down tasks (as well as the constructs used to label the tasks) into functions required to perform the task. In this way, if a child fails a task, hypotheses can be formulated about which *function* or *functions* are responsible for the poor performance. In addition to loading on executive and general attentional functions, performance on the visual figure-ground and visual closure stimuli in TVPS predominantly depends on the visual selective attention functions of zooming in to see detail and zooming out to appraise the whole image, respectively. These tests were designed to evaluate the range of normal visual abilities, and not to probe specific disorders in higher visual functions. In trying to uncover disorders in higher visual functions, the term "visual figure-ground" may contaminate interpretation by assuming that if a child's performance is poor, the child has some sort of visual figure-ground dysfunction—that is, that the child will do poorly at all sorts of figure-ground tasks, which is not necessarily the case. For example, a child who has a dysfunction in local visual selective attention, who is unable to deal with a crowded picture of overlapping lines due to a disorder in local visual selective attention, may be perfectly able to understand the well-known face-vase picture (in which an image can appear to be either a vase or two faces in profile looking at each other), which is also a figure-ground task. In like manner, visual closure is not a function. It consists mainly of two functions: global visual selective attention and the creation of the missing parts by using visual working memory to engage in envisioning visual imagery. To be able to really help a child who performs badly at figure-ground tasks, we need to know which of these functions is impaired, if not both.

In addition, many of the TVPS test items require different abilities than the test intends to measure. For example, many of the visual closure stimuli are fairly crowded. As a result, a child with a disorder in adopting a small visually attended area (that is, to attentionally "zoom in" to details in a crowded stimulus) is very likely to perform poorly, but not because of difficulty "visually closing" the figure. Along the same line of reasoning, the Visual Form Constancy items are often hidden in a crowded picture, and as such do not measure "visual form constancy" (which arguably depends on mental manipulation *functions*, like mental rotation, of the visual material), but again requires the ability to locate and attend to a small visual area. As a result, it can be argued that TVPS fails in construct and test validity for higher-order visual functions, and the potential risk of misinterpretation of the results needs to be recognized.

In sum, assessment needs to be focused on identifying disorders in functions, rather than constructs or stimulus characteristics (such as "figure-ground" or "visual closure"). Tests such as TVPS can at best be used to build hypotheses about the child's visual abilities by extracting the functions needed for the particular items a child has difficulty performing. At worst, misinterpretation can lead to misrepresentation of a child's visual difficulties.

### *Difficulties in Copying Figures*

Children with brain damage often have difficulties with line directions, parallel lines, angles, and pictures composed of several forms that are partially on top of each other. Those with brain damage from birth usually have limited experience with drawing and many do not know how a printed model or sample picture was created, so the child is asked to watch the examiner draw the figures for drawing tasks. The child can then copy the basic form after watching the examiner create it (Figure 13.7). This short test situation is similar to visual tasks in geometry and is a good test of school readiness because it evaluates visual analysis of geometric forms and eye-hand coordination in copying forms with different angles in them.

FIGURE 13.7
**Copying Task**

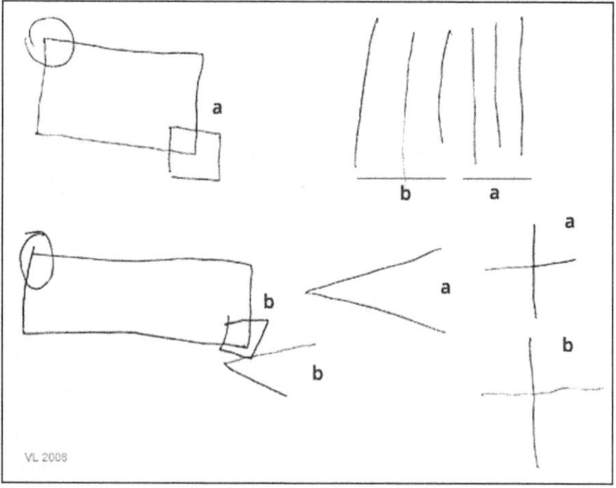


Copying these figures caused no difficulty for one child with CVI. The drawings were copied at the same speed that the tester used when drawing the model pictures. The tester's model drawings are marked with an *a* and the child's drawings are marked with a *b*.

*Source:* Reprinted with permission from Hyvärinen, L., & Jacob, N. (2011). *WHAT and HOW does this child see?* (p. 134). Helsinki, Finland: VISTEST Ltd.

## Summary of Assessment Methods of Higher Visual Functions

Table 13.1 lists the higher cognitive visual functions identified in this chapter, along with suggestions on how to try to assess them, as well as suggestions for some ways

TABLE 13.1

## Methods for Screening Assessment of Higher Visual Functions

*Sander Zuidhoek*

| *Higher Visual Functions* | *Recommended Assessment Method* | *Recommended Intervention (if Amenable to Intervention)* |
|---|---|---|
| **1. Visual Selective Attentional Functions** | | |
| *A. The ability to select big parts of a visual scene as well as small details from a large amount of visual information both at will and as imposed by salient stimuli in the environment (global and local visual attention, in a top-down as well as a bottom-up fashion)* | | |
| 1. Big parts (*Global visual attention*) | Global visual attention *(see figures in Chapter 6)*<br>• Navon Letters (Figure 6.2)<br>• Gestalt Stimuli (Figure 6.3)<br>• Visual scenes | • Decrease the workspace size<br>• Do *not* enlarge visual material<br>• Decrease material size<br>• Encourage concrete reasoning about the details of a scene or object<br>• Only display visual material relevant to the task<br>• Teach the child to keep his or her workspace as empty as possible<br>• Enlarge text and other visual materials<br>• Increase line spacing<br>• Seat child in front of class<br>• Use color coding for the beginnings of paragraphs or chapters<br>• Teach the child to cover parts of a page or picture |
| 2. Small details from a large amount of visual information (*Local visual attention*) | Local visual attention<br>• Follow one line among (many) other crowded lines | |
| 3. Continuous switching between global and local visual attention | Continuous switching between global and local visual attention<br>• Crowded overlapping line drawings<br>• Difficult serial search tasks, such as TEA-ch "Map Mission" (Manly, Robertson, Anderson, & Nimmo-Smith, 1998) | |
| *B. The ability to select information from a visual scene based on visual imagery of color, shape, or identity using mental visual imagery of the desired selective criterion or criteria (see* visual working memory functions*)* | "Can you point to all the red things in this room?" | |
| **2. Perceptual Functions** | | |
| *A. The ability to consciously see and identify/understand whatever has been selected (visual consciousness and visual identification; the "what" pathway)* | | |
| 1. Visual perception/identification of objects and animals<br>2. Visual perception of faces, visual identification of known persons | Try to determine what material a child understands. Go from realistic to more abstract in small steps, and display single objects; present them only visually (i.e., with no accompanying haptic or auditory information). | Change pictures to the level of material the child understands based on assessment results. |

*(continued on next page)*

**TABLE 13.1** *(continued from previous page)*

| *Higher Visual Functions* | *Recommended Assessment Method* | *Recommended Intervention (if Amenable to Intervention)* |
|---|---|---|
| 3. Visual perception/identification of simple well-known two-dimensional geometric shapes[a], such as triangles, circles, squares, ovals, diamonds, rectangles | Ask children to name the stimulus, preferably; matching does not necessarily require actual identification.<br>Use color as well as black-and-white stimuli, use "natural" vantage points. | |
| 4. Visual perception/identification of simple well-known three-dimensional geometric shapes[b], such as triangles, circles, squares, ovals, diamonds, and rectangles, and pictures of these[c] | Use stimuli such as the following:<br>• Real objects/animals/real faces of people known to the child<br>• Smaller and/or larger sized objects/animals/faces<br>• Photographs of objects/animals/faces<br>• Realistic drawings of objects/animals/faces<br>• Abstract drawings of objects/animals/faces<br>• Unconventional viewpoints of objects/animals/faces of different difficulty levels<br>• Pictures of stereotypical, simple, well-known shapes<br>• Pictures of simple shapes of unconventional intrinsic proportions and/or from unconventional viewpoints | |
| *B. The ability to* understand the spatial characteristics *of what is selected by visual selective attentional processes and consciously seen (visuospatial perception; "where" pathway)* | | |
| 1. Understanding where the perceived object(s) are in relation to oneself and other objects *(location perception)* | Location perception (see Figure 13.5) | Locations closest to the frame seem easiest for the children to understand. To improve visual location perception, one may try to teach the child to divide the space into, for example, four equal quadrants to provide the child with more reference lines to help the child learn to interpret the location. |

*(continued on next page)*

**TABLE 13.1** *(continued from previous page)*

| *Higher Visual Functions* | *Recommended Assessment Method* | *Recommended Intervention (if Amenable to Intervention)* |
|---|---|---|
| 2. Understanding how perceived objects are oriented *(orientation perception)* | Orientation perception:<br>• Relative orientation perception—A simple method is to present two lines on a sheet of paper which either have the same or a different orientation and ask the child to respond to the question, "Do these lines point in the same direction?" The difficulty of the task—the difference in orientation, should be varied.<br>• Absolute orientation perception: have the child judge the minute hand on analog clock.[e] | To improve relative orientation perception one may try to teach the child to mentally elongate both lines to see if they would cross. If so, they do not have the same orientation. |
| 3. Knowing whether the perceived object is moving *(movement perception)*, and if so: | Perception of movement of objects:<br>• Pepi the Dalmatian in motion (Hyvärinen & Jacob, 2011)<br>• Johansson's Walking Man (Hyvärinen & Jacob, 2011; Johannson, 1976) | |
| a. how fast (*speed perception*), and<br>b. in what direction (*direction perception*).[d] | No assessment methods available. A suggested method is to devise a computer task in which the movement speed and direction can be systematically varied. The child verbally judges if there is movement (yes/no), direction (to one of a variable number of locations on the screen), and speed (one of a variable number of presented speeds). | |
| **3. Visual-Motor Functions** | | |
| *The ability to perform fast and accurate actions toward a visually selected (part of an) object (visuomotor processing; the "how" pathway)* | | |

*(continued on next page)*

**TABLE 13.1** *(continued from previous page)*

| *Higher Visual Functions* | *Recommended Assessment Method* | *Recommended Intervention (if Amenable to Intervention)* |
|---|---|---|
| Any visually based movement that has a certain direction toward a stimulus (with any body part) involves different transformations from eye coordinates to motor coordinates. In principle, the automatic transformation of visual information for motor use can be disrupted for different body parts, independently of one another. | Have children make, for example, a grasping or kicking movement (or whichever sort of goal-directed movement seems to cause problems and/or limitations) with and without a visual target to try to detect a difference between the one and the other. If, according to a physical therapist, the movement without the visual target is faster and more fluent than with the visual target present, the automatic transformation from "visual coordinates" to "motor execution coordinates" may be disrupted. | The systematic training of visual-motor deficits may not work. Have tools and materials always in the same location in the workspace. The child may learn their locations proprioceptively. Once they do, they do not have to use the visual information to get the desired tool. |
| **4. Visual Consciousness: Emotional Response Functions** | | |
| *Having a feeling about significant images, without cognitively interpreting them.*[f] | No assessment method known to this author. | |
| **5. Visual Memory** | | |
| *The ability to recognize and/or actively recall the identity and/or spatial properties of previously viewed visual targets (short-term, longer-term, and long-term memory)*<br>A. Identity | Present the child with one or more objects or pictures that you are sure she understands by having the depiction identified by the child.<br>Try both *active recall* ("Remember the picture I showed you? What was on it?") and *recognition* ("Have you seen this picture? Which of these pictures did I show you earlier?") directly, or after a few seconds, an hour, a day, and after a few weeks, in order to trigger the different memory systems. | Try to teach the child to categorize the objects (for example, animals or furniture) into different possible classes in order to retain them in memory more easily.<br>Try to teach the child to verbalize the objects in order to retain them in a verbal way. |

*(continued on next page)*

**TABLE 13.1** *(continued from previous page)*

| *Higher Visual Functions* | *Recommended Assessment Method* | *Recommended Intervention (if Amenable to Intervention)* |
|---|---|---|
| B. *Spatial properties* of the formerly perceived object(s) or animals/faces/ spatial scene (The fundamental visual spatial functions are listed above: Perceptual functions, 2.)<br><br>Memory[g] | Spatial properties are either intrinsic (belonging to any visual stimulus) or extrinsic (between visual stimuli), but they encompass the same fundamental properties.<br>Try both *active recall* and *recognition.*<br>Note that in TVPS III (MEM) and TVPS III (SEQ) iconic and short-term only (and maybe longer term) memory is targeted. Note also that the target stimulus is only shown for 5 seconds, which may not be enough for a child to even understand its visuospatial characteristics (because of visual attentional or perceptual dysfunctions, for example), let alone memorize them. | Try to teach the child a route by both presenting it on a map and by traveling it together: point out the landmarks of the route explicitly, again and again. Make a list of the landmarks and have the child try to memorize them by heart. Let the child lead the way. |
| **6. Visual Working Memory Functions** | | |
| *The ability to generate and manipulate a mental visual image*<br>A. Generate visual mental image | Have a child draw something from memory, and try to interpret the developmental level of the drawing, taking into account motor and visuomotor skills. | Try to teach the child to mentally rotate better by slowly showing real rotations, and having her try very small mental rotations. |
| B. Manipulate a mental visual image | Have a child mentally rotate herself using the Standardized Roadmap Test of Direction Sense (Money, 1976).<br>Have a child rotate a stimulus to match that of an example (for suggested material, see, e.g., Shepard & Metzler, 1971).<br>Use different degrees of rotation to assess the child's ability. | |

*(continued on next page)*

**TABLE 13.1** *(continued from previous page)*

| *Higher Visual Functions* | *Recommended Assessment Method* | *Recommended Intervention (if Amenable to Intervention)* |
|---|---|---|
| **7. Being Able to React to and Perceive Visual Stimuli Quickly**[h] | | |
| Visual processing speed | Motor response to the sudden onset of a visual stimulus (FePsy "Visual Reaction Time" [Alpherts & Aldenkamp, 1997]), or comparable task with a verbal response.<br>Verbal successive response to a string of simple visual stimuli: TEA-ch "Opposite Worlds," the "Real World" Condition. Note that these tasks also depend on the time the child needs to form and perform the required responses. | |

[a]Although learning these geometric shapes is likely to initially depend on the "where" pathway, the actual recognition of a known shape probably depends on the "what" pathway.
[b]Although learning these geometric shapes is likely to initially depend on the "where" pathway, the actual recognition of a known shape probably depends on the "what" pathway.
[c]Pictures of three-dimensional shapes are generally called "2.5 dimensional."
[d]Although there are tasks with stimuli that reveal single objects or animals to those observers who are able to detect the movement of dots, this author does not know of tools to assess the actual movement of objects or their speed and direction, which, arguably, would have more ecological validity.
[e]Although a difficult task for most young children, the alternative of having the orientation matched will trigger "relative orientation perception" instead of "absolute orientation perception."
[f]We have not addressed this group of visual functions in the present chapter, since it is not directly related to the role of the executive system in seeing.
[g]In order to be able to assess memory functions, one needs knowledge about what memory is and how it works. This is far beyond the scope of the present chapter; it suffices to say that we have different memory systems for different durations, varying from less than two seconds to a lifetime. In addition, memory comprises many different more implicit and explicit encoding and retrieval processes, entailing different sensory systems. All of these processes can be disrupted independently of one another. Note that visual information may be remembered in a different form, for example, verbally. For example, a visual sequence like "O+O O+" may be remembered as "otoot"; that is, visually presented digits may be encoded verbally.
[h]Some people respond slowly to visual stimuli, without showing a dysfunction in any of the aforementioned visual functional units.

to treat disorders in these functions. For the assessment of the visual selective attentional functions, the first group of higher visual functions, the existing neuropsychological material mentioned in Table 13.1 is suggested, or material based on this; the material and methods are described in more detail in Chapter 6. With respect to the other functions, some neuropsychological tests are suggested in addition to the ones described in the previous sections; in addition, alternative assessment suggestions are listed when neuropsychological assessment tools are not available. The suggestions on how to *treat* the specific visual dysfunctions are, at this stage, speculative.

While reading the table, it must also be recognized that the processing of visual information also depends on attention, attentional control (the executive system) and, therefore, on emotions, urges and motivations, and the salience of visible objects in the physical environment. (See Chapter 6 for a detailed discussion.) Remember that the quality of perception depends not only on the "what" and "where" pathways, but also on the nature and quality of visual selective attentional processes and the quality of the lower visual functions. In addition, note that before one can assess the quality of memory functions, the quality of perceptual (and therefore of visual selective attentional) functions should be clear, as these dictate access to the information to be remembered.

Sidebar 13.1 considers the role of the neuropsychologist in the assessment of children who may have CVI.

SIDEBAR 13.1

## The Role of the Neuropsychologist in the Assessment of Children with CVI

***Sander Zuidhoek***

It is problematic to apply existing neuropsychological assessment tools to assess disorders in higher visual functions directly. One of the reasons is that when these tools were designed, the existence of CVI was only beginning to emerge. The tests were developed to map the normal development of visual *skills*, not to diagnose disorders in specific higher visual *functions*. Our purpose is different from that of the test designers. Our purpose is to habilitate or rehabilitate children with specific visual dysfunctions, in which case it is not enough to know a child's developmental level on a set of visual tasks.

In habilitation it is crucial that we know the disorders in *functions*. Why is that so? A simple analogy can be used to explain this. Consider a child who has difficulty walking. In order to help that child to walk as well and efficiently as possible, a physiotherapist needs to know the exact cause or causes of the difficulty before he or she can start effective treatment. It matters whether the causes of the trouble stem from the functioning of the foot, the ankle, the lower leg, the knee, the upper leg, the hip, the back, the brain, or a combination of these. And after the sites of the difficulty have been identified, the exact dysfunction and its mechanism need to be identified.

The role of helping a child to see better is no different. Moreover, in order to be able to optimally help the child, just as if the child had a physical disorder, the treatment should be designed to fit *that* particular child. Therefore, it is always necessary to know about the quality of the child's other physical as well as cognitive functions and his or her specific compensatory abilities, personality, and socio-emotional development.

Since the cognitive higher visual functions are the domain of neuropsychologists, and the quality of these functions depends on the more general cognitive functions, neuropsychologists are best trained to identify and diagnose the cognitive higher visual dysfunctions.

In an education setting, there are four ways of helping children overcome the problems and limitations that result from their dysfunctions:

- *adjusting* their environment and the material they work with,

*(continued on next page)*

**SIDEBAR 13.1** *(continued from previous page)*

- *educating* members of the social environment (parents, siblings, teachers, etc.),
- *teaching* a child how to use *compensatory techniques*, and
- *training* of visual (or other) skills by focusing on improving the functions that are responsible for the problems and restrictions in daily life.

In order to be able to efficiently treat a child, it is not enough to have "just" a list of *tasks* the child is unable to do well or a list of materials the child does not understand: these lists are endless in principle. In contrast, there are only a handful of identified fundamental functions that significantly impact daily life. In a perfect world, we would be able to assess all the visual as well as the nonvisual functions reliably. Once we knew the quality of all functional units (visual as well as nonvisual) and understood how and what the child sees and why, we could *predict* which tasks and stimuli would or would not be difficult for the child to cope with. We would be able to explain to the parents and teachers how the child sees the world and why, and what they can do to help the child. In addition, we could try to adjust the material in such a way that it eliminates the effects of the specific dysfunction. Moreover, we could make a start at trying to efficiently train the child to overcome the problems and limitations in daily life either by training to overcome the specific dysfunctions, by making use of the child's compensatory abilities, or both.

The world is far from perfect, however. We do not currently have good tests that assess actual higher visual functions. We urgently need these. Before we can design good assessment tools for different functions, we need to identify the higher visual functions. Neuropsychologists are the most likely discipline to succeed in this regard, help us to understand the neurocognitive mechanisms that underlie these dysfunctions, and design tests to assess these. The higher visual functions as identified by this author are listed in Part A of this chapter. Moreover, ways to assess and treat disorders in these functions are suggested.

Until we have reliable and valid tools to seek and measure higher visual dysfunctions directly, we need neuropsychologists to try to assess the higher visual and other functions to allow us to unravel them using the current imperfect tests. Children's neuropsychologists who are specialized in this field should be able to break down any task or test into those particular functions that are necessary for good performance. By following hypotheses based on the complete picture of the child, and having a child perform many selected tasks and tests, the neuropsychologist should be able to identify those functions that are disrupted and relate them to the different problems and restrictions in daily life. The neuropsychologist can thus clear the way for effective treatment and optimally functioning children. Although we are not there yet—neuropsychologists are relatively new to this field—we are making good progress in the Netherlands toward this goal. Those who do not have access to specialized neuropsychologists need a good, holistic view centered around a neuropsychological framework in order to understand seeing and to interpret disorders in visual behavior.

## Identifying CVI in Young School-Age Children

The earlier that CVI can be identified, the earlier measures can be put into place to enhance development. Some aspects of CVI may not be detected in young children until they are early school age. Appendix 13A at the end of this chapter describes an evidence-based screening battery designed for this purpose. It screens for visuo-attentional abilities associated with CVI in children in the general population aged 4 to 6 years who have normal or near-normal acuities and who do not have severe visual, cognitive, or physical limitations.

## Combining Information from a Variety of Sources

It is important to remember that test results alone may not provide sufficient information to explain a child's strategies or problems in daily life situations. Repeated observations in typical environments as well as careful questioning of caregivers and teachers (see Chapters 10, 11, 14) are crucial for assessing children who have CVI. Careful recording of information from parents, teachers, classroom assistants, and therapists through structured history taking is imperative (see Chapter 11). This can be correlated with observations in school, home, and community, along with information from the child's medical rehabilitation team, to reveal the nature of the child's atypical strategies in learning and communication. When combined with medical, optometric, and psychological findings, educational tests, observations and history taking are powerful tools for characterizing and understanding the child's vision and for the development of effective intervention plans, all of which needs to be shared with rehabilitation teams.

# PART C: A Profile of Visual Functioning and Case Studies

*Lea Hyvärinen, Namita Jacob, and Anne Henriksen*

Many children with CVI have changes in all areas of visual processing. Visual processing functions are involved in numerous daily activities, where their role in the child's atypical or adaptive strategies needs to be assessed. Therefore, it is important to carefully observe and discuss students' specific functional abilities for all areas that might be affected by CVI.

## Profile of Visual Functioning

Schools and early intervention teams may find it helpful to use a list of functions to review during a functional vision assessment. The Profile of Visual Functioning presented in this chapter contains a list of measurements and observations that can be used to summarize clinical and functional vision findings in children with multiple disabilities, for educational assessment purposes (Hyvärinen & Jacob, 2011; Hyvärinen, Walthes, Freitag, & Petz, 2012). Figure 13.8 shows a sample profile for a detailed case presented in this chapter. The profile contains a great deal of assessment information, and assessors cannot expect to complete it during a single assessment phase. It is best to complete it over time as the skills and abilities of a child become better known.

In the profile, the standard clinical findings on vision and all other observations are recorded as "normal" (N), impaired but useful (I), or profoundly impaired (P), and marked with three shades of gray to black. This facilitates rapid appraisal of the student's capabilities and challenges. Empty spaces are also provided for observations unique to the child. If a visual processing function cannot be measured due to other conditions (e.g., cerebral palsy), it is marked "not possible."

The Profile of Visual Functioning does not reveal a clinical anatomic diagnosis but helps to highlight the functions that should be investigated further and understood in detail. In the authors' experience, the completed profile usually confirms that many, if not most, of the child's vision-related functions are normal. This is an important finding for parents, therapists, and teachers who

FIGURE 13.8

## Profile of Visual Functioning Completed for Bertil, 9 Years Old

**Key:**
N=normal
I=impaired but useful
P=profoundly impaired

| CLINICAL FINDINGS, OCULAR MOTOR | N | I | P |
|---|---|---|---|
| A Fixation | | | |
| B Following movements | | | |
| C Saccades | | | |
| D Nystagmus | | | |
| E Strabismus | | | |
| F Convergence | | | |
| G Accommodation, compensated | | | |
| **CLINICAL FINDINGS, SENSORY** | | | |
| H Binocularity | | | |
| I Visual acuity, matching | | | |
| J Visual acuity, naming | | | |
| K Grating acuity, detection, not tested | | | |
| L Grating acuity, discrimination, 8 cpd | | | |
| M Gratings, line quality in the center | | | |
| N Contrast sensitivity, optotype | | | |
| O Contrast sensitivity, grating | | | |
| P Color vision | | | |
| Q Adaptation speed, CONE adaptation | | | |
| R Photophobia | | | |
| S Visual field, central | | | |
| T Visual field, peripheral, lower | | | |
| U Motion perception, Pepi Test | | | |
| V Biological motion, Walking Man | | | |
| X Depth perception | | | |
| Y Refraction | | | |
| Z Glasses | | | |

| VENTRAL NETWORK | N | I | P |
|---|---|---|---|
| A Recognition of objects | | | |
| B Recognition of details | | | |
| C Recognition of pictures of objects | | | |
| D Noticing errors and missing details | | | |
| E Recognition of faces | | | |
| F Recognition of facial expressions | | | |
| G Reading body language | | | |
| H Recognition of landmarks | | | |
| I Abstract pictures of objects | | | |
| J Abstract forms, letters, numbers | | | |
| K Increased crowding effect, NO MORE | | | |
| L Comparison with pictures in memory | | | |
| M Recognition in mathematical tasks | | | |
| N Scanning strategy | | | |
| O Cartoons, interpreting the content | | | |
| P Overview of large pictures | | | |
| Q Visual Imagination | | | |
| R Reading, need of magnification | | | |
| S | | | |
| | | | |
| **MIRROR NEURON SYSTEM** | | | |
| A Early eye contact, delayed | | | |
| B Early social smile, delayed | | | |
| C Early Interaction, delayed, supported | | | |
| D Early interest in movements of mouth | | | |
| E Early interest in hand movements | | | |



(continued on next page)

**FIGURE 13.8** *(continued from previous page)*

| **EARLY PROCESSING** | | | |
|---|---|---|---|
| A Length of lines, visual comparison | | | |
| B Orientation of lines, visual comparison | | | |
| C Stereovision | | | |
| D Visual closure | | | |
| E Textures and surface qualities | | | |
| F Objects/figures on patterned background | | | |
| G Short time memory | | | |
| **DORSAL NETWORKS** | | | |
| A Awareness of space, directions, distances | | | |
| B Orientation in space, map based | | | |
| C Orientation in space, route based | | | |
| D Observation of surrounding | | | |
| E Simultaneous perception | | | |
| F Eye-Hand coordination, directions | | | |
| G Eye-Hand coordination, length, not possible | | | |
| H Grasping and throwing objects | | | |
| I Drawing, copying a model, simple | | | |
| J Drawing, from memory | | | |
| K Drawing geometric forms, assisted | | | |
| L Copying from blackboard | | | |
| M Spatial problems in math | | | |

| F Early copying of hand movements | | | |
|---|---|---|---|
| G Interpretation of facial expressions | | | |
| H Recognition of parents at 6–8 months | | | |
| I Effect of image quality on above functions | | | |
| J | | | |
| K | | | |
| | | | |
| **OTHER COMMON PROBLEMS** | | | |
| L Integration of sensory functions | | | |
| M Visual overload | | | |
| N Auditory overload | | | |
| O Specific memory problems | | | |
| P Head control | | | |
| Q Body control | | | |
| R Hand functions | | | |
| S Moving | | | |
| T Hearing | | | |
| U Executive functions | | | |
| V Use of devices | | | |
| X | | | |
| PARTICIPATION | | | |
| ENVIRONMENT | | | |

can modify their interventions to assist the child to incorporate their intact capabilities as strategies to support effective study and participation.

## Case Example of Assessment Using the Profile of Visual Functioning: Bertil

A case example is presented to assist in understanding how evaluations of visual functions and visual processing functions can be used to characterize visual processing functions that may be compromised in children with CVI. This case illustrates that isolated findings from individual tests do not paint a clear picture of children who have CVI. It is important to coordinate information from a variety of sources in order to more fully understand the functional vision of these children.

### History

Bertil, a 9-year-old boy who has cerebral palsy, was known to have normal eyes, periventricular leukomalacia (PVL), impairment of part of the lower visual field, slightly irregular saccades compensated with head movements, mild accommodation insufficiency compensated with glasses, and several visual processing impairments. Reports of observations by the family, therapists, teachers, and O&M instructor were gathered along with clinical findings from the child's ophthalmologist, optometrist, and pediatric neurologist for the first functional assessment at the boy's present school. Figure 13.8 depicts the assessment areas that were discussed for the educational assessment.

### Reported Behaviors

Bertil was reported to have issues in multiple areas of visual functioning. In infancy, he had slower than normal responses to eye contact and facial expressions, even at close distances. His social smile and interest in observing and copying goal-directed hand movements developed late, as well as responses to parents' faces. These functions improved during early intervention activities. Face blindness had been noticed early and was formally diagnosed at the age of 8 months. It was not total, and compensatory information (such as hair color or eyeglasses) was used as well. Other difficulties in recognition functions were diagnosed in preschool. Caregivers also reported difficulty with noticing fast-moving objects.

Despite his many atypical visual and motor processing functions, Bertil had developed well. Motor problems with his hands required the use of a dictation device and computer instead of writing on paper, along with adapted test situations and learning materials. Clinical findings partly explained the cause of the functional problems in moving, that is, the slow shifts of attention to the lower part of the visual field, especially to the lower left, were likely to be an important cause. (This was described in medical reports as being clearly observable during clinical testing and Goldmann visual field measurement.)

### Initial Observations

There was no pediatric clinical test for Bertil's major problem: difficulty in perception of fast-moving objects and body parts—that is, motion perception. Perception of fast movements is important both in communication where lip movements are fast and short, and in traffic and sports. His difficulties with motion perception had been carefully observed in sports, ball games, and in gymnastics. In gymnastics some movements had to be shown using slow modeling. This problem was due to a combination of difficulties in perceiving movement and in copying it. He did not have notable problems in seeing the facial movements accompanying speech. The vision-related parietal functions of being able to see multiple events were especially problematic in soccer (Hess, Hutchinson, Ledgeway, & Mansouri, 2007). Fast-moving players could not always be properly seen and were recognized by their clothing. Often, Bertil did not know at which end of the lawn their goal was. He loved soccer. His peers, having grown up with him, accepted his vision-related adjustments while playing. Bertil was hypersensitive to movement in the peripheral visual field and to auditory noise, and considerable effort was made to reduce this type of distraction in Bertil's environment at school, especially in the classroom.

### *Assessments and Results*

Bertil came to his evaluation session wearing well-fitted filter lenses in comfortable frames. He explained that without his filter lenses, he was severely dazzled in some brightly lit situations. The assessments (see Chapter 12 for details of the various assessment tools) produced the following results:

- ***Visual acuity*** was the same as reported by Bertil's ophthalmologist, a good normal 1.25 (10/8.0 or 3/2.4; equivalent to 20/16 or 6/4.8) with ETDRS, LEA Numbers, and LEA Symbols standard tests (near and distance). Thus the recognition of abstract forms such as letters, numbers, and geometric forms seemed to be normal (Candy, Mishoulam, Nosofsky, & Dobson, 2011).
- ***Grating acuity*** measured with LEA Grating Acuity Test had resulted in a low value, 8 cpd at 57 cm. Bertil could see the grating lines as straight lines at the edges of the test target, but in the middle of the test target, grating lines were seen as blurred and distorted. When the test was brought closer (28cm), he was able to see gratings that were 4 cpd, and he perceived these lines as straight. Based on his optotype acuity of 20/16, the evaluators would have expected a grating acuity of 35 to 40 cpd (Mayer, Fulton, & Rodier, 1984).
- ***Reading acuity*** was also measured. Bertil pronounced letters slowly when reading a usual schoolbook and often had to spell short words twice before saying them. His reading became easier when the text size and/or spacing were increased, consistent with the grating assessment. (Similar problems have also been seen in several children who had atypical severe reading problems despite typical visual acuities. Some children start a line all over again when only half of the line has been read, and, like Bertil, their reading becomes easier when the text size and/or spacing are increased. See the section on Dyslexia in Chapter 7.) Although Bertil had a normal visual acuity, he always chose a 28- to 40-point font to achieve a normal reading speed and to remember the content. The cause of this unusual relationship between good recognition acuity, print size, reading speed, and remembering is not clear but could relate to the difficulties in perception and encoding of fine gratings due to a form of visual crowding similar to although different from amblyopia. His working memory required further examination because it interfered with copying. Bertil said that he finds he forgets the information he has read when he moves his gaze from the blackboard to the paper.
- ***Contrast sensitivity*** was measured with the LEA Numbers chart and was low normal 0.32 (10/32, 3/9). The low-contrast grating acuity (LEA Low Contrast Grating Acuity test) was a very low measure of 3 cpd (see Appendix 12C). The fine low-contrast lines were less disturbed than the fine high-contrast lines, but he was unable to see the horizontal and vertical lines on graph paper.
- ***Color vision,*** when tested with the Panel 16 Quantitative Color Vision Test, was normal as in a previous clinical examination. Bertil had no difficulties in pointing at a colored cap that was "nearly the same color" as the sample, but could not grasp the color cap pieces, so the tester moved the caps into place for him.
- ***Figure-in-motion*** was tested with the Pepi Test (Hyvärinen & Jacob, 2011). Bertil

functioned normally. He recognized the slow movement of the Dalmatian and had normal eye movements.

- ***Perception of biological movement*** in Johansson's Walking Man (Hyvärinen & Jacob, 2011), which is also slow movement, was normal.
- ***Body language*** was difficult for Bertil to interpret as noted in observations.
- ***Length of lines and objects*** was correctly perceived and interpreted in the purely visual part of the Rectangles Game (Hyvärinen, 2014). Bertil could not grasp the rectangles with his limited hand use; thus the eye-hand coordination part of the test could not be used.
- ***Directions of lines*** (Hyvärinen & Jacob, 2011*)* were difficult for Bertil to interpret in the context of the Mailbox Game due to the poor functioning of Bertil's hands, but in the purely visual task, Bertil was quick and exact in his responses.
- ***Depth perception*** was unusual. Bertil said that he did not really know what depth perception was. He related that objects that were said to be far were, for him, in "depth," or "deep as in water" and that objects closer "were floating above them."
- ***Visual imagination*** was weak but had improved slowly. For example, he felt that he could imagine and draw, when assisted, simple pictures of houses. Within arm's length he had normal stereovision with the Titmus Fly Stereotest (Rosenbaum & Santiago, 1999).
- ***Object/background discrimination*** **and *interpreting surface structures at low contrast*** was difficult, so for this reason his orientation and mobility instructor encouraged the use of a cane with a curved lower end that moves smoothly on uneven paths and surfaces.
- ***Recognition of facial features*** was poor in everyday situations, but he sometimes recognized people in photographs quite quickly. Bertil felt that he was good in recognizing typical expressions in pictures because they did not move.
- ***Map-based orientation*** was very weak. Bertil was not aware of how to walk to destinations, and he solved this difficulty at school by walking behind his classmates.
- ***Learning routes*** had been intensively trained, but the order of landmarks was difficult for Bertil to remember. Therefore, he took pictures and videos of landmarks and trained regularly with an O&M instructor. Even with this intensive training, he had not become an independent traveler, even in his local neighborhood, because he did not know in which direction he should look for a landmark or remember which list of landmarks he should consult to find where the landmark was. He dreamed of having a guide dog and the freedom his older friends had in moving with their dogs.
- ***In math,*** Bertil could handle only one task in the middle of a white page, and in examinations, he would work with his assistant in a separate room and tell him what and where to write or draw. He had no mental image of hundreds, tens, and units. This was in surprising contrast to his abilities in languages; he is bilingual (as is his family) and was learning a foreign language with ease.

### *Summary*

The goal of the evaluation was to understand Bertil's visual processing capabilities so that his school team could then plan educational interventions to address any weaknesses and capitalize on strengths. Observation and interviews were used to assess Bertil's motion perception skills, reading behavior, understanding of body language, interpretation of surface structures in the environment, effects of visual clutter on worksheets and in the environment, facial feature recognition, memory for travel routes, and visual attention skills in school tasks. In addition, some visual processing issues became more clearly defined through the use of tests of visual functions and visual perception.

The assessment team identified a number of ways that visual processing might affect Bertil's school work, mobility, skills of daily living, and social interaction skills. Additional assessments required from specialists can now be identified, and instructional methods developed to provide support for Bertil in his school, home, and community. This case highlights a number of features:

- Children with cerebral palsy can have multiple, relatively subtle but fundamental visual difficulties that can easily be overlooked unless actively sought.
- Disorders of perception of fast movement (dyskinetopsia) can accompany periventricular white matter disorders, and can be disabling.
- Visual crowding, elicited in this case by using gratings, can affect function even in the context of normal optotype visual acuities.
- Detailed assessment leads to appropriate intervention strategies for each area of visual functioning.

## Ensuring Identification of Ocular Visual Impairments

It is critical that evaluators correctly determine the underlying cause of visual behaviors, whether they are due to ocular visual impairment, to visual processing problems resulting from damage to the visual brain, or to both of these factors. Children with CVI require careful assessment of visual functions related to ocular vision impairment as well as visual processing. The following case illustrates how ocular issues can be overlooked:

**Jon is a 6-year-old boy who was assumed to have** visual processing problems. He had several behaviors and symptoms typical of children with brain-damage-related vision impairment. Often he did not know where he was and did not learn routes. At a family gathering, Jon became distressed and unable to cope with the many people moving and chatting. He could not recognize his cousins at the gathering and withdrew to a corner to look at picture books. He also stumbled on objects quite often. Jon's visual functioning had been affected for years, probably from birth; his parents had noticed that, as a baby, Jon did not respond to toys in front of him in moderately dim light.

A variety of tests were administered to Jon by different specialists, and their results were collated with observations and reports of behaviors from school and family. Jon's visual acuity was only moderately reduced (0.5 or 10/20; see Appendix 12C) with a full-contrast LEA Numbers chart at 3 meters (10 feet), and most responses on visual processing tasks were within the normal range. The most remarkable results obtained from the test battery were lack of dark adaptation, very poor contrast sensitivity, and a reduced binocular visual field of 7 degrees. The limited visual field and poor contrast sensitivity could explain Jon's difficulties in learning routes, stumbling, and recognizing people. With further testing, Jon was found to show evidence of a nonprogressive retinal condition characterized by an abnormal electroretinogram (ERG). While problems associated with visual processing now appear to be less likely, Jon still needs to be observed at school and tested again in a year to verify the assumption that a retinal condition is the only cause of his atypical behaviors, rather than CVI. Orientation and mobility training was discussed and arranged in the light of Jon's small visual fields.

It is important to note that, as in Jon's case, visual fields are often not measured before school age, not even as a confrontation field; thus his limited visual field was not reported. This can easily lead to incorrect explanations of visual functioning, especially if the child has a large angle esotropia that results in two small visual fields unrelated to each other. Such a child may have to close one eye to be sure to understand where he is looking. Children with very small visual fields have difficulties with many neuropsychological tests because they cannot get an overview of the tasks. However, it should also be noted that visual fields are the most difficult clinical measurements to make in the assessment of children with brain-damage-related vision impairment. Teachers and therapists can contribute important information about visual fields through their observations.

## Conclusion

Disorders causing visual processing problems are common in children with cerebral visual impairment. Structured history taking and careful observation of the child's daily activities can lead to suspicion that such disorders are present and need to be probed further. This chapter has reviewed some of the methods available to evaluate visual processing in children with CVI from a variety of perspectives. A multidisciplinary approach is recommended with a range of evaluation methods sensitive to the many ways in which visual processing can be affected in children who have CVI including those with near-normal visual acuities and those with multiple disabilities.

Selected standardized tests can prove helpful in those children who have sufficient vision to see test items and who can understand and appropriately respond to them, but the results need to be understood within the context of each child's unique set of disabilities and interpreted accordingly. Less rigorous, but nevertheless informative, adapted methods of assessment are used for children who can cooperate. Children with severe multiple disabilities require inferences made from the results of history taking, combined with observation of any progress made when appropriate adaptive measures are put in place. The results of all tests carried out need to be translated into the sets of strategies that the team considers likely to best assist the child. These need to be communicated to teachers and families in ways that are clearly understood so that they can be implemented both at home and school. Since our understanding of higher-order visual processing and how it develops in children is still developing, the information in this chapter can best be used to point the way toward the advancement of future, more refined assessment methods.

## References

Achenbach, T. M. (1991). *Integrative guide for the 1991 CBCL/4-18, YSR, and TRF profiles.* Burlington: University of Vermont, Department of Psychiatry.

Alpherts, W. C. J., & Aldenkamp, A. P. (1997). *FePsy, The iron psyche: Manual.* Heemstede, The Netherlands: Instituut voor Epilepsiebestrijding.

Beery, K. E., Buktenica, N. A., & Beery, N. A. (2010). *Beery-Buktenica developmental test of Visual-Motor Integration* (6th ed.). San Antonio, TX: Pearson Assessments.

Benton, A. L., Sivan, A. B., Hamsher, K. D., Varney, N. R, & Spreen, O. (1994). *Contributions to neuropsychological assessment: A clinical manual* (2nd ed.). New York: Oxford University Press.

Candy, T. R., Mishoulam, S. R., Nosofsky, R. M., & Dobson, V. (2011). Adult discrimination performance for pediatric acuity test optotypes. *Investigative Ophthalmology & Visual Science, 52*(7), 4307–4313.

Cavézian, C., Vilayphonh, M., De Agostini, M., Vasseur, V., Watier, L., Kazandjian, S., . . . Chokron, S. (2010). Assessment of visuo-attentional abilities in young children with or without visual disorder: Toward a systematic screening in the general population. *Research in Developmental Disabilities, 31*(5), 1102–1108.

Cavézian, C., Vilayphonh, M., Vasseur, V., Caputo, G., Laloum, L., & Chokron, S. (2013). Ophthalmic disorder may affect visuo-attentional performance in childhood. *Child Neuropsychology, 19*(3), 292–312.

Corkum, V., Byrne, J. M., & Ellsworth, C. (1995). Clinical assessment of sustained attention in preschoolers. *Child Neuropsychology, 1*(1), 3–18.

Fantz, R. L. (1970). Visual perception and experience in infancy: Issues and approaches. In F. A. Young & D. B. Lindsley (Eds.), *Early experience and visual information processing in perceptual and reading disorders* (pp. 351–380). Washington, DC: National Academy of Sciences.

Ferris, F. L., III, Kassoff, A., Bresnick, G. H., & Bailey, I. (1982). New visual acuity charts for clinical research. *American Journal of Ophthalmology, 94*(1), 91–96.

Flom, R. (2004). Visual functions as components of functional vision. In A. H. Lueck (Ed.), *Functional vision: A practitioner's guide to evaluation and intervention* (pp. 25–59). New York: AFB Press.

Gioia, G. A., Isquith, P. K., Guy, S. C., & Kenworthy, L. (2000). *Behavior Rating Inventory of Executive Function.* Lutz, FL: Psychological Assessment Resources.

Hammill, D. D., Pearson, N. A., & Voress, J. K. (2013). *Developmental Test of Visual Perception* (3rd ed.). Torrance, CA: Western Psychology Services.

Hess, R. F., Hutchinson, C. V., Ledgeway, T., & Mansouri, B. (2007). Binocular influences on global motion processing in the human visual system. *Vision Research, 47*(12), 1682–1692.

Hyvärinen, L. (2012). *Heidi expressions.* Retrieved from http://www.lea-test.fi/index.html?start=en/vistests/instruct/heidiexp/heidi.html

Hyvärinen, L. (2013). *Hiding Heidi low contrast face test for communication distances.* Retrieved from http://www.lea-test.fi/index.html?start=en/vistests/instruct/hidinghe/hidinghe.html

Hyvärinen, L. (2014). *LEA rectangles game.* Retrieved from http://www.lea-test.fi/index.html?start=en/vistests/instruct/pvrectan/pvrectan.html

Hyvärinen, L., & Jacob, N. (2011). *WHAT and HOW does this child see?* Helsinki, Finland: VISTEST Ltd.

Hyvärinen, L., Walthes, R., Freitag, C., & Petz, V. (2012). Profile of visual functioning as a bridge between education and medicine in the assessment of impaired vision. *Strabismus, 20*(2), 63–68.

Johansson, G. (1976). Spatio-temporal differentiation and integration in visual motion perception. An experimental and theoretical analysis of calculus-like functions in visual data processing. *Psychological Research, 38*, 379–393.

Laurent-Vannier, A., Chevignard, M., Pradat-Diehl, P., Abada, G., & de Agostini, M. (2006). Assessment of unilateral spatial neglect in children using the Teddy Bear Cancellation Test. *Developmental Medicine & Child Neurology, 48*(2), 120–125.

Looijestijn, P. L. (2002, July). *Visual activities & participation scales.* Presentation at 7th International Conference on Low Vision, Goteborg, Sweden. Retrieved September 2, 2013, from http://www.visualprofile.info/LinkClick.aspx?fileticket=%2bO9jITFXNNo%3d&tabid=71&mid=482

Looijestijn, P. L. (2007). *Visuele activiteiten en participatie schalen.* Huizen, The Netherlands: Visio.

Looijestin, P. L. (2008, July). An evaluation of 20 years of WHO-ICIDH and ICF-based activities by Royal Visio. Proceedings of the 9th International Conference on Low, Montréal, Canada. Retrieved September 6, 2013, from http://www.visualprofile.info/Articles/tabid/71/Default.aspx

Manly, T., Robertson, I. H., Anderson, V., & Nimmo-Smith, I. (1998). *The Test of Everyday Attention for Children.* San Antonio, TX: Pearson.

Martin, N. (2006). *Test of Visual Perceptual Skills (non-motor)* (3rd ed.). Novato, CA: Academic Therapy Publications.

Mayer, L., Fulton, A. B., & Rodier, D. (1984). Grating and recognition acuities of pediatric patients. *Ophthalmology, 91*(8), 947–953.

Money, J. (1976). *A standardized road-map test of directional sense.* San Rafael, CA: Academic Therapy Publications.

Pavlova, M., Staudt, M., Sokolov, A., Birbaumer, N., & Krägeloh-Mann, I. (2003). Perception and production of biological movement in patients with early periventricular brain lesions. *Brain, 126*, 692–701.

Rosenbaum, A. L., & Santiago, A. P. (1999). *Clinical strabismus management: Principles and surgical techniques.* Philadelphia: W.B. Saunders Company.

Shepard, R. N., & Metzler, J. (1971). Mental rotation of three-dimensional objects. *Science, 171*, 701–703.

Van der Meulen, B. F., Ruiter, S. A. J., Lutje Spelberg, H. C., & Smrkovsky, M. (2002). *Bayley scales of infant development II, Dutch version* (2nd ed.). Lisse, The Netherlands: Swets en Zeitlinger.

Warren, D. H. (1994). *Blindness and children: An individual differences approach.* New York: Cambridge University Press.

Warrington, E. K., & James, M. (1991). *Visual Object and Space Perception battery.* Suffolk, UK: Thames Valley Test Company.

Watson, C. S., Kidd, G. R., Homer, D. G., Connell, P. J., Lowther, A., Eddins, D. A., . . . Watson, B. U. (2003). Sensory, cognitive, and linguistic factors in the early academic performance of elementary school children: The Benton-IU project. *Journal of Learning Disabilities, 36*(2), 165–197.

Wechsler, D. (2012). *Wechsler Preschool and Primary Scale of Intelligence* (4th ed.). San Antonio, TX: Harcourt Assessment.

Williams, C., Northstone, K., Sabates, R., Feinstein, L., Emond, A., & Dutton, G. N. (2011). Visual perceptual difficulties and underachievement at school in a large community-based sample of children. *PLoS One, 6*(3), e14772.

Wraga, M., Creem, S. H., & Proffitt, D. R. (1999). The influence of spatial reference frames on imagined object and viewer rotations. *Acta Psychologica, 102*, 247–264.

# APPENDIX 13A

# Evaluation of Visuo-Attentional Abilities (EVA): A Simple and Rapid Battery to Screen for CVI in Young Children

*Sylvie Chokron*

Despite the fact that "seeing" involves more than just the eyes, the availability of tests for higher-order visual functions (that is, visual cognition) is limited for young children known to be at risk for CVI. The increase in survival rates of preterm children and those who have survived perinatal asphyxia, and their greater frequency of neurological abnormalities, places them at risk of CVI. Moreover, several recent studies indicate that even the general population likely includes children (born preterm or full term, with or without known visual impairment or learning difficulties) with abnormal cerebral functioning leading to CVI. Yet, it is likely that these children remain undetected in the general population (Williams et al., 2011). The paucity of standardized tools, validated and adapted for young children, is largely responsible for this lack of systematic evaluation of their visuo-attentional functions.

## The EVA Battery

To facilitate screening of children at risk of a possible neurovisual disorder, the Evaluation of Visuo-attentional Abilities (EVA), a battery of nine selected simple tests of the principal neurovisual functions, has been assembled.[1] Cutoff scores for each subtest were determined from the performance of a control group of 450 kindergarten children, and the specificity and sensitivity of the battery have been investigated by evaluating the performance of a group of children with ophthalmological disorders, and one with neurovisual disorders. (For a detailed description, see Cavézian et al., 2010, 2013).

When children obtain a score equal to or below the cutoff score, they are considered to have failed the subtest. CVI is suspected if 3 or more of the 9 subtests are failed between 4 and 5 years of age, and 2 or more of the 9 subtests are failed between 5 and 6 years of age. The binocular visual acuity is first tested to ensure that it is higher than the level of 4/10 (20/50), with or without correction, required to perform the tests. (The test battery was standardized with 450 children between the ages of 4 and 6 with normal or near-normal visual acuities, but its use can be extended for older children with CVI and those with acuity deficits. In the latter case, the performance will reflect both acuity deficits and CVI.)

The following are descriptions of the nine subtests:

1. **Gaze fixation:** The child is asked to look at the examiner's eyes and to

[1] The EVA battery is distributed by *Association Recherche Santé Développement* on request at recherchesantedeveloppement@gmail.com. Additional information can also be obtained from l'Unité Fonctionnelle Vision et Cognition at www.vision-et-cognition.com.

FIGURE 13.9
**Visual Field Test**

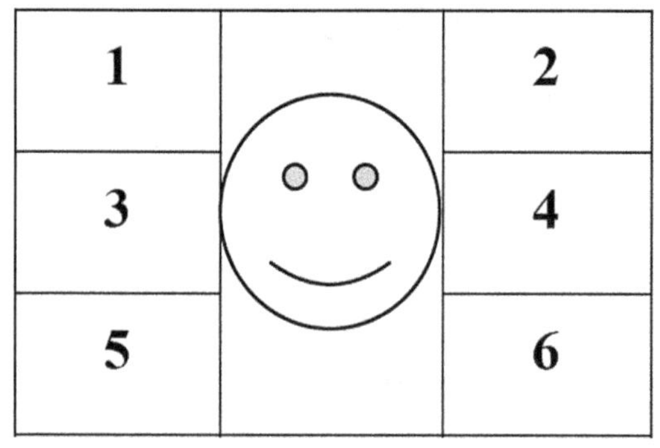


FIGURE 13.10
**Visual Extinction Task**

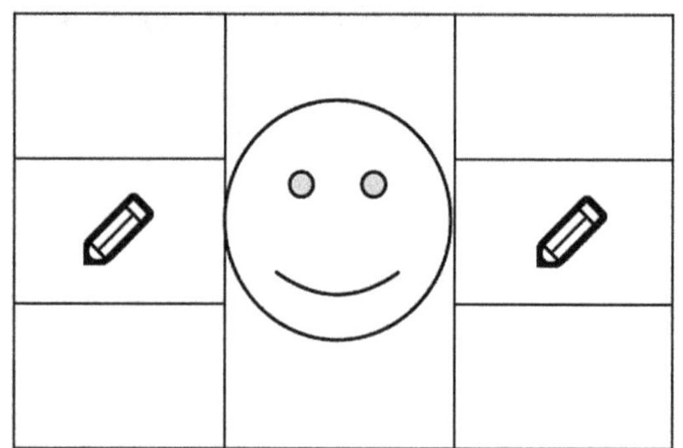

FIGURE 13.11
**Visual Pursuit Task**

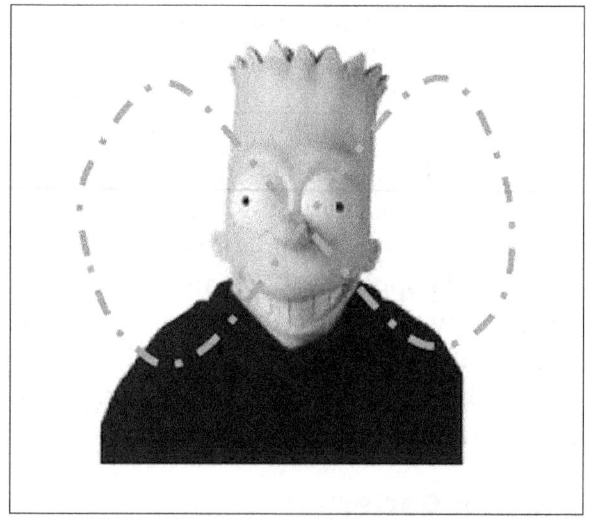

maintain his/her gaze for 10 seconds without moving his/her eyes or head. One point is attributed when no saccade is observed (maximum score, 1; cutoff score: 0, whatever the age).

2. **Visual field test:** The child is asked to close his or her eyes and, when requested by the experimenter, to open his or her eyes to fixate on the experimenter's nose and to grasp or touch the target (a pen held in the experimenter's hand) *without* moving his or her head or eyes (see Figure 13.9). The target is presented at a distance of 30–40 cm from the child, either in the right or left visual field, and in the upper, middle, or lower part of the lateral visual field. Each position is tested twice, giving a total of 12 trials. One practice trial is conducted initially to ensure the child understands the instructions. The number of correct touches *without* head or eye movements determines the score (maximum score, 12; cutoff score: 3 for 4–5 years; 9 for 5–6 years).
3. **Visual extinction task:** As for the previous task, the child is asked to close his or her eyes, then to open them and to fixate his or her gaze on the experimenter's nose. This time the child is required to grasp or touch two pens, each one being presented twice in the three mirror-image visual field locations (see Figure 13.10). If the child is able to grasp or touch the two pens, one point is at-

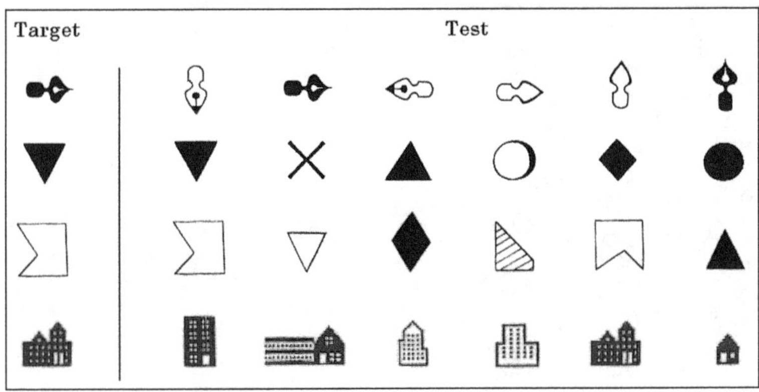


FIGURE 13.12
**Visual Memory Task**

tributed. Trials in which only one pen is presented are control trials and do not contribute to the score of the task. Note that compared to the previous task, eye and head movements are allowed (the same locations as for the visual field are tested) (maximum score, 1; cutoff score: 0, whatever the age).

4. **Binocular visual pursuit:** The participant is asked to fixate on a target (a pencil) and to follow its movement with his or her gaze, without moving his or her head (see Figure 13.11). The target is moved at a speed of 10 cm/sec, in the form of the infinity symbol (∞) crossing at the mid-sagittal plane of the child and extending out to a distance equating with the child's shoulder width. One point is given for each of the following abilities when present (for a total score of 3): (a) the child's eyes are always on the target; (b) no head movement; and (c) smooth pursuit (i.e., no jerking eye movements—that is, nystagmus) (maximum score, 3; cutoff score: 0, whatever the age).
5. **Visual memory task:** The task consists of visually fixating for 7 seconds a visual shape printed on the center of a page and then to find the previously memorized stimulus among six different shapes (the target and five distractors, resembling the target shape) on another page (see Figure 13.12). The child is given two pretest trials (not included in the subtest score) and then four trials. One point is attributed for each target correctly recognized (maximum score, 4; cutoff score: 1, whatever the age).
6. **Teddy bear cancellation test** (Laurent-Vannier, Chevignard, Pradat-Diehl, Abada, & de Agnostini, 2006): The participant is asked to cross out, with the pencil in his or her dominant hand, all of the 15 teddy bears distributed on a sheet of paper (21 × 29.7 cm, or approximately 8.5 × 11.5 inches, landscape orientation) among 60 distractors (see Figure 13.13). The number of correctly cancelled targets constitutes the score (maximum score, 15; cutoff score: 12 for 4–5 years; 13 for 5–6 years).
7. **"A" cancellation task** (Corkum, Byrne, & Ellsworth, 1995): The child is required to cross out all 15 of the upright, upper-case letter *A*'s presented among 45 distractors (the letter *A* in a different orientation; see Figure 13.14). As in the previous task, the number of correctly cancelled targets determines the score (maximum score, 15; cutoff score: 6 for 4–5 years; 10 for 5–6 years).

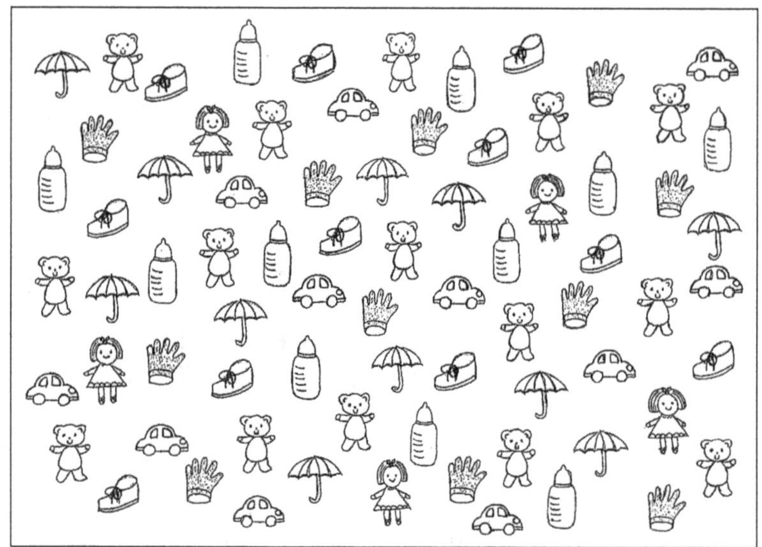

FIGURE 13.13
**Teddy Bear Cancellation Test**

FIGURE 13.14
**"*A*" Cancellation Task**

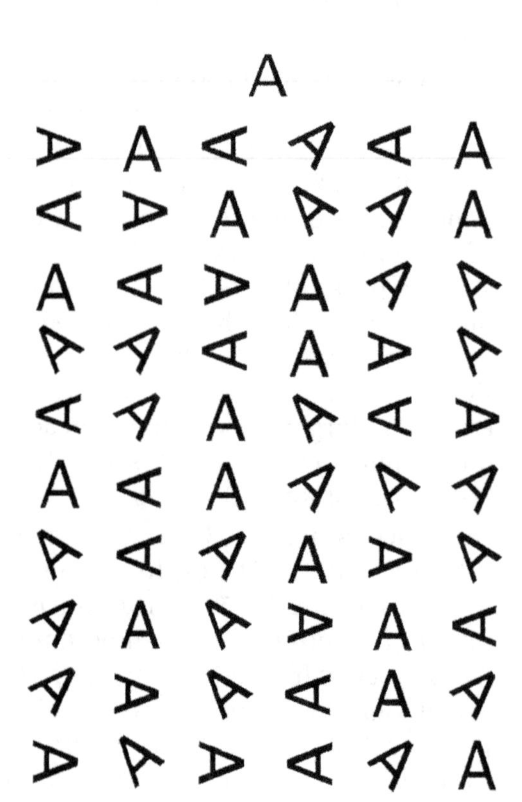

8. **Embedded figures test:** Seven boards are successively presented to the child. Each page presents several drawings consisting of outlines of two or more common objects superimposed upon each other, ranging from 2 to 7 objects with a total of 23 object drawings (see Figure 13.15). Participants are asked to identify as many objects as they can see. One point is attributed for each correct response for a maximum score of 23 points (maximum score 23; cutoff score: 17 for 4–5 years; 20 for 5–6 years).
9. **Matching test:** Eight sheets of paper (21 × 29.7 cm, or approximately 8.5 × 11.5 inches, landscape orientation) with seven black-and-white drawings are individually and successively presented in front of the child (see Figure 13.16). Each child is asked to match the target stimuli to the corresponding shape presented among 6 distractors. The number of correct responses constitutes the score (maximum score 8; cutoff score 4 for 4–5 years; 6 for 5–6 years).

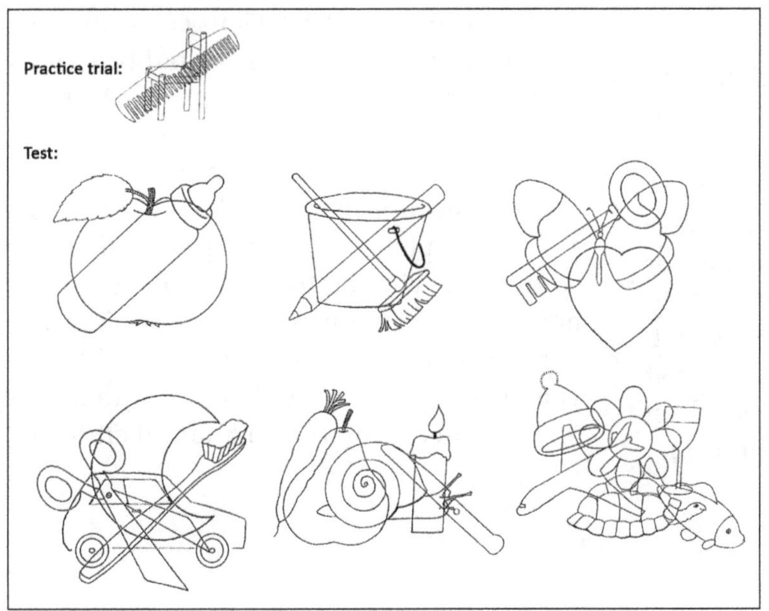


FIGURE 13.15
**Embedded Figures Test**

FIGURE 13.16
**Matching Test**

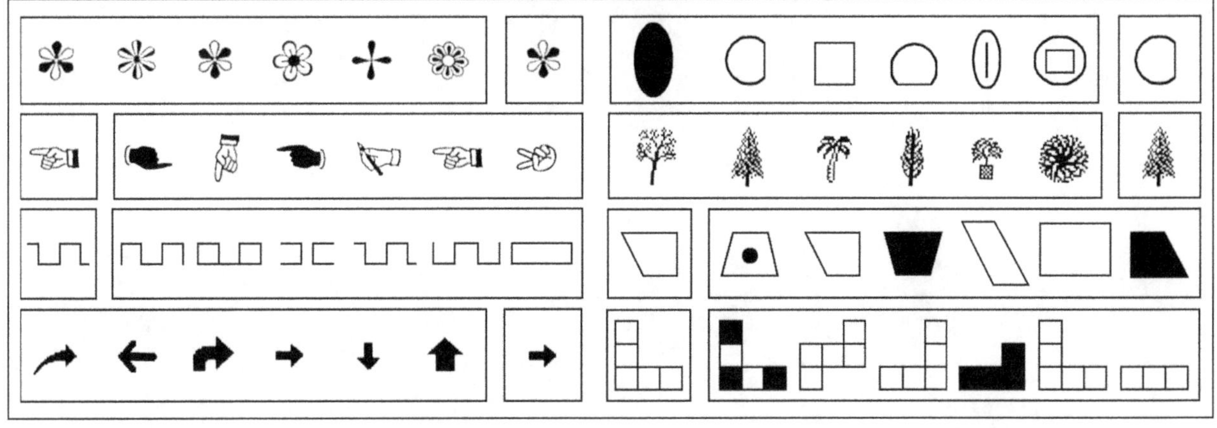

## Total Score

Each subtest that is passed is given a score of 1 point. The maximum total score is 9.

- Children aged 4–5 years with a total score of 6 or less (i.e., a child who has failed three of nine subtests of the battery) may present with CVI.
- Children aged 5–6 years with a score of 7 or less (i.e., a child who has failed two of nine subtests of the battery) may present with CVI.

When CVI is suspected, it should be suggested that the child receive complete ophthalmological and neurovisual examinations that include a history-taking session.

## Conclusion

The test battery described is designed to facilitate assessment of visuo-attentional abilities of young children in the general population without confounding the impairments with those due to ocular dysfunction. Although an ocular visual disorder should always be considered when a child presents with a visual cognitive impairment, our data in school children highlight that even when visual acuity is normal, children can experience impaired visual cognition.

Because of the deleterious consequences of a deficit in higher-order visual functions on learning abilities (Watson et al., 2003), a systematic neurovisual screening test is advocated for young children in addition to the ophthalmologic screening already completed in first grade in many countries. The battery described would not only provide currently unavailable epidemiological information about CVI in young children, but would also facilitate detection and habilitation of affected children.

# 14

# Assessments Linked to Interventions: Observational Assessment of Young Children and Children with Multiple Disabilities

*Marieke Steendam*

Young children and children with multiple disabilities cannot be assessed just by testing all the aspects of their functional vision. Experienced eye care professionals can test for such elements as visual acuity and contrast sensitivity, but many aspects of functional vision cannot be evaluated through formal testing procedures. Ongoing observational assessment is key to determining the level of visual functioning in order to develop and continue to adapt interventions as the child develops.

For young children and those with multiple disabilities, evaluation methods that involve verbal instructions must be at a level the child understands, and may be limited. Therefore, observation during natural activities or activities that have been designed to elicit specific reactions are likely to provide the most useful information about how these children function. These observations focus on what the child *can* see and do rather than what he or she *cannot* see or do. This chapter provides guidance for instructors about a variety of approaches to make best use of observational assessments.

Children with multiple disabilities discussed in this chapter are those with a developmental age between 3 months and 5 years. There can be big differences in the levels attained by a single child within visual, motor, sensory, social, and emotional developmental domains, and it is important each of these areas is addressed at the appropriate level.

Extended observation is necessary to gain insight into the child's visual functioning in familiar and typical situations. Observation demands considerable flexibility, creativity, and methodical thinking from the assessor. How children with cerebral visual impairment (CVI) apply visual behavior in daily life and how they react to specific visual stimuli are important to understand and document.

## Information Prior to Observation

Prior to observation, up-to-date prescriptions for spectacles and low vision devices should be in place. Information about the child's visual acuity, contrast sensitivity, visual fields, timing needs, and lighting requirements is gathered from earlier assessments and background material (see Chapter 12), and baseline knowledge about the child is obtained by in-depth, structured history taking from full-time caregivers (see Chapter 11). Information is gained about the child's likes and dislikes, the caregivers' wishes and concerns for the child, and the details of their observations of the child's visual behaviors (both abilities and disabilities). This information provides guidelines for the evaluator to select the most appropriate observation situations for assessment. Ideally, the evaluator is present at the formal vision assessment by the eye care practitioner and at the time of the interview.

Based on the nature of the information from formal testing and history taking, the evaluator selects the optimal situations in the natural environment to observe and assess the child. Observation of activities within familiar environments is crucial since findings within natural settings are highly relevant to the development of appropriate interventions. Findings in clinical settings or in refined assessment situations may not all be applicable to real-world situations.

## Observation Sessions

Two types of observation are discussed in this chapter:

- Direct observation of spontaneous activities in the child's typical environments.
- Observation following planned modification of materials, environments, positioning, and presentation styles.

Each observation session leads to insights about how vision use can be promoted for the child. As the assessor forms hypotheses about the best methods to promote vision functioning, these methods are systematically incorporated, and subsequently observed, to find out whether they do indeed lead to improved use of functional vision. In this way, visual and other sensory input can be adjusted to find out what works and what doesn't in natural settings. This is a form of diagnostic teaching (discussed further in Chapters 10, 15, 16, and 19). With young children and those with multiple disabilities, observation methods may need to be quickly modified on the spot. Only dates and places to assess can be set beforehand, and the assessor must be ready to adapt precise activities as the observation sessions evolve, as in the following example:

**Monique is a 2½-year-old girl with a syndrome that** includes CVI. During formal visual assessment at home, she was very alert, looked at her environment, and exhibited many visual behaviors. A week later, an observation using specific materials was planned at school. The observation began by showing Monique some suitable colorful toys (age level about 12 months), based on her reactions during the formal visual assessment. However, she hardly reacted visually and kept staring at sunlight coming in from a small, high window, reacting minimally, and only to the assessor rather than the materials. Fortunately, some basic visual

> materials were available, such as cardboard sheets with black-and-white patterns, shiny surfaces, and bright colors. Monique then reacted and started to focus on, and even follow, these strong stimuli. Other basic vision materials were also presented in varying order. After about 30 minutes, Monique was shown the first toys again and this time exhibited a visual interest in them. (Steendam, 2007)

Figure 14.1 shows a child fixating on a black-and-white pattern.

FIGURE 14.1
**Fixating on a Black-and-White Pattern**

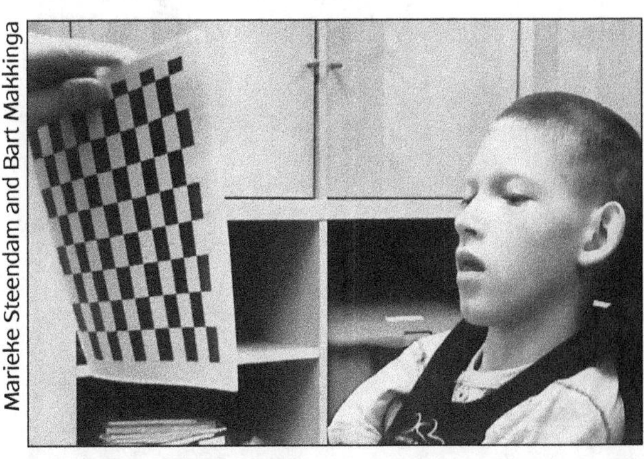

Marieke Steendam and Bart Makkinga

## Interpreting Children's Behaviors during Observations

The assessor must be experienced in observing young children and children with multiple disabilities, but the skills have to be learned on the job. A new colleague can gain such experience by co-observing with an experienced colleague. Assessors need to develop a flexible attitude, a set of skills related to functional vision assessment, a methodological frame of mind, and a mental databank of materials available for use. With these capabilities, they can react appropriately to each child's unique, evolving situation. Aspects of these skills are described in this chapter, but the reader needs to understand that bringing it all together and matching input to the child's capacity to perceive and learn from one moment to the next is what makes an observation worthwhile. It is hard to define and to describe how to do this; observation, empathy, and designing matched effective teaching are not a matter of arithmetic. The best compliment an observer can receive comes when caregivers say that their child and his or her needs have been thoroughly captured in the observational report.

It is important to have one of the child's caregivers attend the observation sessions. Their presence gives the child a sense of security. They know which visual stimuli attract the child, and can clarify the child's reactions if necessary. At the same time it provides an opportunity for the evaluator to point out to the caregivers the reactions of the child to certain stimuli, and allows the caregiver to proceed along similar lines between sessions.

The responses of young children or children with a low level of visual functioning are usually subtle and almost always delayed because these children take a long time to process sensory input and generate a reaction. Moreover, once the children do react, their responses can be either fleetingly short or prolonged since all processing is typically slow. For some, cessation of a response may be difficult. It is important to make sure a response is to a new stimulus and not a response lingering from the previous one.

When observing young children, or those with multiple disabilities who have CVI,

FIGURE 14.2
**Looking Away and then toward Stimulus**

Marieke Steendam

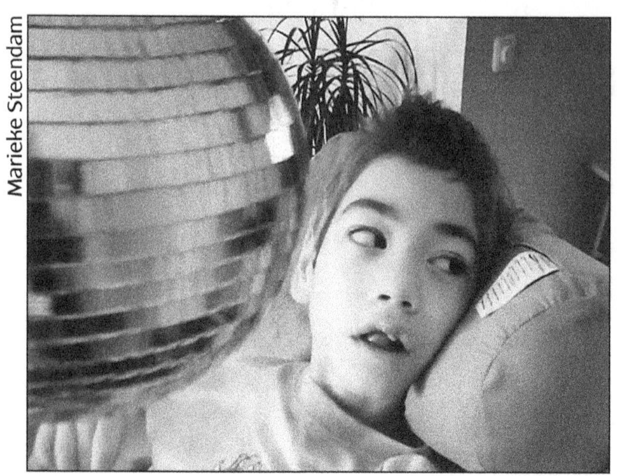

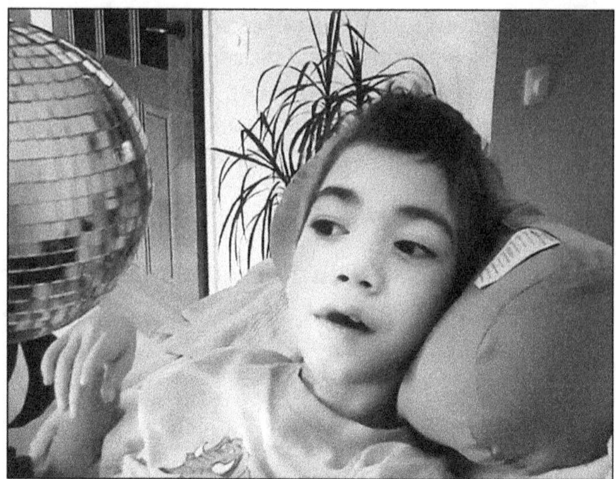

Initially this child looks away from the mirror ball (an indirect sign that it is perceived), but, given sufficient time, he turns his head and eyes and fixates on it directly.

many different reactions to visual stimuli can be seen, including both direct and indirect signs that the stimulus was perceived. The following are direct signs—behaviors that show the visual stimulus was perceived:

- Repeated short fixations in the direction of the stimulus
- Looking past the stimulus, such as looking past a face rather than making eye contact
- Turning the head (and sometimes eyes) toward the stimulus
- Following the stimulus
- Reaching for the stimulus
- Looking away when reaching for the stimulus
- Using the peripheral field of vision rather than the central field

The following indirect signs constitute supporting or acknowledging behaviors:

- Avoiding behavior, such as closing eyes or turning the head away
- Changing posture
- Stilling of movements
- Change in the rhythm of breathing
- Cessation of vocalizations or crying
- Smiling
- Changing facial expression
- Movement of hands or feet

Figure 14.2 shows a child initially looking away from an object, but, given sufficient time, eventually fixating on it.

During direct visual reactions like fixation and following, the observer should focus on the following characteristics:

- Reaction time (e.g., the child needs between 5 to 15 seconds to show a reaction)
- Duration of the reaction (e.g., focusing for 3 seconds)
- Quality of the reaction (e.g., following behavior shows jerky movements; focusing is for very short periods of time, but is repeated)
- Reaction time in relation to viewing distance (e.g., reaction to stimulus at 8

inches [about 20 cm] is quicker than to stimulus at 20 inches [about 50 cm])
- Reaction to repeated stimulation (e.g., reaction time to a new stimulus is longer, or the reaction to a new stimulus is to become alert, but becomes much slower with repetition)
- Duration of attention to an activity

## Questions to Guide Observation Sessions

Observation can have two purposes.

1. The first is to carefully describe how a child responds to specific stimuli or elements in the environment.
2. The second is to describe more general visual behaviors that show how the child approaches his or her visual world.

Within this context, there are three essential observation questions:

1. What visual stimuli does the child react to?
2. What are the child's reactions to these stimuli?
3. How do environments influence the functioning of the child?

Even though these questions initially seem simple, they lead to more complex questions, like branches emerging from the trunk of a tree. Conversely, as the complex questions emerge from the observational data, it is important to remember to return to these basic questions to describe what happens when a child uses his or her vision.

The following questions help lead to an understanding of the important observations regarding stimuli, reactions to stimuli, and the environment.

General visual behaviors:

- Does the child look around to view the room, people, and materials? Does the child show visual curiosity?
- Does the child visually follow the actions of adults?
- Does the child make eye contact with those who are present (familiar, not familiar, or both, and at what distance)?
- Does the child visually monitor his or her own actions in order to perform an activity?
- If the child has a choice (e.g., in play activities), what sort of materials does the child choose (visual or distinctly nonvisual)?
- Is there a difference in reaction or attention span between visual and other stimuli? In other words, is there a general alertness or attention problem, or a specific visual one?

Visual attention:

- Does the child find it hard to *start* looking?
- Is the child able to focus on the stimulus directly?
- Does the child have a fleeting way of using vision, never looking at something longer than a split second?
- Does the child focus on people's faces?
- Does the child focus on light sources?
- At what distance and for what duration does the child fixate on objects or elements in the environment?
- What are the dimensions of targets that actually draw the child's attention, and do these parameters match the measured visual acuities?
- Does the child look away when materials are shown? (Looking away is a form of visual behavior that may not be

constructive in the performance of activities in daily life.)

Global and local attention:

- Does the child have different visual behaviors when shown crowded versus singular pictures or materials? (For example, does the child focus intently on a single stimulus, look past crowded scenes, or look away from certain types of stimuli?)

Sensory motor behavior:

- What is the quality of the child's visually guided motor actions (depending on motor abilities)? (For example, looking away when reaching, or finding it hard to keep looking when manipulating a toy.)
- What role do other senses (touch, proprioception, hearing, olfaction) play when the child examines materials and performs tasks?

## Analyzing Visual Stimuli to Present during Initial Observations

The instructor must analyze visual stimuli in order to be able to choose the right materials for intervention. Objects have different types of properties (such as size, complexity, and emotional meaning for the child), and the assessor can design observations to pinpoint how to manage these properties so that they carry the clearest visual messages to the child. For initial assessments, however, the stimuli must be significantly greater in overall size, detail, and separation, than the minimum that could be perceived according to the measured visual acuity. Sidebar 14.1 shows characteristics to consider when analyzing the influence of visual stimuli and the environment. (See Chapter 12 for additional information.)

For example, if a child has an observable visual reaction to a big, black-and-white ball, the assessor can next choose to show either a *colorful* ball of equal size or a *smaller* black-and-white ball. By changing only one aspect of the visual stimulus at a time, the assessor can isolate which aspect was most important in eliciting a reaction from the child: size, or black-and-white versus color surfaces.

## Determining the Influence of Other Senses on Visual Processing

Another important point of observation is the processing of other sensory information in relation to vision. It is helpful for the assessor to know how well incoming sensory information from all modalities is being received and integrated by the child (sensory integration). However, such information is not always readily available. Many children with brain damage are hypersensitive (extremely sensitive) or hyposensitive (have low or diminished sensitivity) to certain sensory stimuli. Tactile hypersensitivity is often seen. Vestibular stimuli (related to movement and balance) and auditory stimuli can also cause problems. Proprioception (sensing movement and position of muscles and joints) can be insufficiently developed, and as a result, the child may need to divert a lot of conscious attention to maintaining posture. Each of these elements can act as distractors to the use of vision.

Many children with CVI and multiple disabilities can process only one sensory stimulus at a time. If someone is talking to the child, he or she may not be able to view what is being shown. If another student in the class is screaming, the child may not be

SIDEBAR 14.1

### Aspects of Visual Stimuli to Consider and Analyze

The following characteristics of visual stimuli, the environment, and the person who is interacting with the child being assessed will help the assessor or instructor choose and vary visual stimuli:

**Stimulus**

- Source of light: size, intensity, flashing speed*
- Surface quality: shiny material, black-and-white material, fluorescent material, brightly colored material
- Size of object
- Color of object
- Contrast with background or foreground
- Complexity and size of contours and details within an object
- Two dimensional or three dimensional (picture or object)
- Familiarity with specific class of objects in general
- Familiarity with this specific object in particular
- Emotional value of object
- Speed and direction of movement
- Range of ways of presenting stimuli

**Environment**

- Level and type of lighting in general: bright, dim, fluorescent, incandescent
- Level of spotlight on, or underneath, stimulus (use of a flashlight [torch] or light box)
- Viewing distance
- Viewing location (to the left or right, below or above)
- Familiarity with surroundings
- Distraction by visual or other sensory stimuli in surroundings

**Interaction partner**

- Character portrayed (gentle, calm, playful, enthusiastic)
- Speed of communication (matched to child's speed of processing)
- Nature of voice (soft, kind, encouraging, rewarding)

*Flashing lights should not be used with those at risk of epilepsy (photogenic epilepsy).

able to carry out a visual task. On the other hand, some children need a stimulus of sound or touch to motivate them to start looking. So for one child, additional sensory information distracts from looking, while for another, similar information can help support vision and recognition.

Language input to the child must also be optimized in both speed of production and language content. Approaches to promote optimal communication for very young children during assessment and intervention can be found in Chapter 20.

With the questions to guide observations and an understanding of the influences on sensory processing in the back of the assessor's mind, the situations and activities for observation can then be determined.

## Initial Observation of Spontaneous, Familiar Activities Including Activities of Daily Life

For young and multiply disabled children, it is especially important to observe the child in his or her own surroundings, preferably both at home and at school, during spontaneous and familiar activities. Since not all activities can be observed, information from the interview is used to choose the best times to observe the child.

This can be done within the context of activities of daily living, both when the child is active and when being cared for (see Chapter 16). For some young children or those with multiple disabilities, activities of daily living are a time for genuine one-to-one attention from an adult. Often, certain rituals have been developed between the child and caregiver during these activities, and these routines can be developed further to influence visual functioning.

Children with CVI and multiple disabilities preferably should be observed in their everyday activities as they naturally unfold, such as eating at the lunch table in school, dressing after swimming lessons, doing tasks in the classroom, and during playtime according to the class schedule. Additional activities to choose from can include spontaneous play by the child alone, with a caregiver, or with a sibling.

Such observations in natural situations provide a great deal of information about spontaneous functional use of vision and visual perceptual processing. The questions to guide observations mentioned earlier, as well as the visual functions, skills, and behaviors identified in Figure 14.4 (provided later in this chapter), are helpful for organizing the targets of observations and the results. In real-life situations, aspects of vision skills and visual perceptual processing are intertwined. Thus, observational findings must be analyzed afterward, to tease out what factors come into play during each observation session. Video recordings of the observation sessions can be a big help for this purpose.

If being present during the usual time for a critical activity is difficult to schedule, assessors can ask the caregivers to videotape situations that require interpretation.

However, in-person observation allows the assessor to make minor changes to tasks that the child is performing, and to observe whether or not the alterations affect performance. An example would be to take away half of the pictures from a game so as to simplify the visual presentation, or even to present the pictures sequentially. If there is background music playing during class activities, eliminating the music temporarily may result in a better visual performance.

If the child can move independently, be sure to observe the child when mobile to ascertain independent movement capabilities and how the child performs in different sitting situations such as on the floor or at a worktable and chair. Observing how the child interacts with toys also provides useful information about functional vision. For example, how does the child find toys in a cupboard or in a box of toys? How does the child find a ball in the classroom or at home? How does the child react when a ball rolls toward him or her?

## Modifying Activities and Environments to Learn More about the Child's Visual Capabilities

### Setting Up Typical and Atypical Situations

After the observation of use of vision in spontaneous activities, it is important to set up structured situations that answer questions about the child's responses to specific stimuli. Doing this type of assessment in a place familiar to the child, such as at school or at home, will make the child feel at ease. However, the environment can also be purposefully altered in order to determine how the child functions in new situations. When choosing to do this, take into account that a new environment can influence the child's alertness and sense of security.

Some children with damage to the visual brain are often unable to filter stimuli in a typical way. So when conducting this next round of observational assessment, the goal should be to determine how the assessment situation can be modified so that stimuli within it mesh with the child's capabilities for processing them. Optimizing these factors allows the child to achieve the greatest state of alertness to process the stimuli and to mentally organize them. The environment must entice the child to interact, but without overstimulating him or her. When overstimulated, the child may not be able to process anything. Many children can become withdrawn or hyperactive when overstimulated.

## Shaping the Environment for a Structured Assessment

- If possible, start the structured observation in an environment that is decluttered, with no background patterns, and with background sounds eliminated. Remember to look at the environment from the child's view of the room or outdoor space, rather than from the perspective of the attending adult.
- During the observation, add more stimuli, both visual and auditory, in order to see how they influence the child's performance in visual activities.
- Ensure good body posture. Provide sufficient support so that the child does not lose energy by focusing mental and physical energy on maintaining body position. Sufficient support and comfort allows the child to be as active as possible and to be optimally alert.
- Start in a familiar, normally lit room. If there is not a lot of reaction to strong visual stimuli, darken the room and continue the observation using lights, or illuminate the stimuli with the aid of a flashlight (torch) or other spotlight. Be alert to the adaptation time required when changing the light levels; children with CVI may need a much longer time to adapt to lighting changes than children with typical vision. (Sometimes circumstances cannot be changed as described, so be aware of the influence that this may have.)

## Determining the Appropriate Intensity and Visibility of Visual Stimuli

A child who reacts to basic visual stimuli (such as big, bold materials with black-and-white patterns, lights, shiny surfaces, and bright or fluorescent colors) in a limited way—that is, with hardly any response or short moments of fixation and following—will still provide a lot of insight into the level of his or her visual functioning when presented with these materials. Children who are visually more responsive may find such material boring. Basic visual stimuli are offered to them only if there is a need to compare their reactions to these stimuli with more meaningful stimuli, such as toys and objects from daily life.

Basic visual stimuli, such as flashlights (torches), Christmas decorations, and black-and-white striped material, can be used to

FIGURE 14.3
**Elements of SeeSaw**

Marieke Steendam

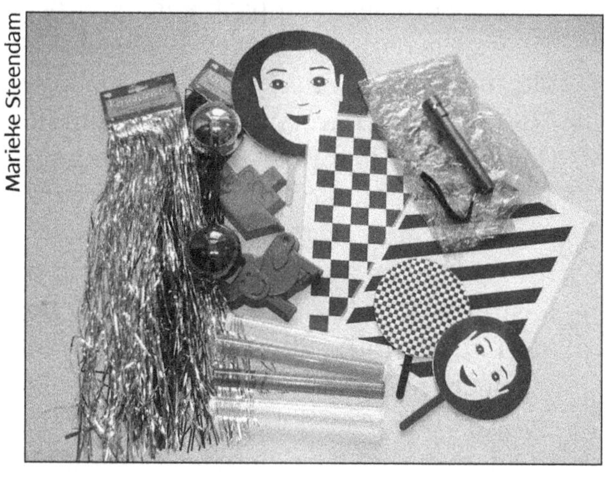

attract and gain attention. For example, at Royal Dutch Visio (a national organization for people who are blind or visually impaired in the Netherlands), a standardized set of basic observation materials, named SeeSaw, has been assembled (see Figure 14.3 and the Resources section at the end of this chapter). Although not a formal test, these materials help to systematize and record observations so that results from the same procedures can be compared over time. When videotaped, comparison of the quality of reactions is made easier.

The Sensory Learning Kit (Smith, 2009; see Resources section) includes vision-related materials and methods that focus on the observational assessment of functional vision. Similar equipment is available in the United Kingdom through Beesneez (see Resources section). Roman-Lantzy has also described an assessment program and assessment scales called the CVI Range (Roman-Lantzy, 2007). Using these alternative approaches may be helpful, noting that there are differences in recommended approaches to the ones discussed in this chapter.

### Determining Stimuli That Are Motivating and Meaningful

Apart from using basic visual materials, it is important to observe the child reacting and interacting with meaningful, functional visual stimuli. Caregivers can suggest potential stimuli so that the child's reactions can be sought to such stimuli as familiar persons; favorite toys that are brightly colored, black-and-white, or shiny; familiar objects from daily life; or favored articles of food.

> **FOR EXAMPLE, LUKE, A 3-YEAR-OLD BOY WITH MULTIPLE** disabilities, did not look at anything during the formal assessment. His mother took a cup with a specific Dutch folklore design out of her bag and said he would usually look best at this cup. Though no formal testing was possible, a lot of information about his visual needs, including distance, field preference, and visual behavior, was determined using the cup.

Such preferred visual stimuli, especially when viewed against a contrasting, plain background, can be significant and have meaning for the child and therefore entice looking. One child may find new toys fun to look at, another child may look only at objects he or she is familiar with, while a third child may prefer to look at food such as a piece of bread with peanut butter. Some children prefer looking at people's faces in preference to any material, no matter how visually stimulating it may seem. Often, a visual focus on faces makes the child appear to have good vision, when in fact the child hardly explores any other stimuli visually.

## Visual Perceptual Processing in Developmental Toys and Games

Observational assessments of children who are less restricted in their visual capabilities must cover many different visual skills and behaviors. Prior knowledge of their visual processing can be gained through developmental testing by a qualified examiner with standardized tests such as the Development Test of Visual Perception (DTVP–3; Hammill, Pearson, & Voress, 2013), the Beery-Buktenica Developmental Test of Visual-Motor Integration (Beery-VMI; Beery, Buktenica, & Beery, 2010), and the Test of Visual Perceptual Skills (TVPS [non-motor]–3; Martin, 2006), if the child's developmental level is within the limits of these tests. Vision tests and visual games by Dr. Lea Hyvärinen—such as the LEA Mailbox game and Pepi, the Dalmatian in motion—can be very useful as observational activities. (See Chapter 13 for a discussion of these tests and their applicability and the Resources section at the end of this chapter for sources.)

Questioning caregivers on the sort of play activities their child enjoys, combined with previous information gathered, allows the assessor to choose toys and games the child already knows. In familiar activities, the strategies the child uses can be observed, and by slightly altering elements that may affect visual processing, their influence can be determined.

When there are developmental activities the child does not like to do (one child may not care for puzzles, for example), make the task an easy one for the child to complete. By choosing the easiest form of the activity—a two-piece jigsaw puzzle or a wooden inset puzzle of only two or three geometric shapes—the child can become successful and the assessor can seek clues to explain the reasons the more complex task is difficult for the child or avoided. There may be indications that there is a vision-related problem for the child. Sorting games and worksheets can be presented in a variable way too, preparing easier ones that have high contrast, with sufficiently large items, and without other visual distractions. Masking sheets can be used to reduce visual clutter.

Many tasks and activities in early education lessons rely heavily on visual processing. The child's performance during appropriately adapted activities needs to be observed carefully during diagnostic teaching to optimize and match the activities to the needs of each child and to gain insights into the nature and degree of any visual processing problems. When a child has a sufficient level of visual functioning to see and understand the details on worksheets, flexibility on the part of the assessor may be less necessary, but thorough preparation before the session may be more necessary, as in the following example:

**In class, Susan, whose simultanagnosia is profound,** cannot finish a worksheet aimed at matching a picture in the left-hand box to the same one out of three pictures on the right-hand side. The assessor can prepare similar worksheets for the next session in different ways: using a plain cardboard sheet with a rectangle cut out to show the row of pictures one at a time, enlarging the worksheet on the photocopier, or cutting out the pictures and pasting them onto a contrasting plain background with similar or greater separation. These can then be tested to find out which adaptation is best for Susan.

A lot of children with severe multiple impairments may never have been given the opportunity to play developmental games such as puzzles or sorting games because their motor functions precluded them doing so in the ordinary way. However, these children can potentially learn adapted communication strategies to play these games. It is worthwhile to offer a child with severe multiple disabilities such games in order to observe this area of development.

**For example, Bram, a 6-year-old boy with severe** quadriplegia and CVI, became energetic and alert when given the challenge of doing a four-piece puzzle. He was taught a specific way of communicating so that he could participate in this activity. When two shapes, chosen to be within his visual acuity, were held in front of Bram, he was taught to look at the matching shape for two seconds (his instructor counting out loud to make it clear) to show that he had chosen that shape. Bram showed he could "solve" the puzzle by using eye gaze to communicate his choice. His mother was amazed at Bram's achievement and by the concentration he so quickly showed. This led to the development of additional communication schemes for Bram.

## Reporting Information from Observational Sessions

### Overview

Observations in familiar and typical situations may be completed in two sessions or more, preferably on different days, to allow for observation of the variability of visual functioning. The evaluator then needs to digest the information gathered both through direct observation and activities captured on videotape.

The fastest and most secure way to record observations and present assessment findings seems to be using predesigned forms and checklists. However, writing a full report ensures that careful observation of the unique responses and needs of the child are fully discovered and documented. Careful review and collation of all the information into a report paints a picture of the child's abilities and strengths and how to make best use of them.

While checklists have a place in collecting information, they should be used with care. For example, checking a box next to the statement "Does the child visually react to an object?" leaves out the following information, which still needs to be gathered:

- Which object?
- Was it familiar or not familiar?
- What was its size, surface, and material?
- At what distance?
- Still or moving?
- What reaction did the child give?
- How long did it take for the child to start focusing?
- For how long did the child maintain fixation?

Often, different reactions to different stimuli must be described.

Even when using the forms from one of the existing assessment systems or other checklists, the assessor needs to combine this information with all other observational data and provide a complete analysis of the child's functional vision. Often, however, the result is a mixture of conclusions leading to additional questions. Visual functioning is so complex that it requires ongoing assessment with new questions to be addressed as interventions are implemented.

The report of the observational assessment is included in the report provided by the entire multidisciplinary team, as described in Chapter 10. However, for young children and those with multiple impairments, the written report needs a more extensive description on the use of visual attention and basic visual skills, as well as the relationship between vision and the child's other impairments.

The assessment report containing the information from the observations can be augmented by two additional forms, to be filled in after the assessment and attached to the multidisciplinary assessment report. They include one that records the level of visual attention and a second that summarizes overall functional vision observations. These forms are meant as tools for the instructor to use when starting interventions. These allow the instructor to choose the appropriate level of activity for the child in specific situations. They provide guidelines to use when preparing instructional sessions.

## Forms for Reporting Observational Assessments

### *Variability of the Level of Visual Attention*

Using the form in Figure 14.4, Level of Visual Attention in Activities (Steendam, 2007), helps to give an indication of the level of visual attention the child can attain in various situations so that instruction can begin at the right level, with suitable materials that are matched to an optimal environment.

Variability in the level of visual attention in children, particularly those who are young or multiply disabled, can be considerable. Visual attention is a key building block for functional use of vision. Recognition of the child's current level of attention provides the starting point for intervention strategies. Figure 14.4 provides a simple method for recording the child's apparent level of visual attention observed during the assessment process. In this scheme, the level of attention is ranked in the context of its influence on the ability to carry out activities of daily living, such as eating and drinking, mobility, communication, playing alone, playing with an adult, and performing tasks. The following categories of visual attention used in Figure 14.4 are derived from careful observation:

- *The child primarily uses other senses in a given activity, and visual attention is minimal or nonexistent:* The child does not look very often. The child uses senses other than vision to obtain information about the world. Often only an experienced assessor sees the brief episodes of visual awareness, evidenced, for example, when the child becomes still when visually stimulated. The visual response of the child can be confusing because, while most of the time the child appears to look right through people, at other moments the child can really be looking at someone and appear to really see them. In addition, some children become obsessed by light sources such as overhead lights, windows, or doorways. They would like to look at them all day.
- *The child fixates briefly and may follow objects momentarily in a given activity:* The child is using vision more. Short moments of fixation on a visual stimulus can be detected. There might even be moments when the child follows a favorite object visually. Looking still takes a lot of energy, and many short moments of visual stimulation are more easily performed than one longer session.
- *The child looks attentively for brief periods independently or with instructor prompts in a given activity, but not for all situations or activities:* The child will look when a situation entices the child or when the child is specifically asked to look. But vision is not the child's favorite sense for exploring the world. When there are too many stimuli, it may cause anxiety or withdrawal. Single stimuli against a plain contrasting background work best. Complex stimuli are often confusing.
- *The child looks attentively and independently in many activities but occasionally uses other senses for exploration and accessing information:* Looking is used spontaneously, but not all the time.

FIGURE 14.4

## Form for Recording a Child's Level of Visual Attention in Different Activities

**Level of Visual Attention in Activities**

**Name:** ________________ **Date of birth:** ________ **Assessment period:** ________________

| | **Level of Visual Attention** | | | | |
|---|---|---|---|---|---|
| **Activity** | ***The child primarily uses other senses in a given activity, and visual attention is minimal or nonexistent*** | ***The child fixates briefly and may follow objects momentarily in a given activity*** | ***The child looks attentively for brief periods independently or with instructor prompts in a given activity, but not for all situations or activities*** | ***The child looks attentively and independently in many activities but occasionally uses other senses for exploration and accessing information*** | ***The child looks attentively and independently in most activities, although visual tasks may still present challenges*** |
| Reacting to basic visual stimuli | | | | | |
| Eating/drinking | | | | | |
| Other skills of daily living | | | | | |
| Communication | | | | | |
| Moving around; mobility | | | | | |
| Playing alone | | | | | |
| Playing in one-to-one situations | | | | | |
| Doing tasks alone | | | | | |
| Doing tasks in one-to-one situations | | | | | |
| **Description of signs of fatigue, including average duration of occurrence** | | | | | |

*Source:* Adapted from Steendam, M. (2007). *Weet jij wat ik zie? Cerebrale visuele stoornissen bij kinderen, een handleiding voor professionals* [Do you know what I see? Cerebral visual disorders in children, a manual for professionals]. Huizen, The Netherlands: Royal Dutch Visio (Koninklijke Visio).

During the day the child obtains information visually, without the need for heightened visual cues. Visual recognition is observed and visual memory is building up.

- *The child looks attentively and independently in most activities, although visual tasks may still present challenges:* The child looks spontaneously throughout the day. The child follows all that is happening around him or her in a visual manner. Visual tasks at school are hard because there are specific deficiencies in visual functioning. Someone who does not know the child will not think that he or she has visual problems, so when the child reacts differently than peers with typical vision, it is attributed to bad behavior and clumsiness rather than being recognized as a result of a visual dysfunction.

Children who mostly manifest one of the first three levels of visual attention described are more likely to be recognized as having issues with visual looking behavior than those in the last two levels.

Fatigue will usually occur for multiply impaired children with CVI after intense use of the visual sense. For children in the last two levels, fatigue may not be so obvious at first, but may result in visual performances that are less than expected. It can also result in avoidance behavior, which may seem to appear for no apparent reason.

### *Identifying Intervention Goals*

Figure 14.5, a form on which to record assessment of visual capabilities, skills, and behaviors in relation to daily activities, shows, in brief, the areas of functional vision potentially affected by CVI. This form identifies key aspects of visual functioning to target for improvement. It should be emphasized that it is a tool to set goals, not to measure improvement. It provides a guide for the instructor to summarize the effects of CVI on the child's performance in daily activities, but it is not sufficiently refined to estimate improvement and does not account for all the variables that can impact a child's visual functioning that need to be considered and applied.

To assist in setting specific goals, the system includes observations of basic visual skills including fixation and pursuit, as well as visual attention and behaviors that can be affected by damage to the dorsal stream and ventral stream (see Chapter 3). These data alone are not sufficient to build an intervention program, but the form provides a useful tool to set goals and to explain the child's visual functioning to his or her caregivers and teachers. It is important to note that, without the data provided by a multidisciplinary assessment report, this scheme is insufficient to work from, as it is a summary and does not paint a complete, realistic picture of what the child can or cannot do. For example, if a child has a very good memory, this may compensate for an inability to recognize pictures. Since the child is already using a good strategy, it may not be a goal for intervention. On the other hand, it needs to be mentioned in the report so that everyone is aware of the child's compensatory strategy because new images, such as pictograms for use at school, must be introduced in a more structured way than would be necessary for a child without CVI.

## Conclusion

After completing the reports and filling in the two charts (shown in Figures 14.4

FIGURE 14.5

## Form for Recording Assessment of Areas of Functional Vision Important for the Performance of Daily Activities

**Assessment of Visual Capabilities, Skills, and Behaviors for Daily Activities**

Name: ________________ Date of birth: ________ Assessment period: ____________________

| **Results from clinical eye examination or low vision clinical examination** | **Prescription** |
|---|---|
| **Spectacles:**<br>Yes _____ No _____<br>Full-time wear _____<br>Wear for near activities _____<br>**Devices to support use of vision** (optical devices, electronic enlargement, computer programs, tablet applications, other):<br>________________________________<br>________________________________ | **OD:**<br>**OS:** |

| *Visual Capabilities (from clinical eye examination, low vision clinical examination, and/or functional vision examination)* | *Assessment results for threshold measures* | *Required size/ contrast for optimum visibility* | *Comments* |
|---|---|---|---|
| Object size at a specific distance (visual acuity) | | | |
| Level of contrast between adjacent stimuli required (contrast sensitivity) | | | |

| | *Assessment results* | *Comments* |
|---|---|---|
| Preferred viewing distance for near tasks | | |
| Preferred viewing distance for far tasks | | |
| Area of vision | | |
| Color vision | | |

| *Visual Skills* | *Adequate* | *Varying, may need intervention* | *Needs intervention* | *Comments* |
|---|---|---|---|---|
| Fixating on visual stimuli | | | | |
| Following, pursuit of visual stimuli | | | | |
| Shifting gaze | | | | |
| Scanning | | | | |

*(continued on next page)*

**FIGURE 14.5** *(continued from previous page)*

| ***Visual Attention*** | ***Adequate*** | ***Varying, may need intervention*** | ***Needs intervention*** | ***Comments*** |
|---|---|---|---|---|
| Awareness of visual stimuli | | | | |
| Sustained visual attention | | | | |
| Selective visual attention | | | | |
| • Global attention: seeing a Gestalt/ zooming out | | | | |
| • Local attention: seeing details/ zooming in | | | | |
| ***Dorsal Stream Functions*** | ***Adequate*** | ***Varying, may need intervention*** | ***Needs intervention*** | ***Comments*** |
| Perception of movement, judgment of speed | | | | |
| Visual guidance of movement<br>• Hands | | | | |
| • Upper limbs | | | | |
| • Lower limbs | | | | |
| Moving through space (judging position of body [parts] in space) | | | | |
| ***Ventral Stream Functions*** | ***Adequate*** | ***Varying, may need intervention*** | ***Needs intervention*** | ***Comments*** |
| Recognition of:<br>• Color | | | | |
| • Shape | | | | |
| • Objects | | | | |
| • Pictures | | | | |
| • Photographs | | | | |
| • Complex pictures | | | | |
| Recognition of:<br>graphic representations:<br>• Letters | | | | |

*(continued on next page)*

FIGURE 14.5 *(continued from previous page)*

| *Ventral Stream Functions* | *Adequate* | *Varying, may need intervention* | *Needs intervention* | *Comments* |
|---|---|---|---|---|
| • Numbers | | | | |
| • Words | | | | |
| • Logos | | | | |
| Recognition of<br>• Faces | | | | |
| • Facial expressions | | | | |
| • Body language | | | | |
| Recognition and memorizing of routes and orientation landmarks | | | | |

and 14.5), the evaluator becomes the instructor, or hands over the assessment information to a colleague to start and manage ongoing intervention. As already mentioned, questions may still be lingering about certain aspects of the visual functioning of the young child or the multiply impaired child. This requires ongoing observational assessment within a diagnostic teaching framework by the instructor during the intervention period.

Each child with CVI has his or her own unique patterns of functioning and set of circumstances that require tailor-made intervention programs, applied for relatively short periods of time, with ongoing assessment leading to careful revision of goals, methods, and programs as needed. The continuous interplay between observational assessment and intervention results in the design of programs that are always relevant and motivating for young children and those with multiple impairments who have CVI.

## References

Beery, K. E., Buktenica, N. A., & Beery, N. A. (2010). *The Beery-Buktenica developmental test of Visual–Motor Integration* (6th ed.). San Antonio, TX: Pearson Assessments.

Hammill, D. D., Pearson, N. A., & Voress, J. K. (2013). *Developmental Test of Visual Perception* (3rd ed.). Torrance, CA: Western Psychology Services.

Martin, N. A. (2006). *Test of Visual Perceptual Skills (non-motor)* (3rd ed.). Novato, CA: Academic Therapy Publications.

Roman-Lantzy, C. (2007). *Cortical visual impairment: An approach to assessment and intervention.* New York: AFB Press.

Smith, M. (2009). *Sensory learning kit.* Louisville, KY: American Printing House for the Blind.

Steendam, M. (2007). *Weet jij wat ik zie? Cerebrale visuele stoornissen bij kinderen, een handleiding voor professionals* [Do you know what I see? Cerebral visual disorders in children, a manual for professionals]. Huizen, The Netherlands: Royal Dutch Visio (Koninklijke Visio).

# Resources for Observational Assessment of Functional Vision

The following information lists sources for obtaining the tests and assessment tools referred to in this chapter.

## ASSESSMENT TESTS

### Beery-Buktenica Developmental Test of Visual-Motor Integration, Sixth Edition (BEERY™ VMI)

Source: Pearson
www.pearsonclinical.com/psychology/products/100000663/the-beery-buktenica-developmental-test-of-visual-motor-integration-6th-edition-beeryvmi.html

### BeesNeez

Source: BeesNeez
www.beesneez.co.uk

### Developmental Test of Visual Perception, Third Edition (DTVP-3)

Source: Pearson
http://www.proedinc.com/customer/productView.aspx?ID=5697

### SeeSaw

Source: Koninklijke Visio (Royal Dutch Visio)
www.visio.org

### LEA Mailbox Game

Source: Good-Lite
https://www.good-lite.com/Details.cfm?ProdID=40

### LEA Vision Test System

Source: Good-Lite
www.good-lite.com/results.cfm?Category=25

### Pepi Test

Source: Lea-Test Ltd.
www.lea-test.fi/index.html?start=/en/assessme/woc/index.html

### Sensory Learning Kit

Source: American Printing House for the Blind
http://shop.aph.org/webapp/wcs/stores/servlet/Product_Sensory%20Learning%20Kit%20(SLK)_1-08611-00P_10001_11051

### Test of Visual Perceptual Skills, Third Edition (TVPS-3)

Source: Academic Therapy Publications
www.academictherapy.com/detailATP.tpl?eqskudatarq=8409-5

## SOURCES OF PRODUCTS

This section lists contact information for the sources of the assessment tools listed in previous section.

### Academic Therapy Publications/High Noon Books

20 Leveroni Court
Novato, CA 94949-5746
(800) 422-7249 or (415) 883-3314
Fax: (888) 287-9975 or (415) 883-3720
www.academictherapy.com

### American Printing House for the Blind

P.O. Box 6085
1839 Frankfort Avenue
Louisville, KY 40206-0085
(502) 895-2405
Fax: (502) 899-2274
www.aph.org
info@aph.org

### Good-Lite Company

1155 Jansen Farm Drive
Elgin, IL 60123
(800) 362-3860
Fax: (888) 362-2576
www.good-lite.com

**Koninklijke Visio (Royal Dutch Visio)**
088 - 585 85 85
www.visio.org
info@visio.org

**LEA-Test Ltd.**
www.lea-test.fi/index.html

**Pearson**
P.O. Box 599700
San Antonio, TX 78259
(800) 627-7271
Fax: (800) 232-1223
www.pearsonclinical.com
clinicalcustomersupport@pearson.com

**PRO-ED, Inc.**
8700 Shoal Creek Boulevard
Austin, Texas 78757-6897
(800) 897-3202 or (512) 451-3246
www.proedinc.com

# 15

# Assessments Linked to Interventions: Literacy and Math

*Lizbeth A. Barclay*

Children with cerebral visual impairment (CVI) possess distinct visual and cognitive characteristics that require educators and family members to become knowledgeable about their individual learning requirements. While some children with CVI and severe additional disabilities may require a program that emphasizes functional skills, others are able to participate in academic programs that emphasize instruction in literacy and mathematics, as well as other core subjects such as science and social studies. Some children with CVI who are able to participate in academic programs may have subtle visual and learning challenges, causing them to struggle academically unless provided the appropriate level of understanding and support. As an assessor for students with visual impairments in a large state for 20 years, the author has observed that many of these students who are participating but struggling in academic programs begin to make good progress when their specific learning requirements are met. Through assessment, educators can skillfully isolate the effects of CVI and resulting requirements for students learning in core curriculum areas such as literacy and mathematics.

As school-aged children with CVI begin to learn to read, write, and demonstrate conceptual understanding of literacy skills and mathematics, regular and careful assessment provides information about their individual visual challenges, development, and requirements over time. This chapter addresses specific literacy and math assessment considerations for school-age (kindergarten through high school) students with CVI who can respond to the assessment techniques and strategies described.

The core curriculum areas of literacy skills—reading, writing, and the closely linked area of listening comprehension—and mathematics have been chosen for emphasis, but guidelines and recommendations can be used when assessing and instructing in other areas of the core curriculum, such as science and social studies. While the emphasis of this chapter is assessment, the techniques for modification described should also be employed during instruction, when found to be appropriate for students with CVI.

The complex nature of the heterogeneous population of students with CVI means that careful consideration must be given to each student's individual constellation of visual and/or visual-perceptual abilities and the assessments needed to address them. Assessment of literacy and math skills of students with CVI will be discussed with regard to the possible effects or consequences of CVI as described by Dutton (2003, 2009) and Lueck (2010) and presented in Chapter 3 of this book. Examples of these effects can be found in Table 15.1, which appears later in this chapter.

## Dominic

The case study of Dominic, a student with CVI, is used throughout this chapter to illustrate some of the issues, assessment strategies, and resulting curricular goals discussed throughout the chapter. The following vignette introduces Dominic and his situation prior to a comprehensive assessment:

**DOMINIC, A FIFTH-GRADE STUDENT WITH CVI SECONDARY TO** cortical insult at birth, had a history of academic challenges. An inquisitive and socially outgoing young man with many interests, Dominic struggled to maintain attention to academic tasks in school. His predisposition for off-task behavior in the classroom and decreasing skill levels in comparison to his peers was making it challenging for him to maintain social connections. While adults enjoyed his quirky personality, peers had begun to stay away from him. Dominic's parents were concerned that he was falling further and further behind his peers.

Although Dominic's distance acuity was measured at 20/80 and his near acuity was 20/114 when viewing single symbols, his near acuity dipped to 20/300 when viewing crowded symbols, indicative of major simultanagnostic visual problems as a result of dorsal stream dysfunction. (As text becomes crowded, the dorsal stream attentional system fails to see the words because there is insufficient capacity for "parallel processing" all of the image data, as discussed in Chapter 3.) He also had reduced depth perception and reduced visual fields. Dominic's vision seemed to fluctuate "without explanation," and his visual-perceptual difficulties affected his fluency in reading. The physical process of using vision seemed to be exhausting to Dominic; this was particularly true while reading print and during handwriting exercises. He had to work unusually hard just to keep his eyes on a line of print. When the text was crowded, it was difficult for him to differentiate letters in words. This made it hard for him to decode words and attend to the overall meaning at the same time.

Although Dominic's expressive language skills were age appropriate and he had much to say, his writing skills were those of a much younger child. It was difficult for Dominic and others to read his handwriting, and because his spelling level was very low (first-grade level), he limited his composition to words he thought he could spell.

Dominic's understanding of basic number concepts was quite strong; however, he made many errors during multistep processes, such as multiplication and division, because he lost his place easily and was not accurate.

Though Dominic received instructional and support services from a teacher of students with visual impairments, it was clear to his parents and teachers that he needed comprehensive assessment to explore, in greater depth, the nature of his instructional requirements resulting from his CVI.

## Information that Informs the Assessment Process

### Vision Examinations and Functional Vision Assessments

As described throughout this book, visual functioning for students with CVI can vary considerably. In order to begin to document and understand students' individual differ-

TABLE 15.1

## Modifying Assessment and Instruction in Response to Identified Effects of CVI

| *Functional Area* | *Information for Assessment/Instruction Preparation and Modification* |
|---|---|
| Visual acuity | Ensure optimal object or print size, letter and line separation (providing the required space between each letter and line when necessary), and optimal distance for placement of materials. This includes pictures, important details, numbers, and operational symbols.<br>Ensure that the student is wearing spectacles if they are prescribed for near viewing and that all low vision devices that the student routinely uses for visual access—such as magnifiers, video magnifiers, laptop computer, or tablet—are available and used as appropriate. |
| Contrast sensitivity | Verify contrast requirements for all testing and instructional materials. |
| Color vision | Determine if color can be reliably used as a visual cue, or if only saturated colors should be used and pastel and light colors avoided. |
| Visual fields | Ensure optimal placement and positioning of materials and of the student during testing and instruction. |
| Hemianopic inattention (common in those with hemiplegia on the same side as the weakness) | Optimal placement of text may be off-center to the attended side from the midline of the page, and chair may be rotated to place text off-center to the attended side of the body (see Chapter 3). |
| Binocular vision/Accuracy of visually guided movement | Determine best placement and contrast of materials, especially when manipulatives are used.<br>Identify how best to employ tactile supplementation of visual guidance of movement; for example, allowing part of the body to be in contact with part of the desk to help locate it. |
| Control of eye movement | Determine the presentation of materials with regard to placement and positioning of materials, word spacing, line spacing, provision of visual support such as pointers, line markers, line length (number of words per line), and alternate presentation (for example, using computer programs with high contrast and well-spaced visual presentation and auditory support). |
| Lighting and glare issues | Make sure that glare does not reflect on testing and/or curricular materials.<br>Provide optimal lighting on testing and/or curricular materials. |
| Visual attention | Observe the amount of detail and clutter associated with loss of attention.<br>Use techniques necessary to encourage visual attention (such as providing movement and pointing to words).<br>For younger students who are learning to write, provide dark-lined paper and dark pencils if they have difficulty maintaining their place while reading.<br>For students who have keyboarding skills, provide access technology during assessment, such as a computer for word processing.<br>Observe the amount of time the student is able to sustain visual attention and do not continue assessment or take breaks when attention to task is not maintained. |

*(continued on next page)*

**TABLE 15.1** *(continued from previous page)*

| *Functional Area* | *Information for Assessment/Instruction Preparation and Modification* |
|---|---|
| Visual search | Observe how easily the student moves to succeeding lines on a page, or to separate sections on a page of text or in a workbook.<br>Provide supports that include L-shaped line markers, vertical anchor lines at the left side of a page, or colored lines around sections to be located, as well as electronic copies of materials that simplify the complexity of the presentations. |
| Visual crowding | Adjust the placement and spacing of print, pictures, and symbols during testing and instruction to increase spacing.<br>Simplify the print environment (provide adequate spacing between and within test items and determine the amount of print on a page that results in an increase of errors).<br>Simplify instructional surfaces.<br>Determine if visual supports such as pointers, line markers, or typoscopes may be necessary.<br>Allow the student to point underneath words while reading, if possible.<br>Ensure the workspace surroundings have minimal pattern and clutter. If testing, keep the testing environment uncluttered. |
| Visual recognition challenges | Observe unusual ways that words or pictures are recognized, such as using a nonsalient feature to remember a picture or word when the picture cannot be recognized (for example, remembering that a picture is of a kitten by the pink color of a bow around its neck, or remembering a specific word because it is written in red rather than black). |
| Other visual perceptual challenges | Observe visual errors, such as calling a picture of a sheep a dog, or reading the word "seat" as "set" or "sat." |
| Visual fatigue factors | Assess the student during the optimal time of day for pursuing visual tasks during testing/instruction.<br>Determine optimal length of testing/instructional sessions while using vision.<br>Watch for physical behaviors indicative of visual fatigue, such as rubbing eyes or tearing.<br>Watch for behavioral signs of visual fatigue or sensory overload, such as looking away or closing eyes. |
| Postural issues | Provide furniture that provides postural support and maximizes visual proximity to testing materials.<br>Make sure the student is well balanced during testing/learning tasks.<br>When working at a desk or table, provide an adjustable reading/writing stand that will enable the student to maintain upright posture when moving close to the material. |
| Visual preferences | Determine the type of visual information that most interests the student and is likely to sustain visual attention. |
| Visual variation | Note and document the optimal time of day for visual curricular tasks, as well as bio-behavioral factors that cause a decrease in visual functioning during curricular tasks. |
| Distraction | Ensure that background noise is not competing for attention. |
| Response time | Allow adequate time for visual processing before a response is expected. |

ences, it is very important to have the most complete and current information from a low vision examination conducted by the student's optometrist, ophthalmologist, or orthoptist (an allied health professional specializing in eye movement and binocular vision disorders), as described in Chapter 12. This information, along with information about functional use of vision, will help to inform the selection and specifications of assessment modes and tools.

In addition to information obtained from clinical low vision examinations, observation and interviews detailing how a student uses vision in different settings is important. This forms the basis for comprehensive assessments in specific subject areas that ideally take place in school and home environments, where the student performs both functional and academic tasks. While vision examinations in clinic settings provide information based on visual measures in a controlled setting, it is through ongoing observation in different environments and for varying lengths of time that parents and educators can gain and document information about a student's use of vision on a day-to-day basis (see Chapter 14). The combination of information from all assessments helps teachers of students with visual impairments choose and prepare additional assessment materials in specific subject areas, such as math and literacy, for their students with CVI.

Table 15.1 lists functional areas commonly affected by CVI, along with considerations and potential adaptations for each that should be reviewed by all assessors and utilized during assessment, as individually appropriate, for students with visual impairments resulting from CVI. Adaptations that prove successful during assessment can then be used for students during instruction.

## Learning/Literacy Media Assessment

Prior to and as part of the assessment of skills in reading, writing, and mathematics, assessment of students' optimal learning and literacy media is essential and should be done early and often throughout their school careers. Described by Koenig and Holbrook as "an objective process of systematically selecting learning and literacy media for students with visual impairments" (1995, p. 1), this type of assessment is designed to determine the most effective method for teaching an individual student or to ensure that the method being used is the correct one. For example, many students with CVI will use vision as their primary modality for learning; other students, although they may use vision for visually guided functional activities and during travel, may utilize tactile learning (braille) or auditory learning (recorded or taped materials) when accessing information. Many students will use a combination of modalities and media to achieve their goals. Because students with CVI may have vision that changes and fluctuates over time, it is important to provide assessment of learning media regularly, especially whenever change of visual functioning has occurred.

Sidebar 15.1 summarizes information derived from the functional vision and learning media assessments of children with CVI that can be used to inform the selection of the most appropriate literacy media. The information obtained needs to be reviewed by members of the collaborative assessment team (including the student and the student's family) to determine the literacy mode

SIDEBAR 15.1

## Determination of Literacy and Learning Media for Children with CVI

*Barry S. Kran and D. Luisa Mayer*

Information from the clinical low vision examination and the functional vision evaluation can be used by educational teams to determine the most appropriate learning media for children who have CVI.

### Clinical Low Vision Examination of Visual Function

The clinical low vision examination, often conducted in a specialized low vision clinic, can provide the following information:

- Spectacle correction for refractive error
- Additional near correction to assist with accommodation for reading or close work
- Contrast sensitivity
- Visual fields:
  - Central scotomas (blind spots)
  - Left hemianopia
  - Right hemianopia
  - Lower visual field impairment
  - Other visual field limitations
- Threshold visual acuity for distance and near tasks
- Effectiveness of eye movements for reading and viewing in general
- Prescription for optical devices for reading

### Functional Vision Assessment and Learning Media Assessment

Functional vision information gathered during the clinical low vision examination and during educational learning media assessments can provide the following information:

- Effects of illumination and glare on literacy tasks, including the use of directional lighting for reading
- Discrimination of color
- Use of low vision optical and electronic devices for literacy and learning tasks
- A guide to begin the determination of optimal print size and working distance for sustained reading tasks

Other information that is most often gathered in a functional vision assessment or learning media assessment by educators includes:

- Use of reading aids such as typoscopes (reading windows), line guides, and anchor lines (vertical lines at the left or right margins of text) while reading (some of this information may be available from the low vision evaluation)
- How to best angle reading material (which may also be assessed at the clinical low vision exam)
- Postural evaluation for reading (which may also be assessed at the clinical low vision exam)
- Student's preferred sensory channels (visual, auditory, or tactile) for different literacy and viewing tasks
- Student's overall readiness for reading in print, auditory, or tactile formats
- Student's reading level, reading speed, and reading fluency
- Observation of the student's performance using alternative print reading delivery methods (such as single words, one line at a time, or full page) to determine ones that are most efficient

For children with CVI, additional information must be gathered to inform the selection of the most appropriate literacy or learning media and to identify the most appropriate formats for visual reading and presentation of other learning materials. This includes:

- Effect of crowded versus uncrowded symbols on reading and picture identification

*(continued on next page)*

**SIDEBAR 15.1** *(continued from previous page)*

(simultanagnosia) (which may also be assessed at the clinical low vision exam)

- Impaired ability to see alignment in rows and columns of numbers without guidelines on the page (which may also be assessed at the clinical low vision exam)
- Impaired letter recognition (literal alexia) (may be acquired)
- Impaired letter and number recognition (as part of integrative agnosia)
- Oblique or vertical reading styles
- Position of material on a page or workspace for students with visual field or visual neglect concerns

or modes and materials best suited for individual students. Reading literacy, math literacy, and writing tasks are the targets for these assessments.

## Choosing Assessment Tools and Modes

In the United States, once a student begins to develop skills in literacy and math, assessment may take place regularly through standardized testing protocols mandated in school districts. Some children with CVI, however, may not be able to participate in standardized school testing because the test design and format are not visually accessible, or because the student's educational team believes that information from such testing does not adequately illustrate the student's strengths, challenges, and learning requirements. Standardized tests, however, may have been inappropriately applied to the many children with CVI not recognized as having this condition in the early grades. Furthermore, in the United States and some other countries or regions, students may have been identified as having learning challenges in a process called Response to Intervention (RTI). Response to Intervention is defined as a process in which additional information about learning needs and progress is acquired through standardized testing for all children (Fuchs & Fuchs, 2006). Since the use of standardized tests is not always optimal for students with CVI, their application must be carefully monitored when used in conjunction with the RTI model. Modes of assessment with regard to students with CVI, including formal and informal assessments, observation, and diagnostic teaching, are described in the following sections.

### Formal Assessments

Standardized tests are formal norm-referenced or criterion-referenced tests. They have been field tested so that standards of performance and standard test items are statistically established and must be administered and scored in a precise manner that is described by each test publisher. The groups of students for whom standardized tests are designed and field tested rarely include students with visual impairments; consequently, when these assessments are used with students with visual impairments, they must be used and interpreted with caution (Barclay, 2003; Lewis & Russo, 1998).

Usually it is not possible to administer a norm-referenced or criterion-referenced test to students with CVI in the manner used to establish test standards; that is, without modifications to font size, spacing, format, or other methods adapted to students' individual needs. Consequently, the comparative or criterion scores derived from tests that have been altered cannot be considered statistically valid. They should never be considered the only source of information, and scores cannot be reported with confidence since the standard test conditions cannot be met. If they are used, they should be interpreted in conjunction with results from informal modes of assessment (Heinze, 2000).

## Informal Assessments

Informal assessments—those that have not been standardized, such as informal reading inventories—can be a valuable mode of reading assessment for students with CVI. Informal reading inventories are individually administered diagnostic assessments designed to evaluate a number of different aspects of students' reading performance. Typically, they consist of graded word lists and passages ranging from pre-primer level to middle or high school levels (Paris & Carpenter, 2003). Word reading and passage reading levels, including decoding, fluency, and comprehension, are tested. Because these are informal tools with no statistically derived scores, the words and passages can be individually modified for each student's learning media needs, and test performance can be interpreted in ways that take into account any individualized modifications. Information can be used to design instruction to address students' strengths and needs and document their reading progress over time (Nilsson, 2008).

## Observation

One of the most powerful modes of informal assessment is *observation* (see Chapter 14). Through observation, a teacher of students with visual impairments can carefully gain information about students' behaviors while they perform literacy and math tasks within the school setting. Such tasks may include shared reading, writing a paragraph, all-class math instruction, or reading during the performance of a functional task (for example, following a recipe or using a calendar). During observation teachers may note the following:

- Idiosyncratic visual behaviors
- Distance from task
- Postural issues
- Signs of visual fatigue
- Willingness to perform tasks within the classroom
- Level of independence in execution of tasks
- Level of organization while approaching tasks
- Literacy and math accuracy and fluency
- Relative performance with and without accommodations such as lines under text during reading and numbers in graph paper (or squares) for math (with a perceptible line thickness matched to acuity)

## Diagnostic Teaching

*Diagnostic teaching*, or prescriptive, individualized teaching that is carefully refined as the teacher finds the best modes of learning for the student, is another type of ongoing assessment. The teaching plan is based on careful and continuous assessment and documentation of the individual's needs, as described in Chapters 10 and 19. Diagnostic teaching enables teachers of students with visual impairments to respond to assessment information and fine-tune instructional strategies to ensure maximum development of literacy skills.

### Ongoing Assessment

*Ongoing assessment* is crucial for children who have CVI. Teachers are often required to assess the literacy and math skills of their students as part of ongoing high-stakes testing where outcomes from standardized tests result in major decisions about a student's progress, placement, or future. As previously noted, students with CVI may or may not participate in regular standardized testing; if they participate, the results may not yield clear information about their reading, writing, or math skills. Regardless of whether or not students participate in their school's standardized testing, it is essential that teachers of students with visual impairments conduct ongoing assessment of their students with CVI using materials that have been modified when necessary, and that are what the student is already reading or likely to read and use during mathematics instruction. It is through ongoing observation, diagnostic teaching, and assessment that teachers of students with visual impairments will be able to respond to assessment information and fine tune instructional strategies to ensure maximum development of literacy skills.

## Literacy Skills Assessment: Reading

As teachers gather assessment information by testing, analyzing student work samples, observing students performing literacy tasks, and interviewing them about their literacy skills and preferences, the following aspects of literacy skills should be evaluated:

- Alphabetics (including phonemic awareness, phonics, decoding, and print awareness)
- Fluency (reading speed)
- Reading comprehension
- Listening comprehension
- Writing (including spelling and writing composition)

It is helpful to understand the typical development of children's early literacy skills, which usually begin as infants gain communication skills, in order to assess whether or not students with CVI possess the foundational skills necessary for progress in literacy skill development, regardless of their visual impairment. Table 15.2 illustrates the link between early communication and early literacy skill development—forming the foundation for learning to read and write.

### Reading Skills

#### *Alphabetics*

There are a number of skill domains within alphabetics:

- ***Phonemic awareness*** is the ability to recognize, manipulate, and use sounds in words, including the ability to hear and discriminate the sounds in language. Typically, children learn to hear and use the sounds in language before attending school, which is usually encouraged and emphasized by parents and caregivers through songs, rhymes, and word play.
- ***Phonics*** is the process of linking sounds to letter symbols and combining them to make words.
- ***Decoding*** is the ability to use phonics skills to translate a word from print to speech, usually by employing knowledge of sound-symbol correspondences. It is also the act of deciphering a new word by sounding it out.

TABLE 15.2

## Developmental Model of Early Literacy

The development of early literacy competencies begins at birth and proceeds through different levels and phases of skill acquisition and accomplishments. The following developmental model for describing early literacy–related skills and accomplishments (Dunst, Trivette, Masiello, Roper, & Robyak, 2006) of infants, toddlers, and preschoolers, birth to 5 years of age, is used at the Center for Early Literacy Learning and illustrates how early communication skills develop into early literacy skills.

| *Months* | *Developmental Levels (Phases)* | *Selected Accomplishments* |
|---|---|---|
| 0–15 | Prelanguage and Early Nonverbal Communication Development | Joint attention, intent to communicate, gestural communication, babbling, mutual vocal play, language/speech perception, phoneme speech stem acquisition |
| 12–30 | Language Onset and Vocabulary Development | First words, vocabulary development, language use, semantic development, early comprehension |
| 24–42 | Language Growth and Emergent Literacy Development | Phonological awareness of sounds, morphological awareness, syntactic development, pragmatic skill acquisition |
| 36–48 | Early Literacy Development and Metalanguage[a] Awareness | Phonological, morphological, and syntactic growth, prewriting, pretend reading, storytelling |
| 48–60 | Literacy and Reading and Writing Development | Phonology refinement, complex syllable use, invented spelling/writing, shared reading |

[a]Metalanguage is defined as the vocabulary used to describe language.

*Source:* Adapted with permission from Dunst, C. J., Trivette, C. M., Masiello, T., Roper, N., & Robyak, A. (2006). Framework for developing evidence-based early literacy learning practices. *CELLpapers, 1*(1), 1–12.

- ***Print awareness*** is basic knowledge about print and how it is typically organized on a page; for example, print conveys meaning, print is read in a specific direction on the page (from left to right in some languages, for example), and words are separated by spaces.

### *Fluency*

Reading fluency is the ability to read a text accurately, quickly, and with proper expression and comprehension. Fluency is important because fluent readers do not have to concentrate on decoding words; they can focus their attention on what the text means (Rasinski, 2009).

### *Comprehension*

Comprehending the content of the text is the reason for reading. Ideally, this occurs when readers actively engage in the complex process of making sense from text; they read with purposes such as learning, understanding, or enjoyment. Readers who truly comprehend what they are reading understand the vocabulary because they have had prior experiences and knowledge of the way texts and authors work (Routman, 2003).

## Assessment Issues for Reading Skills for Students with CVI

### *CVI and Learning Disabilities*

CVI is the "leading cause of bilateral visual impairment in children in Western countries" (Good, Jan, Burden, Skoczenski, & Candy, 2001), and approximately 60 percent of children with visual impairments have additional disabilities (Dote-Kwan, Chen, &

Hughes, 2001; Ferrell, 1998; Hatton, 2001). Children with visual impairments, including CVI, are at risk for additional disabilities, including learning disabilities (Sacks & Silberman, 1998). Learning disabilities are caused by a processing disorder that interferes with a student's ability to comprehend information or demonstrate certain academic skills, such as reading, writing, or math. Learning disabilities may affect attention, memory, auditory processing, conceptualization, and association (Denton & Silver, 2012, p. 375). In addition, children with CVI may experience visual processing difficulties and problems with the organization of skilled action as a result of optic ataxia (impaired visual guidance of movement) and dyspraxia (impaired ability to plan and bring about coordinated movements). These difficulties can impact their ability to find and maintain their place in text while reading and writing (Dutton, 2003; Gillen & Dutton, 2003). See Chapter 7 for a discussion of common features of dyslexia and CVI.

### *Auditory Processing Disturbances and the Development of Phonological Skills*

Students with CVI may have accompanying language impairments and/or auditory processing disorders causing disturbances in phonological skills—the ability to process the sounds of language. If this is the case, children will demonstrate challenges in gaining skills in phonemic awareness, phonics, and decoding. When it is found through assessment that students are not making timely and adequate progress in learning these skills, the list of "Red Flags for Auditory Processing and Phonological Disorders" (Denton & Silver, 2012) found in Sidebar 15.2 can be used by teachers to help determine if referral to the speech language pathologist and/or multidisciplinary team is warranted.

SIDEBAR 15.2

## Red Flags for Auditory Processing and Phonological Disorders

Auditory processing disorders and difficulty with phonological awareness have many characteristics in common. In addition to the overlap between these areas, many of the defining characteristics are not unique to auditory processing disorders or phonological awareness difficulties. Some characteristics may also be noted in individuals with attention deficits, hearing loss, behavioral problems, and learning difficulties.

In general, auditory processing disorders tend to have broader effects than do phonological disorders, particularly related to distinguishing words and creating a clear link with meaning. They generally affect overall comprehension of orally delivered communication. In contrast, phonological awareness skills relate to the ability to manipulate the sound elements: understanding and producing rhymes and segmenting and blending sounds or sound units. For example, an early phonological awareness skill is the ability to recognize each separate word within a sentence or syllables within a word, while a more advanced skill is identification of the individual sounds within a word. The latter of these skills is most directly related to reading and spelling.

The following table lists characteristics of auditory processing and phonological awareness disorders that teachers should watch out for. The table indicates whether the effects of the characteristics might be moderate (M) or strong (S).

*(continued on next page)*

**SIDEBAR 15.2** *(continued from previous page)*

| *Characteristics* | *Auditory Processing Disorders* | *Phonological Awareness Disorders* |
|---|---|---|
| Acts as if a hearing loss is present, despite normal hearing | S | |
| Has difficulty hearing in noisy situations | S | |
| Seems to perceive speech differently; for example, the student cannot distinguish word, phrase, or sentence boundaries; is unable to tell where one ends and the next begins | S | S |
| Has difficulty following speech spoken at a normal or fast rate | S | |
| Has difficulty remembering spoken information | S | |
| May mispronounce words and repeat them as they are perceived | S | S |
| Has difficulty learning sound-symbol associations | M | S |
| Has difficulty with sound blending | M | S |
| Has difficulty with word discrimination | M | S |
| Has difficulty learning to read or spell | M | S |
| Has difficulty following long conversations | S | |
| Has difficulty hearing conversations on the telephone | S | |
| Has difficulty learning a foreign language or challenging vocabulary words | S | S |
| Has a history of chronic otitis (infection or inflammation of the ear) or other otologic or neurologic sequelae | S | S |
| Has significant differences between subtest scores within domains assessed by the speech-language pathologist and psychologist, with identified weaknesses in auditory-dependent areas | S | S |
| Has a verbal IQ that is often lower than his or her nonverbal IQ | S | M |

*Source*: Reprinted from Denton, L. A., & Silver, M. A. (2012). Listening and understanding: Language and learning disabilities. In L. A. Barclay (Ed.), *Learning to listen, listening to learn: Teaching listening skills to students with visual impairments* (pp. 398–399). New York: AFB Press.

### *Visual Attention and Visual Processing Disturbances*

Visual attention and visual processing disturbances may cause difficulties in attaining skills in print awareness. Children with CVI who have disturbances in the processing of visual information may or may not have concomitant low visual acuity (Dutton, 2003); however, they may manifest atypical perception, interpretation, or motor responses in relation to incoming visual information that their eyes transmit to the brain. Often, these children are not aware that they have these problems. Visual processing disturbances that affect the development of reading and print awareness are shown in Table 15.3 (in addition to their effects on math skills, discussed later in this chapter). The visual pro-

## TABLE 15.3

# Possible Effects of Dorsal and Ventral Stream Dysfunctions on Reading and Math Performance

| | *Reading Difficulties That May Result* | *Math Difficulties That May Result* |
|---|---|---|
| **Dorsal Stream Dysfunctions** | | |
| Crowding | Difficulty seeing all of the letters in a word when there is not adequate spacing between them | Difficulty seeing all of the objects, pictures, and corresponding numbers when there is not adequate spacing between them |
| Visual clutter | Difficulty processing more than one or two visual elements at a time when there is too much print information on a page; the presence of surrounding clutter at the workstation or in the room also impairs access to the printed word | Difficulty keeping track of operations in a complex math problem because students may not be able to process more than one or two visual elements at a time; students may have a hard time maintaining place value during operations; students may demonstrate particular difficulty when viewing numbers displayed in charts and graphs |
| Visual sequential memory | Difficulty remembering the sequence of letters in words | Difficulty remembering a sequence of numbers |
| Visual search | Difficulty locating the next line of print on a page or finding sections of a workbook page; for example, as a result of simultanagnosia and the associated disability of easily moving the eyes from one item to another (apraxia of gaze) | Difficulty locating the correct line of numbers on a page when completing math problems or finding sections of a workbook page; for example, as a result of the inability to move eyes easily from one item to another (apraxia of gaze) |
| Simultaneous processing of information | Performance affected by distracting sensory input (e.g., auditory, tactile, visual, olfactory, kinesthetic) or mental or physical discomfort | Performance affected by distracting sensory input (e.g., auditory, tactile, visual, olfactory, kinesthetic) or mental or physical discomfort |
| **Ventral Stream Dysfunctions** | | |
| Shape agnosia | Impaired letter recognition; rarely acquired focal/multifocal damage to the brain can interfere with specific letter recognition (literal alexia) | Impaired number recognition |
| Visual memory | Difficulty matching visual input with the image of letters and words | Difficulty matching visual input with the image of numbers |
| Visual form constancy | Difficulty with letters that are reversed pairs, such as d and b; children usually outgrow this tendency by age 7 | Difficulty with numbers that are reversed pairs, such as 6 and 9 |
| Alexia without agraphia | Inability to read what one has written, despite the ability to write text, as a result of focal damage to specific brain pathways (O'Hare, Dutton, Green, & Coull, 1998) (occurs rarely) | Difficulty reading numbers that they write |

cessing disturbances are categorized into dorsal stream dysfunctions—those that affect the "where" pathway and disrupt visual guidance of movement, visual search, and attention—and ventral stream dysfunctions—those that affect the "what" pathway and disrupt visual recognition (see Chapter 3). In addition, students with visual attention and visual processing difficulties may not use vision to access information, especially when tired, sick or upset, or after taking certain medications, even though they have the ability to see to move around. All these factors greatly affect the acquisition of literacy skills and should be documented during assessment.

### *Challenges to Attaining Fluency*

When students have difficulties with one or more aspects of alphabetics, they will have challenges attaining reading fluency. Challenges in developing alphabetics skills may have to do with the visual processing problems just described, auditory processing problems, or both disorders. Fluency is assessed using reading inventories or grade-level reading passages, timing the student's reading rate, and documenting and analyzing any reading miscues (mistakes). The number of words that the student reads in one minute (wpm) is the reading fluency rate. Reduced reading fluency resulting from issues associated with CVI needs to be differentiated from the slow rate of processing resulting from cognitive difficulties through the multidisciplinary assessment process. The development of adequate reading fluency is important for a variety of reasons, including text comprehension, development and maintenance of the desire to read, and efficiency in academic reading.

Gaining reading fluency skills is very important; children who learn to read fluently develop the ability to fully comprehend text with ease, promoting a greater desire to read. This, in turn, increases the willingness to devote more time to reading. When children read more throughout the day their reading fluency increases, enabling them to engage in academic tasks that require them to read. Likewise, students who struggle while reading are unable to successfully accomplish grade-level academic tasks in a reasonable amount of time.

### *Challenges to Text Comprehension*

Reading comprehension is usually assessed by having students answer comprehension questions about what they have read. Questions should not only assess the student's retention of details from the passage, but also require the student to demonstrate understanding of the main idea of the passage, to make inferences from what has been read, and to demonstrate understanding of the vocabulary used in the passage.

Students who have difficulties in alphabetics, reading fluency, or both will also demonstrate difficulties with text comprehension because they are struggling to decode (read) vocabulary. Working hard to decode the text decreases text comprehension.

When students with CVI who don't have challenges with alphabetics or fluency demonstrate difficulties in reading comprehension, additional language-based learning disorders should also be considered, warranting assessment by a speech-language pathologist. For example, a number of young people with CVI have explained that they tend to think in words rather than pictures, and that descriptive text can therefore be difficult to visualize and remember

(G. N. Dutton, personal communication, January, 2012).

## Assessment of Literacy Skills: Writing

Learning to write primarily involves two broad areas: the mechanics of writing and the writing process. Writing mechanics includes the physical production of text, spelling correctly, and producing accurate grammar. The writing process includes generating and organizing information, planning, and editing. There are many areas of writing that may be assessed as students progress from the earliest stages of learning to write—when they begin to understand that symbols have meaning and that letters represent speech segments—to the most sophisticated aspects of the writing process.

Just as writing skills are taught to children as soon as they begin school, assessment of writing skills begins in kindergarten, with assessment of writing samples as children learn to form letters and begin to approximate writing words. As children progress to learning to spell, their spelling abilities are tested often. As they learn to use vocabulary and grammar to compose sentences, paragraphs, and compositions, these skills are assessed through both standardized and informal assessment modes, primarily by examination of their writing samples.

There are many possible challenges to students with CVI as they learn to write. As with reading, students may be affected by both visual and visual processing challenges that have an impact on their progress. Table 15.4 illustrates the various tasks involved with writing mechanics, the prerequisite skills for each, assessment modes, and some possible effects or disturbances caused by CVI. As the table illustrates, disturbances from CVI are most likely to be observed during the beginning phase of learning to write, such as writing mechanics and learning to spell, making it challenging for some students with CVI to progress to the more sophisticated tasks of writing. Children who have cerebral palsy or other motor challenges resulting from neurological insult in addition to CVI will experience visual-motor challenges, including impaired visual guidance of movement (optic ataxia) (Gillen & Dutton, 2003). Specific visual-motor difficulties that children with dorsal stream dysfunction may have include:

- Difficulty writing horizontally, for which lined paper assists considerably
- Difficulty judging the length of pen strokes and getting them right
- Difficulty judging the direction of pen strokes and getting their orientation right

## Listening Comprehension Assessment

The development of literacy skills is strongly linked to the development of listening skills (Barclay, 2012), and listening is an important mode of curricular access that may support students with CVI. Students' abilities to listen to class directions and instruction, as well as to fiction and nonfiction literature that is read to them, can be assessed through classroom observation and testing. Students with more profound neurological conditions may have slow auditory processing rates; unless the rate of speech is matched to the rate of processing, listening comprehension will be impacted. If it is suspected that students do not fully comprehend what they hear during oral instruction, referral to a

TABLE 15.4

## Assessment of Writing Mechanics and CVI

| *Task* | *Prerequisite Skills* | *Assessment Modes* | *Possible CVI Disturbances* |
|---|---|---|---|
| **Writing Skills (recognition and production of writing)** | | Handwriting and typing samples | |
| | Symbolic understanding (symbols have meaning) | | Cognitive impairment that may be associated with conditions that co-occur with CVI |
| | Alphabetic principle (letters represent speech segments) | | Visual memory tasks |
| | Memory for letters | | Visual memory tasks |
| | Discrimination and recognition of letters, words, and sentences | | Visual acuity and visual fields, control of eye movement, accommodation; visual attention and perception; object, letter, and word recognition |
| | Fine motor skills (handwriting and typing) | | Visual attention and perception; object, letter, and word recognition; visual motor skills |
| **Spelling** | | Standardized and informal assessments, spelling tests, writing samples | |
| | Writing skills (recognition and production of writing) | | Visual attention and perception; object recognition |
| | Sound-symbol connection | | Visual attention and perception; object recognition |
| | Recognition and understanding of spelling conventions and patterns | | Memory task |
| | Memory for regularly and irregularly spelled words | | Memory task |
| **Punctuation/ Capitalization** | | Standardized assessments and informal writing samples | |
| | Memory for punctuation types and capitalization rules | | Visual acuity; visual crowding; visual memory skills |

*Source:* Adapted from Access Center. (2004). *Accessing skills toward successful writing development.* Washington, DC: Author. Retrieved December 30, 2011, from www.readingrockets.org/article/22026/?theme=print.

speech-language pathologist or multidisciplinary team is warranted. Furthermore, some students with CVI demonstrate a lack of visual attention on one side or the other, which can affect auditory attention if they do not realize that someone is talking to them, especially when they are tired. This is particularly true in children with cerebral palsy, for whom subtle hemianopic inattention can occur on the side of the greatest weakness. It is important to determine if this is the case so that communication can be directed to the student's attentive side, especially during assessment.

While assessment of listening comprehension is included in some standardized assessments, it is more often assessed informally by reading grade-level passages to students and asking comprehension questions. As with reading comprehension, not only is it important for students to be able to accurately answer questions about the details of the passage, it is also important that they be able to demonstrate understanding of the main idea, vocabulary, and be able to infer answers from information presented verbally.

Some students with CVI may demonstrate listening comprehension skills that are several grade levels above their reading and writing grade levels. When this is the case, skillful listening will provide a valuable mode of access to the curriculum. In other cases, students with CVI may have concomitant challenges in listening comprehension that may be related to auditory or language processing problems. In any case, it is very important to assess listening comprehension and provide instruction in listening skills (Barclay, 2012; see also Chapters 10 and 23 for more information on instruction in listening skills).

## Mathematics Skills Assessment

Students' skills in mathematics typically are assessed often, beginning in kindergarten and continuing throughout their school years, both formally and informally. Assessments may be administered by a classroom teacher or a teacher of students with visual impairments. Students may participate in math assessment when taking achievement tests with their classmates and during curriculum-based assessment when taking tests that are included in their math textbooks or curricular materials. Aspects of math abilities, such as memory, visuospatial processing, and fluid reasoning, may also be assessed as part of a cognitive assessment.

The effects of CVI will often impact students in their acquisition of math skills, and this should be taken into consideration during assessment. Assessment and curriculum materials can be adapted according to the individual needs of each student with CVI (see Table 15.1).

According to Kapperman, Heinze, and Sticken (2000, p. 373), to be successful in learning mathematics, students must be able to do the following:

- Develop the ability to retain (memorize) facts and data
- Recognize patterns
- Recognize relationships (part to whole and sequential and spatial concepts)
- Categorize and classify
- Organize mathematical information
- Have a basic awareness of when an answer is reasonable or possible
- Think through a problem
- Plan a solution and predict an outcome

TABLE 15.5
### Math Domains

| *Basic Concepts* | *Operations* | *Applications* |
|---|---|---|
| • Numeration (basic number skills)<br>• Rational numbers<br>• Geometry<br>• Algebra | • Addition and subtraction<br>• Multiplication and division<br>• Mental computation | • Measurement<br>• Time and money<br>• Estimation<br>• Interpreting data<br>• Problem solving |

- Differentiate essential information from superfluous and irrelevant information
- Use mental flexibility to identify multiple ways to solve a problem

It is important for assessors to keep these abilities in mind, as well as the specific challenges that may arise as a result of CVI, when reviewing students' assessment results. Domains to consider in the assessment of math skills are shown in Table 15.5. Potential influences of CVI are discussed in relationship to the following skills within those domains:

- Number skills, including counting and computation
- Spatial skills and interpretation of data
- Functional math skills

Challenges arising in these areas as a result of CVI will affect the development of skills in all other aspects of mathematics.

## Number Skills

The foundation for the development of numbers skills is the establishment of number sense. Children may begin to develop number sense, the ability to estimate and judge magnitude as well as the ability to recognize unreasonable results, before entering school (Case, 1998).

Mastering basic number skills involves the ability to learn to count, read numbers, apply numbers to amounts, and learn basic number facts in four operations: addition, subtraction, multiplication, and division. Students with CVI may demonstrate many of the same difficulties when learning to read and write numbers that they experience when learning to read letters, words, and sentences. Visual processing disturbances that may affect the development of number skills can be found in Table 15.3.

When students encounter difficulty learning to recognize and write numbers consistently and have trouble seeing the objects or pictures that they are to count, it will be challenging for them to learn math skills that require basic number skills such as computation, problem solving, and interpretation of data. Some students may learn how to recognize numbers and count objects when their visual requirements with regard to print size, contrast, and spacing are met, but begin to have difficulties with crowding when they encounter computation and data interpretation because of the detailed and crowded formats. Accurate counting of sequentially presented elements can demonstrate that counting is intact if the data/numbers are not presented simultaneously, but rather sequentially revealed.

Because brain injury can result in CVI in addition to other neurologically based processing difficulties, it is important to determine if the student's difficulties with memory of numbers for computation tasks are because of the effects of CVI, memory difficulties, or both. Further assessment by a psychologist in collaboration with the teacher of students with visual impairments and the classroom teacher will be essential in this case. This information will be beneficial in designing the most appropriate curricular modifications and adaptations—for instance, the provision of computation charts or other memory aides—if the difficulty has to do primarily with memory.

## Visuospatial Skills and Data Interpretation

Many aspects of math are represented by pictorial, diagrammatic, or graphic explanation. These graphic representations are very common in both formal and informal assessments of math skills. Some students with CVI will struggle with the visuospatial aspects of math. Consequently, direct and explicit attention and modification to assessment materials should be provided. When students encounter such difficulties during assessment, the following questions should be considered:

- Has the student had explicit, sequential instruction in the use of graphically represented information?
- Does the adaptation, such as providing extra spacing and simplification of format, improve the student's ability to interpret information visually?
- Can the student use tools, such as a line marker or typoscope (card with a cutout reading window) to visually isolate pertinent information?
- If the student can read the information presented, can the student recognize the part to whole relationships represented in the chart or graph?
- If the student cannot visually interpret the information, can the information be presented in concrete modes (using objects such as three-dimensional forms of two-dimensional images)?
- Can the student learn two-dimensional images by (a) first exploring a three-dimensional representation of the shape tactilely; then (b) associating that tactile experience of shape with a two-dimensional image; and (c) later recalling that three-dimensional shape when the two-dimensional image is seen once again?

## Functional Math Skills

Most students with CVI will be instructed and assessed in their functional use of mathematic skills—the applied math skills of being able to use time, money, and measurement in everyday life—and for some students, functional math skill development will eventually be the primary math curriculum of choice. Functional math skills require the application of number skills, including one-to-one correspondence and basic computation skills (addition, subtraction, multiplication, and division), and the ability to use tools of time and measurement such as clocks, calendars, measuring cups, and rulers.

Assessment of functional math skills will be included in many formal and informal math assessments, and can be regularly assessed through observation and by using checklists. Development of number sense is essential to the development of functional math skills. When assessing this area it is important to discern if a student's challenge in functional math skills has to do with a basic lack of number sense or issues related to CVI. In addition, many of the common tools of functional math skills, such as clocks and rulers, are not easily adaptable for day-to-day use. It is important to determine what adaptations can be made during and after the assessment process that will enable students to participate in important everyday tasks involving functional math skills.

## Using Assessment Results to Inform Curricular Goals and Modifications

The goal of assessment is to provide information that will help teachers plan for their student's curriculum needs and necessary modifications with regard to CVI. The case study of Dominic, the fifth-grade student with CVI introduced earlier in this chapter, continues with a synopsis of his assessment results and recommended learning strategies in reading, listening comprehension, writing, and math, illustrating how the principles discussed in this chapter are put into practice.

**Dominic was assessed, over a period of several days,** by a collaborative, multidisciplinary team, including a teacher of students with visual impairments, an orientation and mobility specialist, a psychologist, and a technology specialist. Results from the cognitive assessment revealed that Dominic had the ability to be an academic student—a thinker and learner; his scores on measures of verbal comprehension, perceptual reasoning, and memory were all within the average range.

During assessment of Dominic's literacy skills, he acknowledged that reading was difficult for him. When asked what part was most challenging, he answered, "Sometimes just figuring out what the letters are." At all grade levels tested, Dominic read very slowly; it was very difficult for him to sustain print reading while using either large print text with double line spacing or while using a video magnifier.

A standing reading light was provided and placed at Dominic's side to lessen the effect of the shadow cast as he bent over the print. He yawned and rubbed his eyes as he read, making it apparent that reading was very exhausting. He read the words and passages very slowly from a distance of 6 inches from the print, using his finger as a guide from time to time. He turned his head to dampen his nystagmus (as indicated in his eye reports). When not using his finger to point, he frequently lost his place on the line of print.

Dominic easily decoded words at the second-grade level. When he was reading at his own fifth-grade level and had to decode new words, he didn't always know all of the phonetic sounds that he encountered. Also, when attempting to read new words, he seemed to encounter problems with simultanagnostic crowding. For instance, he read "manga" instead of "manage" and "unsal" for "unusual." It is a great challenge to learn to decode new words when there are both visual acuity and visual processing problems. His reading comprehension while reading a fifth-grade passage at 33 words per minute was at 70 percent, but when listening to alternate fifth-grade passages read to him, his comprehension level was at 90 percent.

Dominic's challenge and fatigue while handwriting were very evident. He said, "Whenever I do much writing I get tired." His letters were large, irregular, and hard to read. He spelled at the second-grade level on the spelling assessment, and his writing sample was short and immature, containing many errors.

Although Dominic said that math was his least favorite subject in school, his basic number skills were quite good when he didn't have to record his responses. It was necessary during testing to point out certain missed details, such as the hair color on an illustration in which hair color was pertinent to the question, and the type of animal, when all were brown, four-legged creatures. For Dominic, it was clear that his visual interpretation of the graphical aspects of math was often inaccurate. Writing his answers and keeping track of place value as he worked were also problematic.

Dominic's assessment revealed that many aspects of CVI, particularly profound simultanagnosia, were affecting his progress in literacy and math skills. Assessment results should lead to curricular modifications and goals that can help improve students' progress over time. In addition to the recommendations from a low vision clinical evaluation with regard to print size and spectacle use, the following recommendations were made for Dominic, based on his assessment results.

## General Vision and Access Recommendations

- Shift the focus of instruction to provide greater emphasis on helping Dominic develop his curriculum access skills, especially listening skills, use of technology within the classroom, and beginning braille instruction.
- Provide ongoing teaching and support in the use of low vision devices. Dominic will need systematic instruction before he can be expected to use them independently.
- Experiment with providing better lighting with a standing movable lamp.

## Assistive Technology

- Provide access to and training in the use of a video magnifier for viewing information in the distance (such as on the board, walls, and presentations during instruction) and at near (books and worksheets at Dominic's desk).
- Provide access to and training in screen magnification and screen reading programs with a document reader, one that uses the "ticker setting" that isolates one line of print and highlights each word while reading. Bring the computer with these programs into the classroom for Dominic to use regularly.
- Shift from handwriting to word processing as soon as Dominic's keyboarding skills become proficient. Spelling word practice might be a good place to start.
- Have Dominic use a scanner and optical character recognition (OCR) software to scan his worksheets and download them to the computer, enabling him to enter answers right on the document with his word processing program.

## Literacy Skills

- ***Introduce braille and provide daily braille reading instruction.*** Presently, Dominic's print reading is inefficient. His visual abilities may improve over time, but until they improve to the point that he is able to efficiently access visual curricular information, he should receive braille instruction in addition to reading instruction using print. Give this at least a year, charting progress to help the Individualized Education Program (IEP) team determine if adequate progress is being made. Instruction should be given daily.
- ***Conduct an ongoing learning media assessment.*** It will be very important to regularly assess Dominic's progress in print and braille reading, utilizing a reading inventory that will help document his growth in reading fluency in both media. This will help the IEP team to determine which learning medium will be his primary one (the one in which most learning will take place).
- ***Provide print fluency exercises.*** Dominic can develop print reading fluency and speed through repeated readings of materials that are just below his reading grade level. A tactile chart with a variety

of tactile markers might be a fun way for Dominic to chart his progress as his reading speed increases. This should be done regularly, but for a short duration (no more than 5 minutes each day), with care taken to make sure that Dominic's visual system is not overly stressed.

- ***Continue to provide reading instruction that includes phonetic skill development.*** Because Dominic has not yet gained reading fluency in any medium, it will be important to continue to teach him the rules of decoding new words. He is still "learning to read," while his peers are "reading to learn."

## Listening Comprehension

- ***Provide instruction and guidance in the development of listening skills.*** Given the fact that so much of Dominic's information will be obtained using audible materials, he will benefit from instruction in how to listen effectively to books that have been recorded or read aloud by a screen reader. It would be beneficial if some of his textbooks (such as social studies or literature) were made available in audible form. He will also require direct instruction in classroom listening strategies, including note-taking during group instruction, identifying and recording important details, and paraphrasing.

## Dictation

- ***Develop dictation skills.*** Dictation is another tool that Dominic can learn to use to provide a curricular response. Although he will often use his computer technology skills to produce much of his schoolwork, once he has gained comfort and ease in their use, there will be times when it may be beneficial for him to dictate his answers for a worksheet or test. This should be considered another acceptable choice for accommodation.

## Writing Skills

- Place emphasis on daily keyboarding instruction; as soon as possible allow Dominic to use a computer for all writing tasks. While it is convenient that Dominic can use handwriting to sign his name or make a short list, it is inefficient for assignments. It is very important that time be given each day at home and school to help him develop keyboarding skills.
- Provide support in writing composition that will encourage Dominic to expand his writing.

## Mathematics

- Provide direct explicit instruction in interpretation of diagrammatic and graphically presented math problems. Instruction should include teaching Dominic to request visual support when he may be confused about the illustrations essential to understanding the problem.
- Teach Dominic to use graph (or squared) paper to help maintain place value during multiplication and long division calculations.
- Teach Dominic to use a systematic approach while completing math worksheets and on tests.
- Teach Dominic to use a piece of heavy card stock as a placeholder and to occlude nonpertinent information as he works on math problems.
- Teach Dominic about appropriate times to use the video magnifier for math work and provide opportunities for regular

practice until its appropriate use becomes automatic.

## Conclusion

There is much to be discovered to assist students with CVI as they participate with their classmates in literacy and math, as well as other core curriculum areas. Dominic, as do all students with CVI, required adaptations to assessment strategies that took into account his unique constellation of visual and learning requirements. His assessment outcomes led to the development of appropriate and effective recommendations for interventions that addressed his specific literacy and math needs.

Through an ongoing process of careful and regular assessment, teachers of students with visual impairments and other professionals can determine students' individualized learning requirements. In turn, understanding students' learning needs results in the formulation of instructional goals and modifications that foster continued curricular growth and development.

## References


Access Center. (2004). *Accessing skills toward successful writing development.* Washington, DC: Author. Retrieved December 30, 2011, from www.readingrockets.org/article/22026/

Barclay, L. A. (2003). Expanded core curriculum: Education. In S. A. Goodman & S. H. Wittenstein (Eds.), *Collaborative assessment: Working with students who are blind or visually impaired, including those with additional disabilities* (pp. 94–149). New York: AFB Press.

Barclay, L. A. (Ed.). (2012). *Learning to listen, listening to learn: Teaching listening skills to students with visual impairments.* New York: AFB Press.

Case, R. (1998, April). *A psychological model of number sense and its development.* Paper presented at the annual meeting of the American Educational Research Association, San Diego, CA.

Denton, L. A., & Silver, M. A. (2012). Listening and understanding: Language and learning disabilities. In L. A. Barclay (Ed.), *Learning to listen, listening to learn: Teaching listening skills to students with visual impairments* (pp. 372–453). New York: AFB Press.

Dote-Kwan, J., Chen, D., & Hughes, M. (2001). A national survey of service providers who work with young children with visual impairments. *Journal of Visual Impairment & Blindness, 95*(6), 325–337.

Dunst, C. J., Trivette, C. M., Masiello, T., Roper, N., & Robyak, A. (2006). Framework for developing evidence-based early literacy learning practices. *CELLpapers, 1*(1), 1–12. Retrieved December 30, 2011, from *www.earlyliteracylearning.org/cellpapers/cellpapers_v1_n1.pdf*

Dutton, G. N. (2003). Cognitive vision, its disorders and differential diagnosis in adults and children: Knowing where and what things are. *Eye, 17,* 289–304.

Dutton, G. N. (2009). "Dorsal stream dysfunction" and "dorsal stream dysfunction plus": A potential classification for perceptual visual impairment in the context of cerebral visual impairment? *Developmental Medicine & Child Neurology, 51*(3), 170–172.

Ferrell, K. A., with Shaw, A. R., & Dietz, S. J. (1998). *Project PRISM: A longitudinal study of developmental patterns of children who are visually impaired.* Greeley, CO: University of Northern Colorado.

Fuchs, D., & Fuchs, L. S. (2006). Introduction to Response to Intervention: What, why, and how valid is it? *Reading Research Quarterly, 41*(1), 93–99.

Gillen, J. A., & Dutton, G. N. (2003). Balint's syndrome in a 10-year-old male. *Developmental Medicine & Child Neurology, 45*(5), 349–352.

Good, W. V., Jan, J. E., Burden, S. K., Skoczenski, A., & Candy, R. (2001). Recent advances in cortical visual impairment. *Developmental Medicine & Child Neurology, 43*(1), 56–60.

Hatton, D. D. (2001). Model registry of early childhood visual impairment: First-year results.

*Journal of Visual Impairment & Blindness, 95*(7), 418–433.

Heinze, T. (2000). Comprehensive assessment. In A. J. Koenig & M. C. Holbrook (Eds.), *Foundations of education: Volume II. Instructional strategies for teaching children and youths with visual impairments* (pp. 27–60). New York: AFB Press.

Kapperman, G., Heinze, T., & Sticken, J. (2000). Mathematics. In A. J. Koenig & M. C. Holbrook (Eds.), *Foundations of education: Volume II. Instructional strategies for teaching children and youths with visual impairments* (pp. 370–399). New York: AFB Press.

Koenig, A. J., & Holbrook, M. C. (1995). *Learning media assessment of students with visual impairments: A resource guide for teachers* (2nd ed.). Austin: Texas School for the Blind and Visually Impaired.

Lewis, S., & Russo, R. (1998). Educational assessment for students who have visual impairments with other disabilities. In S. Z. Sacks & R. K. Silberman (Eds.), *Educating students who have visual impairments with other disabilities* (pp. 39–72). Baltimore, MD: Paul H. Brookes Publishing Co.

Lueck, A. H. (2010). Cortical or cerebral visual impairment in children: A brief overview. *Journal of Visual Impairment & Blindness, 104*(10), 585–592.

Nilsson, N. L. (2008). A critical analysis of eight informal reading inventories. *The Reading Teacher, 61*(7), 526–536. Retrieved November 28, 2012, from www.readingrockets.org/article/23373/

O'Hare, A. E., Dutton, G. N., Green, D., & Coull, R. (1998). Evolution of a form of pure alexia without agraphia in a child sustaining occipital lobe infarction at 2 ½ years. *Developmental Medicine & Child Neurology, 40*(6), 417–420.

Paris, S. G., & Carpenter, R. D. (2003). FAQs about IRIs. *The Reading Teacher, 56*(6), 578–580.

Rasinski, T. V. (2009). *Essential readings on fluency.* Newark, DE: International Reading Association.

Routman, R. (2003). *Reading essentials: The specifics you need to teach reading well.* Portsmouth, NH: Heinemann.

Sacks, S. Z., & Silberman, R. K. (1998). *Educating students who have visual impairments with other disabilities.* Baltimore, MD: Paul H. Brookes Publishing Co.

# 16

# Assessments Linked to Interventions: Independent Living Skills

*Carlene Creamer O'Brien and Angela Martyn*

Students with visual impairments have less opportunity to observe other people performing everyday tasks than do fully sighted individuals. For students with cerebral visual impairment (CVI), fluctuating vision and visual processing differences can further impair these opportunities to learn from visual observations and modeling. This inability to access typical incidental learning opportunities diminishes the acquisition of independent living skills.

The assessment and instruction of functional independent living skills can be viewed in the context of the expanded core curriculum (ECC) for students who are blind or visually impaired. The ECC, as originally defined by Phil Hatlen (1996, 2003; see also Allman & Lewis, 2014; Sapp & Hatlen, 2010), outlines specific skill areas that must be deliberately taught to blind and visually impaired students over and above the core curriculum needed for graduation from high school. The ECC promotes increased access to the core educational curriculum and facilitates the acquisition of additional skills that promote independence for students who are blind and visually impaired. The specific skill areas of the ECC include communication modes, orientation and mobility, social interaction, independent living, recreation and leisure, career education, use of assistive technology, sensory efficiency, and self-determination. This chapter focuses on one of the nine areas of the ECC, independent living skills, as performed by school-age students with CVI who use vision in their daily lives.

"The term *independent living skills* is a broad label that encompasses every skill that an individual needs to have at some time in his or her life to be as independent as possible" (Kelley & Smith, 2000, p. 570). The two areas typically focused on within independent living skills are personal management and home management. Personal management includes eating, grooming, hygiene, the care and identification of clothing, medical care, the identification and management of money, telling time, and time management. Home management includes food and diet management, cleaning, basic household repairs, measurement, shopping, and gardening (Kelley & Smith, 2000).

High-quality assessment of independent living skills is imperative in order to be able to plan and provide appropriate instruction. The ultimate goal is to determine ways to facilitate students' learning by providing motivating activities and environments that lead to successful, independent task performance. Tasks need to be meaningful and functional for each individual student and take into account that student's sensory, cognitive, and physical capabilities. Students with CVI are a heterogeneous group and are placed in a variety of school settings, from self-contained special day classes that focus on functional skills to fully mainstream academic classes, in which concentration is a key educational issue. The type of placement affects the priority given to functional skills within the school day. Regardless of the degree of emphasis placed on independent living skills as a part of their curricula, the independent living skills of all students with CVI need to be assessed to inform the level of intervention and the development of appropriate instruction, so that the students are motivated to learn these important skills.

## Planning an Individual Assessment

Sidebar 16.1 provides an overview of the process of conducting an assessment of a student's independent living skills, including students with CVI. The preparation for an individual assessment begins by gathering available educational, family, and medical background information. Sidebar 16.1 gives examples of information that should be included in this review.

The specialists involved in conducting an assessment of independent living skills may include a teacher of students with visual impairments, an orientation and mobility specialist, an occupational therapist, a rehabilitation specialist, or any combination of these professionals. The scope of specific independent living skills areas for assessment can be found in Figure 16.1. During the interview with the family and student, the student's current level of independence within particular skill areas is determined. If the student performs a particular skill independently, no assessment is required. Skill areas that have not yet been mastered are then ranked according to their priority for instruction. Further assessment will be required in high-priority areas that have yet to be mastered.

When planning for this type of assessment, a variety of issues must be carefully considered, including vision functions and visual processing capabilities (see Chapter 10), as well as factors particularly relevant to daily living skill performance such as:

- Family and cultural expectations as they relate to functional independent living skills
- Language fluency (for example, an interpreter may be needed to conduct a detailed interview with parents)
- Pace of the student (important when allotting time for assessment)
- Physical and cognitive abilities or limitations of the student
- Location of assessment (home, school, or community)
- Comfort of the student in performing functional skills with non-family members present

When formulating a plan for assessing independent living skills, the student's phys-

SIDEBAR 16.1

## Summary of the Independent Living Skills Assessment Process

### Review of Medical, Educational, and Family Records

***Medical and Educational Records***

- Medical information that affects school performance
- Current vision report from optometrist or ophthalmologist
- Functional vision assessment and reports
- Learning media assessment and reports
- Most recent educational plan
- Psychological assessments and reports
- Other educational assessments and reports such as:
  - Orientation and mobility
  - Speech and language
  - Occupational therapy

***Family Background Information***

- Outcome the family would like to obtain from the assessment
- Assessment concerns listed in order of priority
- Behavioral concerns
- Current home life, family members living in the home
- Interaction with family members, peers, and other adults
- Family report of health history and current medications
- Contact information and release of information from current physicians

### Formulation of Assessment Plan

***Determination of Independent Living Skills to be Assessed***

- Independent Living Skills
  - Personal management
  - Home management

***Consideration of Family and Student's Specific Circumstances***

- Language
- Communication style
- Respect of cultural requirements

***Identification of Anticipated Effects of CVI on Skills to be Assessed***

- Visual functioning
- Visual processing
- Physical abilities of student
- Cognitive abilities of student

### Selection of Assessment Tools and Implementation of Assessments

- Educator interviews
- Parent interviews
- Checklists and rating scales
- Observational assessment
- Performance assessment
  - Category
  - Task
  - Effects of CVI on task
  - Functional observation
  - Suggested intervention/hypothesis
  - Outcome of intervention/hypothesis
  - Revisions as necessary

### Compilation of Assessment Results

- Provide an overall picture of the student and the effects of CVI
- Develop specific recommendations within each skill area
  - Write measurable goals for the student with interval measurements
  - Devise a chart or other measurement system for tracking student progress toward the goals

FIGURE 16.1
## Independent Living Skills to Assess

| *Skill Area* | *Independent (Yes/No)* | *Comments* |
|---|---|---|
| **Personal Management** | | |
| ***Personal Hygiene*** | | |
| Showering/bathing | | |
| Hair care | | |
| Skin care | | |
| Care of teeth | | |
| Nail care | | |
| Shaving | | |
| Care of menses | | |
| ***Dressing*** | | |
| Identifying front/back of clothing | | |
| Dressing self | | |
| Using buttons (or other fasteners) | | |
| Tying laces | | |
| Selecting appropriate clothes for various occasions | | |
| ***Care of Clothing*** | | |
| Laundry | | |
| Ironing | | |
| ***Organization of Closets and Drawers*** | | |
| Using hangers | | |
| Folding clothing | | |
| Having method for identifying colors | | |
| **Home Management** | | |
| ***Cleaning Skills*** | | |
| Sweeping | | |
| Vacuuming | | |
| Mopping | | |

*(continued on next page)*

FIGURE 16.1 *(continued from previous page)*

| Skill Area | Independent (Yes/No) | Comments |
|---|---|---|
| Dusting | | |
| Washing windows | | |
| Throwing out trash/recycling | | |
| Scrubbing (bathtub, floors, appliances, counters, walls) | | |
| Care of bed (making the bed, changing sheets/pillowcases) | | |
| ***Cooking*** | | |
| Planning | | |
| Shopping | | |
| Labeling, storing, opening containers | | |
| Measuring (liquids and dry goods) | | |
| Using various utensils and small appliances | | |
| Preparing meals | | |
| Eating | | |
| Dishwashing | | |

ical and cognitive abilities must be taken into consideration, as well as the nature of the skills to be assessed. The same procedures outlined in this chapter can be applied to determining a student's present level of functioning, regardless of the student's physical or cognitive abilities. Many aspects of independent living skills are difficult to assess at school because the natural environment for performing skills such as dressing, personal hygiene, clothing care, and food preparation is in the home. For these skills, interviews with family members combined with observation of skills in the natural environment are required to determine a student's current level of functioning.

## Choosing Assessment Tools

There are very few formal tools available for the assessment of independent living skills for students who are blind or visually impaired. Most of the assessments used are informal and include a combination of observation, educator interviews, parent interviews, checklists or rating scales, and performance assessment to target specific skills. If students cannot independently carry out all the steps required to successfully complete a specific functional skill, they may still be able to perform some of the steps and be partial participants in the process. Through careful observation, the student's level of participation can be established and the requisite steps for instruction identified. (See Chapter 19 for a discussion of partial participation.)

Observation of the student in typical environments provides a snapshot of how the student functions in everyday activities. Observations of this kind may take place at school, in the home, or in the community. Data can be collected about the types of tasks the student is required to perform in typical settings, the environmental circumstances within which tasks are performed, and the visual and other sensory demands of tasks in these settings. The information gained from the natural environment will help guide the evaluator in developing future assessments that focus on the development of specific visual or other sensory adaptations to promote successful task performance.

When gathering assessment information through observation or interview, a checklist can be used as a guide to ensure that all topics are covered. Figure 16.2 shows the example of an assessment checklist for tooth brushing. If the skill is directly observed, details can be documented in the comments section. However, if it is not possible to observe a skill, and the information is obtained solely through a parent interview, it may be necessary to ask additional questions. One entry on the skills checklist reads, "Brushes all teeth." If the assessor asks, "Does the student brush her teeth?" it will often lead to a "yes" or "no" response. One way of obtaining more detailed information is to say, "Tell me more about the way your daughter (or the student's name) brushes her teeth." Wait for a response and listen carefully to the information provided by the parents. Another approach to the interview may be to break the

FIGURE 16.2

**Sample Checklist for Assessing Tooth Brushing**

**Tooth Brushing Assessment Checklist**

**Directions:** Document the child's performance on two different dates. For each assessment date, enter a plus sign if a skill is independently performed and a minus sign if it is not.

| ***Steps in Skill*** | ***Date*** +/– | ***Date*** +/– | ***Comments*** |
|---|---|---|---|
| 1. Locates brush and toothpaste (or powder) | | | |
| 2. Uses toothpaste or powder | | | |
| 3. Brushes all teeth | | | |
| 4. Adjusts faucet (tap) of the sink and rinses brush | | | |
| 5. Locates and uses cup to rinse mouth (optional) | | | |
| 6. Uses mouthwash | | | |
| 7. Flosses teeth | | | |
| 8. Returns all items to their original location | | | |

task down into steps and ask specific questions about tooth brushing. For instance, "Can she locate her own toothbrush? Who puts toothpaste (or toothpowder) on the brush (or finger)? Is she systematic with the brush; does she brush all her teeth? How does she rinse, and does she put the toothbrush away?"

Checklists that can be used for assessment are recommended at the end of this chapter. While many include age ranges, grade-level equivalencies and chronological ages are provided as a general guideline only. It is also important to note that most formal assessments have not been normed on a population of children with visual impairments. When conducting assessments for students who have CVI, it is best to establish a student's current level of functioning, indicating the tasks a student can perform, and use that as a baseline for establishing next steps.

As noted earlier, a *performance assessment* may be conducted after observation in typical settings so that the assessor has the opportunity to develop hypotheses about which adaptations to try during this phase of the evaluation process. For the performance assessment, information obtained about the student's use of vision and other senses is utilized, and the assessor designs and fine-tunes the environment. Providing adaptive tools and methods for a specific activity may optimize the student's performance and lay the foundation for success. All interventions made by the assessor are documented to determine whether each one appears to help or hinder a student's performance. This phase of assessment uses an approach similar to diagnostic teaching in that additional adjustments are made to the environment, to materials, and to teaching strategies based on feedback from the student as tasks are performed during the assessment process. This results in the identification of optimal interventions to be incorporated into a student's curricular plan or independent living tasks. (See Chapters 10 and 19 for more information on diagnostic teaching.)

## Dominic's Assessment of Functional Skills

The following vignette describes Dominic, the fifth-grade student with CVI previously introduced in Chapter 15. It serves to illustrate the assessment process, including observational assessments in school and at home, followed by a sample performance assessment in the home. General background information was provided by parents and teachers through interviews and written questionnaires and gathered prior to the observation.

### School-Related Functional Skills Assessment

**Dominic, a fifth-grade student with CVI secondary** to cortical insult at birth, had many challenges related to his CVI. His distance binocular visual acuity was measured at 20/80; his near acuity was 20/114 when viewing single symbols, and dropped to 20/300 when viewing crowded symbols. He also had constricted visual fields and diminished ability to detect curbs and drop-offs. Dominic's vision seemed to fluctuate "without explanation," and his visual-perceptual difficulties affected his reading fluency. The physical process of using vision seemed to be exhausting to Dominic. Some of the challenges noted by his teachers at school were the organization of his backpack, desk, and books. Information was also obtained during observation of Dominic's personal organization skills at school.

Based on an earlier review of reports and interviews, some of the effects of CVI on Dominic's vision that the assessor was alerted to were reduced contrast sensitivity, reduction of vision in heavily shadowed or low-light areas, difficulty finding an object within a visually cluttered space, lack of ability to simultaneously look straight at an object and reach for it, and significant reduction of vision as a result of glare from windows or lights.

## Preparation for the Observation

After a review of the educational records, an observation of classroom organization skills was conducted. Given the prior comments about poor organization and the possible effects of CVI on his vision, the assessor was looking for evidence that vision might be interfering with Dominic's ability to locate classroom materials in a timely manner. The assessor was looking at the type of systems already in place to make the organizational process easier for Dominic, and for any potential visual distractions or limitations such as too much glare in the environment, a less than optimal seating arrangement, visual clutter, and his proximity to necessary information.

## Observation in the Classroom

**Dominic walked into the classroom and put his** backpack on top of his desk. He reached in, and, without looking, pulled out his lunchbox. He took it over to the yellow bin marked with his room number and dropped it in. He returned to his desk and proceeded to glance into his backpack for his homework. Unable to see into it, he looked away and reached in to try and find the loose papers. Quickly giving up, he walked up to his teacher and said that he couldn't find his homework. Another student was asked to look in Dominic's backpack to help him; the student looked into the backpack and pulled out some crumpled papers from the bottom. He handed them to Dominic, who walked over to the homework tray and quickly tossed them in. Leaving his backpack unzipped, Dominic carried it to his locker and shoved it into the bottom along with his jacket. He closed the locker door and returned to his desk.

Once everyone was settled, the teacher asked the students to take out their daily journals and copy the sentences from the board as they were written, then rewrite them with corrections for spelling and grammar. Dominic opened the top of his desk to look for his black felt-tip marking pen. Inside his desk were loose colored pencils, three number 2 pencils, colored markers, two black medium-tip markers, two purple glue sticks, a multicolored fuzzy rubber ball, several pencil erasers, last week's corrected spelling test, a dome magnifier in a black cloth bag, and a monocular telescope in a green plastic casing. Dominic quickly scanned the contents, looked up to the lights in the ceiling, and reached in for the black marker. He pulled something out, held it up close to his eyes, and saw that it was a red marker. He threw it back into his desk, quickly scanned the contents again, looked once more up to the lights and reached in for the black marker. This time he was successful. Closing his desktop, he placed the marker on top of his desk and got out of his seat to look for the journal in the built-in shelf underneath his seat. Inside the dark storage space under his desk were papers in disorder, some gray folders with black printed labels, three black-lined notebooks with black covers, library books, and art projects to take home. By the time he found what he was looking for and walked up to the board at the front of the classroom to copy the sentences, more than half the class had finished the corrections and were preparing for the next assignment.

Dominic needed to position himself to one side of the print on the whiteboard to minimize the glare from the sun shining in from the side windows. The words on the board were written with a blue marker in cursive writing and close together. Dominic was starting to feel rushed and frustrated as he tried to copy words and spell them correctly.

Counter space in the classroom was minimal. Dominic did not have enough room in his desk for the oversized large-print textbooks. His teacher had made room for him to store his books on the counter under a window, between the current science projects, on the opposite side of the room from his desk. When it was time to retrieve a book, he walked to the counter and, shielding his eyes from the glare of the window with one hand, searched through the disorganized stacks of books, 20 in all, to find the one he needed. By the time Dominic found and carried the large book to his desk, the rest of the class had already started to read the assignment.

Figure 16.3 provides an example of the types of notes the assessor might have recorded—using a form for observational assessment of independent living skills—after this observation of Dominic in the natural environment of his classroom. In recording such observations, it is important to keep in mind the effects of CVI when looking at a list of skills appropriate for a fifth-grade student. The recommendations for intervention provided on the form are discussed later in the chapter.

## Home-Related Functional Skills Assessment

### *Preparation for the Observation*

During an interview, Dominic's parents shared that at home he had challenges organizing his room, in particular, his clothing and shoes. Dominic was interested in and enjoyed being involved in food preparation with his parents, but had difficulty keeping track of the tools he needed and staying on task without distraction. The following describes information obtained during observation of Dominic's personal and home management skills.

### *Observation at Home in the Kitchen*

**UPON ARRIVING AT HOME, DOMINIC QUICKLY TOOK OFF HIS** backpack, jacket, and shoes near the front door and dropped them on the floor. He walked straight to the kitchen to look for a snack. Opening the refrigerator, he faced a visual jumble of jars and plastic bins. Unable to immediately see his favorite smoothie drink, which was located behind a large jar of pickles, he closed the refrigerator and opened the cupboard door, pulling out a bright blue and red packet of cookies. After finishing several cookies, Dominic went to his room and lay on his bed listening to his iPod with his eyes closed.

After a short rest, his mother came into the room and asked if he would help with dinner preparation. Dominic appeared animated and happy to help in the kitchen. A plain, pre-prepared pizza crust was on the kitchen island. His mother left the kitchen to answer a phone call, so he went to the cupboard and looked for a jar of pizza sauce. He became frustrated with the dark interior of the cupboard and the crowded shelves and decided to go to the refrigerator to get out the cheese instead. Since the clear bag of white shredded cheese was in a drawer on top of a red package of bacon, he found it quickly and set it on the counter next to the refrigerator. He then looked for the package of pepperoni. The pepperoni was located under the package of bacon, and, since both packages were similar in color, he did not see it. He started pulling items out of the refrigerator to find the pepperoni, when he located the smoothie he had searched for earlier. By the time he found the pepperoni, many jars and packages were piled on the counter next to the refrigerator. He tried to hurriedly put everything back into the refrigerator before his mother returned, but it was disorderly and did not all fit. When Dominic went to find the white cheese that he had placed on the white countertop, it seemed to have disappeared, causing him additional frustration.

During the preparation of the pizza, Dominic placed ingredients and utensils down randomly and forgot where he put them. He left trash on the counter instead of placing it in the trash bin, knocked over a clear glass of water as he reached for the pizza sauce, and generally appeared clumsy and disorganized.

Figure 16.4 presents an example of one way to record information gathered in observing the scene just described. Careful attention is given to the effects of CVI on accomplishing the task.

FIGURE 16.3

## Record Form for Observational Assessment of Independent Living Skills: Personal Management

### Observation of Independent Living Skills

**Student's Name:** Dominic **Date:** February 16, 2015

**Observer's Name:** Jodi Cameron **Environment:** Classroom

| Personal Management Skill: Organization | Task | Effects of Visual Impairment/ CVI | Functional Observation | Suggested Intervention Approaches | Outcomes of Intervention Hypotheses and Revisions |
|---|---|---|---|---|---|
| Locating personal belongings | Taking homework papers out of backpack | Difficulty looking at a specific object and reaching for it; object had low to no contrast against background | Dominic was unable to locate loose homework papers in his backpack and asked for assistance | Place homework papers in a bright yellow folder, and place folder in a separate zippered section of backpack | Initial visual location of yellow folder in single section and ability to remove folder without vision, using touch |
| Desk organization | Locating black felt-tip pen | Difficulty with visual perception in a crowded environment; looking away when reaching for a specific object | It took two tries for Dominic to visually locate the pen, look away, and grasp the intended object | Organize the inside of Dominic's desk with small, separate colored containers for specific objects; place two or more black felt-tip markers in one narrow orange pencil basket in the lower right corner of his desk | Pencil basket often tipped over, spilling the contents; small clear zippered bag replaced the basket, keeping the contents together |
| Desk cubby organization | Locating class materials | Inefficient organization; use of color and lighting to locate classroom materials | It took extra time, and Dominic exhibited frustration in locating one journal | Provide notebooks of different bright colors for each subject, colored or patterned folders for each subject matter to hold papers to keep or take home, and a small LED flashlight to use when looking in the storage area under his chair | Dominic needed daily reminders to place papers in the appropriate folders, but the notebooks were more easily accessible, helping him complete class projects in a more timely manner |

FIGURE 16.4

## Record Form for Observational Assessment of Independent Living Skills: Home Management

### Observation of Independent Living Skills

**Student's Name:** Dominic **Date:** February 18, 2015

**Observer's Name:** Jodi Cameron **Environment:** Home

| Home Management Skill: Food Management | Task | Effects of Visual Impairment/ CVI | Functional Observation | Suggested Intervention Approaches | Outcomes of Intervention Hypotheses and Revisions |
|---|---|---|---|---|---|
| Locate snack | Find desired beverage in refrigerator | Difficulty with visually crowded area | Dominic could not see the drink he wanted | Specify the location in the refrigerator for beverages | Requires buy-in from other family members, who will all have to put the drink in the same location |
| Prepare pizza | Locate ingredients | Lack of color contrast between cheese and the counter | "Lost" the cheese on the counter | Use a tray to define the workspace and possibly contrast with the ingredients | |
| Maintain organization | Keep utensils within reach | When utensils are placed in random places, they can become visually "lost" in the clutter | Dominic set down utensils and forgot where he put them | Use a nonskid rubber mat of a bright color or a narrow low bin to hold all utensils during food preparation | Utensils that are always placed in the same location are easy to find, making food preparation more enjoyable |
| Clean up | Throw trash away | Pieces of trash left on the counter add to clutter, making it more difficult to find needed tools and ingredients | Trash was left on the counter | Place a small trash container with a bright rim or lid within easy reach of the food preparation area | Reducing unnecessary clutter on the counter improves visually locating needed items |

### *Observation of Personal Organization at Home*

**Dominic went to his room to get his backpack to do** his homework. His backpack was not in its usual location. When he asked his mother where his backpack might be, she suggested he look by the front door. He found it under his jacket and took it to the kitchen table, leaving his jacket and shoes on the floor. He removed his assignment book and tried to read what he had written down for homework. Finding it difficult, he took the book over to a table lamp for better lighting and turned it sideways to read it. With the television on in the family room and his parents talking about their day, he had difficulty focusing on his assignment and quickly filled in his worksheet without much thought. He looked in his backpack for the gray homework folder but did not see it, so he put the paper loose in his backpack.

### *Performance Assessment: Pizza*

After careful examination of the challenges noted during an observation, such as Dominic's pizza preparation, a performance assessment can be set up at school or in the home, depending on availability. Based on observations of Dominic in the kitchen and taking into consideration his CVI, the following elements were deliberately assembled to evaluate what accommodations would enhance his visual functioning:

- Uncluttered, clean, flat surface
- Adequate overhead natural lighting
- A large tray with a small upturned edge to contain spills, set on top of a slip-resistant mat
- Pizza crust and pizza sauce located toward the front of the pantry shelf, with a "stick-up" light above the shelf and a small LED flashlight within easy reach
- The refrigerated ingredients organized on one shelf within easy reach
- A separate bin that could be removed from the cupboard and set next to the preparation area containing red-handled scissors, a bright orange ladle-style spoon, and a yellow pizza cutting wheel
- Two or three colorful flat plastic cutting sheets on the countertop on which to set ingredients and to provide high contrast
- Five-fingered ovenproof gloves set by the oven
- Small open container on the counter for collecting food waste or trash
- Sequential steps for constructing the pizza printed in large black print on a yellow card with nonglare plastic protection
- Large-print timer

**Once the food preparation area was set up, Dominic** familiarized himself with the equipment and organization of the workspace, offering suggestions about placement of the materials. The assessor used a checklist to easily record the effectiveness of the adaptations put into practice. Dominic stated that he did not need the card with the sequential steps printed on it for making pizza, but set it next to the workspace anyway. Dominic's enthusiasm for cooking was evident when he began searching for the ingredients he needed to make the pizza. He enjoyed using the small flashlight to spot cans and jars in the cupboard, and found the pizza sauce right away. After placing the sauce on the counter to the left of the large pan, he went to the refrigerator for the cheese. He was happy to find the cheese and pepperoni together in the front of the shelf. He chose to place the white cheese on a red mat and the pepperoni on a blue mat. He found locating the scissors in the bin to open the packages easy, and after he finished using them, he placed the scissors back into the bin. After opening the jar of sauce, he liked using the ladle-style spoon to scoop out the sauce and pour it onto the pizza crust. He asked what he should put on next, and the assessor referred him to the instruction card. After reading the card, he found the grated cheese, opened it with the scissors, and sprinkled it on the pizza crust with his fingers. The assessor noted that Dominic had missed the very top section of the pizza crust. He then opened the pepperoni and placed the pepperoni randomly on the crust. Again, he missed the same top section of the pizza crust. After sliding the pizza onto the baking pan, he put on the ovenproof gloves and carefully placed the pizza pan onto the oven shelf. He asked how long it should bake and was again referred back to the instruction sheet. He set the large-print timer for 20 minutes.

During the assessment, the assessor took notes on the effectiveness and usefulness of the adaptations for Dominic. In addition, notes were taken on his level of frustration and the amount of time it took him to complete each step. Later, the details recorded on the checklist were used to formulate comprehensive results.

## Use of Assessment Results

Results from all facets of the assessment are compiled to obtain an overall picture of the student. This overview of the results creates a basis for composing overarching recommendations to help the student make accommodations for the effects of CVI.

Once the overview of results is compiled, specific recommendations within each skill area are developed. Educational specialists use this information when formulating individual goals for the student as part of the educational program plan. The following examples show recommendations provided for Dominic.

### Overview of Skills

Dominic struggled to maintain organization of his personal items at home, at school, and while preparing food. Because of the nature of his visual impairment, color, optimal lighting, and contrast are important factors to maximize his visual function.

#### *Recommendations for Organization*

- Set up an organizational system for school paperwork with Dominic. Involve him in the process to ensure that the system makes sense to him and to provide the expectation that he take ownership of his belongings.
- Use brightly colored folders for school to divide paperwork. Encourage him to choose the colors and create labels for each folder.
- To maintain the newly developed colored folder system, provide guided maintenance at regular intervals (possibly once a week at first). Teach Dominic to maintain this new system and create an accountability chart.
- Place a small flashlight in Dominic's desk, and attach a flashlight key chain to his backpack to allow him to visually search for items in those dark spaces.
- At home, establish a bin or basket for his shoes.
- Collaboration between home and school will be required to help Dominic maintain organizational skills.

#### *Recommendations for Cooking*

- Provide a dark tray or mat for the kitchen counter that can be used to visually define the workspace against the light counter.
- Mount lights under the cabinets to improve illumination of the workspace.
- Establish a shelf in the refrigerator for Dominic to keep his snacks.
- Group ingredients required for his planned cooking activities in a box or tray within the refrigerator so that ingredients can be located quickly and with minimal frustration.

- Provide a set of bright, multicolored measuring cups.
- Encourage the use of a small trash bag or bowl on the counter that can be used throughout the cooking process so that Dominic does not scatter trash on the counter. Keep the workspace clear of clutter to help minimize frustration.

## Conclusion

Assessment of independent living skills for students with CVI requires careful planning, with consideration of the effects of CVI on specific skills. Many functional skills, such as dressing, occur with greater frequency in the home environment. Assessment within the home and at school is optimal. Interviews with parents, caregivers, and teachers are essential for documenting baseline information. Combining information from interviews with results from observations within the natural environment provides the basis for establishing a student's baseline performance in functional independent living skills.

Taking into consideration a student's strengths and weaknesses, performance assessments can be designed to establish the effects of adaptations and subsequent modifications on a student's level of proficiency for specific independent living skills. As a result of the unique needs of a student with CVI, all recommended interventions must be highly individualized for each student. Based on the student's baseline information and the results of the performance assessment, realistic goals can be written and implemented as part of the student's Individualized Education Program plan, with measurable intervals to chart the student's progress.

## Assessments for Independent Living Skills

### Formal Assessments

Formal assessments are typically administered by a psychologist in collaboration with a teacher of students with visual impairments regarding accessibility.

Bruininks, R. H., Woodcock, R. W., Weatherman, R. F., & Hill, B. K. (1996). *Scales of Independent Behavior–Revised (SIB-R).* Rolling Meadows, IL: Riverside Publishing.

Harrison, P., & Oakland, T. (2003). *Adaptive Behavior Assessment System (ABAS-II)* (2nd ed.). San Antonio, TX: PsychCorp.

Sparrow, S. S., Cicchetti, D. V., & Balla, D. A. (2005). *Vineland adaptive behavior scales* (2nd ed.). San Antonio, TX: PsychCorp.

### Informal Assessments

Anderson, S., Boignon, S., Davis, K., & deWaard, C. (2007). *Oregon Project for visually impaired and blind preschool children* (6th ed.). Medford: Southern Oregon Education Service District.

Kelley, P., & Smith, P. (2000). Evaluation of independent living skills for a student with a visual impairment. In A. J. Koenig & M. C. Holbrook (Eds.), *Foundations of education: Vol. II. Instructional strategies for teaching children and youths with visual impairments* (2nd ed., pp. 594–609). New York: AFB Press.

Loumiet, R., & Levack, N. (1993). *Independent living skills: A curriculum with adaptations for students with visual impairments.* Austin: Texas School for the Blind and Visually Impaired.

## References

Allman, C. B., & Lewis, S. (Eds.). (2014). *ECC essentials: Teaching the expanded core curriculum to students with visual impairments.* New York: AFB Press.

Hatlen, P. (1996). The core curriculum for blind and visually impaired students, including those with additional disabilities. *RE:view, 28*(1), 25–32.

Hatlen, P. (2003, December). *Impact of literacy on the expanded core curriculum*. Paper presented at the Getting in Touch with Literacy Conference, Vancouver, BC.

Kelley, P., & Smith, P. (2000). Independent living skills. In A. J. Koenig & M. C. Holbrook (Eds.), *Foundations of education: Vol. II. Instructional strategies for teaching children and youths with visual impairments* (2nd ed., pp. 569–615). New York: AFB Press.

Sapp, W., & Hatlen, P. (2010). The expanded core curriculum: Where we have been, where we are going, and how we can get there. *Journal of Visual Impairment & Blindness, 104*(6), 338–348.

# 17

# Assessments Linked to Interventions: Orientation and Mobility

*Marion Felder and Darick Wright*

Being able to orient oneself and move safely and efficiently through the environment is an essential part of independence for an individual, as well as for inclusion in school, the community, and society. To get from a point of origin to a destination, a person must have orientation and mobility (O&M) skills adequate for the mastery of the route and its reversal. This ability requires coordination of both ocular, oculomotor, and other brain functions and, therefore, may be affected in children who have cerebral visual impairment (CVI).

To understand the implications of CVI on O&M, it is necessary to describe some of the foundations for successful O&M in children whose visual impairments are caused primarily by a sensory-based visual field or visual acuity impairment. It is also necessary to provide understanding of the roles of O&M specialists, the goals of O&M training, and current assessment tools in order to give insight into O&M instruction for children with CVI.

## Role of the O&M Specialist

The ultimate goal of O&M training is to enable the individual to become as independent as possible when navigating through various environments. Equally important, however, is the understanding of the characteristics of the environment that have a direct impact on safe, efficient, and independent travel such as contrast, the visual and sensory complexity of pattern and clutter, and the organization of the environment.

Ideally, O&M training and environmental adaptations in a child's environment are provided by certified O&M specialists who are trained to teach children and adults with various degrees of visual, physical, and cognitive abilities. They provide direct instruction in O&M to the child and also consult with the child's educational team (teacher of students with visual impairments, classroom teacher, parents, and other related service providers) and eye care providers (optometrists, ophthalmologists, and orthoptists). It is essential that skills taught in a lesson are also carried out by other team members, such as the child's classroom teacher, the teacher of students with visual impairments, teaching assistants, and parents. There are also circumstances when an O&M instructor is not available or is only available on a consultative basis. In some countries, the roles of service providers may differ, and the role occupied by an O&M specialist may be filled by a teacher of students with visual impairments or other professionals. It is crucial, however, that the child receives structured assessment and intervention by a trained professional if the goal is safe and independent travel for the child. The authors feel strongly that there needs to be a highly trained and qualified person responsible for the child's O&M needs on the child's educational team.

## Basic Principles and Goals of O&M Instruction

For sighted individuals, visual perception plays a crucial role in orienting and moving through space. Objects, places, streets, and signs can be visually identified, organized, and used as landmarks for orientation. Cognitive processes such as attention, memory, perception, and decision-making skills are fundamental for orientation (Iaria & Barton, 2010). To navigate through space safely and efficiently, an individual needs to be able to gather and process sensory information in order to identify objects and to determine his or her own position in space and in relation to surrounding objects. Some environments are more complex than others, and the level of skill required to manage an environment varies accordingly. The sighted traveler with intact visual-motor control uses efficient visually guided movements to update his or her position in space and in relation to objects in it, employing continuous, coordinated, and automatic eye movements. Furthermore, selective visual attention determines the size of the area that is seen. A traveler needs to have an overview of both the environment (global visual attention) and specific landmarks within it (local visual attention). The seemingly simple task of crossing a room to get a book off a shelf is in fact a highly complex task, requiring many different areas of the brain to work together.

A blind or visually impaired traveler who has a visual acuity or visual field impairment with additional perceptual and cognitive impairment may be unable to use visual information or may not be able to rely on visual information alone. Thus, visual information needs to be substituted or supported by other sensory information—for example, sound, touch, knowledge of body movement (kinesthesia), and smell—so that these travelers can learn to orient themselves and move through space independently.

Children who are blind or visually impaired usually compensate for the lack of vision by learning a cluster of skills, described as the five-point travel system (Jacobson, 2013) to stay oriented in an environment. This travel system includes the use of route patterns or shapes, landmarks and cues (auditory, kinesthetic, tactile, and olfactory), compass directions, names of hallways and streets, and the application of these points on the reversal of the route (Jacobson, 2013). In addition to those skills, children with functional vision learn how to use their vision in a systematic manner (by fixating, tracking, and scanning, for example) to locate and identify landmarks and to use assistive technology (including optical and electronic devices).

Use of these complex cognitive, motor, and visual skills requires specialized instruction, practice, and motivation. Children who are blind or visually impaired must be able to access salient sensory information in a systematic manner (to differentiate between pertinent landmarks and other less significant objects or to determine the direction of a sound, for example) and to process the information and make decisions based on current information and past experiences and knowledge. Organizing incoming sensory information by forming a "mental map" of a route or area facilitates independent and efficient orientation.

In the absence of sufficient visual information, individuals may also use a long cane, a dog guide, or a human guide (a person assisting the visually impaired or blind traveler) to detect landmarks and avoid obstacles, such as stairs, curbs, drop-offs, and the like. These tools involve varying degrees of motor control and accuracy—for example, holding the cane and walking in a straight line, keeping the cane at a certain height, maintaining an appropriate cane arc width for safety, maintaining grasp of a sighted guide's arm, or holding on to the harness of a dog guide.

In summary, it can be said that to move safely and efficiently through an environment, a complex set of skills is necessary. When an individual is blind or visually impaired, systematic training is necessary to teach compensatory skills in addition to improving the individual's ability to use available vision. Even though skills may be taught in isolation at first, such as practicing how to walk with a cane, eventually that skill has to be integrated with other skills, such as maintaining orientation in a specific environment.

## Aspects of CVI That Affect O&M

CVI poses significant problems related to O&M. It may affect visual attention, visual memory, visual perception, oculomotor control, orientation to the environment, and the ability to move safely and efficiently (McKillop & Dutton, 2008; see also Chapter 3). As is described elsewhere in the literature (Dutton, 2003) and this book, CVI may also cause an individual to have inaccurate reach and grasp, problems in the estimation of depth, variations in functional visual field, difficulties identifying moving targets or only being able to see stationary objects, difficulties moving through space, difficulties seeing boundaries on the floor, difficulties negotiating curbs and stairs, and motor planning problems. In addition, visuospatial attention may be disrupted in children with damage to the parietal lobes and inferior and middle frontal lobes (Smith & Chatterjee, 2008; see also Chapter 6). This may result in an inability to attend to objects and people in a given space and may affect the ability to travel safely around them.

Dorsal stream dysfunction (see Chapter 3) can interfere with O&M by impairing visual guidance of movement and causing impaired perception in crowded scenes at a subconscious level (McKillop & Dutton, 2008). Children with dorsal stream dysfunction may have difficulties visually attending in visually complex or crowded environments. If visual attention is impaired, independent travel in the school or community environment may be difficult, and safety concerns may arise. In addition, children may bump into other people or objects since movements under visual control are impaired. This issue may be particularly challenging in children with cerebral palsy as it can be difficult to assess the cause of the difficulties.

Ventral steam dysfunction (see Chapter 3), on the other hand, is rarer and causes impaired object and person recognition and impaired orientation in surrounding and extended space (topographic agnosia) (McKillop & Dutton, 2008; see also Chapter 3). Akinetopsia is a very rare disorder, causing an inability to see moving objects. However, impaired perception of movement (dyskinetopsia) or slow overall visual and mental processing are not uncommon, resulting in failure to see rapidly moving targets, such as automobiles, until they slow down. A reduced ability to process multisensory information and to direct visual attention, as well as a reduced ability to estimate the speed of moving objects contribute to this problem. Children who exhibit these difficulties may be unsafe when crossing any hallway or street. They may also bump into people or be unable to catch a ball on a playground (Zihl, von Cramon, & Mai, 1983).

All these functional impairments can have a significant impact on moving safely through the environment. A child may not be able to visually locate and track a moving vehicle while crossing a street. Reaching for a railing while navigating stairs and efficient integration of sensory information obtained through use of a long cane may be difficult. Stairs, drop-offs, and curbs may be particularly challenging since the automatic estimation of depth to guide movement, which comes so naturally to most people, can be impaired. Moving through an unfamiliar room may be frightening and unsafe, particularly when the environment is visually complex. Since eye movements (specifically visual pursuit movements) may be impaired, an individual may not be able to visually follow a moving object or person, such as a teacher or classmate.

Hemispatial neglect (or inattention) can sometimes coexist with CVI. This is a complex disorder with many different facets and symptoms (Chokron et al., 2002; Farnè, Ponti, & Làdavas, 1998; see also Chapter 6). For the purpose of O&M, neglect can be described as inattention to the field that is contralateral (opposite) to the side where the brain injury occurred (Trauner, 2003). Only rotation of the body will bring neglected items to attention. Thus, unlike hemianopia, visual neglect cannot be compensated for by head or eye movement. It is quite common and often intractable in adults after a stroke (Marsh et al., 2009). Hemispatial neglect can have a devastating impact on a person's O&M abilities, since half of the body, a room, or an object may be neglected (not attended to) and its existence sometimes simply denied. This can lead to bumping into walls, objects, and people. In terms of route completion, a person may get lost on a simple I-shaped route (straight line). Hemispatial neglect of variable degree does occur in children, though research on the topic is scarce (Marsh et al., 2009; Trauner, 2003). It may also not be as long-lasting as in adults after brain damage (Marotta, McKeeff, & Behrmann, 2003; Marsh & Hillis, 2008; Marsh et al., 2009), perhaps as a result of greater neuroplasticity in childhood.

If other parts of the brain that facilitate orientation are also damaged, a person can get lost in the environment, even on a simple route. Topographic disorientation (disorientation in the environment) is an impairment that is seen as a result of ventral stream damage (Milner & Goodale, 2006). In addition, there are various types of visual problems related to the inability to identify objects, pictures, and scenes. Children may not be able to identify single objects or more than one object at a time. They may perceive certain elements of a visuospatial layout, but not the whole scene. The inability to recognize objects or the overall layout of a room or hallway can lead to significant disorientation.

Formalization of O&M instructional strategies for individuals with CVI is only now beginning to develop. More work is needed to develop strong research-based methods of instruction. In the meantime, the following are some ideas that the O&M specialist many find useful in working with students with CVI.

- Educate the staff of educational agencies, such as schools and early intervention programs, about children with CVI and their associated O&M problems. It is critical to promote an understanding of the behavioral hallmarks of CVI and the fact that CVI is a brain-based problem.
- Employ a structured history-taking approach (Dutton, 2003). This may help identify some core O&M problems in children with CVI. The interview process, normally part of a typical educational assessment protocol, should always include questions about the child's learning style, strengths and weaknesses, and interests and motivation. (See Chapter 11 for more on structured history taking.)
- Use of alternative language-based approaches such as poetry and song to remember the sequence of specific routes (see, for example, Fazzi & Petersmeyer, 2001) can prove very effective for children with CVI who have profound difficulty with orientation (topographic agnosia).
- Objects and pictures can give valuable cues for initial orientation and for maintaining orientation on a route.
- A team approach to assessment and instruction is important. Collaborate with the student's physical or occupational therapist to differentiate whether the problems result from lack of physical coordination or lack of vision.

## O&M Assessment for Children with CVI

O&M specialists follow a number of steps when assessing a child with a visual impairment. Given the complexity and variety of ways CVI can manifest itself with each individual, a thorough and specialized assessment must be conducted by the vision professional to develop appropriate goals and implement effective instructional plans. It is crucial to develop an O&M assessment battery that includes review of records, interviews with the student, teachers, and family members, and structured observation of the student's skills in real-life environments. Ideally, this assessment battery would include formal tools developed and used by other related professions.

### Referral Process

Children are usually referred to O&M specialists through their early intervention or school programs, low vision clinics, or medical or ophthalmological professionals. Most often the referral is based on an eye report stating that a visual field or visual acuity impairment is present. The process of referral for children with CVI can be more difficult and may not follow a protocol, as some of the children may not have any visual field or visual acuity problems, despite profound visual difficulties. Teachers, parents, and perhaps even ophthalmologists may attribute the problems the children exhibit while moving through space to overall cognitive functioning, behavioral problems, and lack of motivation or even to general "clumsiness," not to lack of vision. The awareness that these problems may be attributable to vision problems needs to be raised through a variety of initiatives, such as working with ophthalmologists, neurologists, general education teachers, school administrators, and others who are responsible for referring students.

## Record Review

An important aspect of O&M assessment is the review of the child's records. The relevant records may include reports, assessments, and evaluations from other related service providers: medical and ophthalmological reports, educational reports, as well as reports by occupational therapists, physical therapists, and others working with the child. Record review is also important to obtain the child's ophthalmological status and to clarify whether the child has additional ocular visual impairments that may contribute to the lack of vision. Visual acuity and visual field information contained in an eye report are critical pieces of information for developing an instructional plan. In addition, reviewing records can also provide insight into the child's receptive and expressive language and communication abilities, interests, strengths, and weaknesses.

One discipline often overlooked as a part of record review for O&M is neuropsychology. The integration of information from a qualified neuropsychologist into an education plan and advocacy for a comprehensive neuropsychological assessment can yield critical pieces of information for the O&M specialist in the areas of attention, motor planning, self-regulation, problem-solving ability, and visual perceptual weaknesses. Since children with CVI may have complex disorders and needs, it is imperative that educational professionals work together with neurologists, neuropsychologists, and other professionals to provide the best service for the child.

Sometimes children have conditions such as seizure disorders, the risk of which needs to be considered in planning O&M instruction. Some children have movement disorders that may mask the visual impairment, or vice versa. All team members need to know about the impact medications have on a child's ability to move safely and independently through an environment. Children with brain damage may have additional problems, such as impulse control, attentional issues, and, sometimes, behavioral problems that contribute significantly to the child's ability to travel. The child may also experience impaired short-term or long-term memory and may have limited comprehension for language. A state-of-the-art neuropsychological evaluation conducted by a qualified clinician can often contribute to knowledge about a child's learning style, verbal and visual strengths and weaknesses, as well as the design of optimal teaching strategies. (See Chapter 13 for additional discussion of neuropsychological assessment.)

## Interviews with Caregivers, Teachers, and the Child

Interviewing caregivers and teachers about the child's problems may be either the first or second step after the child has been referred for services by an O&M specialist. Often, the interview process begins as records are still being obtained. The child should also be included in the interview process as much as possible, as the child is the one experiencing the difficulties. It is therefore crucial that the O&M specialist is able to communicate with the child in the mode used by the child. Care also has to be taken to ask questions that are appropriate to the child's developmental level.

O&M specialists usually use structured intake questions (Pogrund et al., 2012), but they may also develop their own questions. For students with CVI, a structured history-taking approach (Dutton, 2006) may also be applied to solicit more information about the child's problems (see Chapter 11). The interview process should conclude with some goals that a teacher, parent, or child may want to accomplish as the outcome of O&M training (for example, finding the bathroom in the school building or crossing a street in the neighborhood).

### Structured Observation of the Child through an Observation Protocol

As a next step, the O&M specialist usually observes the child in his or her natural environment. The specialist should see the child at home and at school. Sometimes perspectives of parents and teachers are different, based on the different relationship they have with the child. It is therefore important to observe the child in both environments. (See Chapter 14 for additional discussion of observational assessment.) O&M specialists need to get a holistic view of the child in various environments and assess him or her in multiple environments. Current observation screening tools examine O&M skills for children who have visual impairments in general (see Pogrund et al., 2012). Sidebar 17.1 provides an observation protocol that may be used specifically to observe a student with CVI in a more structured way.

SIDEBAR 17.1

## O&M Observation Protocol for Students with CVI

1. **How does the child move in the most familiar environment (home)?**
   - **a.** Does the child find all rooms and areas in a familiar environment such as the home?
   - **b.** Does the child move through a visually complex home environment independently and with consistency?
   - **c.** Is the child able to ascend and descend stairs without problems?
   - **d.** Can the child identify common objects from around the house?
   - **e.** Can the child identify objects that are motivating to him or her?
   - **f.** Can the child identify colors, shapes, and pictures?
   - **g.** Is the child able to find pertinent objects in his or her own bedroom?
   - **h.** Is the child able to find pertinent objects in other places of the house?
   - **i.** Is the child able to find highly motivating objects in his or her room or house?
   - **j.** Can the child describe, in his or her communication mode, where rooms and objects are located in the house?
   - **k.** Can the child draw a picture or map of his or her room?

*(continued on next page)*

- **l.** Does the child hesitate or become overly cautious at door thresholds and flooring changes?

**2. How does the child move in less familiar places (school)?**

- **a.** Does the child travel to and from important places or areas at school (such as the bathroom, cafeteria, or classroom) at a similar pace to his or her peers?
- **b.** Does the child move independently through classrooms, hallways, elevators, the school campus?
- **c.** Can the child visually locate objects in his or her path and navigate around them without contact?
- **d.** Does the child inadvertently contact objects on one side or the other?
- **e.** Is the child able to ascend and descend stairs in the building without difficulty?
- **f.** Can the child identify pertinent objects/landmarks in classrooms, hallways, and throughout the building?
- **g.** Can the child locate specific areas in the classroom?
- **h.** Can the child locate his or her own seat in the classroom?
- **i.** Does the child ever hesitate or become overly cautious at door thresholds and flooring changes?
- **j.** Does the child move through classroom space with ease? Describe any awkward or atypical behavior regarding navigation through space.
- **k.** Does the child bump into things or peers?
- **l.** Does the child visually attend to pertinent activities even if the environment is complex (visually or auditorily)?
- **m.** How much time does it take for the child to move through space during activities or to locate objects as compared to peers? (This may be a question for the child's teachers.)

**3. How does the child move in the community environment?**

- **a.** Does the child find and get to and from relevant places in the neighborhood, such as a neighbor's or friend's house?
- **b.** Does the child move through the outdoors with ease (thinks about curbs and uneven pavement)?
- **c.** Is the child able to recognize certain routes when driving in the car with an adult? (Does the child anticipate the destination? Does the child recognize pertinent landmarks on the way?)
- **d.** Does the child find his or her way around in a small store/convenience store?
- **e.** Is the child able to find certain objects in a small store/convenience store?
- **f.** Does the child independently find his or her way in a busy supermarket?
- **g.** Can the child reverse a familiar route inside a store to locate the entrance/exit?
- **h.** Is the child able to find a certain object in a busy supermarket?
- **i.** Could the child draw a map of the store?
- **j.** Does the child appear to "get lost" in the community even though the route seems simple? Please describe.
- **k.** Does the child visually attend to pertinent activities, objects, landmarks, or traffic in the community environment even in the presence of visual and auditory distractions?
- **l.** Does the child bump into people or objects when traveling?
- **m.** Does the child show signs of dependency when traveling with others?
- **n.** Does the child remain oriented in familiar and unfamiliar community environments?
- **o.** Is the child able to use and interpret information from a map or diagram efficiently?

## Formal O&M Assessments for Students with CVI

Even though originally developed for students with traditional visual impairments (visual field and visual acuity impairments), some of the currently used O&M assessments contain items that can also be used for students with cerebral visual impairments. Table 17.1 provides a list of some tests developed for children with visual impairments that are applicable for children with CVI.

*TAPS (Teaching Age-Appropriate and Purposeful Skills)* (Pogrund et al., 2012) is a checklist that is widely used by O&M specialists. It includes some visual perceptual items such as body planes, body awareness, body in space, geometric shape, and basic spatial awareness, which are all prerequisites for successful orientation. The *Hill Performance Test of Selected Positional Concepts* (Hill, 1981) specifically tests spatial and positional concepts and is standardized. However, it relies heavily on receptive understanding (verbal directions) of the test items. Aspects of Roman-Lantzy's CVI Orientation and Mobility Resolution Chart (Roman-Lantzy, 2007, pp. 206–208; 2010) may also be used to assess a child's ability to respond to moving or stationary targets, colors, and processing time of visual information. It may yield valuable information about how a child responds and attends to certain stimuli in the environment. There are also subtests on the Oregon Project Curriculum and Skills Inventory (part of the *Oregon Project for Preschool Children Who Are Blind or Visually Impaired* [Anderson, Boigon, Davis, & deWaard, 2007]) that include items such as visual recognition and visual motor perception and pre-mobility tasks. The *Barraga Visual Efficiency Program* (Smith, in press) includes a test battery and full program to teach visual perceptual skills to children with a visual impairment. All these tests or assessments were developed for children with low vision.

TABLE 17.1

**O&M Assessment Tools and Their Applicability to Students with CVI**

| *Name of Test/Assessment and Description* | *Assessment Items Included* | *Applicability for CVI* |
|---|---|---|
| *TAPS: Teaching Age-Appropriate and Purposeful Skills: An Orientation & Mobility Curriculum for Students with Visual Impairments* (Pogrund et al., 2012)<br>Age group: 0–22 years<br>Designed for children and adults with visual impairments and blindness | Orientation and mobility at home, at school, and in the community<br>General attention<br>Auditory abilities<br>Receptive and expressive language<br>Posture and gait<br>Body awareness<br>Directionality<br>Laterality<br>Color and shape concepts<br>Spatial awareness<br>Recognition of landmarks and clues | All components can be used with children with CVI<br>Good tool to assess concepts the child has about him- or herself and the environment<br>Assesses posture and gait, body awareness, directionality, laterality, color and shape concepts, spatial awareness, recognition of landmarks, and cues and clues<br>Offers goals and objectives<br>Offers structured teaching and ongoing assessment in compensatory methods such as trailing with the hand and use of long cane |

*(continued on next page)*

**TABLE 17.1** *(continued from previous page)*

| ***Name of Test/Assessment and Description*** | ***Assessment Items Included*** | ***Applicability for CVI*** |
|---|---|---|
| *Hill Performance Test of Selected Positional Concepts* (Hill, 1981)<br>Age group: 6–10 years<br>Designed for children with visual impairments | Object-object relationships<br>Body awareness<br>Position of body in space and in relation to object<br>Knowledge about spatial concepts | All components can be used with children with CVI if they have the ability to follow verbal directions<br>Assesses body awareness, object-object, and object-person relationships<br>Assesses body in space<br>Assesses spatial concepts |
| The Oregon Project Curriculum and Skills Inventory, in the *Oregon Project for Preschool Children Who Are Blind or Visually Impaired,* Sixth Edition (Anderson, Boigon, Davis, & deWaard, 2007)<br>Age group: 0–6 years<br>Designed for preschool children with visual impairments | Pre-mobility and mobility skills<br>Ability to recognize pictures, colors, shapes, and objects<br>Communication skills | All components can be used with children with CVI<br>Assesses discrepancies in visual and other abilities<br>Assesses fine and gross motor skills, communication skills, cognitive skills, and visual skills such as recognition of pictures |
| CVI Orientation and Mobility Resolution Chart (Roman-Lantzy, 2007, 2010)<br>Age group: 0 and up<br>Designed for children with cortical visual impairment | Light responsiveness, color preferences, responsiveness to moving or stationary objects<br>Time to visually respond to stimuli<br>Reaching ability for visual stimuli | Can be used for children with CVI, particularly children with multiple disabilities<br>Assesses color preferences, which could be used to highlight landmarks<br>Assesses responsiveness to stationary and moving targets, which is important for O&M<br>Assesses ability of child to respond to visual information in the presence of auditory, tactile, and other competing visual stimuli |
| *Barraga Visual Efficiency Program: Evaluation* (Smith, in press)<br>Age group: cognitive developmental skills at or beyond level of 3-year-old<br>Designed for children with low vision | Visuospatial perception skills such as color, shape, size, internal detail, closure, figure-ground, visual memory, constancy, and part-whole relationships | Although not developed for children with CVI, some aspects of the assessment can be used for children with CVI if appropriate accommodations are in place<br>Assessment is conducted with objects, pictures, and graphic symbols<br>Assess visual perception and visual closure<br>Contains a Developmental Sequences Chart |

## O&M Interventions with Students with CVI

As mentioned earlier, a blind or visually impaired traveler may use nonvisual compensatory skills to navigate through the environment, such as using tactile or auditory landmarks and cues and clues to stay oriented while traveling. Brunsdon, Nickels, Coltheart, and Joy (2007) point out that investigation into topographical disorientation, or the inability to find one's way around environments in a normal manner, is rare in children and that there has been no known description of a treatment program for children.

To avoid obstacles, travelers who are blind or have low vision often use a long cane and other special techniques (such as sighted guide, trailing, and protective techniques) to move safely through the environment. If needed, children with low vision are systematically taught to fixate, track, and scan while moving through the environment. Other mobility strategies include environmental modifications such as keeping the environment obstacle free, highlighting pertinent areas with colored markers or tape (for example, on thresholds), and creating an environment free of visual and other distractions, particularly when visual attention to a task is required. Some of these strategies may also be useful for certain students with CVI.

The following case studies of three children with CVI highlight some of the critical issues surrounding O&M intervention.

### A Child with Ventral Stream Dysfunction

**CA**, A 6-YEAR-OLD CHILD WITH TOPOGRAPHICAL DISORIENTATION related to ventral stream dysfunction, was the subject of a detailed study by Brunsdon et al. (2007). CA was first assessed in detail, and then a systematic O&M training program was developed, involving identification of landmarks and relevant pictures. Her strong verbal skills were used to teach orientation systematically. Implementation of an instructional plan occurred after extensive neuropsychological testing and the development of two baseline measures of CA's ability to travel certain routes. The first baseline was conducted after the child was in school for three weeks, traveling the routes. Then a second baseline was conducted three weeks after that, to see if the child made progress just by being exposed to the route. Her scores on photo and landmark recognition and route finding were compared to those of a classmate. In all areas, CA exhibited significant problems as compared with a peer.

The instructional method consisted of various stages. In Stage 1, the team focused on teaching CA to recognize the school building and pertinent landmarks. They did this by taking photographs of the relevant sites and practicing identifying those photographs with her through drill and repetition (two exercises every day until she accomplished the task). In Stage 2, the target route was broken into small steps, such as (1) to red wall; (2) down stairs to tree; (3) to fourth tree. This verbal script was practiced in addition to walking the same route with CA. Each step in the sequence was kept as simple as possible. Data were collected over time, and the child's progress carefully evaluated.

Clear benefits from the training could be seen (Brunsdon et al., 2007). It was found that everyday exposure to the routes did not cause the progress the child made, as evidenced by comparison of the two baseline measures. Instead, systematic teaching, practice, and verbal scripting, in addition to walking the routes, appeared to make the difference. CA made progress in photo recognition and landmark training, route finding, total number of hesitations, and total amount of time needed to complete a route. The authors of the study state that CA was not only able to complete the taught routes but she also mastered them with greater efficiency.

### Child with Dorsal Stream Dysfunction

**CLARA IS A 12-YEAR-OLD GIRL WITH CEREBRAL VISUAL** impairment as a consequence of shaken baby syndrome at age 3 months. Despite extensive ophthalmological testing, her significant problems in recognizing pictures, faces, and particularly visual scenes cannot be explained by ocular visual impairment (pale optic nerves) alone. Her inability to navigate safely through the school environment seems particularly puzzling. MRI study has revealed bilateral occipito-parietal lobe damage.

Clara also has a diagnosis of cerebral palsy and uses a wheelchair to move around in her environment. She is beginning to propel the chair more independently. Clara is a verbal student, and language (receptive and expressive) is identified as a relative strength. Formal neuropsychological testing revealed large discrepancies between verbal and visual abilities. She is highly motivated by anything visual, loves books, but every picture has to be explained to her over and over again, as she cannot generalize. She has excellent verbal memory and appears to use verbal cues to find certain objects in a scene.

Clara underwent nine years of weekly O&M training, which was reinforced by her classroom team. The focus was on teaching her the layout of the classroom and hallway in school and being able to reach regular destinations such as the cafeteria, the bathroom, or the elevator as independently as possible. The language used during instruction was simple and repetitive. With practice and repetition she was able to identify landmarks from her home base to multiple destinations. Since she could not identify photographs, only verbal scripts could be used for teaching. Rewards were built into the activity to motivate her.

Clara is still not an independent traveler. In unfamiliar settings she will bump into obstacles. She may also bump into objects or furniture in her classroom unless the environment is kept clear of obstacles and remains consistent in its arrangement. She is most independent in her home environment since she knows this layout the best. She has no concept of drop-offs, nor can she perceive them. When traveling, she relies completely on the assistance of sighted people. In the future, a long cane or sensors detecting obstacles attached to her wheelchair may have to be considered. Over the years, she has been systematically taught to attend to and identify sounds and smells to remain oriented in her environment, as well as using some large visual landmarks.

## Child with Unilateral Brain Absence Leading to Homonymous Hemianopia and Mild Neglect

**Peter, an 8-year-old boy, had a right hemi**spherectomy (removal of the entire right hemisphere) at age 3 as a result of an intractable seizure disorder. Peter has homonymous hemianopia and some residual neglect of the left side. He has received O&M training from the time he was 4 years old and has used a long cane for the past three years. He orients in his environment very well, but is not always safe when walking through crowds. Peter has good visual perceptual skills.

A psychological evaluation revealed discrepancies in visual and verbal abilities and great difficulties in processing speed related to visual information. He recognizes pictures, photographs, and scenes. He is a great mapmaker and describes every route he travels in detail. Peter can be very distracted by sounds and people, which may not always leave him safe while traveling. Since he misses his left field in both eyes, he has to be particularly attentive to his left side, which is not always easy, given that he is 8 years old and has attentional problems. As a compensatory strategy, Peter uses head turns, and sometimes turns his whole body to the left, in order to use his intact right visual attention more efficiently.

Observation of his eye movements revealed that he experienced difficulty tracking objects smoothly to the left and making return saccades to the midline and right side. This method of observation utilized Peter, one of his classmates, and two adults. One adult, sitting behind Peter, ensured a stable and still head position while the adult in front of Peter presented the stimuli and observed his eye movements. In order to get a better idea of what typical eye movements look like, one of Peter's classmates in his inclusion classroom was asked to do the same task. The observed difference in eye movements was astounding, and this was verified by multiple observers as the procedure was repeated.

By stabilizing his body in a supine position on the floor, Peter was able to increase his ocular motility ability to the left when pursuing targets. Given the observation of his eye movements, it seems essential that Peter use a long cane for safety while walking, in addition to using slight head movements which still enable him to keep focused on obstacles in front of him and to the left and right sides. The use of the long cane makes Peter more aware of his left side and helps him focus his attention to that side. It also appears to give him a "break" from constantly having to turn his head all the way to the left, since the cane protects his left side and provides information through alternatives to the visual and auditory sensory channels. This seems to be very important, since he can be visually and auditorily distracted. Specific and consistent verbal prompts, such as "eyes out front," are used during traveling in order to remain safe. Other children and adults are asked not to talk to Peter while he is traveling to help him maintain focus and safety. He is placed either in front of a line of children, or at the back, so that he can use his cane while moving through the hallways during transitions. This also is the safest method for all other students, as they may otherwise trip and fall over the cane. When entering the classroom, the cane is stored in a consistent place, and Peter retrieves it from that location when leaving the classroom. Caring for the cane also teaches Peter responsibility for his own safety and taking care of his belongings. At the end of each lesson, the instructor and Peter both summarize what occurred during the lesson and talk about it. Problem solving is an integral part of the process.

Peter is now progressing from indoor travel to traveling in his neighborhood, such as finding his friend's house and identifying pertinent landmarks on the route. Peter enjoys O&M training. It gives him self-confidence in moving through the environment.

These case studies highlight the importance of systematic training and using a child's strengths to compensate for lack or loss of vision. They also highlight the fact that some children with CVI face additional problems—physical and cognitive—which need to be considered during the teaching process. As the cases of Peter and Clara in particular illustrate, there are no "quick fixes" when teaching O&M to children with CVI. Each child needed specific and individualized instruction methods that consider the following options:

- Use of a total sensory approach
- Ensuring body stability for increased visual attention and oculomotor control
- Creating a simple, consistent, and barrier-free environment
- Use of a long cane for additional tactile input and protection
- Periodic physical assistance (human guide)
- A highly structured approach to teaching and learning
- Consistent use of verbal prompts and terminology
- Use of photographs to establish and recognize landmarks
- A reward system

Teaching of O&M skills to children with CVI must be ongoing as the child gets older and demands for travel to different destinations increase. Some children may become independent travelers. Others may be independent at home or in a familiar classroom, but not outdoors.

## Conclusion

The topic of CVI has received much debate and concern in the O&M professional community because of the great variability of its impact on function and lack of specific, formal O&M assessments in this area. Some children with CVI may exhibit significant problems in orienting and moving through the environment (McKillop & Dutton, 2008). Some children cannot recognize objects or pertinent landmarks in their environment and get lost on the simplest route. Other students appear to have intact orientation and recognition ability but are unable to guide their movements in the desired direction when using visual control (McKillop & Dutton, 2008). In some students a combination of problems occurs. Other children may have a multitude of diagnoses, including visual field and visual acuity impairments based on ocular anomalies as well as damage to the visual brain and other impairments. In some parts of the world, there is a concern that children with CVI "fall through the cracks," as they might not necessarily be eligible for, or even be referred to, O&M specialists because they often have relatively good visual acuity and visual fields.

There is currently no single assessment tool or battery available to assess these students. Practitioners in the field report that they are often puzzled by how these children present and are in need of better assessment and intervention tools. As a first step, an observation protocol was outlined that attempts to focus on items that may be useful in assessing children with CVI.

Children with CVI have specific and often long-term needs that affect their O&M, education, and general quality of life. The difficulties for O&M specialists in terms of assessment lie in the fact that they rarely have access to neuropsychological information as part of the intake process. For example, TAPS (Pogrund et al., 2012) includes a comprehensive intake form, including interviews with caregivers and students, as well as medical and ophthalmological history. However, it does not include neuropsychological information. Reviews of neuropsychological information are not usually part of the O&M intake process, even though this information may yield some additional clues to a child's behavior.

Children with CVI constitute an extremely heterogeneous population. Thus, care should be taken with "cookie-cutter" prescriptions or prognoses. What works for one child may not work for another child. More research is needed to create a "toolbox" of intervention methods. Each tool could then be tested systematically, within a given time frame, and its success assessed by the child's team in the natural environment of the child.

In the future it will be necessary to revise training programs for O&M specialists to include topics such as CVI and the needs of children affected by it. The referral and eligibility process for O&M services needs to include children who do not necessarily have a visual field or visual acuity impairment but who have other visual deficits. O&M specialists must work closely with neuropsychologists, teachers of students with visual impairments, occupational therapists, and other professionals to identify these children. They may also want to educate teachers and administrators they already work with about CVI to increase awareness and highlight the need to refer affected children for O&M services.

## References


Anderson, S., Boigon, S., Davis, K., & deWaard, C. (2007). *The Oregon Project for preschool children who are blind or visually impaired* (6th ed.). Medford, OR: Southern Oregon Education Service District.

Brunsdon, R., Nickels, L., Coltheart, M., & Joy, P. (2007). Assessment and treatment of childhood topographical disorientation: A case study. *Neuropsychological Rehabilitation, 17*(1), 53–94.

Chokron, S., Colliot, P., Bartolomeo, P., Rhein, F., Eusop, E., Vassel, P., et al. (2002). Visual, proprioceptive and tactile performance in left neglect patients. *Neuropsychologia, 40*(12), 1965–1976.

Dutton, G. N. (2003). Cognitive vision, its disorders and differential diagnosis in adults and children: Knowing where and what things are. *Eye, 17*(3), 289–304.

Dutton, G. N. (2006). Discussion paper. In E. Dennison & A. H. Lueck (Eds.), *Proceedings of the summit on cerebral/cortical visual impairment: Educational, family, and medical perspectives, April 30, 2005* (pp. 27–34). New York: AFB Press.

Farnè, A., Ponti, F., & Làdavas, E. (1998). In search of biased egocentric reference frames in neglect. *Neuropsychologia, 36*(7), 611–623.

Fazzi, D. L., & Petersmeyer, B. A. (2001). *Imagining the possibilities: Creative approaches to orientation and mobility instruction for persons who are visually impaired.* New York: AFB Press.

Hill, E. W. (1981). *The Hill performance test of selected positional concepts.* Wood Dale, IL: Stoelting.

Iaria, G., & Barton, J. J. (2010). Developmental topographical disorientation: A newly discovered cognitive disorder. *Experimental Brain Research, 206*(2), 189–196.

Jacobson, W. H. (2013). *The art and science of teaching orientation and mobility to persons with visual impairments* (2nd ed.). New York: AFB Press.

Marotta, J. J., McKeeff, T. J., & Behrmann, M. (2003). Hemispatial neglect: Its effects on visual perception and visually guided grasping. *Neuropsychologia, 41*(9), 1262–1271.

Marsh, E. B., & Hillis, A. E. (2008). Dissociation between egocentric and allocentric visuospatial and tactile neglect in acute stroke. *Cortex, 44*(9), 1215–1220.

Marsh, E. B., Newhart, M., Kleinman, J. T., Heidler-Gary, J., Vining, E. P., Freeman, J. M., . . . Hillis, A. E. (2009). Hemispherectomy sustained before adulthood does not cause persistent hemispatial neglect. *Cortex, 45*(5), 677–685.

McKillop, E., & Dutton, G. N. (2008). Impairment of vision in children due to damage to the brain: A practical approach. *British and Irish Orthoptic Journal, 5*, 8–14.

Milner, A. D., & Goodale, M. A. (2006). *The visual brain in action* (2nd ed.). New York: Oxford University Press.

Pogrund, R., Sewell, D., Anderson, H., Calaci, L., Cowart, M. F., Gonzalez, C. . . . Roberson-Smith, B. (2012). *Teaching age-appropriate purposeful skills (TAPS): An orientation and mobility curriculum for students with visual impairments* (3rd ed.). Austin: Texas School for the Blind and Visually Impaired.

Roman-Lantzy, C. (2007). *Cortical visual impairment: An approach to assessment and intervention* (pp. 206–208). New York: AFB Press.

Roman-Lantzy, C. (2010). Teaching orientation and mobility to students with cortical visual impairment. In W. R. Wiener, R. L. Welsh, & B. B. Blasch (Eds.), *Foundations of orientation and mobility: Vol. II. Instructional strategies and practical applications* (3rd ed., pp. 667–711). New York: AFB Press.

Smith, M. (in press). *Barraga visual efficiency program.* Louisville, KY: American Printing House for the Blind.

Smith, S. E., & Chatterjee, A. (2008). Visuospatial attention in children. *Archives of Neurology, 65*(10), 1284–1288.

Southern Oregon Education Service District. (2007). *The Oregon Project curriculum and skills inventory* (6th ed.). Medford, OR: Author.

Trauner, D. A. (2003). Hemispatial neglect in young children with early unilateral brain damage. *Developmental Medicine & Child Neurology, 45*(3), 160–166.

Zihl, J., von Cramon, D., & Mai, N. (1983). Selective disturbance of movement vision after bilateral brain damage. *Brain, 106*(2), 313–340.

# 18

# Assessments Linked to Interventions: Computers, Tablets, and Other Assistive Technology

*James Carreon, Adam Wilton, and Amanda McKerracher*

Assistive technology related to computers and tablets can be essential for all students with visual impairments, but it can be particularly critical to support the education of and specific interventions with a child who has cerebral visual impairment (CVI). In addition to adjustments to accommodate vision needs related to size, color, and contrast issues, many students with CVI can have additional visual concerns, such as sensitivity to the crowding effects of pictures, words, and letters; location of materials within a visual display; and speed of presentation. These children can benefit greatly from alternative methods of presentation that take this range of concerns into account to provide access to educational materials and design appropriate instruction programs related to vision use.

Assessment for computer technology must address the questions many teachers and parents first think about in relation to setting up a system for a student with visual impairments:

- What constitutes an accessible computer?
- What modifications to my current computer system should I make?
- What peripheral devices should I use in order to get the most from the computer?
- Doesn't my child need to learn to use the same computers as everyone else?

But technology questions for students with CVI go beyond these basic hardware concerns, and their technology solutions must include consideration of a range of devices, software options, formats for presenting content, and response methods that best meet students' individual needs.

The right technology to meet the unique needs of the student can only be determined by a team of parents and professional educators who are aware of the wide variety of options available. When selecting any assistive technology for a student with a cerebral visual impairment, the team must consider not only the child's visual difficulties related to ocular and cerebral visual impairment, but also any gross and fine motor issues, as well as additional cognitive and processing issues. As with most visually impaired students, a unique set of problems requires a unique set of devices, software, and strategies tailored to the specific needs of the student.

This chapter begins by summarizing the main types of computer options that are available for all students with visual impairments to provide the background for considering the special technology needs of children with CVI. It first focuses on computers and the options for making them accessible. Then screen magnifier and screen reader programs are considered, as these are used by many visually impaired students to access the information on their computers. Keyboards are crucial as the main link between the user and the computer. Other assistive technology software includes word prediction and voice recognition software and optical character recognition systems. Video magnifiers are a type of hardware that can be used separately or in conjunction with computers. Finally, touch tablets are a relatively recent addition to the array of assistive technology tools for students with visual impairments. Then specific considerations and strategies are presented for assistive technology assessment and for formulating recommendations for the use of technology that are specific to students who have CVI.

## Accessibility and Computers

A computer that is accessible is possibly the most powerful single educational tool available to many students with CVI, enabling them to participate more fully in inclusive school settings. A computer system provides access to an almost unlimited range of programs, from the most basic cause-and-effect applications to simple games, word processing, Internet access, e-mail, and access to electronic books. The computer can run programs that convert print documents into electronic text, or recognize the spoken language and convert it to text or commands that control the computer. In addition, it provides accessibility options, including magnification of the computer screen for students with low vision, and screen-reading programs for students with little or no vision. Objects on the screen can be manipulated with a keyboard, a mouse, joystick, voice commands, or a touch screen.

### Operating Systems

An accessible computer starts with one running a mainstream operating system, either Apple or Windows. While there are other operating systems available, they are not often found and supported in most schools. Both the Windows and Apple operating systems include the basic tools and modifications needed to be accessible by a student with visual impairments. They go about it, however, in significantly different ways.

***The Apple operating system*** (referred to as iOS) provides a built-in screen magnification program for students with low vision and a robust screen reader for students with severe visual impairments. These programs are bundled with the operating system at no additional cost. Since they may go a long way toward meeting the access needs of blind and low vision students, there are few, if any, similar programs available from third-party vendors for Apple systems. If you don't like the Apple screen reader or screen magnification programs, you really have no alternative options that can be used with Apple products.

***The Windows operating system*** has a basic screen magnification program and a very rudimentary screen reader. Neither should be considered a full-featured product. The screen magnification program may prove adequate for some students with CVI; however, the screen reader in no way provides the necessary access for a student who is blind. As a result, there are a number of third-party companies that have filled this gap by developing much more robust screen access software programs. If the programs bundled with the Windows operating system are not adequate for the student's needs, there are a number of other options available. (See the Resources section at the end of this chapter for more information.) The cost of adding a full-featured screen magnification program or screen reader to the Windows operating system can be significant, however. (Screen magnification programs are discussed in more detail later in the chapter.)

When selecting an operating system, it is important for the child to sit in front of the computer and "try it out for size." This process should include a full technology assessment from a qualified assistive technology specialist who is knowledgeable about the features and options in both operating systems and who understands the issues related to visual impairment (Presley & D'Andrea, 2009). They must also know software options and peripheral devices that may help a child with CVI meet his or her unique educational needs and that mesh with existing school resources.

## Selecting a Computer

A computer for a child with CVI must be able to run the basic operating system, all mainstream programs, the access software, the Internet, and all peripheral hardware, such as a printer and scanner. That means it must be at least as powerful and as functionally versatile as those used by typically sighted students in school. It is not acceptable to have a computer system in a classroom for students who are visually impaired that has been handed down from a classroom for students with typical vision. A child with CVI needs to use the same programs as his or her sighted peers, but also requires an additional layer of specialized software to make those programs accessible. If the computer is obsolete for a sighted student, it is certainly obsolete for the visually impaired student!

## Components of the Computer

A student who is visually impaired must have a reasonably new computer that meets the minimum set of specifications, which is constantly changing. Rather than providing baseline numbers that will be obsolete before the ink dries, some key components are described here. Teachers should discuss this set of specifications with the school information technology department or knowledgeable salesperson before purchasing a new computer and make sure they understand how the computer will be used.

***The central processing unit (CPU)*** is the "brain" of the computer. How fast the computer processes calculations is measured in gigahertz (GHz) per second. Generally speaking, the higher the number associated with the CPU, the faster the processor.

***Random access memory (RAM)*** is temporary memory. When the computer is turned off, anything stored in RAM disappears and is lost, unless it has been saved to a storage device such as a hard drive. One should never skimp on RAM. It is relatively cheap and vital to a good running computer.

***A hard drive or other storage device*** is required to permanently save programs and data. Most computers come with adequate storage, but if additional space is needed, an external hard drive can easily be added. Files can also be saved to a portable storage device such as a memory card or USB flash drive. This gives the student the ability to easily move files from one device to another and from school to home. Files can also be saved on an Internet site (cloud storage). This has the added advantage of storing information at a location that cannot be lost or corrupted and is available anywhere there is Internet access.

***The video graphics card and sound card*** are also very important. The video card refreshes the monitor's screen. Its speed is also measured in GHz; again the higher the number the faster the processor. Most video cards also have their own RAM, which helps speed up the video processing. A good, mid-level video card will probably meet the needs of most students. A standard sound card is needed to play music and listen to audio books and is used by a screen reader or screen magnification program when producing synthesized speech.

***The monitor attached to a computer system*** is a critical component, especially for a child with CVI. The most popular type of monitor is the flat-screen liquid-crystal display. This type of monitor provides a light, thin, bright display with good contrast and excellent resolution. Screen sizes are measured diagonally in inches across the screen. Typical sizes include the 13-inch monitor for a small laptop computer up to a 20- or even a 24-inch monitor for a full desktop computer. Monitors also come in a standard aspect ratio of 4:3 (width to height) and a wide-screen aspect ratio of 16:9.

Current Windows operating systems support touch screen monitors. A student can select and open applications by pointing at and "double tapping" them with a finger. This is a more natural way of selecting objects on the screen for most students than using a mouse or other pointing devices and can be particularly helpful to students who have problems with hand-eye coordination related to CVI. The number of programs available for the Windows operating system that take advantage of this feature, however, still lags behind those available for touch tablets, discussed later in this chapter.

The first instinct when purchasing a monitor for a student with low vision is to get the largest one available. This is not always the best decision, especially for a student with a visual field impairment. It may take far longer for a student with tunnel vision to find and select a particular icon on a larger screen than on a smaller one. On the other hand, a child with CVI who has no significant field impairment would probably benefit from a full-size, wide-screen monitor of about 18 to 20 inches, so that icons on the desktop can be enlarged and spread out for ease of viewing and so that opened software programs can have displays with larger print and pictures.

## Modifications to the Computer

Alterations made to the default configuration of the computer when it is purchased can change the appearance of text and images on the monitor and make them more accessible to the viewer. This is done in the

Control Panel in the Windows operating system or System Preferences in the Apple operating system.

One decision to make is what screen resolution to use to display the image on the monitor. Screen resolution is the number of "dots" or pixels on the screen, as measured horizontally and vertically. A typical resolution for a wide-screen monitor may be 1920 x 1200 or 1280 x 800. Notice that the ratio of width to height (dividing 1920 by 1200 or 1280 by 800) is 1.6:1. This is the screen resolution ratio found on most wide-screen monitors. A screen resolution of 1024 x 768 produces a ratio of 1.3:1. This default screen resolution ratio of 1.3:1 is found on most standard (non-wide) screen monitors. Using the wrong resolution can result in stretching of the image, either horizontally or vertically.

The higher the resolution, the smaller the contents of the screen will appear, but with more fine detail. A lower resolution will provide a relatively larger image but with less detail. At lower resolutions the image will often appear "fuzzy" around the edges; however, this may not be evident and is usually not an issue for those with low visual acuity.

The correct resolution for any student depends on the student's vision, but also whether the student will use a separate screen magnification program to enhance the screen. If the student intends to use a full-featured screen magnification program, then accepting the default screen resolution recommended by the operating system for the attached monitor will almost certainly meet his or her needs. This is because a screen magnification program modifies the image sent to the monitor and can be adjusted to meet the needs of the child. However, if the student does not use a separate screen magnification program, the student will want to try out several resolution settings and other modifications to the desktop and icons to find a compromise between size and detail.

Other modifications include choosing a larger mouse cursor, enlarging the icons on the Desktop and Start menu or the Dock (Apple), selecting a larger text size for the Internet browser, and selecting a "zoom" or magnification level within an application such as a word processor when available.

These changes may result in a more functional computer for a student with CVI. However, it is important to understand that these changes are static. Once set, they are not easily changed for a specific need and then changed back to their default setting. If the student's needs change, someone will need to go back to the Control Panel (Windows) or System Preferences (Apple) to make these modifications. Using a separate screen magnification program, even the one built into the operating systems, may alleviate the need to make constant changes to the computer's settings.

## Screen Magnification Programs

### Windows Magnifier

The screen magnification program found in Windows is called Magnifier. This program allows the user to dynamically change the level of magnification with simple keystrokes. Magnifier can display the magnified image in full-screen mode, a lens view (similar to a handheld magnifier), and docked mode, in which the portion of the screen that is enlarged is located in a fixed position (or docked). There are a number of other modifications available in the Magnifier toolbar, including zoom level, lens size, color inversion, and tracking. Many of these settings have a keyboard command that allows the student to make changes to Magnifier without opening the toolbar or taking their hands off the keyboard to use the mouse. For example, holding down the Window key (two keys to the left of the spacebar on a standard keyboard) followed by the plus key will increase the amount of magnification; Window key and the minus key reduces magnification.

### Apple Zoom

The Apple operating system includes a screen magnification program called Zoom. It can magnify the screen contents from 2 to 20 times (2x–20x) and can display a full-color or high-contrast screen. VoiceOver, the screen reader bundled in the Apple operating system, can add text-to-speech while Zoom is running.

Pixelation becomes more apparent with the use of Zoom and Magnifier at higher magnification levels. Pixelation is the blocky appearance of graphics or text. It is most noticeable on letters with diagonal lines, such as *k* or *y* and on lower-quality graphics.

Magnification levels and basic navigation can be accomplished with "gestures" on an Apple multitouch trackpad, found on all Apple laptop computers. The so-called Magic Trackpad can be purchased separately and added to any Apple desktop computer. Using one, two, or three fingers with taps and swipes across the trackpad, the student can navigate the Apple environment and manipulate zoom levels without using a key command or touching the mouse. VoiceOver and Zoom in the Apple operating system are similar to their counterparts found on the Apple touch tablet and phone.

### Other Screen Magnification Programs

As noted earlier, if the Magnifier program proves inadequate for the needs of students who are using Windows computers, there are a number of screen magnification programs available through third-party companies. These options range from free or low-cost Internet downloads (usually not much better than Magnifier) to full-featured screen magnification software from well-established assistive technology companies (see the Resources section at the end of this chapter).

There are many advantages to using one of these full-featured screen magnification programs. They provide a number of zoom levels, viewing options, availability of technical support, training materials, and a community of users who share program tips within the educational field and through online forums. Magnification levels in these programs range from 1x (no magnification) through 24x or more. Some provide for smaller, incremental magnification at lower levels such as 1.5x or 1.75x. Many have the ability to greatly reduce the effects of pixelation on text and allow a high degree of customization that can be saved as a profile and opened as the need arises. This comes in handy when a computer is used by more than one low vision student or a single student uses different settings depending on the application. For example, a student may choose a negative image (black background with white letters) with 2x magnification when working in a word processor. However, that same student may choose a full-color screen with 2.5x magnification when on the Internet. Each profile can be saved and opened, depending on which application the student is using.

Adjustment of the space between characters is also an important feature of a good screen magnification program used by a child with CVI. Increasing the space between letters, words, and lines can help to reduce visual clutter.

Another feature of a screen magnification program is color enhancement. The student can choose from an almost infinite number of combinations for background and font color. Often there are a number of preset color combinations to choose from as well. The color and shape of the mouse and typing cursors can also be modified. Increasing the size of the cursor, selecting a color, and choosing a flashing or blinking cursor can help students locate their position on the screen.

Many screen magnification programs have the option of adding speech. This speech includes *typing echo,* in which every letter is spoken as it is typed, every word is spoken after pressing the spacebar, or both are spoken, depending on the user settings. *Mouse echo* is also available to speak the text as the mouse cursor moves over the screen. Finally, the program can speak the information found in menus, dialogue boxes, and other areas of the computer.

The teacher and student must be aware of the proper level of magnification, along with the requisite separation of letters, words, and lines to promote reading. A student with CVI may have the ability to recognize letters and words with 12-point font and no magnification. However, if this setting requires the student to hunch over the keyboard, move his or her face to within a few inches of the screen, and become fatigued after a few minutes of reading, reevaluation of the level of screen magnification may be needed. It is important to be aware of this "threshold" level of magnification that a student can use, but also the larger magnification level and spacing requirements needed to support sustained reading, without compromising speed by overmagnification.

Any screen magnification program with speech is capable of reading a document using standard navigation keystrokes. For example, Ctrl-right arrow (Command-right arrow for Apple) moves the cursor to the next word in a document. With the correct speech settings, the speech synthesizer can read that word. A down arrow moves the cursor to the next line of text and the speech synthesizer can vocalize that line.

A unique feature of some screen magnification software is the ability to read text copied from a document or website in a separate document reader tool. Reading speed, font size, and color enhancements can be adjusted within the document reader.

There are some students who use extreme magnification levels to try to read text on a computer screen. In some cases they can only display a single word on the screen at a time. This does not promote good reading habits or efficient computer navigation. For these students, a screen magnification program, even one with speech, should be replaced with a screen reader, as discussed in the next section.

## Screen Readers

A screen reader provides speech and enhanced keyboard commands to navigate most applications, including the Internet, without relying on the student's vision. Screen readers can be used on computers, tablets, and mobile phones. Typically, a user will navigate the device with keyboard commands, gestures on a touch screen, or voice commands. A screen reader must provide more information than just reading the text on the screen. It must be able to identify the location of the cursor's focus, such as a dialogue box, edit field, link, and a host of other elements displayed on the screen. This information is presented to the user through a speech synthesizer in the form of synthesized speech. It should allow the user to connect a refreshable braille display, if desired, so the user not only hears the information but can also read it in braille.

If a child with CVI requires a very high level of magnification to work on a computer or other device, then a screen reader may be warranted. At extreme levels of magnification, it is probably better to view the student as functionally blind and rely solely on a screen reader. Knowing when to use screen magnification software, a screen reader, or both, is not always easy to determine but is a decision that should be made by the student, teacher of students with visual impairments, and an assistive technology specialist.

## Keyboard Shortcut Commands, Keyboarding Instruction, and Adapted Keyboards

### Keyboard Shortcut Commands

It is important for a student using a screen reader or screen magnification program to use standard keyboard shortcut commands whenever possible. There is no reason to use the mouse to click on the printer or disk icon when Ctrl-P will open the print dialogue box or Ctrl-S will open the save dialogue box. Using these common key commands helps the student become a much more efficient computer user. Lists of keyboard shortcuts can be found in various places on the Internet (see the Resources section).

Learning to use a computer keyboard is one of the most important skills any student can gain. Speed is important, but accuracy is critical. A student who is constantly looking for a key or backspacing over mistakes is usually less efficient than a student who types more slowly but makes fewer mistakes. For a visually impaired student, knowing the standard computer keyboard means knowing all the keys: letters, numbers, arrows, "six-pack" (six keys found above the arrow keys), modifier keys (Ctrl, Alt, Esc), numeric keypad, and function keys (F1, F2, etc.). Visually impaired students need to know these other keys because they are used to navigate around the Internet or a document, modify access technology (for example, zooming in or zooming out), and open tools with keyboard commands. Knowing these keys helps them to eliminate the need to take their hands off the keyboard to use the mouse.

### Keyboarding Instruction

Learning to type accurately is central to the use of a computer, especially for someone with visual impairments. The best way to teach keyboarding skills is through a well-designed typing program. The best way to choose that program is to download a demonstration copy from the Internet and allow the child with CVI to try it out. Most commercial and low vision typing programs work well for students with CVI if they do not require screen magnification. It is necessary to make sure that the text prompts and student responses are large enough for the student to see. Some programs come with speech, so the letter is displayed on the screen along with a typing echo. If screen magnification is used along with the typing program, the entire screen may not be displayed. As a result, the responses typed by the student may eventually drift off the screen. The usual tracking of the typing cursor does not work because the program often displays only a picture of letters, not true letters. This is mostly true of commercially available typing programs.

There are two programs designed specifically to teach keyboarding to students with visual impairments from the American Printing House for the Blind that are both low in cost and effective in teaching typing in English: Learn Keys and Talking Typer (see the Resources section at the end of this chapter).

## Adapted Keyboards

Some students may have difficulty with fine motor control of one or both hands. If the small finger of the left hand does not work well, it is acceptable to use the ring finger to press the *q, a,* and *z* keys if it is more efficient for the student. Some students may use only the index finger of each hand to type. Again, if it is the most efficient way for the student to type, then modifying the typing process is acceptable. Guides are available on the Internet for teaching one-handed typing on a regular keyboard. In each case it is important to make the attempt to allow the student to type using a standard QWERTY computer keyboard. Adaptations should only be made when necessary. However, the ultimate goal is consistent, efficient, and accurate typing.

If it becomes apparent that a student may never become efficient with a standard computer keyboard, there are many other options. (See the Resources section at the end of this chapter for vendors of these and other assistive technology products.) There are keyboards with very large, high-contrast keys in both the standard QWERTY layout and in alphabetical order. The alphabetical layout is significantly different from a standard keyboard so a student may need to have one at school as well as at home. One-handed keyboards are available in many layouts from vendors of assistive technology. There are keyboards with a limited number of keys, requiring the student to press combinations of keys to make each character. This is similar to a braillewriter, where a combination of six keys can produce any letter. Other keyboards have all the keys within reach of either the left or right hand. This is done by packing all the keys onto a curved surface. Another approach is to provide only half a keyboard to the student. A modifier key is used to change the left-hand keys to the right-hand keys. It is important to remember there is a significant learning curve with each of these adaptive keyboards. Training is critical and requires constant adult supervision and guidance until the student is familiar with the product.

Programmable membrane keyboards are also available for students requiring additional adaptations. There are no keys on the keyboard until programmed. A standard overlay is slid into the keyboard; its layout is recognized and configuration sent to the computer. There are a number of standard layouts to choose from including a QWERTY, alphabetical, and math layout. If you do not like any of the standard layouts that come with the keyboard you can create a custom overlay. Each key can contain a letter, number, whole word, short phrases, or even computer commands such as "Ctrl-p+Enter" to print the current document. This makes any programmable keyboard a potentially powerful tool for a student with CVI and physical disabilities.

## Word Prediction and Voice Recognition Software

***Word prediction software*** is another tool available for a student who has limitations in typing or spelling skills. It is found in many programs designed for students with learning disabilities and as an add-on to any existing word processor. As a student types one letter at a time into a word processor, a list of words is continually updated on the screen. When the desired word appears in the list, the student can select and enter it into the document by typing a corresponding number or with a mouse click. (For some information about word prediction software, see the National Center to Improve Practice website at www2.edc.org/ncip/library/wp/toc.htm; see also the Resources section.)

***Voice recognition software*** has been around a long time and is now becoming a mainstream writing tool. Students can speak into a head-mounted microphone or the microphone of the laptop computer and have that speech recognized and the resulting text entered into a word processor. However, voice recognition programs (of which there are many) are very complicated and are not perfect. The makers of much voice recognition software claim it can achieve "up to 99 percent recognition accuracy right out of the box." That means, at its best, it will make 1 mistake for every 100 words spoken, and it probably makes many more mistakes than that. As a result, the student must be able to recognize those mistakes and have the ability to correct them efficiently either by voice or with the keyboard. Voice recognition programs require a significant amount of training and constant practice to use efficiently; many students may never learn to use them well enough.

Another problem to consider is the classroom environment. Background noise can make it difficult for the microphone to pick up the student's speech. In addition, voice recognition software requires a significant amount of processing power and cannot be run on an older computer or one that barely meets the software's minimum requirements. Moreover, not every student is capable of composing a document in his or her head and speaking those thoughts into a document. It is, however, a skill that can be taught by a teacher and learned by a student with CVI.

Voice recognition software is compatible with screen magnification software, but text may move off the edge of the screen and will require adjustments by the student to keep it on screen. A student who requires a screen reader, however, has added a whole new level of complexity to the process. Now the student is using voice recognition (speech-to-text) to enter text into a document and using a screen reader (text-to-speech) to review and edit the document. This additional complexity requires additional training for the student, in addition to a head-mounted microphone with in-line volume control and a mute button. The student can then speak into the voice recognition software, hear feedback from the screen reader, adjust the volume, and mute the microphone as needed when editing his or her document.

## Optical Character Recognition

Optical character recognition (OCR) is the process used to provide electronic access to a printed document to a student with visual impairments. There are three major steps in this process:

1. taking a picture of the printed document,
2. recognizing the proper reading order, and
3. recognizing each shape on the page as a letter, number, or punctuation mark.

The first step, taking a picture of the text, is typically done with a scanner or camera. A paper document is placed face down on a flatbed scanner with the edge of the paper lining up with the paper guides. This is not always easy for some students with CVI and may require some training. A student who has difficulty lining up the paper correctly may benefit by using an automatic document feeder that allows the student to place a single page or multiple pages and have them fed automatically onto the scanning bed. Once a print document is converted to an editable electronic text document, it can be saved in a number of file formats including .doc or .docx (MS Word), .txt (plain text), .rtf (rich text format), and .pdf (portable document format), among others.

Some OCR software is designed specifically for use by students who are blind or have low vision, with features that are particularly helpful to a child with CVI. They are, first of all, extremely easy to use. The entire process is automated and accomplished with a single keystroke. They come with a speech engine that converts the text document into synthesized speech. As the program reads the document, the text is highlighted, allowing the student to follow along visually as well. The student has the option to stop the reading at any point to enter text into the document. This allows the student to listen to a scanned worksheet and answer the questions. The entire finished worksheet can be printed and handed in to the teacher.

The low vision features of these programs include adjustments to the background and font colors and adjustment of the text size and spacing between letters and words. The programs can be bundled with a camera system that significantly speeds the process of capturing the original document and making it easier to eliminate skew. They can also convert the spoken text into an MP3 file and export the audio document to any MP3 player. However, since the entire process is automated, these programs do not allow the user to eliminate unwanted text and graphics or to select the desired reading order of the text. As a result, errors may be introduced into the final product that will require additional editing.

Other OCR programs can assist students with CVI who are able to best access the printed word presented sequentially in the same location on a computer screen. The words can be made to appear automatically at a preset rate (known as rapid serial visual presentation or RSVP), or at a rate controlled by the student (elicited sequential presentation) (Arditi, 1999; Kreuzer & King, 2004).

## Video Magnifiers

During the school day a teacher may present information to her students in any of a number of ways. The teacher may write on a whiteboard at the front of the room or use a projector to present audio-visual information. The teacher may ask the student to read a passage in a book and answer questions on a worksheet. Whether located in a special education or a regular classroom, the student with CVI must have access to all the information presented throughout the classroom if the student is to be successful. For students with poor acuity, the video magnifier can help provide that access through its ability to zoom in on distant objects and make small text appear large enough for the low vision student to read it.

A typical video magnifier consists of a color camera connected to a monitor. The size of the monitor will vary depending on its intended use. A small 3-inch monitor can be found on a portable handheld video magnifier not much larger than a paperback book, small enough to carry in a backpack or purse. In contrast, a desktop video magnifier (also known as a closed-circuit television system or CCTV) can have a 24-inch or larger monitor and would typically be located in a resource room. Some desktop and handheld video magnifiers have the ability to zoom in on distant objects, like the whiteboard at the front of a classroom.

Of course there are advantages and disadvantages to both types of video magnifiers. The desktop video magnifier provides a large, high-quality monitor with plenty of user controls, auto-focus lens, and a movable table (known as an X-Y table) on which to rest a book, but it is not portable. The desktop model provides a steady platform for the camera, allowing the student to locate and zoom in on a distant object and keep that object in view indefinitely.

The small paperback-size video magnifier is portable, but will have a limited battery life, a very small screen, and fewer controls and features. The portable video magnifier is typically handheld. It is much less steady, more difficult to use to locate the desired distant object and to keep it in view for any length of time. However, portability and smaller size may be desirable characteristics for some students with CVI since devices with these features are similar in appearance to general-use smartphones and small touch tablets.

There are video magnifiers that aim to find a compromise between the stationary desktop and the portable handheld models. These devices use a variety of strategies to get the best features of both types of video magnifier. Some devices provide a camera and means to connect it to a laptop screen or external monitor, allowing students to carry only the portable camera from class to class and connect it to a prepositioned monitor or to their own laptop screen. Other models provide a camera with a detachable 12-inch monitor. The camera and monitor are transported in a small suitcase. It can be considered a semiportable video magnifier.

Some desktop video magnifiers have the unique ability to capture an image of a document and rearrange the text. As the student increases the zoom level, words on the screen "wrap," or move down, to the next line. In addition, text can be displayed one word at a time, in a column, or streamed across the screen like a news crawl or "zipper." These options provide the child with CVI the ability to remove clutter and present text in a format conducive to a natural reading style.

It is important for students to understand what they need in the way of a video magnifier. Features to consider are the need for portability, the size of the monitor, the presence of an X-Y table, auto focus, battery life, and distance viewing. A video magnifier cannot realistically be selected from a catalog. The student, parent, and teacher must try out different models and explore the many different combinations of features available. Hands-on sampling of different video magnifiers at a conference or showroom is required to select the magnifier best suited to the student's unique needs.

## Touch Tablets

In recent years, the touch tablet has come to rival the computer as an accessibility tool, at least in certain aspects. It is not a traditional computer but a computing device that provides many of the same capabilities in a new package. The tablet provides an on-screen keyboard, the mouse is replaced with a touch-sensitive screen, and software is replaced with "apps" (short for applications), small, often simple programs that typically allow the user to accomplish only a single set of tasks. These apps are low- or no-cost programs designed for the specific tablet's operating system, taking full advantage of the touch-sensitive screen. The system comes on quickly, the student can interact with this device easily, and learning takes place easily as a result of the immediate feedback received when interacting with the touch screen.

The tablet is a game changer for some students with CVI. They may find the touch screen display more compelling than a traditional computer and keyboard due to its brightness, interactive capabilities, ease in altering the position and distance of the display, and the wide variety of applications available, all of which make tablets very versatile. The child with CVI no longer needs to learn to use a mouse to select items on the screen, which may be difficult for children with hand-eye coordination issues or those who have difficulty shifting gaze from mouse or keyboard to screen. He or she can find the item on the touch screen and simply do what comes naturally: touch it. This is also true of the on-screen keyboard. The student can select a letter and see it appear in the document on the same screen as the keyboard. If the student is capable of touch-typing, an external wireless keyboard can be paired to the tablet. More information on touch tablets for children who are learning to use their vision can be found in Appendix 18A. The variety of material available to students with CVI is increasing rapidly and can accommodate the learning needs of students with a range of functional vision.

Assistive technology for touch tablets is available as part of the operating system on some devices and can be added as an app to others. The iPad from Apple (and other devices that use the Apple operating system) ships with Zoom screen magnification software and the VoiceOver screen reader fully integrated into the tablet's operating system. Zoom provides a magnified image of the screen and can be adjusted with a three-finger double tap and drag, up or down, to adjust the level of magnification. The enlarged view, however, will now be too big to fit on the touch screen, requiring the student to scroll around to locate all available items and text. Not all apps are compatible with Zoom, however. While Zoom may magnify the screen, the screen may no longer respond to the user's touch.

VoiceOver provides text-to-speech access to all parts of the regular screen but may not provide access within some apps. The student can place a finger on the screen, and as his or her finger moves over text, buttons, and icons, VoiceOver identifies the object and reads the text. If the student wants to select the object, he or she can double tap anywhere on the screen. Similar screen-reading apps can be purchased for other tablets and phones.

Screen reader access to apps is variable. Some apps have a picture of text, not true text. A tablet's screen reader cannot read pictures of text. Other apps will not run at all when the screen reader is active. For example, one app requires the student to "pop" a colored balloon. The screen reader does not announce the color of the balloon (there is no text for the screen reader to read) and the balloon will not pop when selected until the screen reader is turned off. So, while the assistive technology can provide access to and navigational support for basic applications, not all apps have the ability to take advantage of the assistive technology.

There are over one million apps available for touch tablets (Statista, 2014) divided into several categories, including games, business, entertainment, and education. Within the education category, there are apps covering every subject, language development, and special education. With so many to choose from, the difficulty is finding just the right app for a student's needs. Before setting out to find an app, it is critical to have vision-related assessment and learning goals in mind for a particular student. Only then can the search begin for apps that can help facilitate those specific goals. A multitude of goals can be addressed using apps. They can be related, for example, to noticing movement of bright objects on the screen; completing puzzles that require different levels and types of visual facility; identifying pictures, letters, numbers or the special ways to highlight visual elements in them (for example, making a letter red or highlighting a part of an illustration to make it stand out); and reading words presented one at a time or words presented within a full sentence on the screen, combining vision with audio output. One of the simplest ways of finding an app for a specific purpose is to search for it on the Internet. For example, an online search for "cause-and-effect iPad apps"—apps that help children understand the concept of cause and effect by responding to the child's actions—results in a variety of links, including one leading to a website listing 10 free app downloads. Another source of information on the use of touch tablets for visually impaired students is AppleVis (www.applevis.com), a website for visually impaired users of Apple's iOS devices, which provides reviews and recommendations for apps that work with the assistive technology built into Apple's iOS devices.

Two critical issues must be addressed when tablets are used in a school setting. First, these devices must have wireless access to the Internet. Without it, teachers are not able to download new apps and some apps, already installed, will not function. This requirement can provoke tension between the school's information technology (IT) staff and those who support the assistive technology (AT). The goal of IT is to protect the school's network and provide a safe web-surfing environment for students and staff. The goal of AT is to provide access to the largest array of learning tools, the ability to install new software, and transfer files from one device to another. To protect the network, IT staff may not want to allow administrative access to the tablet for AT staff, but without it, they will be not able to fulfill their goals for their students. A dialogue between the two camps must be ongoing to meet the educational needs of a child with CVI. Teachers and AT specialists must support IT staff in maintaining a safe network and IT staff must understand and support the critical role of the computer and tablet devices in the education of the child with CVI.

The second issue that must be addressed regarding tablet devices is the ability to purchase and download new apps and books. Purchases made from tablets require an account that has been activated with a credit card or gift card, but school business offices generally don't work that way. Again, open communication between the business office, administrator, and teacher is required in order to allow AT staff the ability to purchase apps that help to meet the child's educational needs.

## Considerations for Technology Assessment and Instructional Programming Use

Students with CVI vary considerably in their visual and cognitive functioning, while the breadth of functionality in assistive technology—from low-tech to high-tech devices and programs—offers a wide range of options. Faced with an abundance of technology options available for students and to make recommendations for the technology that will be most helpful for a particular student, practitioners need to gather assessment data across several domains relevant to a student's use of assistive technology (perceptual, cognitive, physiological, environmental, and so forth). There are numerous sources of important data and recommendations related to the student's access to learning materials and instruction. These include more formal sources such as functional vision assessments, learning media assessments, clinical reports (such as ophthalmology and occupational therapy reports), and orientation and mobility evaluations. Informal sources of data, such as interviews with parents and teachers, anecdotal notes, and running records or checklists, also provide valuable insights into the student's functioning (Chapters 10 through 17 discuss relevant assessment methods).

### Specific Assessment and Intervention Strategies for Students with CVI

Considerations and strategies for assistive technology assessment and use need to be uniquely tailored to students with CVI, as informed by the extant research literature devoted to this population. Assistive technology assessment for students with CVI is a third-tier assessment according to the Assessment Model for Vision and Visual Processing Tied to Behavioral Indicators (Table 10.1) and is conducted in the context of functional tasks and situations in the student's learning environments. As mentioned earlier in the chapter, assessment for high-tech assistive technology goes beyond evaluation of specific hardware and software options because this evaluation must take into account a student's vision needs, physical and cognitive requirements, educational goals, personal preferences, availability of instructional and technical support, and funding. Gathering this information from multiple sources, followed by collaborative decision-making among assessment team members, including the family and the student, are critical. Comprehensive guides to assistive technology assessment for students with visual impairments are available (see, for example, Presley, 2010; Presley & D'Andrea, 2009).

Table 18.1 provides specific suggestions for assistive technology assessment and use tied to specific potential effects of CVI (listed in the first column). The table provides examples of how students may experience each effect of CVI in the learning environment, unique considerations for selecting appropriate strategies and materials for the assistive technology assessment, and suggestions

TABLE 18.1

## Behavioral Manifestations of Cerebral Visual Impairment with Corresponding Considerations for Assistive Technology Use

| *Potential Effect of CVI* | *Related Pattern of Behavior in the Learning Environment* | *Considerations for Assistive Technology Assessment* | *Considerations for Assistive Technology Solutions* |
|---|---|---|---|
| Impaired inferior visual field (Jacobson, Flodmark, & Martin, 2006) | The student finds it difficult, or is unable, to locate items or displays in situations where the student must accommodate the impaired inferior visual field. | Observe the student's eye and head movements as he or she writes or uses a keyboard. Ensure that the height of any computer display is adjustable, and record the student's responses at variable heights. Consult the functional vision assessment for any information on visual field testing. | The use of a stand will bring the page closer to the student when writing by hand, enabling him or her to maintain better posture while writing.<br>Computer monitors should have adjustable stands so that the monitor can be raised to a point where the student can comfortably view the entire display. Consider instruction in touch-typing. This will reduce the need for vertical head and eye movements as the student moves visual attention from the keyboard to the monitor and back again. |
| Right or left hemianopia or hemi-neglect (McKillop et al., 2006) | The student is reading from left to right and he or she finds it difficult to read the next word in the line of text (right hemianopia or right hemi-neglect). | Consult the functional vision assessment and eye examination reports for information on visual field loss. Observe and record as the student reads continuous text on a computer monitor, taking note of any words that the student may miss (especially at ends of lines on the right side of the display). Adjust the positioning of the display to the better functioning side, and observe the student's interactions with the technology. Record the relative location of input devices that the student consistently misses or ignores (e.g., a switch or joystick). | A thick, bold anchor line down the right margin of the text display will provide the student with a clear finish point for each line of text.<br>Moving an index finger or pointer along with the text until the anchor line is reached will decrease the likelihood that the student will miss words in a line.<br>Some students are more effective when reading words vertically upward (as opposed to the typical horizontal, left-to-right orientation; McKillop et al., 2006). Tactile markers can be used to indicate the right side of the display for younger students (e.g., for a student using a tablet computer). |

| | | | |
|---|---|---|---|
| | The student is reading from left to right and he or she finds it difficult to quickly locate the next line of print (left hemianopsia or left hemi-neglect). | Same as above. | A thick, bold anchor line down the left margin of the text display will provide the student with a clear starting point for each line of text.<br>Moving an index finger or pointer down the left anchor line after each line is read will decrease the likelihood that the student will miss the next line.<br>Some students are more effective when reading vertically downward (as opposed to the typical horizontal, left-to-right orientation; McKillop et al., 2006). Tactile markers can be used to indicate the left side of the display for younger students (e.g., for a student using a tablet computer). |
| Impaired ability to make accurate visually guided movements (optic ataxia) (Dutton et. al., 2004) | The student over-reaches or under-reaches for objects or input devices. | Provide ample time and opportunity for the student to reach for the target.<br>Consider the use of touch screen technology (such as the iPad) to provide students with tactile feedback as they interact with the technology, to motivate visually guided reaching and manipulation of the device.<br>Note: Visually guided reaching behavior should be assessed in and of itself and not be ascribed to any domain of cognitive or perceptual functioning. Visually guided reaching and manipulation is a skill in which some students may need explicit training (for an example, see Lueck, Dornbusch, & Hart, 1999). | Technology should remain in a relatively fixed, consistent location for the student's use. This will enable the student to develop expectations of his or her position in space relative to the technology (e.g., distance from seat to a touch screen). If hand-eye coordination and mouse use is an issue for the student, consider instructing the student to use shortcut keys to minimize the "point and click" required to execute commands (e.g., CTRL-A to "select all" in a PC environment). |
| | The student is hesitant to experiment with or use peripheral devices (e.g., portable scanner, USB storage devices). | Provide the student with a chance to touch and interact with peripheral devices. Record his or her preferences (e.g., prefers manipulating a larger DAISY file player than a smaller handheld player). Repeated practice may improve students' visually directed reaching and manipulation of objects (McKillop et al., 2006). | Make the boundaries of important visual targets highly salient by using color and texture cues (e.g., framing the control panel of the scanner with brightly colored tape). The student can use his or her pinky finger as a means to judge the position of his or her hand in relation to the device or computer (Lam, Lovett, & Dutton, 2010). The pinky finger provides the student with tactile feedback that relays the position of the student's hand in space relative to the device. |

*(continued on next page)*

**TABLE 18.1** *(continued from previous page)*

| *Potential Effect of CVI* | *Related Pattern of Behavior in the Learning Environment* | *Considerations for Assistive Technology Assessment* | *Considerations for Assistive Technology Solutions* |
|---|---|---|---|
| | The student finds it difficult to write quickly and legibly. The student prefers to use a scribe or to express him- or herself through oral language. | Review samples of the student's writing from diverse sources for legibility (such as creative writing exercises or a journal). Ask the student to copy words and sentences, as well as write words and sentences from dictation (Presley & D'Andrea, 2009).<br>Gather data on the student's typing speed. Consult the student's functional vision and learning media assessment reports for information relevant to the student's use of a word processing program, such as optimal font size and screen magnification. | Provide the student with an ergonomic keyboard and a seating arrangement that optimizes comfort as well as good head and body posture (Anderson, 2003).<br>Instruction in keyboarding will help the student to increase his or her written expression through word processing.<br>If keyboarding proves too slow and taxing for the student, consider the use of speech-to-text software and related peripheral devices (such as a microphone headset). |
| Impaired auditory search ability (G. N. Dutton, personal communication, April 17, 2012) | The student may have difficulty isolating the voice of a single speaker in an auditory stream. Students may not be able to attend to a story if there are extraneous voices and sound effects. | Texts in auditory formats (e.g., digital talking books) may not be appropriate for the student. These texts may contain some background noise (such as background music or sound effects). Assess the student's comprehension of the story to determine if the noise has a deleterious effect on the student's understanding of the text. | Select texts in auditory formats with little to no extraneous background noise (such as a cacophony of voices on a pirate ship). Preview the text with the student and match the student's interests and instructional programming to texts that the student can easily follow. |
| Oculomotor concerns | Nystagmus is present. Nystagmus is commonly found among students with periventricular leukomalacia (PVL) (Jacobson, Ygge, & Flodmark, 1998). | Refer to the student's functional vision assessment report, as well as any ophthalmological, orthoptic, or optometric reports, to determine the documented impact.<br>Determine optimal head and eye position (the null position in which nystagmus is minimized and vision is enhanced). | Assist the student to adopt his or her habitual head position to optimize vision when he or she is using a given device or computer to determine optimal placement (e.g., when seated at a laptop computer).<br>Ensure that the student can be seated comfortably while using the technology, taking his or her posture at null point positioning into account. For example, a reading stand may be required to raise a student's tablet computer so that it sits on an incline. |

| | | | |
|---|---|---|---|
| | Student has difficulty following along a line of symbols or print as a result of impaired eye movements. | Same as above to determine documented impact. | If the student has issues with eye movements when reading print, consider alternative presentation formats. Using rapid serial visual presentation (RSVP), individual words are presented in sequential order at a consistent location on a display. This minimizes the number of letters or words the student must take in per eye movement (visual span; see Legge et al., 2007). Other adaptations include allowing the student to control the rate of visual presentation (elicited sequential presentation; see Arditi, 1999), presenting text in a line-by-line orientation, and serial highlighting of single words along a line of print. |
| Low visual acuity | Student requires reading materials to be enlarged and/or closer. | See considerations for oculomotor concerns to determine optimal strategies. | Use a screen magnification program to enlarge the visual display. Simply increasing the size of the font may not result in the level of magnification that is required; dialogue boxes and icons may remain in their original size (although icons can be enlarged). When determining font size, note that different fonts of the same nominal point size will not be equivalent in actual size (Rubin, Feely, Perera, Ekstrom, & Williamson, 2006). |
| Poor contrast sensitivity | Student demonstrates poor sensitivity to materials that are in low contrast to their background (Watson, Orel-Bixler, & Haegerstrom-Portnoy, 2007). | Consider the assessment materials in advance and determine if testing materials have sufficient contrast. For example, if obtaining a writing sample, ensure the line guides on the page are thick and bold. Consult the student's functional vision assessment and reports from previous eye examinations. Determine if the student prefers dark symbols on a light background or vice versa to optimize viewing. | High contrast, sometimes with specific colors, can be of assistance for an individual child rather than black on white or white on black. This can help the student compensate for poor visual acuity.<br><br>Note that contrast sensitivity has been shown to improve somewhat with age, and so responses to contrast should be assessed throughout instruction (using diagnostic teaching methods) to detect any changes in the student's capacity to discern contrast (Watson et al., 2007). |

*(continued on next page)*

**TABLE 18.1** *(continued from previous page)*

| *Potential Effect of CVI* | *Related Pattern of Behavior in the Learning Environment* | *Considerations for Assistive Technology Assessment* | *Considerations for Assistive Technology Solutions* |
|---|---|---|---|
| Difficulty shifting visual fixation (Fazzi et al., 2007) | The student has difficulty shifting his or her gaze between two visual targets. | It may be helpful to minimize the frequency with which the student needs to shift his or her gaze to complete a task in class (such as copying from the board), and to make adjustments to accommodate different distances at which the student needs to focus. Consider assessing the student's ability to make use of a rotating camera (i.e., room-viewing system), enabling the distant visual target to be displayed on a computer monitor. | Copying notes may be difficult for the student. Consider providing the student with his or her own copy of class notes, overheads, etc. Place the student's computer in front of a blank wall or blank bulletin board, so that visual attention is not divided between the monitor and extraneous targets behind the monitor. |
| Simultanagnostic visual dysfunction (Lam, Lovett, & Dutton, 2010) | The student has difficulty distinguishing visual targets from complex or cluttered backgrounds (Stiers et al., 2001). | Consider adjusting the size of the visual span through sequential presentation of text (see RSVP above) and/or enlargement and recording the student's subsequent reading speed. Small increases in the spacing between characters may reduce clutter in the visual display and result in higher reading speeds in young readers with low vision (McLeish, 2007). However, research with sighted adults has shown that larger increases to spacing between characters can have a deleterious effect on reading speed, since it contracts the size of the visual span required for reading (Yu, Cheung, Legge, & Chung, 2007). Conduct reading speed assessments to determine what intercharacter spacing is optimal for the student. | Students with CVI have been shown to demonstrate improved behavior and attention in environments with minimal visual clutter (Dutton et al., 2004). Situate the student's assistive technology (e.g., desktop computer) in an area where there are few wall decorations or fixtures.<br><br>Some class materials, particularly in elementary grade levels, may have superfluous designs and images that are not directly related to the intended use of the material (e.g., stylized decorations or borders). Critically assess what features are necessary for the student to complete the task, and what features can be discarded in order to simplify the visual display. |

| | | | |
|---|---|---|---|
| Impairment of visual perception (van den Hout et al., 2004) | The student has difficulty recognizing familiar shapes, objects, etc. (McKillop et al., 2006; Stiers et al., 2001). | Young children with hypoxic-ischemic brain damage (including those with PVL) are less able to identify common objects under suboptimal conditions (e.g., incomplete contour lines, overlapping images) than typically developing peers (Fazzi et al., 2009; Stiers et al., 2001). Therefore, materials intended to assess the student's visual object recognition should be presented under optimal conditions. | Ensure that the target images in software programs are unobstructed, complete in form, and as typical as possible (i.e., avoid obscure variants of an object that the student may have difficulty recognizing).<br>Encourage the student to recognize peripheral devices and hardware using a multisensory approach by combining tactile, visual, and auditory inputs. |
| | When using materials such as maps or diagrams, the student has difficulty processing spatial information (Fazzi et al., 2009). | Consult the student's functional vision assessment and any psychoeducational reports that refer to the student's visuospatial abilities. Observe and note the student's ability to solve puzzles as well as locate and arrange various images and dialogue windows on a computer display. Assess how effectively the student interacts with interfaces of varying complexity. For example, a DAISY player has a simple interface compared to other devices. | Orient the student to the various menus and dialogue boxes required to use a given program or operating system, drawing special attention to spatial relationships (e.g., the "Recycle Bin" is located above the "Start Menu" on the desktop).<br>Encourage the student to maintain an organized workspace when using assistive technology.<br>Keep the student's assistive technology in a consistent location in relation to other technology and classroom fixtures. |

for formulating effective recommendations for students, all of which can be included in the assistive technology assessment report.

## Conclusion

Matching appropriate assistive technology to the unique needs of particular students with CVI requires an understanding of the range of technology options, how they operate, their strengths and weaknesses, and their applicability to students with different specific visual and learning needs. This chapter reviewed basic operations of such options and how they might be of assistance to children who have CVI. Potential effects of CVI that need to be addressed when selecting and designing technology solutions have also been presented.

Technology options are constantly expanding and becoming more sophisticated, with increased application to students who have CVI. It is hoped that the information summarized in this chapter provides the reader with some basic information as these expanding options are considered and understanding of the effects of CVI grows.

## References

Anderson, J. (2003). Expanded core curriculum: Technology. In S. A. Goodman & S. H. Wittenstein (Eds.), *Collaborative assessment: Working with students who are blind or visually impaired, including those with additional disabilities* (pp. 237–263). New York: AFB Press.

Arditi, A. (1999). Elicited sequential presentation for low vision reading. *Vision Research, 39*(26), 4412–4418.

Dutton, G. N., Saeed, A., Fahad, B., Fraser, R., McDaid, G., McDade, J., & Spowart, K. (2004). Association of binocular lower visual field impairment, impaired simultaneous perception, disordered visually guided motion and inaccurate saccades in children with cerebral visual dysfunction—A retrospective observational study. *Eye, 18*(1), 27–34.

Fazzi, E., Bova, S., Giovenzana, A., Signorini, S., Uggetti, C., & Bianchi, P. (2009). Cognitive visual dysfunctions in preterm children with periventricular leukomalacia. *Developmental Medicine & Child Neurology, 51*(12), 974–981.

Fazzi, E., Signorini, S. G., Bova, S. M., La Piana, R., Ondei, P., Bertone, C., . . . Bianchi, P. E. (2007). Spectrum of visual disorders in children with cerebral visual impairment. *Journal of Child Neurology, 22*(3), 294–301.

Jacobson, L., Flodmark, O., & Martin, L. (2006). Visual field defects in prematurely born patients with white matter damage of immaturity: A multiple-case study. *Acta Ophthalmologica Scandinavica, 84*(3), 357–362.

Jacobson, L., Ygge, J., & Flodmark, O. (1998). Nystagmus in periventricular leucomalacia. *British Journal of Ophthalmology, 82*(9), 1026–1032.

Kreuzer, D. T., & King, J. (2004). Guidelines for customizing visual displays for students with visual impairments who have severe speech and physical impairments. In A. H. Lueck (Ed.), *Functional vision: A practitioner's guide to evaluation and intervention* (pp. 343–350). New York: AFB Press.

Lam, F. C., Lovett, F., & Dutton, G. N. (2010). Cerebral visual impairment: A longitudinal case study of functional outcomes beyond the visual acuities. *Journal of Visual Impairment & Blindness, 104*(10), 625–635.

Legge, G. E., Cheung, S.-H., Yu, D., Chung, S. T. L., Lee, H.-W., & Owens, D. P. (2007). The case for the visual span as a sensory bottleneck in reading. *Journal of Vision, 7*(2), 1–15.

Little, S., & Dutton, G. N. (2015). Some children with multiple disabilities and cerebral visual impairment can engage when enclosed by a "tent": Is this due to Balint syndrome? *British Journal of Visual Impairment, 33*(1), 66–73.

Lueck, A. H., Dornbusch, H., & Hart, J. (1999). The effects of training on a young child with cortical visual impairment: An exploratory study. *Journal of Visual Impairment & Blindness, 93*(12), 778–793.

Lueck, A. H., & Heinze, T. (2004). Interventions for young children with visual impairments and students with visual and multiple disabilities. In A. H. Lueck (Ed.), *Functional vision: A practitioner's guide to evaluation and intervention* (pp. 277–352). New York: AFB Press.

McKillop, E., Bennett, D., McDaid, G., Holland, B., Smith, G., Spowart, K., et al. (2006). Problems experienced by children with cognitive visual dysfunction due to cerebral visual impairment—And the approaches which parents have adopted to deal with these problems. *British Journal of Visual Impairment, 24*(3), 121–127.

McLeish, E. (2007). A study of the effect of letter spacing on the reading speed of young readers with low vision. *British Journal of Visual Impairment, 25*(2), 133–143.

Presley, I. (2010). The impact of assistive technology: Assessment and instruction for children and youths with low vision. In A. L. Corn & J. N. Erin (Eds.), *Foundations of low vision: Clinical and functional perspectives* (2nd ed., pp. 589–654). New York: AFB Press.

Presley, I., & D'Andrea, F. M. (2009). *Assistive technology for students who are blind or visually impaired: A guide to assessment.* New York: AFB Press.

Roman-Lantzy, C. (2007). *Cortical visual impairment: An approach to assessment and intervention.* New York: AFB Press.

Rubin, G. S., Feely, M., Perera, S., Ekstrom, K., & Williamson, E. (2006). The effect of font and line width on reading speed in people with mild to moderate vision loss. *Ophthalmic and Physiological Optics, 26*(6), 545–554.

Statista. (2014). Number of apps available in leading app stores as of July 2014. Retrieved November 17, 2014, from http://www.statista.com/statistics/276623/number-of-apps-available-in-leading-app-stores

Stiers, P., van den Hout, B. M., Haers, M., Vanderkelen, R., de Vries, L. S., van Nieuwenhuizen, O., et al. (2001). The variety of visual perceptual impairments in pre-school children with perinatal brain damage. *Brain & Development, 23*(5), 333–348.

van den Hout, B. M., de Vries, L. S., Meiners, L. C., Stiers, P., van der Schouw, Y. T., Jennekens-Schinkel, A., . . . van Nieuwenhuizen, O. (2004). Visual perceptual impairment in children at 5 years of age with perinatal haemorrhagic or ischaemic brain damage in relation to cerebral magnetic resonance imaging. *Brain & Development, 26*(4), 251–261.

Watson, T., Orel-Bixler, D., & Haegerstrom-Portnoy, G. (2007). Longitudinal quantitative assessment of vision function in children with cortical visual impairment. *Optometry and Vision Science, 84*(6), 471–480.

Yu, D., Cheung, S-H., Legge, G. E., & Chung, S. T. L. (2007). Effect of letter spacing on visual span and reading speed. *Journal of Vision, 7*(2), 1–10.

# APPENDIX 18A

# Touch Tablets and Applications for Children Learning to Use Their Vision

*Hubertine Burgers*

**Sam is a 2½-year-old boy with CVI. Because he showed** limited visual attention, his therapist and his parents have been encouraging him to use his vision to see lights and shiny objects for about six months. He has been making some progress visually fixating, but still does not follow objects consistently.

Sam seems to have better visual attention when watching things on a device that uses a screen, such as a television or laptop. On the laptop he loves to look at cause-and-effect games and is able to follow the objects on the screen with more ease. He can press a switch himself to make changes on the screen, but when he does, he cannot look at the screen at the same time. This problem, along with the fact that Sam is more attentive when he is lying down, gave rise to the idea of using a touch tablet for him.

A touch tablet was put on a stand on the floor, right next to where Sam was lying. It was placed so that the screen of the touch tablet was in his intact upper visual field. An app (application) was started that contained a lot of stars and twinkling sounds (see Figure 18.1). Sam was lying on his back, and as soon as the app started, he turned his head around to see what was happening on the screen. The therapist took his hand and guided Sam to touch the screen. The touch made the stars fly away with a funny sound. Sam's eyes widened and he started laughing. He touched the screen again, and the same thing happened. He couldn't get enough of it. Sam touched the screen over and over while he watched what was happening on the screen with a lot of concentration.

FIGURE 18.1
**App with Stars**

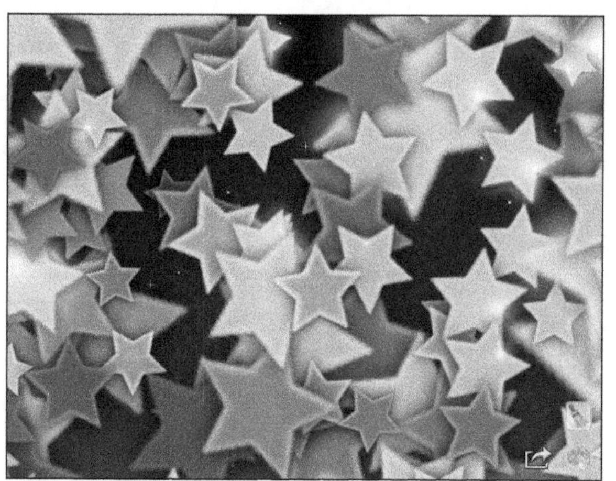

---

**Anna is a 5-year-old girl with CVI. She loves looking** at several cause-and-effect games on a laptop with an adaptive switch. She presses the switch herself, but this seems more accidental than purposeful. Anna didn't seem to make the connection between pressing the switch and what was happening on the screen. She started to use a touch tablet with an app in which shapes were moving across the screen. When she accidentally touched the screen, a color was displayed at the spot she had touched, accompanied by a sound (see Figure 18.2). Using this app made her realize that she was the one creating the color and sound, and she could control the app herself.

Although interventions for children who have CVI have traditionally been conducted with light boxes and, more recently, computers, touch tablets have presented new opportunities for vision intervention. Many

FIGURE 18.2
App with Moving Shapes

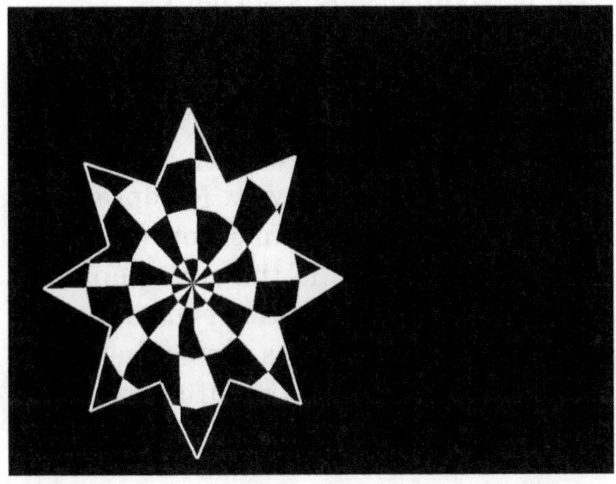

children with CVI find it easier to see lights and objects in high contrast (Lueck & Heinze, 2004; Roman-Lantzy, 2007). Touch tablets, like light boxes, have a bright, high-contrast screen, yet their interactivity and sounds, like computers, are a great deal more engaging for children with CVI.

## What Is a Touch Tablet?

A touch tablet is a small, thin, flat computer that has many of the key features of a full-size personal computer. A touch tablet is essentially a small laptop computer with a built-in keyboard (although it is possible to connect an external keyboard), and it is equipped with a touch screen as an input device. It is used like touch-screen smartphones, and runs via an adapted operating system, such as the Apple iOS or Android.

The software programs that are used on touch tablets are called apps. Touch tablets from different manufacturers have different "app stores" or online retailers where users can download apps. Apps made for iOS cannot be used on an Android touch-screen tablet and vice versa.

## Benefits of Touch Tablets in Vision Intervention Programs

Touch tablets have a lot of benefits over traditional computers (or laptops) for vision intervention programs. The most important benefits are explained below.

### Screen

Most touch tablets have a very bright screen that provides high-contrast colors that are attractive for children with CVI to view. This effect can be increased even more by working in a quiet semi-dark environment for those children with simultanagnostic difficulties because other visual stimuli cannot be seen in the darkness. The same effect can be gained by constructing a makeshift tent that encloses the child and therapist or teacher. Limiting peripheral auditory and visual distraction allows the child to perform better (Little & Dutton, 2015).

The touch tablet can be used in both portrait mode (with the longer side of the tablet as the height measurement) and landscape mode (the longer side as the width measurement). The screen adjusts automatically as soon as the tablet is turned, but it is also possible to lock the screen for one presentation mode.

### Size and Weight

The most used touch tablets have an average weight of 1.1–1.5 lbs (0.50–0.70 kg) and are very thin. This make them easy to carry and use wherever needed.

### Positioning

Touch tablets are easy to position at any angle that is beneficial for the child. They can be placed on wheelchair tables and can even be used when a child is lying down. This makes it easy for a child to see the screen at close range in a posture that works best.

There are different kinds of stands available to assist in positioning tablets. For example, one line of accessories provides a stand for the touch tablet as well as rubber frames that surround the device, protecting it and making it easier to grasp. There are also stands that attach the touch tablet to a wheelchair table with a suction cup. These and other accessibility accessories can be found through an Internet search.

### Controls

The controls of touch tablets are intuitive. With a traditional computer, the child has to press a switch to make things happen on the screen. For some children, it is hard to understand the connection between pressing the switch and what is happening on the screen (such as Anna in the example presented earlier). Using touch tablets makes this concept of cause and effect much easier to understand; the child touches the screen and something happens immediately on the screen right at the place that was touched. Also, children who experience difficulties pressing the switch while looking at the screen at the same time (such as Sam from the earlier example) benefit a lot from the touch technology. Children are motivated to keep looking at their hands while they touch the screen since the resultant visual and sound effects happen immediately.

Most touch tablets have one small button to end the app and return to the main menu. It is is not very likely the child will press this button by accident. Last but not least, touch tablets are easy for the therapist, teacher, or caregivers to control. They are much easier to control compared to traditional computers. In fact, a lot of computer experience is not needed to control a touch tablet. Even downloading required apps is not hard.

### Apps

Applications downloaded from an app store or online retailer will be installed on the touch tablet right away. Except for the need to have a wireless Internet connection to download an app to the tablet, no other implements are needed to start using an app with the child. Most apps can be used without an Internet connection after they have been downloaded.

### Cost

Most apps used for vision intervention are free or very inexpensive, compared to most of the traditional computer software used for this purpose. Many apps that may cost a few dollars for the full version have a free "lite version." Although these lite versions are "demonstration versions," they can often be used successfully with children.

### Choices

Apps have a wider range of choices for a specific child than available traditional computer software, and more are becoming available every day. However, this variety of choices can also make it harder to find the right apps.

## Finding Apps

### App Store or Online Retailer

To download an app onto a touch tablet, access to the Internet is required to go to the app store or online retailer to make a selection. Apps can be searched by category or by a keyword. As stated above, because there are so many apps, finding the right one for a particular intervention requires some investigation.

Apps can be used to encourage an array of rudimentary vision skills. They can engage visual attention and promote visual following, shift of gaze, and awareness of color or shape, for example. Once rudimentary skills are elicited and sustained, then more complex visual skills can be introduced, such as color, shape, and object identification, promotion of hand-eye coordination, and matching of visual targets. As vision skills increase, learning activities in other areas can be promoted through use of vision, depending on the learning capabilities of individual children.

Given these uses, the following list offers some good keywords for finding vision apps for early intervention that promote basic visual skills:

- fireworks
- bubbles
- fluid
- glitter
- stars
- glow
- cause and effect
- shapes
- colors
- moving
- paint
- draw
- baby
- infant
- early intervention
- early learning
- special education

For more advanced apps, in which the child has to do more, such as touch the screen on a specific point, or perform skills such as matching, sorting, and making puzzles, the following are some additional keywords:

- toddler
- matching
- sorting
- puzzle
- letters
- numbers
- alphabet

Keywords can be used to access apps from the app store or online retailer via the touch tablet, but it is also recommended that an Internet seach be conducted in order to read about the experiences of other people who have used specific apps. To do this, the word "apps" can be paired with one of the previously mentioned keywords—for example, "puzzle apps"—when performing the Internet search.

### Social Media

Social media is also a great way to find information about apps and read reviews by parents, teachers, and therapists. A good way to find these social media groups is to search for general topics related to touch tablets such as "special needs apps," special education apps," "early learning apps," or "iPad+CVI."

### Websites

Websites in the fields of visual impairment and special education are monitoring iPad apps for children with special needs that will make it easier to find appropriate apps. Keep in mind that not all apps are available in all countries, but a good many of them of them are available internationally. Some recommended websites for finding appropriate apps to use with children who have CVI are listed in the Resources section at the end of this chapter.

## Afterword

The author has found that many children with CVI reacted very well to the touch tablet. Children who weren't interested in more conventional materials, such as lights, black-and-white patterns, or glitter materials, for a long period of time seemed to have a longer attention span with the touch tablet. This made them experience the joy of looking and also stimulated them to look at other things for a longer period of time. Working with a touch tablet may stimulate the child's brain to make connections that aid in the understanding of what the eye is seeing and assist in developing the ability to interpret images.

# Resources for Assistive Technology

The following listing comprises a representative sample of assistive technology products that can be useful when working with students with CVI. For additional information about assistive technology and resources and a more complete listing, visit the American Foundation for the Blind's searchable Product Database at www.afb.org/prodMain.asp.

## KEYBOARDS

### *Keyboard Shortcuts*

**Apple Keyboard Shortcuts**
Source: Apple
http://support.apple.com/en-us/HT201236

**Windows Keyboard Shortcuts**
Source: Microsoft
http://windows.microsoft.com/en-us/windows/keyboard-shortcuts

### *Keyboarding Instruction*

**Learn Keys: Verbal Keyboard Feedback**
Source: American Printing House for the Blind
http://shop.aph.org/webapp/wcs/stores/servlet/Product_Learn%20Keys:%20Verbal%20Keyboard%20Feedback_1090193P_10001_11051

**Talking Typer for Windows**
Source: American Printing House for the Blind
https://shop.aph.org/webapp/wcs/stores/servlet/Product_Talking%20Typer%20for%20Windows_1088609P_10001_11051

## APPS

### *iPad Reviews and Articles*

**Recent iPad App Reviews and Articles**
Source: Wonder Baby
www.wonderbaby.org/articles/ipad-apps

**Care and Modification of iPads**
Source: Paths to Literacy
www.pathstoliteracy.org/care-and-modification-ipads-students-multiple-disabilities

### *Sources of Apps*

**AppleVis**
(Source for apps that work with Apple devices' assistive technology)
www.applevis.com

**Educational Technology and Mobile Learning**
www.educatorstechnology.com/2012/12/a-list-of-all-best-ipad-apps-teachers.html

**Paths to Literacy: Technology**
www.pathstoliteracy.org/technology

**Teaching Learners with Multiple Special Needs**
http://teachinglearnerswithmultipleneeds.blogspot.nl/2011/08/android-apps-for-our-kids.html

## SOFTWARE

### *Word Prediction Software*

**Co:Writer Universal**
Source: Don Johnston
http://donjohnston.com/cowriter

## SOURCES OF ASSISTIVE TECHNOLOGY PRODUCTS

The companies listed in this section distribute a wide variety of assistive technology products described in this chapter.

**ABISee, Inc.**
30 Sudbury Road, Unit IB

Acton, MA 01720
(978) 637-2900 (Local)
(253) 595-3623 (Fax)
(855) 354-4080 (Toll-Free); (800) 681-5909 (Toll-Free TDD/TTY)
http://www.abisee.com/
info@ABiSee.com

**American Printing House for the Blind**
1839 Frankfort Avenue
Louisville, KY 40206-0085
(502) 895-2405
Fax: (502) 899-2274
www.aph.org
info@aph.org

**Independent Living Aids**
200 Robbins Lane
Jericho, NY 11753
(516) 937-1848 or (800) 537-2118
Fax: (516) 937-3906
www.independentliving.com
can-do@independentliving.com

**LS&S Group**
145 River Rock Drive
Buffalo, NY 14207
(847) 498-9777 or (877) 498-1482
Fax: (877) 498-1482
www.lssgroup.com
info@LSSproducts.com

**Magnifying Aids**
4760 East Bay Drive Ste. E
Clearwater, FL 33764
(727) 526-2020 or (866) 691-2450
(866) 691-2450 (Toll-Free)
Fax: (727) 531-7224
www.MagnifyingAids.com
Sales@MagnifyingAids.com

**MaxiAids**
42 Executive Boulevard
Farmingdale, NY 11735
(631) 752-0521 or (800) 281)3555
Fax: (631) 752-0689
www.maxiaids.com
sales@maxiaids.com

**SightConnection**
9709 Third Avenue NE, #100
Seattle, WA 98115
(800) 458-4888
www.sightconnection.org

# PART IV

## Intervention for Children with CVI

# 19

# Intervention Methods: Overview and Principles

*Amanda Hall Lueck and Gordon N. Dutton*

The complex web of abilities, skills, and behaviors that can be affected by early damage to the visual brain, causing CVI, are uniquely expressed in each child. The behavioral expressions are identified through appropriate assessments that seek a variety of possible effects, as discussed in Part 3 of this book. A skilled team of professionals can then work with the child and the child's family to identify areas to target for intervention.

Comprehensive instructional programs differ depending on the age of the child, the salient visual issues, and other impairments, as well as educational and overall life goals. Interventions motivate engagement and participation in activities that promote learning, independence, and self-esteem. They may involve a variety of approaches, including:

- Direct teaching of skills and behaviors.
- Systems to ensure access to educational materials and instruction that are matched to, and do not exceed, a child's skills and abilities (for example, enlarged print or high-contrast material for reading; slower presentation time for verbal material).
- Approaches to task requirements that promote successful completion and a sense of self-efficacy and accomplishment (asking for a verbal response rather than a written one).
- Changes to the general environment to promote interactivity and learning that minimize the need for direct instruction, special materials, or special techniques (reduction of visual clutter in a common play area; addition of high-contrast stripes to stairs to increase visibility; reduction of background noise).

While children with CVI may require interventions specific to the visual and behavioral sequelae of damage to the visual brain, at the heart of intervention for all children are good teaching practices. For children with CVI, it is important to address these general strategies in addition to targeting their needs for special interventions. For this reason, some comprehensive teaching methods will be mentioned briefly to highlight their importance prior to a discussion of specific intervention methodologies associated with the effects of CVI.

The authors thank Mary Morse and John Morse for their contribution of some of the material appearing in the Presentation Style and Format section of this chapter.

## Self-Determination as a Goal for All Students with CVI

Self-determination is central to current philosophies of teaching and learning. Interventions promote and support self-determination and further the capacities that individuals bring to the decision-making processes in their daily lives. They also provide the environmental support needed to promote the individual's use of personal choice (Research and Training Center on Community Living, 2008). In the expanded core curriculum for children with visual impairments, self-determination is one of nine educational areas believed to encourage and empower students to inform, set and reach their personal goals, and participate fully in the world around them throughout their lives (Allman & Lewis, 2014; American Foundation for the Blind, 2011; Hatlen, 2003). The areas of the expanded core curriculum are:

- career education
- self-determination
- compensatory or functional academic skills, including communication modes
- sensory efficiency skills
- independent living skills
- social interaction skills
- orientation and mobility
- use of assistive technology
- recreation and leisure skills

Strategies to promote self-determination give students of all ages opportunities to choose their learning activities, facilitate their acquisition of decision-making skills, encourage independent exploration and investigation, promote self-worth through activity, mastery, and positive feedback, and provide instruction in self-advocacy skills.

For practitioners, this type of teaching for the full range of children with CVI requires respect for and understanding of a student's abilities, needs, and wishes. It also requires teachers to exercise patience, restraint, flexibility, and informed creativity in instructional design, as they avoid giving unneeded external assistance by gently, consistently, and wisely encouraging the unfolding evolution of self-determination. Self-determination evolves from a variety of developing skills and behaviors into a more sophisticated, integrated system of self-advocacy and independent living unique to each student. Interventions for children with CVI need to be delivered within the framework of a knowledge-based curriculum that encourages the progressive development of self-advocacy and independent living to whatever degree possible, given a child's capabilities.

This conceptual framework applies to the full range of children with CVI, from the very young with severe visual, cognitive, and physical challenges who are learning to use their vision systems in functional tasks, to older children with near-normal binocular functional visual acuity, who are learning academic and independent mobility skills, and to teenagers ready for transition to work or higher education. According to Wehmeyer (1998, p. 10), "There is almost always some aspect of even the most complex activities or tasks, from decision making to goal setting, in which people with significant cognitive disabilities can participate with adequate support and accommodations." Self-determination is fostered by opportunities to exercise and learn self-determination skills, promote maximum participation at home, in school, and in the community, and ensure that appropriate supports and accommodations are in place (Wehmeyer, 1998). Self-determination skills are intertwined with all curricular areas and are addressed throughout a child's school career from early education through high school and beyond.

## Equitable Instructional Practices

### Principles for Optimal Access to Learning

Two frameworks to guide the design of curricula have been developed around principles that are pertinent to the needs of the wide range of children who have damage to the visual brain: universal design and differentiated instruction.

#### *Universal Design*

Universal design can be thought of as design with sufficient flexibility to meet the needs of all users, whether able bodied or having any type of disability. Initially these principles were applied to architectural design. Soon after, they also became associated with the development of technological hardware, software, and other products and systems for use by all. A core tenet is that everyone benefits from approaches that address the diverse needs of the whole population, including people with disabilities (Rose & Meyer, 2002).

Universal design practices that complement the educational goals of curricula and promote self-determination emphasize the following (Connell et al., 1997):

1. Flexible and alternative methods that can accommodate a wide range of preferences and abilities.
2. Designs that are simple and intuitive.
3. Information that is perceptible under a variety of conditions.
4. Methods that readily promote targeted functional actions and minimize hazards.
5. Designs that optimize physical comfort to minimize fatigue.
6. Methods that conform to space and size requirements of specific situations.

In addition, McKillop and Dutton (2008) recommend designs that minimize sensory distractions to be particularly relevant for children with CVI.

#### *Differentiated Instruction*

Children are different and learn in different ways, and a variety of methods and options for learning need to be easily accessible to all children in a classroom. Meshing instruction to each child's readiness, interests, and learning profiles, rather than requiring the whole class to adjust to a fixed presentation format, is the guiding principle of differentiated instruction (Tomlinson & McTighe, 2006). According to Tomlinson (2000), four elements needed to meet the diverse learning needs of students and engage them in learning can be differentiated:

- Content—what is learned and how information is accessed
- Process—activities leading to content understanding and mastery
- Products—projects that review, apply, and extend what has been learned
- Learning environment

Differentiation of instruction is intimately connected with a curriculum that facilitates self-determination since differentiated instruction furthers and supports a learner's basic capacities, provides supportive learning environments, and offers options for personal choice. These methods also align with the goals of universal design for learning (UDL), which incorporates a system that broadens the concept of universal design to include learning material, curricula, and activities for children (Hall, Strangman, & Meyer, 2011).

### Equitable Access to Curricula, Materials, and Activities

Individualized instruction, a hallmark of special education, tailors instruction and learning environments to meet the unique needs of each child. Differentiated instruction goes beyond the design of instruction for individual students and shapes the entire classroom climate such that intervention and environmental options are available to all children in a classroom.

Around the globe there is a movement toward inclusive education, where children with special needs are taught alongside general education peers rather than in more segregated settings. As part of this educational trend, it is important to consider environmental design, and the incorporation of curricula, materials, and activities that contain options to enhance learning, not only for children with special needs, but also for all children in typical school placements. This is particularly relevant for the large numbers of children with CVI who are expected to participate in standards-based, general education curricula. These children would most certainly benefit from the availability of learning options within general education, and from environmental modifications that provide full access to media, curricula, and activities (Williams et al., 2011).

### Equitable Access to Learning Environments

While modifications for children with disabilities to participate in learning have often focused on curricular content, organization, materials, and activities, both differentiated instruction and universal design principles emphasize the role of environmental influences on teaching and learning (Hall et al., 2011). This is especially important for children with CVI since environmental factors can exert a strong influence on their access to the curriculum and to learning. In addition, the mode, degree, and amount of varied sensory input can affect learning processes for these children. Elements such as ambient background sound, sound levels, visual distraction and clutter, lighting and glare, visibility of terrain features (surface changes, stairs, drop-offs), and the visibility of school or classroom features (decorations, signs, posters) can all pose barriers to learning for children with CVI when not optimally designed.

Environmental factors that can be potential barriers to perception, attention, and learning need to be adjusted in ways that turn them into potential learning supports for all children including those with CVI. Methods to provide optimal environments for children with CVI as well as measures to minimize the impact of negative environmental influences are discussed throughout this book, and are found specifically in Chapter 22.

## Development of Optimal Instructional Strategies

Instructional strategies to promote success in learning, as well as participation in activities in school, at home, and in the community, now and in the future, require careful foresight and planning by educational teams involving the children and their families. Methodologies particularly applicable to children who have CVI are highlighted in this section.

## Diagnostic Teaching

Little is known about the types of skills and behaviors most amenable to training for children with CVI, but there are indications that direct teaching of basic skills and behaviors can lead to positive outcomes for children (Brunsdon, Nickels, Colthear, & Joy, 2007; Lanners, Piccioni, Fea, & Goergen, 1999; Love, 1994; Lueck, 2006; Lueck, Dornbusch, & Hart, 1999; Malkowicz, Myers, & Leisman, 2006; Roman-Lantzy & Lantzy, 2010; Werth & Seelos, 2005). Since the evidence base for the effects of intervention is just beginning to emerge, it is, at this time, recommended that a simplified form of diagnostic teaching, an approach that integrates assessment with intervention (Valencia & Wixson, 1991), is used as the cornerstone for the development of appropriate instructional strategies for these children. (The guiding principles of diagnostic teaching [Koenig & Holbrook, 1989, 1995] are discussed in Chapters 10, 15, and 16.) In addition, since different strategies work for different children, and strategies may not continue to be effective over time, constant monitoring and evaluation of the effectiveness of the solutions and strategies applied is also recommended (Macintyre-Béon et al., 2010), consistent with a diagnostic teaching approach.

In diagnostic teaching, hypotheses are formulated about ways to promote students' performance based on available assessment data. Interventions are then designed, based on these hypotheses, as in the following example:

**FIVE-YEAR-OLD STEVIE HAS DIFFICULTY LOCATING OBJECTS** within groups of items because of simultanagnosia (the inability to pick out and thus recognize multiple elements in a visual presentation) resulting from CVI. He also does not often ask for assistance since he does not want to stand out from his peers in class. Moreover, he cannot know to ask questions about things he has not seen. The following intervention hypothesis has been formulated for Stevie based on these behaviors:

> *In the classroom, Stevie will read for longer durations during free-reading time, when storybooks at his reading level that he can readily access are placed on a separate shelf so that he is able to find them without help.*

This desired teaching method is implemented, accompanied by observation and data collection to evaluate the outcome. This method allows constant review of outcomes, promoting refinement of further procedures to accord with Stevie's learning needs.

Observations include an examination of factors related to both the learner and all aspects of the learning environment. Data may be quantitative or can be running logs of student outcomes and environmental conditions, depending on the activities under scrutiny. Results can be entered on data-collection record sheets (such as, for Stevie, a table that includes columns for day, time, how long Stevie reads, and how often he accesses books on the special shelf), or results can be entered as a running text log of events by date, for example:

> On Monday, Stevie read for two minutes when he tried to read a book that he found on the floor. He spent a lot of time looking around at what other students were doing. On Tuesday, Stevie read for seven minutes when he chose to read a book of interest on his special shelf. He occasionally glanced at other students but returned to his book until free reading time was over.

If the new approach does not lead to improved outcomes for students, the data collected along the way can be used to help reformulate hypotheses and revise the intervention protocols. These "experiments" in teaching, when systematically analyzed, lead to methods that optimally promote learning. (Additional examples of diagnostic teaching can be found in Chapter 15 related to literacy and math instruction, Chapter 16 related to independent living skills instruction, and Chapter 21 related to instruction in the use of functional vision for young children and those with multiple impairments.)

## Functional and Meaningful Activities

The provision of instruction that facilitates a child's completion of tasks that contribute to successful performance of functional and meaningful activities in usual environments—school, home, community, and workplace—is also a part of a curriculum to promote self-determination. Successful completion of functional and meaningful tasks is another key to independence and sense of self-worth. Functional and meaningful activities are determined by a child's needs and preferences, and also take into account cultural and family values.

Such activities need to be age appropriate for children who have cognitive delays. For example, a teenager who needs to learn to sort by shape can learn this skill by sorting cups and plates onto shelves in a kitchen cabinet after they have been washed and dried at the end of lunch. To promote this goal of sorting, skills and behaviors targeted for instruction have been embedded into this functional and meaningful activity to increase the teenager's motivation to engage in a sorting experience. A focus on critical tasks (tasks that a child must perform during typical activities) provides opportunities for the child to practice skills and behaviors as they arise naturally during typical daily routines and increases the chances of successful task completion.

It is critical that caregivers and school personnel coordinate their efforts through careful discussions with much give-and-take, so that the strategies used in critical tasks are optimal. Care must be taken to ensure that strategies used in one setting for a particular routine are applied in similar ways in other settings to reinforce desired behaviors and to reduce conflicting signals to a child. Routines or activities at school or in the home in which instruction can be infused include the following:

- playtime or leisure time routines at school or home
- playground routines
- personal hygiene routines including bath time for young children
- reading and math activities
- classroom routines
- transition routines from one activity to the next at school and home
- school cafeteria routines
- travel routines at school and home
- eating routines at school or home
- vocational education routines
- sporting activities
- music activities

**In another example, learning to select and sort** red and yellow cubes is one way to teach color discrimination and matching to a 15-year-old student, Joseph, who has CVI and developmental challenges. But this may not be the most motivating activity that could be devised for him, as it is not tied to a meaningful activity. Furthermore, practice with cubes is not an everyday activity and may not generalize to other tasks requiring color discrimination and matching as critical elements for successful completion.

A more powerful instructional design for Joseph, who enjoys helping in the school office, is one that involves a daily activity there. As a consequence, he is asked to sort red and yellow student passes that permit students to leave class for special projects. Here Joseph is learning to discriminate, match, and sort on a regular basis. He is also completing a pre-vocational task in which he learns responsibility, gaining a sense of accomplishment and connection with the school office staff and other students. Other such tasks that include color discrimination, matching, and sorting to further extend Joseph's use of color are warranted.

Interventions to deal with the effects of CVI need to be incorporated into functional and meaningful activities as soon as possible, as in the following examples:

**A 3-YEAR-OLD CHILD, IRINA, LEARNED TO FOLLOW A** favorite, self-illuminated toy in a dimly lit room, and later learned to follow a favorite toy that did not light up in typical lighting conditions as her skills increased. Visual following skills, as they developed, were quickly embedded into functional and meaningful activities throughout the school day for Irina to practice, generalize their application to a variety of tasks, and reinforce learning. For example, visual following was encouraged as Irina watched a light-colored spoon against a dark, contrasting background as it is moved from her applesauce to her mouth by her teacher during daily snack time. The spoon, at its furthest viewing distance, was wider than the size of the equivalent stripe on the Teller Acuity Card at that same distance that Irina could see; therefore Irina was likely to see it. The teacher knew to vary the location from which the spoon moved from the side to Irina's mouth in order to reduce Irina's habituation to the path of the spoon's movement. Visual following was also encouraged as Irina followed the movements of a large puppet in a daily puppet show presented 4 feet away in her preschool class. Each of the puppet's facial features were matched in size to those that Irina could readily see at that distance.

---

**ROBERTO, A 16-YEAR-OLD WITH CVI, HAS 20/60 (6/18)** visual acuity in both eyes and loves to read. His reading speed slows down considerably, however, in his history class when he has to read crowded text material for an extended period of time. He is now learning to use line markers and typoscopes (reading windows cut in a piece of cardboard or plastic) to facilitate his reading efficiency. He started using these adaptations with one-page handouts in his classes, an immediate functional task. He then applied the techniques to more lengthy text material in his recreational reading and his school textbooks. He later learned to read textbooks and leisure reading material with the assistance of electronic devices that have built-in mechanisms to underscore, highlight, and section off print.

## Task Analysis to Promote Learning

Task analysis has been found to be an effective, systematic tool for analyzing and teaching skills and behaviors that are naturally embedded into functional and meaningful activities to address learning goals and objectives. This process has been shown to facilitate learning outcomes for children who have learning disabilities (Swanson, 1999) and is also a basic component of instruction for students who have multiple disabilities (Udvari-Solner, Causton-Theoharis, & York-Barr, 2004). To facilitate teaching and learning via task analysis, tasks can be broken down into their component parts. This is done systematically by identifying a sequence of task components needed to complete a specific task efficiently by typical students.

Once tasks have been analyzed, the next step is to determine which of the subtasks a child with CVI can perform independently and which of the subtasks will require assistance. This process is called *discrepancy analysis* (Brown, Shiraga, York, Zanella, & Rogan, 1984; Falvey, 1995). While discrepancy analysis was developed for students with moderate to severe impairments, it is useful to apply the methods in this system to children with CVI who might have subtle performance constraints that can be addressed using adapted methods or materials. Discrepancy analysis enables the practitioner to pinpoint precise task components that are presenting difficulties and that might inadvertently be overlooked as targets for instruction. This may include such variables as the visibility, order, or cognitive or physical demands of task elements. In task analysis, task components are ones that are observable and lend themselves to objective measurement. Here is an example:

**TEN-YEAR-OLD MING-YU HAS 20/100 (6/30) VISUAL** acuity with both eyes viewing. She experiences difficulty walking through crowded areas and seeing fast-moving objects. She wants to walk from her classroom to the slide equipment on the playground at recess when there are many children and much activity. An abbreviated analysis of the observable tasks that typical peers complete to reach the slide is as follows:

1. Go out the back door of the classroom and turn right.
2. Travel along the walkway along the school building.
3. Stop when the opening in the playground fence is reached on the left and enter the playground.
4. Walk about 50 feet (about 15 meters) at a 45-degree angle toward the play equipment through open space.
5. Enter the play equipment area and negotiate through the equipment toward the slide at the far end.

When the playground was empty, Ming-Yu learned the route from beginning to end and was able to complete the task without external assistance.

This process, moving through the stages at the beginning of a task, one by one, to the end stage, is called *forward chaining*. Learning the stages from the end toward the beginning is call *backward chaining*. Backward chaining can be used with a child who cannot readily learn the full sequence of tasks from beginning to end. The child can experience immediate success by learning and performing the last step independently and then achieving the overall goal. Later, the child can learn the additional steps, moving backward in the sequence, learning one step at a time.

**MING-YU DOES NOT NEED ASSISTANCE WHEN THE PLAY**ground is empty, but she does need assistance when the walkway and playground areas are crowded, noisy, and full of children who are running in different directions and playing ball games. At these times, Ming-Yu is overwhelmed by all the noise and activity, cannot anticipate moving hazards along the route, and cannot see fast-moving targets—all behavioral consequences of her form of CVI. A long cane for mobility was considered, but it was found that Ming-Yu was still unable to sort out the cacophony of sounds and sights to operate safely with the long cane in the noisy playground setting. For safety and to instill confidence, she now walks with a classmate directly to the playground equipment area, the last task in the sequence, in order to play on a slide at recess.

The situation changes, however, when the children on the playground "freeze" at the sound of a whistle from a playground monitor at the end of recess and quietly walk back to class in a single line. Now, Ming-Yu can complete the slightly altered return route to her classroom on her own. She can reach the edge of the playground equipment, walk at an angle through the open space to join the line of quiet children, and follow the line toward her classroom. Ming-Yu has learned the sequence of the return route to her class and can complete every step independently at the end of recess.

For the route from her classroom to the playground during recess, Ming-Yu cannot complete all the steps of the task, and requires assistance. This process is called *partial participation*, and it occurs when a student can participate in a task but cannot complete all of its component parts independently. In Ming-Yu's situation, assistance is required at some times but not others. A careful review of Ming-Yu's abilities, task requirements, and environmental conditions led to instructional strategies that provided the appropriate amount of assistance at the right times—neither too much nor too little. This allowed Ming-Yu to participate in a favorite activity with her peers, even when she could not complete all the component parts of a task to reach the activity independently. Along with the instruction for Ming-Yu, her peers have also had instruction in order to learn when Ming-Yu needs assistance and how to offer help when needed and in a respectful way.

## Incorporating Skills and Behaviors into Intervention Goals

To achieve students' successful performance of functional and meaningful tasks, activities must be evaluated to determine the underlying abilities, skills, and behaviors needed to perform them and whether the complex interplay of visual, physical, cognitive, and psychosocial capabilities that the child brings to each task in an activity is sufficient to complete them independently (see Figure 19.1). When a

FIGURE 19.1

**The Intervention Process to Develop Complex Skills and Behaviors in Functional and Meaningful Activities**

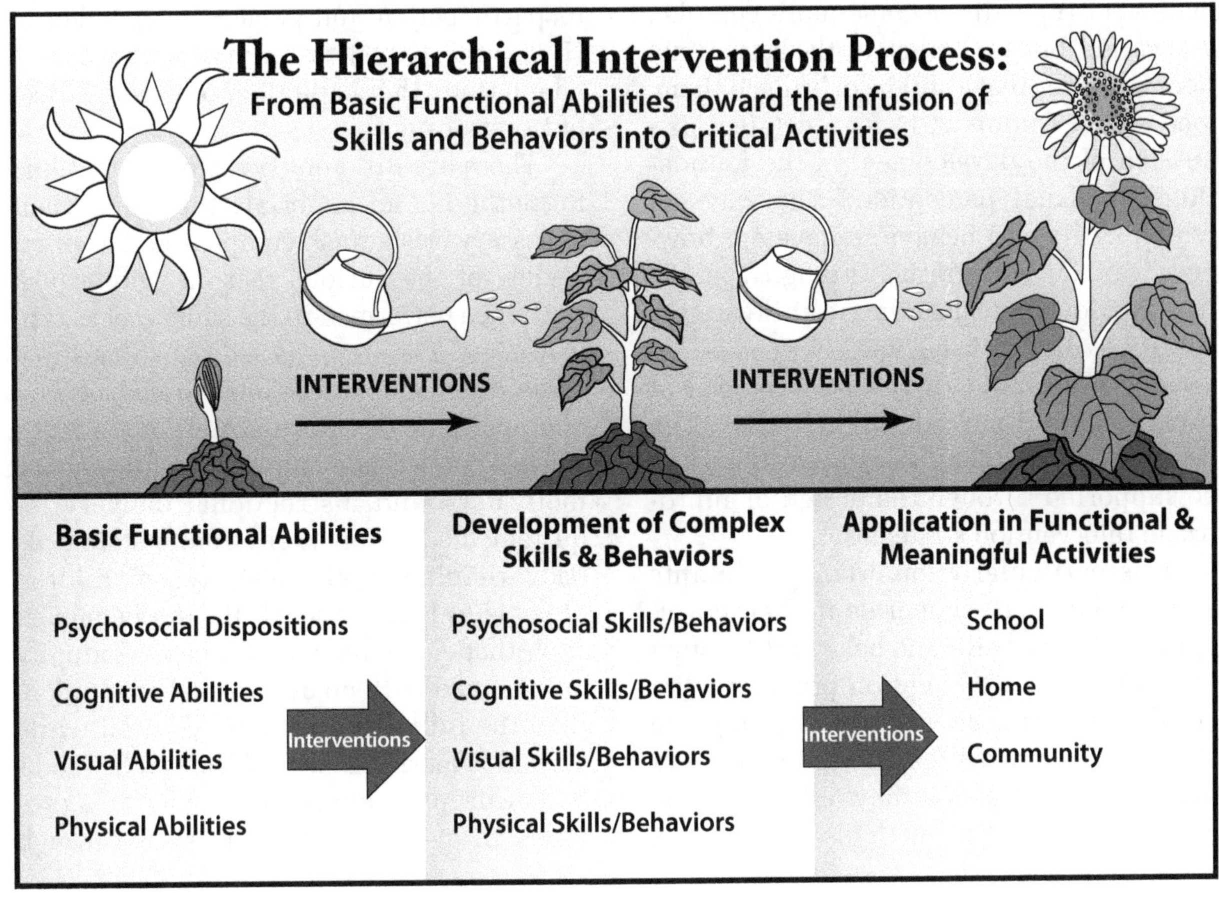

child does not have the underlying abilities, skills, and behaviors to complete a desired task, the task can be modified, the requisite materials adapted, or assistance provided to complete it, as described in the next section. Some children who have the necessary psychosocial, cognitive, visual, and physical capabilities to complete a task can learn specific basic skills and behaviors through well-conceived interventions without adaptations along the way or use of alternative methods, materials, or physical assistance as long-term solutions (Lueck, 2004a).

Basic functional abilities are psychosocial, cognitive, visual, and physical traits that a child can draw upon in the performance of basic skills and behaviors needed to interact in a meaningful way in the world. As a child grows and learns, these skills and behaviors typically become more complex and varied, but are limited by the basic functional abilities that a child can bring to them. (See Zihl & Dutton, 2015 for a detailed discussion of the development of the foundations of visual perception.) The ways in which skills and behaviors develop, however, can be encouraged through specific intervention strategies. Once a child attains specific skills and behaviors, they can be applied by the child in the performance of functional and meaningful activities. The depth and breadth of these applications can be supported through the design of appropriate intervention strategies.

It is particularly important for infants and toddlers to be supported in their development of basic skills and behaviors through intensive early intervention programs. If a child is making progress in learning the skills and behaviors that are components of more complex tasks, it may only be necessary to use adaptive methods or materials or to provide direct assistance in the short term until the requisite skills are acquired. Methods to promote the acquisition of basic skills and behaviors for all children with CVI are presented throughout Chapters 15 to 24 of this book.

## Use of Adaptations

Adaptations to educational tasks or the environment are changes that enable a student to participate in classroom activities. Many interventions for children with CVI involve changes that optimize delivery of methods, materials, and response modes. Others result in alteration of the content of lessons or lead to the addition of more instructional or technological support. When training to improve skills or behaviors is not feasible, use of adaptations is the key to participation and greater independence. Hyvärinen (2003) recommends the use of adaptations that capitalize on strong areas of functioning.

There are different types of adaptations to methods and materials that can, when necessary, assist task completion, based on review of the various reasons why a task cannot be performed in the same way as typical peers. For students who have multiple disabilities, adaptations are chosen based on characteristics associated with a student's learning preferences, physical requirements, motivators, and instructional delivery requirements, as well as environmental needs (Udvari-Solner et al., 2004). When children are able to learn basic skills and behaviors such that elements of a task can eventually be executed with no or minimal adaptation, then the initial adaptations required while a child is learning basic skills can be modified or dropped altogether. Figure 19.2 provides an overview of the process through

FIGURE 19.2

**Development of Adaptations for Children with CVI**

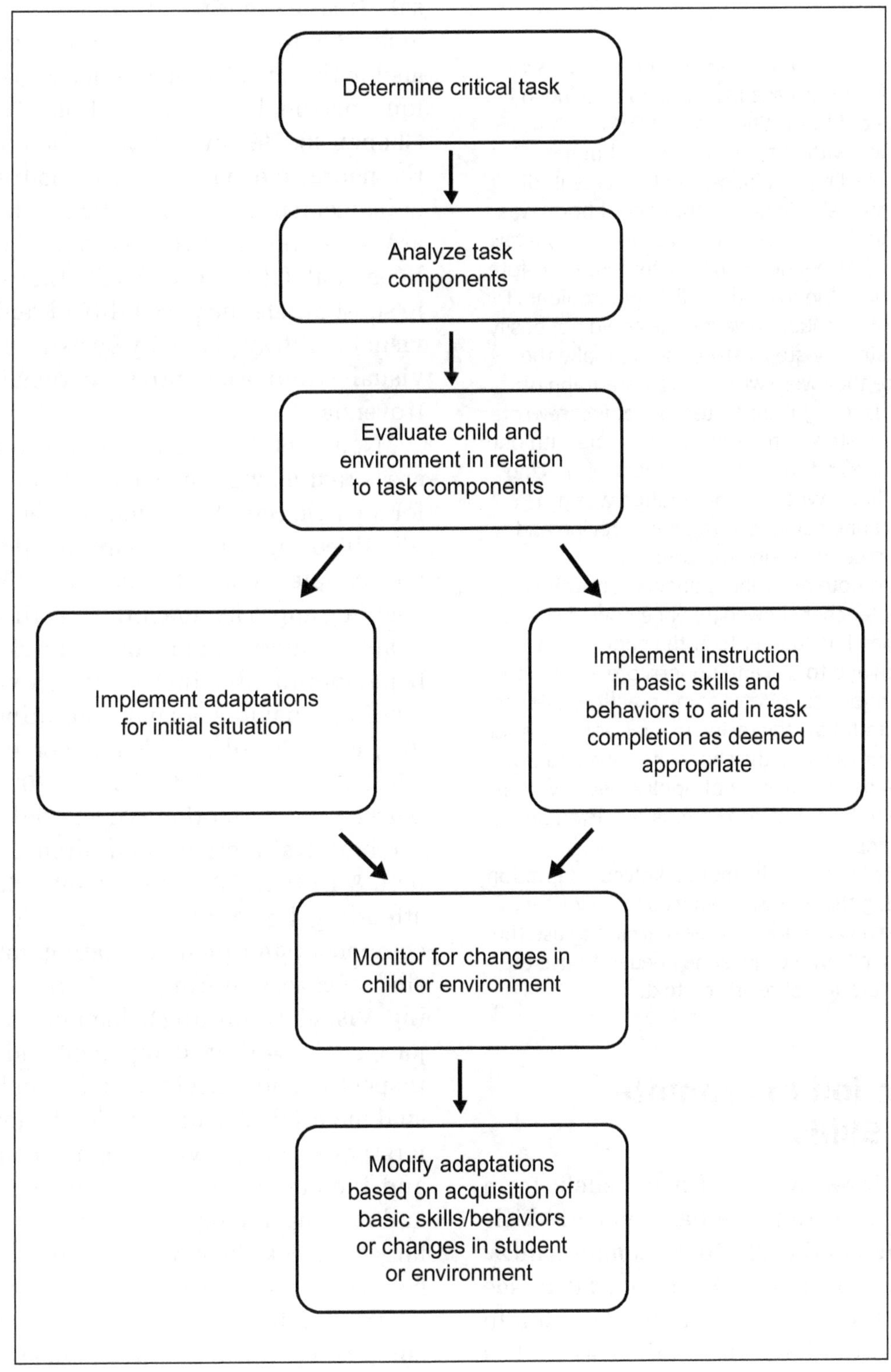

which adaptations are developed, implemented, evaluated, and modified. Here is an example:

**When she was 14, Julienne wanted to learn how to** make a chocolate cake from a simple recipe in her mother's cookbook. She has 20/60 (6/18) functional vision with both eyes viewing, but has difficulty reading continuous text as a result of CVI. The print size in her mother's cookbook was large enough for Julienne to read when only a few words per line needed to be processed. Therefore, Julienne was able to read the list of ingredients for the chocolate cake. However, she could not easily read the step-by-step instructions to make the cake since they were written in a paragraph of continuous text. Julienne's teacher at first rewrote the step-by-step instructions for Julienne with one step per line and with a large amount of spacing between lines. When this adaptation was provided, Julienne could read the entire recipe and had no difficulty making the cake.

To promote more independence, however, Julienne's teacher showed Julienne how to create an L-shaped line marker to fit the page of the cookbook and to use it to underscore and follow the continuous text. After some practice, Julienne was able to follow the recipe in the book using the line marker to make the chocolate cake and other recipes in her mother's cookbook as well, without the need to have the instructions rewritten one step per line.

In this instance, the more involved adaptation of rewriting the text was replaced by a simpler one using a line marker. While learning to use the line marker, however, Julienne needed to use the initial adaptation of rewritten text.

## Instruction to Promote Visual Skills

Some children with CVI may benefit from instruction to improve basic visual skills and behaviors (Lueck, 2006; Roman-Lantzy & Lantzy, 2010; Zihl & Dutton, 2015; see Chapter 5). This is particularly important to explore with infants and toddlers as well as children who have experienced recent neurological injury. Areas associated with dorsal stream function are likely to be more amenable to instruction than areas associated with ventral stream function (G. N. Dutton, personal communication, 2013; see Chapter 3). However, it must be noted that the neural mechanisms responsible for the enhancement of visual skills and behaviors are still under investigation. Macintyre-Béon et al. (2010, p. 176) state that evidence to substantiate the possibility of "enhancing visual pathway plasticity by using a specific visual stimulation program remains controversial."

Nonetheless, it is important to identify areas that may be responsive to instruction for a particular child. Once target areas are identified, instruction can be developed and coupled with the use of a diagnostic teaching approach mentioned earlier in this chapter. Interventions in basic skills and behaviors involve instruction in visual attending behaviors, visual examining behaviors, and visually guided motor behaviors (Hall & Bailey, 1989; Lueck, 2004b). Impaired visual attention is commonly seen in cerebral dysfunction in children (Das, Bennett, & Dutton, 2007; see Chapter 6). Visual attending behaviors have a major visual component and include fixating, following, shift of gaze, scanning, localizing, and tracing. Visual examining behaviors have a major visual-cognitive component and include inspecting, identifying, and matching visual material. Visually guided motor behaviors have a major visual-motor component and include reaching for, turning toward, and moving among obstacles toward visual targets (Lueck, 2004b). For examples of these behaviors, see Figure 19.3.

Instruction in visual skills can be accomplished through (1) changes to the

FIGURE 19.3

**Visual Behaviors of Visually Impaired Children from Birth to Age 2**

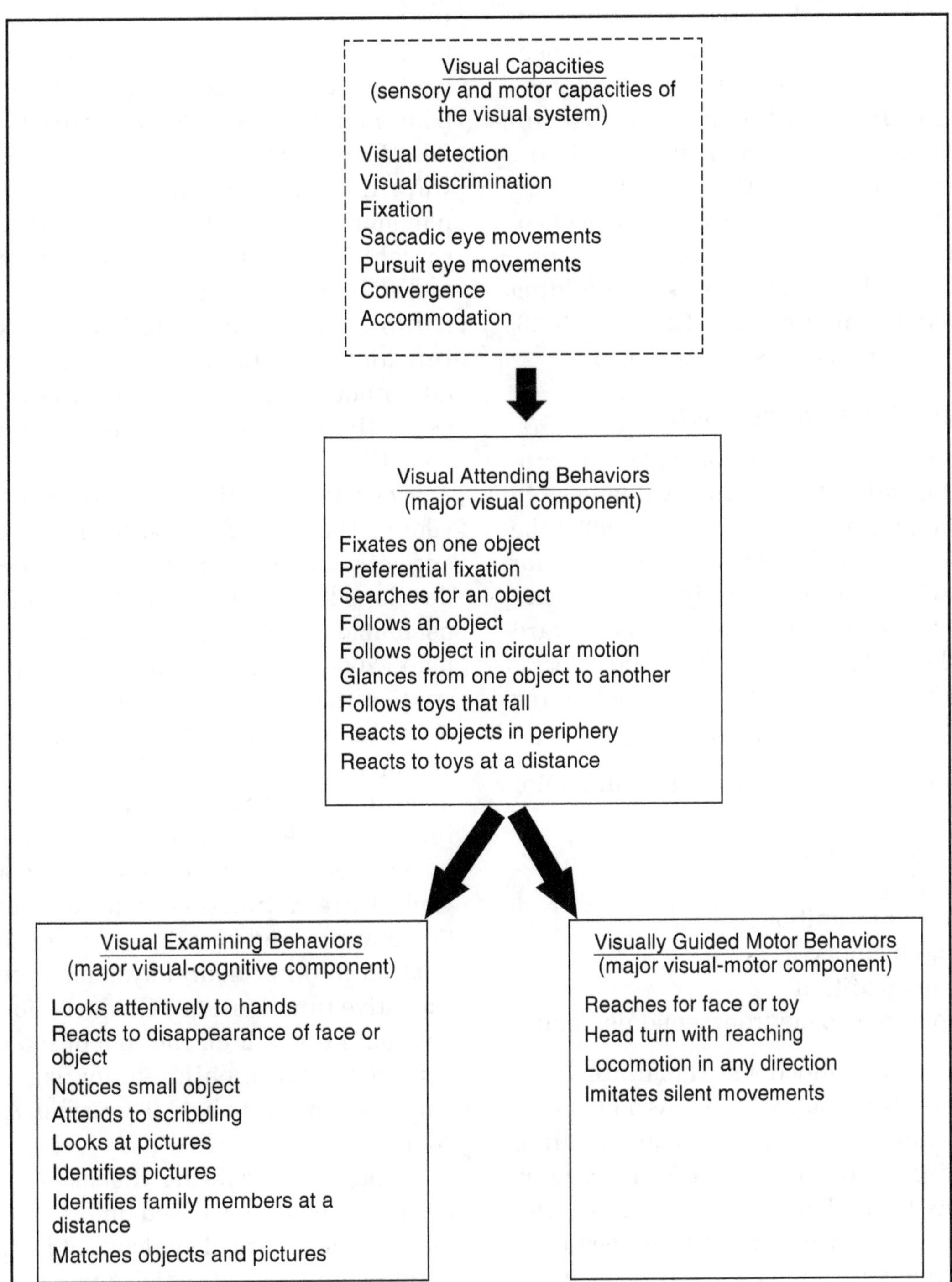


*Source:* Adapted from Hall, A., & Bailey, I. L. (1989). A model for training vision functioning. *Journal of Visual Impairment & Blindness, 83*, 390–396.

visual environment that engage the child and foster the use and development of visual skills, (2) direct instruction in visual attending skills required for the development of more complex visual skills and behaviors, and (3) visually dependent task instruction which applies the use of existing visual skills to tasks the child is to perform. Table 19.1 summarizes key aspects of these three approaches. (Interventions to promote visual skills and their use in children are covered in more detail in Chapters 15, 16, 20, and 21 and in adults in Chapter 24.)

## Models of Vision Instruction

Models of vision instruction have been proposed for individuals who have damage to the visual brain. One by Warren (1993), the Visual Hierarchy Model, was developed for adults with acquired brain injury. Warren's model theorizes that instruction toward higher-level skills evolves from the integration of lower-level skills in the following order from lower to higher:

1. visual acuity, visual field, oculomotor control
2. arousal and attention
3. scanning
4. pattern recognition
5. visual memory
6. visual cognition
7. adaptations to environmental demands

To these can be added visual planning.

Warren's model, which was not tested with children, focuses on visual attending skills linked to accurate shifts in gaze as the basis for higher-order visual skills and behaviors. Scanning training has been used extensively with adults with acquired brain injury as proposed in Warren's model. Adults point to or name individual or patterns of lights in an array in order to learn compensatory head turns to areas of visual field deficit and to identify patterns made by the array of lights. In one example, training then moves on to pencil-and-paper tasks as well as dynamic training in travel tasks (Kingston, Katsaros, Vu, & Goodrich, 2010). See Chapter 24 for more information. The ways in which this approach can be implemented in children needs further research for clarification of systematic methods and outcomes. Zihl and Dutton (2015) present some detailed case reports in which systematic training in scanning and other basic visual skills has been successfully implemented with children who have CVI.

For children with CVI, models of intervention that align fully with current knowledge of visual brain function have yet to be developed, although initial attempts have been made (see Malkowicz, Myers, & Leisman, 2006). This is not surprising since studies that investigate the child's developing brain in the context of holistic use of vision have only recently picked up momentum. Proposed models need to take into account how vision functions develop, as well as the development of dorsal and ventral stream functions. and the coordination of visual and visual processing skills in relation to other neural systems including executive functions. See Chapter 6 for a discussion. Research on the role of the mirror neuron system in children, for example, is only now coming to light (Hyvärinen & Jacob, 2011).

Familiarity training (Lueck & Heinze, 2004) is a technique based on best practices rather than empirical evidence. It is used for children with visual search and recognition difficulties to facilitate a child's ability to discriminate, recognize, and select desired items more accurately from a field of choices.

TABLE 19.1

## Characteristics of Instructional Programs to Encourage Use of Vision

| Description | Target Population | Methods | Examples |
|---|---|---|---|
| ***Visual Skills Instruction*** | | | |
| Instructor-directed training of visual attending behaviors:<br>fixating<br>shifting gaze<br>scanning<br>localizing<br>tracking/following<br>tracing | Students who do not have or have rudimentary visual skills<br>Students recovering from neurological insult (Erin & Paul, 1996)<br>Students who have experienced sensory deprivation (Erin & Paul, 1996) | In isolated setting with intention to fade isolated setting and generalize to usual settings where skills will be applied<br>In functional activities | Training to increase complexity of visual elements in targeted tasks<br>Eccentric viewing training<br>Increasing print-reading efficiency |
| ***Visually Dependent Task Instruction*** | | | |
| Integration of vision into tasks using existing visual skills and behaviors (visual cognitive or visual-motor tasks) | Students who have developed visual skills | Identify key tasks where vision is efficient means for task completion<br>Heighten stimuli as necessary; fade stimuli gradually if possible<br>Direct teaching to encourage application of vision in specific task, pointing out methods and cues for efficient task completion<br>Plan for fading teacher-directed instruction<br>Plan generalization to other settings | Scanning for recipes in cookbook<br>Finding words in dictionary<br>Locating house numbers<br>Using vision to catch a ball |
| ***Visual Environmental Management Instruction*** | | | |
| Within functional tasks<br>In visually altered, naturally occurring environments | Students whose visual skills and behaviors are still developing<br>Students with recent vision loss who are learning to use their visual capabilities | Select or control visual cues to encourage desired visual behaviors<br>Heighten cues or decrease in intensity, depending on training goals<br>Fade heightened cues whenever possible<br>Provide a variety of environmental opportunities to learn skills | Increasing visibility of pictures in books used at free reading time to encourage visual attending<br>Reduce visibility of ball in rolling ball game to increase visual following to low-contrast target and to promote use of non-adapted target for socialization |

*Source*: Adapted from Lueck, A. H. (2004b). Overview of intervention methods. In A. H. Lueck (Ed.), *Functional vision: A practitioner's guide to evaluation and intervention* (pp. 266–267). New York: AFB Press.

It involves instruction in knowing what to look for (salient features) in order to identify objects, pictures, or symbols based on repeated experience with visible targets matched to visual acuity levels. Recognition of critical elements of objects and environments in order to facilitate visual identification is the defining feature of this approach. At higher skill levels, it includes teaching where to look for visual targets as well as features of targets for a visual search. Initial presentations are best in ideal, uncluttered environmental conditions with gradual modifications made as instruction shifts to natural settings (Lueck & Heinze, 2004).

Activities for familiarity training can be integrated into daily routines. For example, working with a child to identify his or her jacket from an array of jackets on hooks in the classroom can begin with a small number of jackets and the identification of critical features that define the child's specific jacket (for example, red jacket). Then a visual search can be made for that one distinctive feature. The number of jackets can be increased as skills improve.

Roman's (2010) CVI Complexity Sequences program for young children and children with major developmental delay involves the identification of images based on their salient features. This program encourages children to identify images that are presented against increasingly complex backgrounds. Familiarity training and the CVI Complexity Sequences program both take into account the associative effects of learning and experience on vision development to teach visual search and recognition strategies, and call for consideration of top-down paradigms for vision instruction that begin with more complex skills and behaviors (Jones, Sinha, Vetter, & Poggio, 1997) as compared to bottom-up strategies that begin with basic visual functions, as proposed in the model by Warren (1993).

## Psychological and Social Implications of CVI for Children

Children with CVI experience their worlds in unique ways. To understand how these children's worlds are constructed is a major goal of interventionists. Only then can they possibly understand why these children operate in atypical ways that are functional for them, and how their behaviors can easily be misunderstood. Children's behaviors may be confounding to teachers, family, and peers who may not be aware of the often subtle, and sometimes not so subtle, effects of CVI. Children's inappropriate actions or words may, for example, be ascribed to maladaptive behavior or simple misbehavior, cognitive impairments, or learning disabilities. As a result, it is extremely important for any intervention program for children with CVI to include instructional strategies that help the child, family, school staff, and peers understand the behavioral consequences of CVI and to teach the child methods to inform others about themselves in socially appropriate ways. Such interventions are specifically addressed in Chapter 23. Sacks (2010, p. 67) has generated some excellent basic points to consider related to the psychological and social implications of low vision, which are adapted here for children with CVI:

- Children who have CVI have varying psychosocial experiences depending on the severity and nature of their CVI as well as the reactions of family and the public.

- The general public may not understand the functional characteristics of CVI and may misinterpret behaviors and needs.
- In most situations, children's ability to communicate clearly to others about their CVI needs will result in more effective social experiences and environmental access; however, children with CVI should carefully consider when, where, and how to disclose this information.
- Family members and professionals who understand the psychosocial needs of children with CVI can facilitate the adjustment process for these children.
- Family members and professionals can promote and support the positive self-identity of children with CVI.

## The Planning Process for Intervention

In planning and implementing interventions for children with CVI, it is critical to have family input and follow-through. All members of the team, including the family, must work toward similar goals for a child and use consistent methods and materials. Instruction must be implemented in consistent ways by the coordinated team, and expectations must also be realistic and consistent. If a method, material, or activity is not working well, this needs to be communicated to all team members, and appropriate adjustments to intervention methodologies need to be made by everyone working with a particular child.

### Comprehensive Overview of How the Child Functions

Assessment results, pulled together by the educational team (see Part 3 of this book), paint a summary picture of ways in which a child functions that address such questions as these:

- What does the child perceive, and what does he or she miss?
- How does the child prefer to interact with his or her world?
- How does the child react in different environments and under different environmental conditions?
- How do internal states affect function (for example, discomfort, sickness, hunger, fatigue, emotions)?
- How are the environments in which the child operates constructed?
- What activities motivate the child?
- What are the child's likes and dislikes?
- What are the child's and family's understanding of CVI and the child's condition?
- What are the child's and family's immediate and future concerns?

This picture is used to better understand how the child functions in different settings and how best to design matching interventions so that they are multidimensional and address the complex interplay of vision and vision processing with other areas of function.

As with assessment of children with CVI, interventions may also need to be multidisciplinary to address diverse learning and environmental needs (Lueck, 2004b). Furthermore, interventions can also address the design of general learning environments to minimize distraction and reduce stress from competing sensory stimuli. Such learning environments, with or without adaptations, can render key elements perceptible for all children in order to promote active participation, interaction, and learning.

## Components of the Instructional Planning Process

All the elements of good teaching enter into the process of intervention. For children with CVI, however, there is a special need to develop strategies that focus on particular abilities and skills, identified through the comprehensive assessment. The components of the intervention planning process can be found in Figure 19.4.

The process of planning for intervention begins once the assessment of functional vision and other sensory abilities has been undertaken to determine perceptual thresholds, limitations in function, and adaptive requirements for methods, materials, and environments. The identification of critical tasks that are meaningful and functional for a specific child is another integral component of the educational assessment process that must be completed. Once critical tasks are identified, each is broken down into its component subtasks via task analysis. The functional demands that each subtask places on the child are determined, then evaluated to find out whether or not the abilities and skills a child brings to it are sufficient. If they are not, then interventions are required. Interventions are selected that promote perception, attention, motivation, understanding, and the coordinated application of skills and behaviors. They are implemented as soon as possible within critical activities and are used to guide the design of optimum general learning environments. Interventions include the following (Lueck, 2004b):

- *Instruction to promote visual skills and their use* (for example, teaching a 4-year-old to visually follow a large, bright ball in a game of catch).
- *Instruction to use and integrate information from all sensory systems* (for example, teaching a 10-year-old child to listen for the rustling of papers of other students in class to know when a silent workbook period is nearly over or teaching a 17-year-old during a mobility lesson to get ready to look for a visual landmark when he smells bread baking from a bakery along the travel route).
- *Instruction in the selection and use of visual adaptations*—changes to the environment that promote the effective use of vision (such as use of large print, color coding, or increased contrast).
- *Instruction in the selection and use of sensory substitutions for vision or supplements to vision* (such as use of the long cane, auditory material, or braille; simultaneous use of vision and audition for reading).
- *Instruction in the application of assistive technologies to maximize vision use* (for example, low-tech line markers or high-tech electronic magnification devices).

The types of interventions chosen will vary with the capabilities of each child and task demands. Here is an example:

**BILLIE JEAN IS A 10-YEAR-OLD GIRL IN FIFTH GRADE WHO** has 20/200 (6/60) visual acuity, reduced lower visual fields, and substantially reduced contrast sensitivity perception. Billie Jean also has problems deciphering visually crowded materials, impaired perception of fast-moving targets, and impaired recognition of facial expressions even when close enough to compensate for her reduced visual acuity. She is a print reader and is enrolled in a regular education class. She identifies people by their voices and salient features such as hair or eyeglasses. She loves art lessons and drawing. Consequently, her assessment team identified her art lesson as a meaningful functional activity for Billie Jean.

Table 19.2 shows an abbreviated analysis of Billie Jean's art lesson made by her teacher

FIGURE 19.4
**The Planning Process for Intervention**

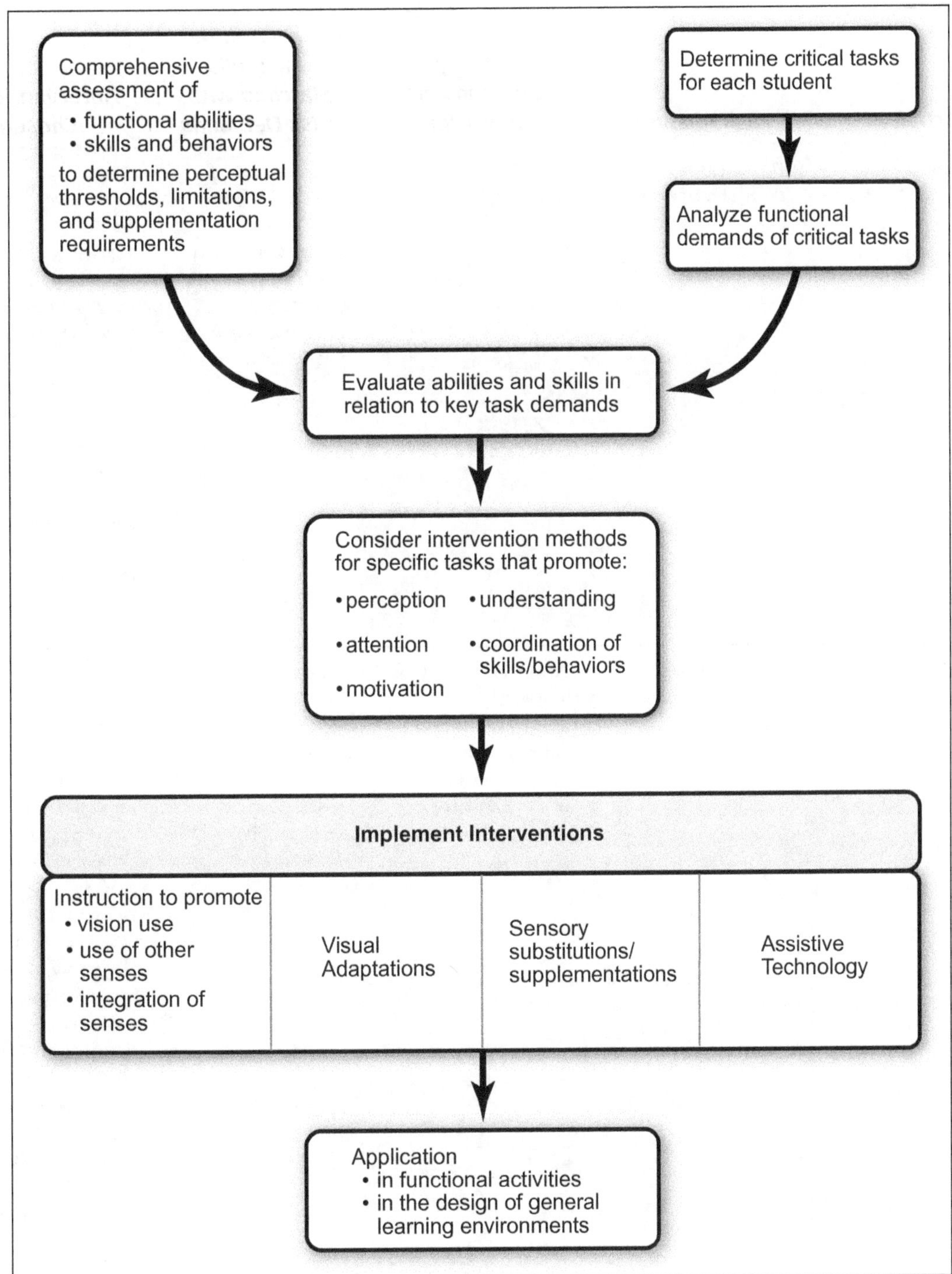

TABLE 19.2

**Identification of Needed Interventions in an Art Lesson for 10-Year-Old Billie Jean**

| *Activity* | *Task Analysis* | *Sensory Demands of Subtasks* | *Child's Abilities and Skills Matched with Task Demands* | *Interventions Chosen* |
|---|---|---|---|---|
| Draw with colored chalk during art lesson | Watch teacher demonstration | View moving target from 3 feet away | Sees faces and facial expressions from 1 foot away<br>Sees slow-moving visual targets only<br>Understands directions when spoken slowly | Student will sit 1 foot away from teacher<br>Teacher will stay in one position rather than moving back and forth in front of class<br>Teacher will summarize directions slowly for all children in class<br>Classroom paraprofessional will move around room to review directions non-intrusively with specific students |
| | Locate and open cupboard with art materials | Walk from desk to cupboard<br>Locate handle on door of cupboard; cupboard and handle are same color as wall | Has reduced lower visual field and often trips on materials left on floor<br>Locates large, single objects readily<br>Has reduced contrast sensitivity | Student's desk will be located at left end of row<br>Walks around desks rather than in between them to avoid tripping on children's items left on floor<br>Bright picture of a paint palette is placed on cupboard to identify it as art cupboard<br>Student is taught to search for handle of cupboard on the right side of palette picture and to trail down the right side of door with right hand until handle is detected tactually |

*(continued on next page)*

**TABLE 19.2** *(continued from previous page)*

| *Activity* | *Task Analysis* | *Sensory Demands of Subtasks* | *Child's Abilities and Skills Matched with Task Demands* | *Interventions Chosen* |
|---|---|---|---|---|
| | Finding art materials in cupboard | Locating small materials in cluttered cupboard | Does not see individual objects within a group of objects visually | Materials in cupboard are spaced apart<br>Areas of cupboard labeled with clear, large letters<br>Student taught words on the labels during previous lessons |
| | Return to seat at desk with art materials | Walk from cupboard to desk<br>Locate desk and chair | Has reduced lower visual fields and often trips on material left on floor<br>Sees desk and chair as a single object | Desk located at left end of row<br>Walks around desks rather than in between them to avoid tripping on children's items left on floor<br>Taught to face right side of room when locates desk, then to locate top of desk tactually to search for chair with left hand |
| | Draw representa-tional picture | Select colored chalk<br>Hand-eye coordination to draw | Picks out desired chalk with primary colors even when they are in a cluster; may not see chalk as individual objects but can see colors<br>No difficulty with hand-eye coordination for drawing | No specific interventions required |

after her functional vision assessment. It reviews the tasks required, the sensory demands of each subtask that may impact Billie Jean's skills and abilities in relation to the sensory demands of each subtask, and the interventions chosen to promote their successful completion. To implement these interventions, Billie Jean's educational team included her general education classroom teacher, a teacher of students with visual impairments, an orientation and mobility specialist, and a paraeducator (classroom assistant) assigned to the general education class.

To maximize Billie Jean's participation in the art lesson, the following strategies were implemented:

- Ensuring that strategies in the task were within her visual acuity capabilities and therefore perceptible
- Direct teaching of vocabulary words so that she could read the labels in the classroom art cupboard
- Direct instruction to both optimize mobility and to locate items within the classroom
- Specific physical placement within the classroom to maximize her independent visual performance
- Occasional assistance by the paraprofessional (classroom assistant) to review her teacher's directions
- Modifications by her general education teacher in the delivery of the lesson (reduced movement, slower pace of verbal directions, all group presentation material rendered visible)
- Modifications to the general classroom environment (bright picture to identify art cupboard)
- Removal of obstacles to mobility on the floor

## Presentation of Lessons

The delivery of instruction requires sensitivity to the many ways to optimize the presentation of lessons to children with CVI so that they are optimally supported to participate fully in learning activities. Interventionists need to choose lessons that are engaging, enjoyable, and motivating. The activities should be pleasurable for both the student and the interventionist! Furthermore, activities need to have content that children with CVI can comfortably perceive and need to be presented in ways that readily enable them to assimilate, understand, and react to the material. Features of formal lessons or constructive play situations must be individualized to meet the needs of each child. The provision of appropriate activities and materials facilitates successful inclusion for children who are in mainstream settings. Some points to consider in the design of learning activities follow.

### Environmental Supports

#### *Examine the Environment*

Is the environment crowded, disorganized, overly colorful with numerous wall hangings, and with many objects hanging from the ceiling? If so, consider adapting to an environment with stations; minimal patterns; cabinets with closed doors or nonpatterned, noncontrasting curtains covering the shelving; nonpatterned rugs on the floor (if allowed) to reduce acoustic feedback; and plain window coverings (shades) to reduce glare from light or snow, and, simultaneously, create an atmosphere of calm. Diffuse lighting is optimal as it minimizes glare and additional patterns resulting from shadows.

### *Categorize Materials*

Place loose items such as markers, scissors, and so forth in closed containers that are all the same color. The containers may be marked on the outside with an object that references the contents, a clear photograph of one of the objects, or a printed word, depending on the students' reading levels.

### *Wear Solid-Colored Shirts without Patterns*

Wearing solid-colored shirts without patterns will help to minimize the difficulty students with CVI may have in separating something the adult is holding from the visual background of his or her clothes. Color-coding staff (having a person significant to the child wear a consistent color scheme so that they are readily identified by clothing color) in school environments for identification purposes is effective only if restricted to one or two staff members who provide major direct services as perceived by the student (such as feeding, changing, or comforting). Such color-coding is restricted by time, place, and routines. It is also important to remember that there is no control outside the classroom in regard to such color-coding of clothing, so children can only be taught to use this system in specific areas for specific people.

### *Eliminate Artificial Aromas*

Artificial aromas (perfume, aftershave lotion, and scented materials) tend to distract students with CVI. They should be avoided, since these students require help to maintain focus rather than additional distractions.

### *Control Type, Intensity, and Duration of Sensory Information*

Students with CVI must be calm and alert so that they are ready to pay attention for the purpose of learning. It is very difficult for many students with CVI to listen, look, and simultaneously plan and implement motor movements. Difficulty with such sensory-motor demands may even extend to reading out loud for those students who have difficulty coordinating the movement of their lips (called oral-motor apraxia). It also is important for adults to keep their own arousal at an appropriate level to establish and maintain the appropriate level of arousal for their students.

## Making Visual Sensory Input Perceptible

To promote engagement in learning activities, it is crucial to use materials that can be readily perceived, given a child's sensory profile. If children cannot see and/or hear a lesson, they do not know what they have missed, and they cannot participate fully in it. For children who have CVI, it is critical to consider not only the actual teaching materials, but also the ways in which the surrounding learning environment may affect perception and attention.

Factors to consider that affect the visual presentation of lessons vary with the needs of each child and include the following:

- size
- color
- movement
- contrast
- lighting and glare
- positioning of the student and materials to maximize use of available visual fields
- arrangement of objects, pictures, or print
- adjustments for insufficient accommodation
- use of icons

### *Size*

Learning materials need to be presented at a size that is readily visible at required viewing distances. Materials should be approximately 2 to 5 times above the child's visual acuity limit (called threshold acuity; see Chapter 12) to ensure that viewing of visual tasks is comfortable and attention to them can be sustained (Topor, Lueck, & Smith, 2004). The size of print above visual acuity threshold that each child requires (referred to as *visual reserve*) is individually determined.

For example, it is determined that, under typical classroom lighting conditions, the *smallest* high-contrast object 4-year-old Nila can see at a distance of 12 inches (30.5 centimeters) has a height of 2 inches (5 centimeters). The size of this object at that distance is at her visual acuity threshold. To see things without straining, Nila's teacher has determined that materials presented to Nila should be at least 3 times larger than her visual threshold so that she sees them easily. As a result, materials held at a 12-inch distance for Nila need to be at least 6 inches high (3 x 2 inches = 6 inches, or 15.25 centimeters) for comfortable viewing to promote learning. (See Table 19.3 for additional examples of the relationship between object size and viewing distance.) If Nila's learning materials are too small, she will tire from her learning task very quickly. If they are too large, she will not be able to work with them efficiently.

It is important to remember that the size of material to be presented must be related to viewing distance. If Nila's learning material is held at 24 inches (61 centimeters) or twice as far, then the size of the material presented to Nila must also be doubled to ensure that Nila can still see it, as shown in Table 19.3. If viewing distance is tripled, then the object size must also be tripled.

This rule of thumb related to size and distance also holds when considering optimal print size for reading, as in the follow-

TABLE 19.3

**Relationship between Object Size and Viewing Distance for Nila**

| | *Object Size* | *Viewing Distance* |
|---|---|---|
| **Part 1: Determination of optimal size for viewing from visual threshold for Nila** | | |
| Visual threshold at 12 inches for Nila | 2 inches (5 cm) | 12 inches (30.48 cm) |
| Optimal size for viewing by Nila is determined to be 3 times visual threshold by Nila's teacher | 6 inches (15.25 cm) | 12 inches (30.48 cm) |
| **Part 2: Size changes when viewing distance changes for Nila's optimal size of 6-inch object viewed at 12 inches** | | |
| Viewing distance doubled, so object size is doubled for Nila | 12 inches (30.5 cm) | 24 inches (61 cm) |
| Viewing distance tripled, so object size is tripled for Nila | 18 inches (46 cm) | 36 inches (91 cm) |

ing example. (See Appendix 12A for print size equivalents in different measurement units such as M-notation, which signifies the print size in metric units and is a consistent way to represent letter height for measuring reading acuity [Greer, 2004].)

**RONALD'S TEACHER DETERMINES THAT HIS VISUAL ACUITY** threshold for reading is 1M (9 point) Times New Roman print held at 6 inches (15.25 centimeters) when both size and distance are considered. She also determines that Ronald requires 2 times the visual threshold size to read comfortably at any viewing distance. As a result, Ronald is given 2M (18 point) Times New Roman print that is held at 6 inches. If Ronald's reading material is held at twice the distance of 12 inches (30.5 centimeters), then the most comfortable print size of 2M must be doubled to 4M (36 point) to arrive at the optimal size print for that longer distance. At 18 inches, or 3 times the original distance (3 x 6 inches = 18 inches), Ronald's optimal print size is 6M or 54 point (3 x 2M = 6M print).

It should be noted that the size of print above visual threshold that each child requires (called *visual reserve*) is individually determined. For example, another child, Marcus, may function optimally with print that is three times greater than his visual threshold.

### *Color*

The ability to see color is often spared in children with CVI (Good et al., 1994). Many practitioners, in anecdotal reports, indicate that children with CVI have specific color preferences, particularly for red and yellow, but it is best to determine any color preferences on an individual basis. The use of color has been shown to attract and maintain attention in one study for children with CVI (Cohen-Maitre & Haerich, 2005), but preference for one color over another was not noted in the forced-choice preferential looking tasks administered by these researchers. The use of consistent color-coding of learning materials was recommended, however, so that children can differentiate items by their prominent color (Cohen-Maitre & Haerich, 2005). In addition, color-coding or outlining visual targets in color has been encouraged as a best practice to help students locate words on a page of text or pictures on a worksheet.

### *Movement*

In addition to color, and perhaps more compelling than color, movement has also been found to attract and maintain attention for many students with CVI (Cohen-Maitre & Haerich, 2005). Simultaneous presentation of color and movement cues may further attract a child's attention. However, there are also some children with CVI who have difficulty attending to objects that are moving quickly (Dutton, 2003; see also Chapter 3).

Since the ability to see movement of visual targets (either stationary or fast-moving) can be a concern for children with CVI, it may be necessary to adjust the presentation of visual targets with respect to movement: (1) targets may need to be moving to optimize the use of vision (or the child may need to move, or move his or her head while looking), (2) the rate of speed of moving objects may require adjustment, or (3) objects may need to be stationary to engage the visual system. If any of these adjustments are to be implemented to optimize visual presentations, they must be individually determined. If a child has specific stimulus requirements related to movement, then these must be incorporated into learning strategies and be explained to the child, peers, family, educational team, and others.

### *Contrast*

The ability to detect differences between the brightness of two adjacent surfaces is called contrast sensitivity. Black on a white background or white on a black background have the highest contrast. This visual function can be affected in some children with CVI. These children require that objects, pictures, or printed matter have intrinsic high contrast, and they must be presented against a high-contrast background in order for the children to see them readily. Not all children with CVI require high-contrast materials; this needs to be determined via the assessment process.

### *Lighting and Glare*

Good lighting helps all children, but it can be especially important for children who have CVI. Lighting should be sufficient to view learning materials and also minimize the effects of glare. This means that light from a directional lamp should not be directed into the eyes of a child, nor should it dazzle by reflecting from a surface directly into a child's eyes. Lighting in general should be diffuse, such that it reflects off surfaces in many directions. In addition, some children may function best in bright light conditions without glare, leading to increased acuity or speed of visual processing. Others have found that children with cortical visual impairment see better in dim light conditions (Good & Hou, 2006). Some children may also have difficulty adapting to changes in light levels (going from a dark area indoors to a sunny area outdoors or vice versa).

Glare may be uncomfortable to all children but can be especially troublesome for some children who have CVI with light sensitivity. Outdoors, glare can be a major issue in orientation and mobility (Ludt, 1997; Smith & Geruschat, 2010). Sunshades (filters) can be used to limit the effects of some forms of glare outdoors (and sometimes indoors), as can hats with wide brims. Since filters or sunshades reduce the amount of light in general, it is important to work with the eye care specialist to choose the best type of filter or sunshade. Methods to optimize lighting and reduce the effects of glare in indoor environments include the following:

- Use directional lamps with opaque shades for viewing learning materials that are positioned so the light rays do not shine directly into children's eyes
- Position children facing away from windows
- Reduce glare from windows with the use of curtains, shades, or blinds
- Position young children or those with mobility problems who spend time on their backs so that they are not directly under bright ceiling lights
- Place light-colored learning material on a dark surface that absorbs light
- Use paper that does not reflect light; consider cream or buff colors with a matte finish
- Use sunshades (filters) indoors after consultation with an eye care specialist
- Work in north-facing classrooms (in the Northern Hemisphere, and vice versa in the Southern Hemisphere)

### *Positioning the Student and Material to Maximize Use of Available Visual Fields*

Children with CVI may have reduced fields of vision or they may pay reduced attention to certain quadrants of their visual field (their "fields of visual attention"). As a result, they may need to be positioned or have their viewing material placed in ways that maximize the field of vision that they commonly use. If children have a left or right visual field or attentional deficit, desktop school materials, for example, should be placed more toward the side of their functional visual field. If a child has a reduced left visual field then the child should sit toward the left side of the classroom to maximize use of the right visual field. Many children with hemianopias will move their head or eyes to compensate for their field loss, and they will function quite well with this biobehavioral adaptation.

The occipital lobes serve the visual field with respect to the eyes. This is often not the case for children who have reduced visual attention on one or the other side. In such cases, the posterior parietal lobes serve visual attention with respect to the body, and it is these children who have greatest need for visual information to be presented off-center to the functioning side (see Chapter 3), perhaps rotating the chair at the desk so that the attended visual field is widened (as shown in Figure 3.3). Appropriate positioning is therefore extremely important for children who experience visual inattention. Mixed visual field impairment with inattention is not uncommon.

In addition, if a child has a reduced lower visual field affecting reading, then reading material should be elevated so that it is within the available field of vision. This especially applies to children who have cerebral palsy accompanied by lower field impairment, difficulty with head control, and are in wheelchairs. These children need to work with physical and occupational therapists to determine methods to position learning materials on their wheelchair trays or to determine special adaptations to their trays that make optimal use of their sighted areas, preventing presentation of material in locations where it is not accessible.

### *Arrangement of Objects, Pictures, or Print*

Children with CVI who exhibit simultanagnosia or similar problems may have difficulty operating within complex visual scenes (see Chapter 3). When there is such "visual clutter," a child may not see single elements in a group of adjacent visual targets. For these children, it is important to separate or spread out visual elements in learning materials so that children can distinguish the individual elements. For example, play areas with toys on shelves may need to be simplified to a few toys spread out along the shelf. Workbooks may need to be simplified by eliminating some nonessential lines in pictures or nonessential print to make individual elements easier to discriminate. A piece of dark-colored construction paper can be used to cover portions of a page or diagrams to reduce the visible elements on a worksheet, book, or drawing. A typoscope (reading window) can be used to show sections of print as the child reads. Optical magnifiers also reduce the amount of material that is viewed at one time. Settings on electronic magnifiers can be arranged so that only a small segment of text, a line of text, or a section of a line of text is visible to the child at one time, thereby reducing visual clutter. Words or sentences can also be presented in a serial format (see Chapter 18).

### *Adjustments for Insufficient Accommodation*

Children with CVI may have difficulty focusing on material that is held at close range as a result of accommodation insufficiency (inability to maintain clear focus as viewing distance varies) (see Chapters 9 and 12). Without the proper spectacle correction, these children must be presented with near range material at a greater distance than typical children of the same age so that their eyes can focus on it and the material is not blurred. An optical prescription for viewing at close distances (reading eyeglasses) has the advantage of bringing near material into focus and magnifying it somewhat, both by its proximity and as a result of the properties of the spectacles themselves. This also diminishes visual crowding.

If a child requires both a distance and near prescription, it is important to work with the ophthalmologist or optometrist to determine if the near prescription should be provided in the form of a separate pair of eyeglasses, as part of a bifocal prescription, or as varifocal (progressive) lenses that also facilitate optimal intermediate viewing (see Chapter 9). If children have head or eye movement control issues or severe cognitive challenges, a separate pair of eyeglasses for near work may be the best solution. If children cannot wear eyeglasses, then the best distance for reading material at close range needs to be determined so that it is not blurry and is an optimal size to facilitate viewing and learning.

#### *Use of Icons*

Icons are visual symbols that reference an activity, object, action, or emotion. Some icons are used as universal signs (stop sign, or images on roadside signs for railroad tracks or curvy road) while others become communication systems for people who cannot use speech and do not read in a traditional manner. With students who have CVI, it is important to be cautious in using icons as they are visually complex and tend to be very small and crowded together with a kaleidoscope of colors that can add to the visual complexity. Use clear photographs and print that are known to be within the child's visual and cognitive capabilities (see Sidebar 12.2 for guidelines).

### Making Auditory Sensory Input Perceptible

As with the visual aspects of lessons, materials, and the environment, it is important to consider auditory factors such as the following and adjust them to each child's needs:

- pace of auditory input
- modulation of voice
- adjustments for competing auditory stimuli

#### *Pace of Auditory Input*

If a child has difficulty assimilating vocal input, verbal information or instructions need to be presented at a pace that promotes perception, understanding, integration, and response. That pace will depend on the abilities of the child, the type of information to be conveyed, environmental circumstances (level of visual and auditory distractions), and the child's biobehavioral state (fatigue level, illness, hunger, emotions, interest in task).

Many students with CVI have difficulty when presented with a barrage of language, especially multiple and extensive verbal directives. These students do better when attention is gained and directives are at the right speed, kept simple and short, and perhaps, repeated exactly the same way a second time. Allow a respectful and uninterrupted amount of time for auditory processing and for the student to plan and execute a response. Repeating the direction too quickly may result in a loss of what the student partially processed, as attention is drawn to what appears to be "new" information. Should confusion be apparent, it might help to ask the student to repeat what was heard to be the direction before automatically repeating it. This will highlight where confusion may be found. It is important to match communication speed to the child's information processing speed.

### *Modulation of Voice*

It often also helps to heighten modulations (changes) in speed, pitch, cadence, and emphasis for young children or children with cognitive challenges to attract and maintain their interest in and attention to a task or activity.

### *Adjustments for Competing Auditory Stimuli*

Some children with CVI may have auditory processing issues in addition to visual processing issues (Morse, 2012). For these children, it is important that the amount of competing auditory information be kept to a minimum. This can pose a problem at home, for example, when a television is on during family conversations, or at school in busy classrooms, school cafeterias, hallways during class change time between periods, and on active, boisterous playgrounds. When competing auditory input cannot be reduced, alternative ways for children to access their learning materials and environments can be considered, depending on each child's needs and the situation.

## Duration and Speed of Presentation

How quickly material is presented and for how long also affects the ability of children with CVI to process what they are seeing and hearing. Adaptations can include the following:

- Reducing the duration of presentation
- Providing breaks during instruction
- Increasing time to respond
- Slowing the pace of overall presentation

### *Reducing the Duration of Presentation*

Children with CVI may tire more quickly from visual tasks than typical peers. High demand from the visual system in unfamiliar tasks or visually complex tasks can reduce the time children with CVI can work on some tasks compared to typical peers. Children may also tire more quickly on tasks that demand integration of vision with movement, audition, or a high degree of cognitive processing. Sensory distractions (sound, touch, vision, movement) in the environment can also affect the length of time a child can focus on a particular task. When children are uncomfortable, in pain, ill, hungry, tired, fearful, or upset, the length of time spent on a specific learning activity can also be diminished. If any of the above factors are in operation, the interventionist must be sensitive to them and make adjustments to the duration of lessons to accommodate the moment-to-moment needs of each child.

### *Providing Breaks during Instruction*

Children with CVI who do tire of instruction easily for whatever reason can benefit from frequent breaks during instruction. This may mean providing some quiet time within a lesson or a change of pace to a different type of lesson, depending on the child, the environment, and the learning activity. The frequency, format, and durations of breaks will vary with individual situations. For some children, a separate quiet room can prove helpful for some activity breaks. For others who are unable to express that they are feeling overwhelmed, some practitioners have found that teaching children to display a special card (for example, a red card) at such times can be a useful way to communicate to the teacher that a break is needed before continuing the lesson.

### *Increasing Time to Respond*

Some children with CVI may be slower to integrate incoming information from the visual system with information from other senses or with auditory, motor, and cognitive output. This means that they will require more time to process information and to respond. This may require adjustments to reduce the number of elements within a learning activity. Translated into practice this could mean that less is taught during a single time period, or fewer items are given for practice to accommodate the length of response time each child requires. Longer response times also necessitate patience on the part of interventionists, who must wait for children to organize their input, processing, and output systems in order to respond. The results are often well worth the wait. Hastening ahead, on the other hand, is counterproductive.

### *Adjusting the Pace of Presentation*

Some children benefit from a reduction in the overall speed of lesson presentation so that they have time to take in and digest what is happening in order to respond appropriately. To maintain a child's interest in a lesson, the interventionist may need to vary the pace of lessons going from a fast pace to a slower one, and then back to fast pace once again. The interventionist needs to be sure, when trying this strategy, that the child maintains attention as the pace changes. If a child is very tired, ill, hungry, fearful, or upset then a slow pace may be necessary throughout. A faster pace can be used for material or methods in which the interventionist knows the child is competent, while the slower pace may be needed to facilitate the development of new skills and convey new knowledge. While this is a universal rule, the need for such adjustments can be more marked in those with CVI of all types.

## Other Variables to Consider When Presenting Activities

The following suggestions for adaptations and interventions highlight a variety of additional factors that may affect the ability of children to participate in learning activities. Additional suggestions for interventions with infants can be found in Chapter 20.

### *Present Learning Activities at or Slightly above Child's Present Level of Performance*

Activities presented to children for comfortable independent work or recreational pursuits should be at a level that children can complete without special learning assistance or unfamiliar environmental supports. This is the child's *independent level.*

Activities to promote growth in skills, behaviors, understanding, and performance will involve tasks that are slightly above a child's current capabilities. These tasks lead to outcomes that interventionists and families believe children can achieve with guidance.

Tasks to promote development and learning are ones that children can accomplish with proper educational support—also called *scaffolding* (Vygotsky, 1978)—to reach that next level in the learning sequence.

Myriad variables affect the performance of children who have CVI. These are examined during the assessment phase of children's programs and also during the intervention phase through diagnostic teaching. All this information leads to an understanding of the child's present level of functioning and the next levels. This information contributes to the optimal design of educational programs. In the design of programs, interventionists must consider where children are, where they want them to go, and the incremental steps that lead to those ultimate goals. Taking things one step at a time, and providing lessons that promote success by understanding the series of steps in a learning sequence for a particular child, are critical program elements for children who have CVI.

### *Use Favorite Activities and Materials*

Activities that children find enjoyable and that use favorite materials, colors, themes, and strategies promote learning. Children's favorites are ascertained during the comprehensive assessment process and during diagnostic teaching activities. Family input, gathered systematically via interviews, observations, and written surveys, is invaluable to gain this information.

### *Provide Clear Structure to Activities with Prominent Cues*

Some examples of ways to provide structure include the following:

- Structure activities at a specific time, specific place, or with a specific person
- Structure events within activities so that sequences, materials, and participatory routines can be anticipated
- Use defined areas such as work boards, placemats, or cookie sheets, or mark off an area with carpenter's tape
- Space presented stimuli so that objects, photographs, letters of the alphabet, words, and so forth appear as distinct entities against a plain background
- Use relevant color, but avoid a kaleidoscope of colors that may be visually confusing

### *Use Memory Aids*

Most students with CVI tend to have difficulty with organizational skills. Starting early in their education career, begin to teach students with CVI how to use a variety of memory aids as, for example, a half-day schedule, a full-day schedule, and subschedules related to events that will occur within each of the activities referenced on the main schedules. Once this process is learned, the more advanced systems of the weekly schedule may be introduced, and so forth (Blaha, 2001).

### *Involve Child in Task Analysis Process for Key Activities*

Task analysis, discussed earlier in this chapter, will help the student grasp the important steps in each functional activity and reduce confusion. This is essential for many students with CVI so they can perceive what is expected, learn the motor aspects of the activity, and better understand what they see.

### *Provide Positive and Frequent Feedback*

Positive and meaningful interactions with instructional staff, family, and peers can promote learning for children with CVI. For example, supportive feedback and modeling for children has been found to contribute to successful outcomes for children with learning disabilities (Swanson, 1999). For children with CVI, who may not understand why they are not functioning in ways similar to sighted peers, this type of feedback can help them appreciate ways to address learning tasks and how to succeed in them.

### *Provide Familiarity and Consistency in the Environment*

Children with CVI who have cognitive delays may respond more readily to familiar people, settings, and materials. For all children with CVI, too much novelty to be processed is confusing, often difficult, and frequently stressful. Discover the amount of novelty that each student can tolerate and arrange the student's activities accordingly. It is important, however, to gently guide children slowly toward greater variety while at the same time providing familiarity and consistency in their environment to optimize the learning process. If the environment is to be modified, allowing the child to "help" assists in gaining familiarity with any changes from the outset.

### *Alternate Activities of High and Low Sensory-Motor Demand*

Some students with CVI tire very quickly when required to visually fixate (watching TV), track (reading), scan (looking for a specific letter, picture, number among many others), and shift visual gaze (copying from the whiteboard to a computer). This does not mean the student can have a nap. Rather, the student might straighten the desk, put books away, or perform some other alternate task. This is an area in which the teacher of students with visual impairments may be able to take baseline information on how long the student can engage in these varying visual tasks, what adaptations might help to increase the time, and techniques that make the tasks easier for the student.

### *Vary Types of Activities to Address Arousal Levels*

It is often helpful to provide a gross motor activity to increase a child's level of alertness prior to an activity that requires quiet and sustained attention. And often, it helps to vary active and quiet activities to maintain arousal levels and promote a climate conducive to constant learning.

### *Use Methods of Focusing Visual Attention to Promote Visual Inspection*

Children with CVI may require assistance to focus on single items or to single out one item in a larger visual array. The precise methods chosen depend on the profile of the individual child and the instructional objectives to be addressed. Be sure that the item of visual regard is perceptible to the child in terms of size, contrast, visual field, color, and amount of detail. Methods that encourage visual attention toward a single item or to one item in an array of items can be found in Table 19.4.

### *Vary Activities to Reduce the Effects of Habituation*

Habituation occurs when stimulus targets or activities are repeated multiple times, resulting in children's decreased interest in the stimulus. This is an important area to understand for infants and toddlers with CVI and for children with CVI who have cognitive challenges. Smith (2009) suggests that eliciting an initial visual orienting response to

TABLE 19.4

## Methods of Encouraging Visual Attention to a Single Item or to One Item in an Array of Items[a]

| *Methods of Encouraging Visual Attention* | *For Children with Profound Visual Impairment Resulting from CVI* | *For Children with CVI Who Have Functionally Useful Vision and Cognitive Challenges* | *For Children with CVI Who Have Functionally Useful Vision and Work at or Near the Expected Academic Level for Their Age Group* |
|---|---|---|---|
| Shine a directional light on a single object or one item in an array (care must be taken to keep the light from shining or reflecting directly into the child's eyes) | X | X | |
| For a child who responds to movement, move or shake the object to be viewed | X | X | |
| Use a sound source paired with the object (or as part of the object) to engage the child's attention to a single object or to one item in an array | X | X | |
| Use a pleasant scent that can be associated with a single visual target (for example, pierce an orange to engage the child's visual attention toward the orange; eating the orange can then be a reward) | X | X | |
| Use a readily visible pointer to draw attention to a single object or an item in an array (in addition, tapping with the pointer may provide the additional assistance of a sound cue) | X | X | |
| Instruct the child verbally where to look at a single object or an item in an array | X | X | X |
| Highlight a single picture with a child's favorite color or draw a colored outline around it | | X | X |
| Make a single item with a favorite color or mark an item in a different color from other items in an array | X | X | X |

[a]Boxes have been left blank when a strategy either exceeds the capabilities of children in that category, or the strategy is not necessary because the children can be expected to operate well without its use.

*(continued on next page)*

**TABLE 19.4** *(continued from previous page)*

| *Methods of Encouraging Visual Attention* | *For Children with Profound Visual Impairment Resulting from CVI* | *For Children with CVI Who Have Functionally Useful Vision and Cognitive Challenges* | *For Children with CVI Who Have Functionally Useful Vision and Work at or Near the Expected Academic Level for Their Age Group* |
|---|---|---|---|
| Cover extraneous visual material surrounding an object, picture, or letter (with construction paper in workbooks or with cloth for objects on a desk) | X | X | X |
| Have the child point with a finger to single out letters or words when reading | | X | X |
| Highlight print or pictorial material to be viewed with color or by an outline around the material | | X | X |
| Have the child use a typoscope (reading window) that shows single letters or words on a page | | X | X |
| Have the child use a line marker to single out sentences on a page of text | | X | X |
| Encourage the child to use a prescribed magnifier to single out words or phrases in text; the magnifier delimits the field of view | | X | X |
| Have the child use special electronic hardware or software that enables the presentation of single words at a time (serial presentation of text) or highlighting words as they are to be read | | X | X |

a stimulus using a cue that a stimulus or change in the environment is about to happen serves to alert children so that they then attend to what comes next in the lesson sequence. However, children do not maintain interest in repeated presentations of the same stimulus within a short time span. There must be some variation in presentation, otherwise children get used to (habituate to) the stimulus, do not continue to orient to it, and subsequently lose interest in the learning task. (This was an early concern about vision stimulation programs for students with visual impairments that focused solely on the presentation of vivid visual stimuli to promote the development of visual skills and behaviors [Lundervold, Lewin, & Irvin, 1987].)

Repetition of visual stimuli without embedding the stimuli into meaningful activities or without varying their presentation to recapture the children's attention will create situations in which attention to and engagement in learning tasks wane. For example, habituation has been shown to affect the detection of stimuli for children who have blindsight (awareness of moving targets, lights, and colors in a non-seeing area of vision). These children did not follow a moving target if the direction of movement remained the same. If the target was moved in a different direction, the visual following response was temporarily renewed until habituation again arose (Boyle, Jones, Hamilton, Spowart, & Dutton, 2005). The authors give the example of bringing a spoon to a child's mouth from different directions to maintain visual attention to the spoon when eating.

### *Provide Optimal Positioning for Children with Physical Disabilities*

Children with CVI who also have motor impairments may function better visually when in specific body positions. Minimizing distractions related to discomfort can enhance attention. Some children are more visually alert in standers, others while seated, and others on their backs. It is important to consult with physical and occupational therapists to determine the best positioning for students during lessons to promote the use of vision.

### *Present Lessons at Optimal Times of Day*

Many children with CVI must exert a great deal of effort to sustain attention to tasks with strong visual components. Educationally taxing tasks need to be presented when children are alert and comfortable. Children are often most alert when fully rested in the mornings, for example. Right after lunch may not be a good time to present tasks that require strong concentration. If children have just taken a medication with immediate side effects that affect learning, these times should also be avoided for educationally intense activities. If children are tired after recess, they should be given time to recoup before activities with high learning demands are instituted.

### *Alternate Easy and Demanding Activities*

It is often helpful to vary demanding activities with ones that are less demanding so that children have time to recuperate from the intense experiences, relax with some pleasant activities, and then return to a lesson that again includes high learning demands.

### *Utilize Activity Sequence Setups*

Utilizing activity sequence setups helps a student understand visual and tactile events that need to be performed in an activity. To implement this technique, sequence the materials that will be used in the activity in a left to right order and in a defined area (on a work tray, cookie sheet, or placemat). Do this *with* the student. For example, in a cooking activity, the ingredients might be lined up, from the student's left to right, in the order they will be used according to the recipe.

### *Make Appropriate Adaptations for Discrete Trial Training*

A variety of disciplines that are trying to develop the most effective ways of managing behaviors of concern have actively promoted *discrete trial training* as a process that has benefit with students diagnosed with autism and those who demonstrate significant learning and behavior difficulties (Lovaas, 1987; Smith, 2001). In this approach, which is often used as part of the applied behavior analysis approach, tasks are broken down into short, simple steps called trials. In the beginning, each trial is usually very short with a reward provided at the end. A particular trial may be repeated many times, over and over again, before the child learns to perform the components of a short task sequence independently.

If discrete trial training is part of the program for a student with CVI, the pace of presenting tasks needs careful consideration. Visually, the student may be unable to maintain a speedy presentation of the materials or a requirement for a speedy response. Students with CVI usually require more time to perceive what needs to be done, plan, and then execute responses. (For more information, a web search for *applied behavior analysis* or *ABA*, in addition to *discrete trial training,* will be helpful.)

### *Generalization of Skills*

For children with CVI who have cognitive challenges, it is important to remember that they may not generalize skills and behaviors learned within the context of one activity performed in a certain location with specific people to other activities, locations, or other people. Lessons may need to be devised that assist the child to generalize learned skills and behaviors into other contexts. For example, a child who learns to put a straw into a small milk carton during lunchtime at school with a favorite teacher may not automatically be able to place a straw into a cup of milk at dinnertime at home with a family member. The child may require more direct instruction and practice to accomplish the latter task.

### *Use Consistent Language Input*

Ensure that the child's known vocabulary is used in context both at home and at school. Children with limited vision capabilities and few words need consistency of language usage throughout their day. (Additional intervention suggestions for infants related to language input can be found in Chapter 20.)

## Conclusion

Interventions that facilitate self-determination for children with CVI help these youngsters understand their own functional needs, gain competence in explaining these needs to others, and develop advocacy skills that increase independence and help them establish meaningful life goals. A team approach to interventions leading toward self-determination is essential since the needs of children who have CVI can be complex and must draw on the combined and coordinated expertise of a variety of professionals. Input, support, and follow-through by family members are invaluable components of the instruction process.

Instructional activities, methods, and strategies for children with CVI are ones that engage, motivate, and sustain students' interest and attention within a framework of instruction that highlights the use of appropriate adaptations to maximize their active participation. Instruction in the basic skills needed to perform more complex tasks can be considered for some children with CVI. This instruction is especially important for infants and toddlers, but may also apply to older children who have CVI and who have additional learning challenges.

Since the evidence base for successful interventions for children with CVI is just beginning to develop, diagnostic teaching is recommended as a way to evaluate the effectiveness of instructional approaches in a systematic way. With this approach, methods and progress are monitored regularly, and successful interventions are developed, maintained, and expanded. Intervention protocols are revised when they do not work or no longer apply, as children grow and change, or as their learning environments alter.

Instructional elements to promote learning are presented slightly above a child's independent level of functioning with sufficient support and assistance to minimize frustration and ensure success over time. Intervention approaches for children who have CVI must take into account a variety of influences specific to each child. They most often require collaboration by a team of professionals from a variety of disciplines who work in tandem with the child's family to maximize development and learning.

## References


Allman, C. B., & Lewis, S. (Eds.). (2014). *ECC essentials: Teaching the expanded core curriculum to students with visual impairments.* New York: AFB Press.

American Foundation for the Blind. (2011). *The expanded core curriculum for blind and visually impaired children and youths.* Retrieved June 28, 2011, from http://www.afb.org/Section.asp?SectionID=44&TopicID=189&SubTopicID=4&DocumentID=2117

Blaha, R. (2001). *Calendars for students with multiple impairments including deafblindness.* Austin: Texas School for the Blind and Visually Impaired.

Boyle, N. J., Jones, D. H., Hamilton, R., Spowart, K. M., & Dutton, G. N. (2005). Blindsight in children: Does it exist and can it be used to help the child? Observations on a case series. *Developmental Medicine & Child Neurology, 47*(10), 699–702.

Brown, L., Shiraga, B., York, J., Zanella, K., & Rogan, P. (1984). Ecological inventory strategies for students with severe handicaps. In L. Brown, M. Sweet, B. Shiraga, J. York, K. Zanella, P. Rogan, & R. Loomis (Eds.), *Educational programs for students with severe handicaps: Vol. XIV* (pp. 33–41). Madison, WI: Madison Metropolitan School District.

Brunsdon, R., Nickels, L., Colthear, M., & Joy, P. (2007). Assessment and treatment of childhood topographical disorientation: A case study. *Neuropsychological Rehabilitation, 17*(1), 53–94.

Cohen-Maitre, S. A., & Haerich, P. (2005). Visual attention to movement and color in children with cortical visual impairment. *Journal of Visual Impairment & Blindness, 99*(7), 389–402.

Connell, B. R., Jones, M., Mace, R., Mueller, J., Mullick, A., Ostroff, E., . . . Vanderheiden, G. (1997). *The principles of universal design. Version 2.0.* Raleigh: North Carolina State University, The Center for Universal Design.

Das, M., Bennett, D. M., & Dutton, G. N. (2007). Visual attention as an important visual function: An outline of manifestations, diagnosis and management of impaired visual attention. *British Journal of Ophthalmology, 91*(11), 1556–1560.

Dutton, G. N. (2003). Cognitive vision, its disorders and differential diagnosis in adults and children: Knowing where and what things are. *Eye, 17,* 289–304.

Erin, J. N., & Paul, B. (1996). Functional vision assessment and instruction of children and youths in academic programs. In A. L. Corn & A. J. Koenig (Eds.), *Foundations of low vision: Clinical and functional perspectives* (pp. 185–220). New York: AFB Press.

Falvey, M. A. (Ed.) (1995). *Inclusive and heterogeneous schooling: Assessment, curriculum, and instruction.* Baltimore, MD: Paul H. Brookes Publishing Co.

Good, W. V., & Hou, C. (2006). Sweep visual evoked potential grating acuity thresholds paradoxically improve in low-luminance conditions in children with cortical visual impairment. *Investigative Ophthalmology & Visual Science, 47*(7), 3220–3224.

Good, W. V., Jan, J. E., DeSa, L., Barkovich, A. J., Groenveld, M., & Hoyt, C. S. (1994). Cortical visual impairment in children. *Survey of Ophthalmology, 38*, 351–364.

Greer, R. (2004). Evaluation methods and functional implications: Children and adults with visual impairments. In A. H. Lueck (Ed.), *Functional vision: A practitioner's guide to evaluation and intervention* (pp. 177–253). New York: AFB Press.

Hall, A., & Bailey, I. L. (1989). A model for training vision functioning. *Journal of Visual Impairment & Blindness, 83*, 390–396.

Hall, T., Strangman, N., & Meyer, A. (2011). *Differentiated instruction and implications for UDL implementation. Effective Classroom Practices Report.* Peabody, MA: National Center on Accessing the General Curriculum. Retrieved January 31, 2015, from http://ok.gov/sde/sites/ok.gov.sde/files/DI_UDL.pdf

Hatlen, P. (2003, December). *Impact of literacy on the expanded core curriculum.* Presentation at the Getting in Touch with Literacy Conference, Vancouver, British Columbia, Canada. Retrieved June 28, 2011, from http://www.tsbvi.edu/national-agenda/1213-impact-of-literacy-on-the-expanded-core-curriculum

Hyvärinen, L. (2003, November). *Assessment of CVI.* Lea Hyvärinen's lectures at San Francisco State University. Retrieved from http://lea-test.fi/en/assessme/sfracvilect/index.html

Hyvärinen, L., & Jacob, N. (2011). *WHAT and HOW does this child see?* Helsinki, Finland: VISTEST Ltd.

Jones, M. J., Sinha, P., Vetter, T., & Poggio, T. (1997). Top-down learning of low-level vision tasks. *Current Biology, 7*(12), 991–994.

Kingston, J., Katsaros, J., Vu, Y., & Goodrich, G. L. (2010). Neurological vision rehabilitation: Description and case study. *Journal of Visual Impairment & Blindness, 104*(10), 603–612.

Koenig, A. J., & Holbrook, M. C. (1989). Determining the reading medium for students with visual impairments: A diagnostic teaching approach. *Journal of Visual Impairment & Blindness, 83*(6), 296–302.

Koenig, A. J., & Holbrook, M. C. (1995). *Learning media assessment of students with visual impairments: A resource guide for teachers* (2nd ed.). Austin: Texas School for the Blind and Visually Impaired.

Lanners, J., Piccioni, A., Fea, F., & Goergen, E. (1999). Early intervention for children with cerebral visual impairment: Preliminary results. *Journal of Intellectual Disability Research, 43*(Pt 1), 1–12.

Lovaas, O. I. (1987). Behavioral treatment and normal educational and intellectual functioning in young autistic children. *Journal of Consulting and Clinical Psychology, 55*(1), 3–9.

Love, C. (1994). The effect of specific vision enhancement on the functional vision of children with cortical visual impairment (Doctoral dissertation, The University of Texas at Austin, 1994). *Dissertation Abstracts International, 55*, 1527.

Ludt, R. (1997). Three types of glare: Low vision O&M assessment and remediation. *Re:View, 29*(3), 101–113.

Lueck, A. H. (2004a). Optimizing interventions for students with low vision. *Vision Impairment Research, 6*(1), 45–52.

Lueck, A. H. (2004b). Overview of intervention methods. In A. H. Lueck (Ed.), *Functional vision: A practitioner's guide to evaluation and intervention* (pp. 257–275). New York: AFB Press.

Lueck, A. H. (2006). Issues in intervention for children with visual impairment or visual dysfunction due to brain injury. In E. Dennison & A. H. Lueck (Eds.), *Proceedings of the summit on cerebral/cortical visual impairment: Educational, family, and medical perspectives, April 30, 2005* (pp. 121–130). New York: AFB Press.

Lueck, A. H., Dornbusch, H., & Hart, J. (1999). The effects of training on a young child with cortical visual impairment: An exploratory study. *Journal of Visual Impairment & Blindness, 93*(12), 778–793.

Lueck, A. H., & Heinze, T. (2004). Interventions for young children with visual impairments and students with visual and multiple disabilities. In A. H. Lueck (Ed.), *Functional vision: A practitioner's guide to evaluation and intervention* (pp. 277–351). New York: AFB Press.

Lundervold, D., Lewin, L. M., & Irvin, L. K. (1987). Rehabilitation of visual impairments:

A critical review. *Clinical Psychology Review, 7*(2), 169–185.

Macintyre-Béon, C., Ibrahim, H., Hay, I., Cockburn, D., Calvert, J., Dutton, G. N., et al. (2010). Dorsal stream dysfunction in children: A review and an approach to diagnosis and management. *Current Pediatric Reviews, 6*(3), 166–182.

Malkowicz, D. E., Myers, G., & Leisman, G. (2006). Rehabilitation of cortical visual impairment in children. *International Journal of Neuroscience, 116*(9), 1015–1033.

McKillop, E., & Dutton, G. N. (2008). Impairment of vision in children due to damage to the brain: A practical approach. *British and Irish Orthoptic Journal, 5*, 8–14.

Morse, M. T. (2012, October 1). *Cerebral/cortical visual impairment*. Paper presented at the Educational and Conference Center Series of the Southeastern Regional Education Service Center (SERESC). Retrieved December 15, 2012, from http://www.seresc.net/cerebral-cortical-visual-impairment

Research and Training Center on Community Living. (2008). *Self-advocacy/self-determination*. Retrieved June 28, 2011, from http://rtc.umn.edu

Roman, C. (2010). *CVI complexity sequences kit*. Louisville, KY: American Printing House for the Blind.

Roman-Lantzy, C. A., & Lantzy, A. (2010). Outcomes and opportunities: A study of children with cortical visual impairment. *Journal of Visual Impairment & Blindness, 104*(10), 649–653.

Rose, D. H., & Meyer, A. (2002). *Teaching every student in the digital age: Universal design for learning*. Alexandria, VA: Association for Supervision and Curriculum Development.

Sacks, S. Z. (2010). Psychological and social implications of low vision. In A. L. Corn & J. N. Erin (Eds.), *Foundations of low vision: Clinical and functional perspectives* (2nd ed., pp. 67–96). New York: AFB Press.

Smith, A. J., & Geruschat, D. (2010). Orientation and mobility for adults with low vision. In A. L. Corn & J. N. Erin (Eds.), *Foundations of low vision: Clinical and functional perspectives* (2nd ed., pp. 833–870). New York: AFB Press.

Smith, M. (2009). *Sensory learning kit*. Louisville, KY: American Printing House for the Blind.

Smith, T. (2001). Discrete trial training in the treatment of autism. *Focus on Autism and Other Developmental Disabilities, 16*(2), 86–92.

Swanson, H. L. (1999). Instructional components that predict treatment outcomes for students with learning disabilities: Support for a combined strategy and direct instruction model. *Learning Disabilities Research & Practice, 14*(3), 129–140.

Tomlinson, C. A. (2000). Differentiation of instruction in the elementary grades [ERIC_NO: ED443572]. *ERIC Digest*. Retrieved June 30, 2011, from http://www.eric.ed.gov/ERICWebPortal/contentdelivery/servlet/ERICServlet?accno=ED443572

Tomlinson, C. A., & McTighe, J. (2006). *Integrating differentiated instruction: Understanding by design*. Alexandria, VA: Association for Supervision and Curriculum Development.

Topor, I., Lueck, A. H., & Smith, J. (2004). Compensatory instruction for academically oriented students with visual impairments. In A. H. Lueck (Ed.), *Functional vision: A practitioner's guide to evaluation and intervention* (pp. 353–421). New York: AFB Press.

Udvari-Solner, A., Causton-Theoharis, J., & York-Barr, J. (2004). Developing adaptations to promote participation in inclusive environments. In F. P. Orelove, D. Sobsey, & R. K. Silberman (Eds.), *Educating children with multiple disabilities: A collaborative approach* (4th ed., pp. 151–192). Baltimore, MD: Paul H. Brookes Publishing Co.

Valencia, S. W., & Wixson, K. K. (1991). Diagnostic teaching. *The Reading Teacher, 44*(6), 420–422.

Vygotsky, L. S. (1978). *Mind in society: The development of higher psychological processes*. Cambridge, MA: Harvard University Press.

Warren, M. (1993). A hierarchical model for evaluation and treatment of visual perceptual dysfunction in adult acquired brain injury, Part 2. *American Journal of Occupational Therapy, 47*(1), 55–66.

Wehmeyer, M. L. (1998). Self-determination and individuals with significant disabilities: Examining meanings and misinterpretations. *Journal of the Association for Persons with Severe Handicaps, 23*(1), 5–16.

Werth, R., & Seelos, K. (2005). Restitution of visual functions in cerebrally blind children. *Neuropsychologia, 43*(14), 2011–2023.

Williams, C., Northstone, K., Sabates, R., Feinstein, L., Elmond, A., & Dutton, G. N. (2011). Visual perceptual difficulties and under-achievement at school in a large community-based sample of children. *PLoS One, 6*(3), e14772.

Zihl, J., & Dutton, G. N. (2015). *Cerebral visual impairment in children: Visuoperceptive and visuocognitive disorders.* Vienna: Springer-Verlag Wien.

# 20

# Cerebral Visual Impairment and Cerebral Blindness in Very Young Children: Connecting Assessment to Intervention

*Gordon N. Dutton and Amanda Hall Lueck*

Developmental changes can occur rapidly in some infants and very young children who are affected by cerebral visual impairment (CVI); thus their assessments need to be an ongoing process. Their evolving developmental or sensory capabilities need to be systematically ascertained and immediately taken into account so that the design and implementation of intervention approaches evolve, along with each child's growth and learning. For this reason, some basic principles of functional vision assessment and intervention with infants and very young children who have CVI are considered together in this chapter, and those terms are used interchangeably to refer to all of these children.

The chapter addresses issues related to the population of children who have evident CVI or cerebral blindness. These are the children most often identified at early ages as a result of their more prominent and severe vision deficits or blindness. Milder vision deficits are often not detected until children reach school age. As a rule, the earlier a child with CVI is identified as having a problem with vision, and the more extensive the damage to the brain, the more profound the visual disability.

Profound damage to the visual cortex and the incoming pathways causes this form of CVI, or if more severe, cerebral blindness (defined as profound impairment or absence of vision, due to bilateral damage to the visual pathways posterior to the lateral geniculate bodies, which may be accompanied by damage to other regions of the brain that serve vision). The most common cause in the very young infant is lack of oxygen and blood supply to the brain causing a stroke before, during, or shortly after birth; other causes are described in Chapter 3.

The child with cerebral blindness has occipital lobes (the area at the back of the brain) that function poorly. This rarely occurs in isolation. More commonly other brain areas (for example, the frontal lobes that serve intellectual processing or the parietal lobes in the middle of the brain that bring about body movement, and hear, interpret, and formulate language; see Chapter 2) are affected so that each child is unique in the nature of his or her disabilities, abilities, and needs. Very early onset damage has been shown to be followed by profound reorganization of the neural networks in the visual brain (a function of brain plasticity; see Chapter 5), but this major restructuring has not been identified in children with later-onset brain damage (Tinelli et al., 2013). Since the brain structures of young children can, in fact, recover and rearrange in response to injury, intact functions and their limitations must be identified and addressed through medical and educational interventions as early as possible to achieve optimal development and learning. The key facilitators of this process are caregivers who need to be well supported, well informed, and provided with guidance in ways to attain the best outcomes for their child.

## Functional Visual Assessment for Infants and Very Young Children with Damage to the Visual Brain

Functional vision assessment in infants follows three major steps that are described in the sections that follow:

1. An initial screening through careful observation of the child's behavior to learn how the child behaves and reacts through vision and hearing.
2. Structured history taking to elicit information from caregivers and teachers.
3. Careful assessment of functional vision.

Functional vision is assessed when the infant is awake and attentive, so it may precede history taking, or may have to be rescheduled for the infant who is fast asleep.

## Initial Screening Observations of the Behavior of the Infant and Very Young Child

Initial screening observations are completed within the first minute or two of seeing the infant or young child if he or she is awake and attentive, or by seizing the opportunity if the infant wakes from sleep and becomes aware later on. In this way, if the child later goes back to sleep or becomes inattentive during the assessment process, the child's capabilities have been captured, and this break provides a welcome opportunity to elicit the history from the caregivers without distraction.

The observations discussed in the following sections are used to estimate, if possible, the practical everyday thresholds of clarity, speed, and intensity of visual and auditory stimuli needed to promote communication. This rapid "pattern recognition" evaluation process is repeated at each meeting as the child grows and develops. The observations are compared with past assessments.

### Preparation of the Infant or Young Child and the Environment (Home, Clinical, or Educational Setting)

- Ensure that the room has been prepared. Minimize clutter and limit the amount of decoration. Limit background auditory noise. Have all the tests at hand.
- Make sure the child is comfortable so that discomfort and pain do not distract.

- Throughout the interview and assessment, watch to see what the child looks at, how big the object is, and how far away.

### Eye Contact, Facial Expression, and Eye and Head Movements

- Give a big, animated silent smile, and approach the child to see if he or she looks at your eyes. Observe the distance at which this occurs, and if it happens, record the maximum distance of consistent eye contact.
- Move your head a little from side to side and watch for eye and head movements. Watch to see if your smile is returned.

### Detection, Following, and Reaching for Objects

- Provide a favorite toy against a contrasting background. Wait and watch for any responses.
- Is the toy observed, tracked, or reached for? If so, what size is it?
- To gain the child's visual attention, does the toy need to be static or moving; in the central or peripheral visual field; in a specific quadrant of the visual field; silent or noisy?

### Attention to Vocalization

- Is attention given to your voice? If so, at what volume, clarity, and speed of enunciation of words, consonants, and vowels?
- What degree of variation in pitch and cadence is needed to attract and maintain attention? (Vary your voice to become slower and more distinct, and watch for the reactions of stilling and attention.)
- Demonstrate to caregivers the voice features needed for the infant to attend to vocalization.

## Structured History Taking for Infants and Very Young Children

Structured history taking elicits information related to functional vision from parents and other caregivers (see Chapter 11). The questions are asked after the initial screening observations, and if the child was attentive on arrival, it is best to take the history after the assessment of vision. The information obtained is remarkably informative for both caregivers and practitioners. It gives feedback about the child's visual capabilities so that they can be used to best advantage. Questions are asked about person, place, and time (see Sidebar 20.1).

More information on how to frame questions to obtain a structured history can be found in Chapter 11. In addition, Roman-Lantzy (2007) provides some excellent sample questions for taking a history of young children who have limited functional vision as a result of CVI.

## The Vision Assessment Process

Information gathered in the initial encounter through the screening observation and structured history taking can be used to determine elements to evaluate systematically in an assessment of functional vision (or can complement any assessment already carried out). This section explains some methods that can be used to estimate the functional vision of infants and very young children.

### Normal Infant Visual Function

Knowledge of normal visual development is needed to interpret findings. Infants' vision

SIDEBAR 20.1

## Questions to Ask During Structured History Taking

During a structured history taking for a child with CVI, caregivers are asked questions such as those listed here in the broad categories of person—that is, the nature of the child's experiences and behaviors—place and time, to obtain information about the child's visual capabilities.

### Person

- Tell me about your child's vision?

*If caregivers report that there is vision, ask the following questions*:

- What does your child see?
- Does your child:
  - Follow people's movements?
  - React to someone who is approaching?
  - React to lights being turned on and off?
  - Return a silent smile?
  - React to food through vision?
  - Reach for a drink?
  - React to a reflection of himself/herself in a mirror?
  - React to and reach for silent objects?

*If responses to any of the above are positive, a measurable visual acuity, using preferential looking methods, is likely to be elicited (McCulloch et al., 2007).*

- What kinds of distraction interfere with vision? *(These may include pain, discomfort, auditory noise, and visual clutter. Give examples as needed, to clarify this question.)*
- Can your child pay attention to silent or noisy, static or moving targets?
- What are the features of the targets that bring about and keep attention?
- What does your child know and understand about what he or she sees?
- What are your child's favorite targets?
- Does vision vary from hour to hour, or from day to day?

*If caregivers report limited or no vision, questions can be formulated to address the following possible instances of vision:*

- Mouth opening when a spoon is brought toward the mouth from the side, but not when brought from straight ahead. *(This behavior can be variable and less evident when the activity is repeated.)*
- Occasional reflex smiling to a moving, large smile from close range when there appears to be little or no other evidence of vision. *(This is called affective blindsight and may result from automatic subconscious visual functions coming into play [Pegna, Khateb, Lazeyras, & Seghier, 2005].)*
- Improved visual function in darkened conditions (Good & Hou, 2006).
- Discomfort in bright lighting conditions.
- A tendency to stare at lights (Jan, Groenveld, Sykanda, & Hoyt, 1987).

*For the child who shows any evidence of visual functions, the following additional questions can be posed:*

### Place

- In what locations does your child give the best visual performance?
- Do some parts of the area of vision (visual field) give better responses than others?
- Where and in what situations do visual responses occur? Ask for examples.

### Time

- When does your child see best and when is vision/attention lost?
- For how long can visual attention be maintained?
- Does your child's vision function some times but not others? If so, when is it best and when are visual responses least?

improves progressively (see, for example, Ferrell, 2010, 2011). Visual acuity, contrast sensitivity, color discrimination, visual fields, visual search, visual attention, recognition, and visual guidance of movement all develop over time. Visual acuity, as measured using preferential looking cards (Moseley, Fielder, Thompson, Minshull, & Price, 1988; Teller, Dobson, & Mayer, 2005), improves so that, as a rule of thumb, the acuity measured in cycles per degree (see Chapter 12) approximates to the age in months. Thus, at one month, it is around 1 cycle per degree, and at 12 months it is around 12 cycles per degree (Atkinson, 2000, Chapter 4). (See Appendix 12C for table of visual acuity equivalences.)

## Interacting while the Child Is Awake and Attentive

The speed of visual and attentional processing can be slow, so it is important to give sufficient time for the infant to respond. This information can be correlated with information provided by the caregivers during the structured history taking.

- Does the child see and respond to a face and to his or her own image in a mirror? If so, at what distance? (See the discussion later in this chapter regarding the mirror test.)
- Are large targets or toys seen in the peripheral areas? If so, how large do they need to be and in which quadrants of the child's visual field?
- Does the child see and respond to a central target? If so, what was the response and how long did it take?
- Does the child use central vision or peripheral vision to identify and reach for things? (The head and eyes can be turned so that the object of regard is reached for consistently when it is in the peripheral visual field.)
- If the child attends with peripheral vision, which quadrants of the visual field afford the greatest visual attention?

## Eliciting an Estimate of Visual Acuity by Preferential Looking

### *Standard Preferential Looking Method*

The standard methods of measuring visual acuity in infants are described in Chapter 12. To recap in brief, visual acuity is measured with preferential looking methods using such tests as the Teller Acuity Cards (Teller et al., 2005), Keeler Cards (Moseley et al., 1988), or LEA Grating Paddles that present a graduated series of stripes (known as gratings) that go from wide to thin. A child's consistent eye or head movement toward the stripes on a card indicates that the stripe width presented can be seen. The educational aim of doing this is to find the width of the line the child can consistently see at a preferred viewing distance, and to use this line width or wider (as well as spacing between lines, in the creation of images), for all salient elements of any picture or item initially presented at this distance to the child. If items are shown at greater or lesser viewing distances, the width of the line must be adjusted accordingly (for example, a line must be twice the width at twice the preferred viewing distance, or can be half the width at half the preferred viewing distance).

This assessment needs to be repeated regularly as vision develops, to re-evaluate the line widths and spacing required. For some children, such measurements prove ineffective and measurement of the visual acuity and contrast sensitivity by a technique that measures brain function, called visual evoked potentials (if available), can be both reliable and helpful (see Chapter 12; Good, Hou, & Norcia, 2012; Hou, Good, & Norcia, 2007; Mackay, Bradnam, Hamilton, Elliot, & Dutton, 2008).

### *Responses to Unusually Placed and Moving Preferential Looking Targets*

If no visual response is obtained to static, horizontally held grating cards (the standard method), hold the cards with the widest gratings horizontally in the upper visual field of the child, and then the lower field. A response in the upper field suggests lack of lower visual field function and vice versa. Then, hold the cards vertically in the child's left and right visual fields and seek responses. If responses are evident on one side or the other, this suggests either lack of vision or visual inattention on the side where there are no responses.

When no response is obtained, slowly move the card to and fro along its long axis. Watch to see if an eye movement response to the moving target can be generated, and if so, for which thickness of stripes. If moving the card generates a response, then there is evidence of a degree of visual function for moving targets, for the thickness of stripe observed, and in the area in which this happens. Everyone working with the child can then make use of the visual ability that has been noted.

## Estimating the Ability to See Details Using the Mirror Test

A practical method of estimating central visual function in infants and young children who show some evidence of vision is to use a large wall or wardrobe mirror and a tape measure (Bowman, McCulloch, Law, Mostyn, & Dutton, 2010). An infant held up to the mirror will look attentively at his or her own face. When the child is moved back from the mirror, attention tends to be lost at the same distance each time. As the child grows older, the child maintains attention at a little bit greater distance from the mirror (known as the *mirror distance*) each day, as the child's ability to see his or her mirror image increases, as a result of progressively improving visual acuity. The *actual distance* at which the infant or young child is able to see his or her image is equivalent to *twice* the mirror distance (since the image is the same distance behind the mirror as the child is in front of the mirror), and can be used to estimate the child's visual acuity. The improvement in visual acuity in infants over time is shown in Figure 20.1, with estimates of the visual acuities that correspond to the child's distance from the mirror when he or she loses interest. This means that the visual acuity of an infant or very young child who can attend to his or her own reflection can be estimated using a tape measure and a large mirror. Thus, the distance at which eye contact can be established across a room, progressively increasing with age, can be used as an indicator of improving visual acuity as the child gets older.

## Estimating the Area of Visual Field and Visual Attention

Infants and very young children with severe CVI commonly lack functional vision in one, two, or three quadrants of their visual fields. This may result from occipital lobe damage causing lack of visual field, posterior parietal damage causing lack of visual attention, or a combination of both (see Chapter 3). However, in a young child, it is usually not possible to tell the difference, and what one is seeking is the area where the child sees

FIGURE 20.1
## Estimation of Visual Acuity Using the Mirror Test

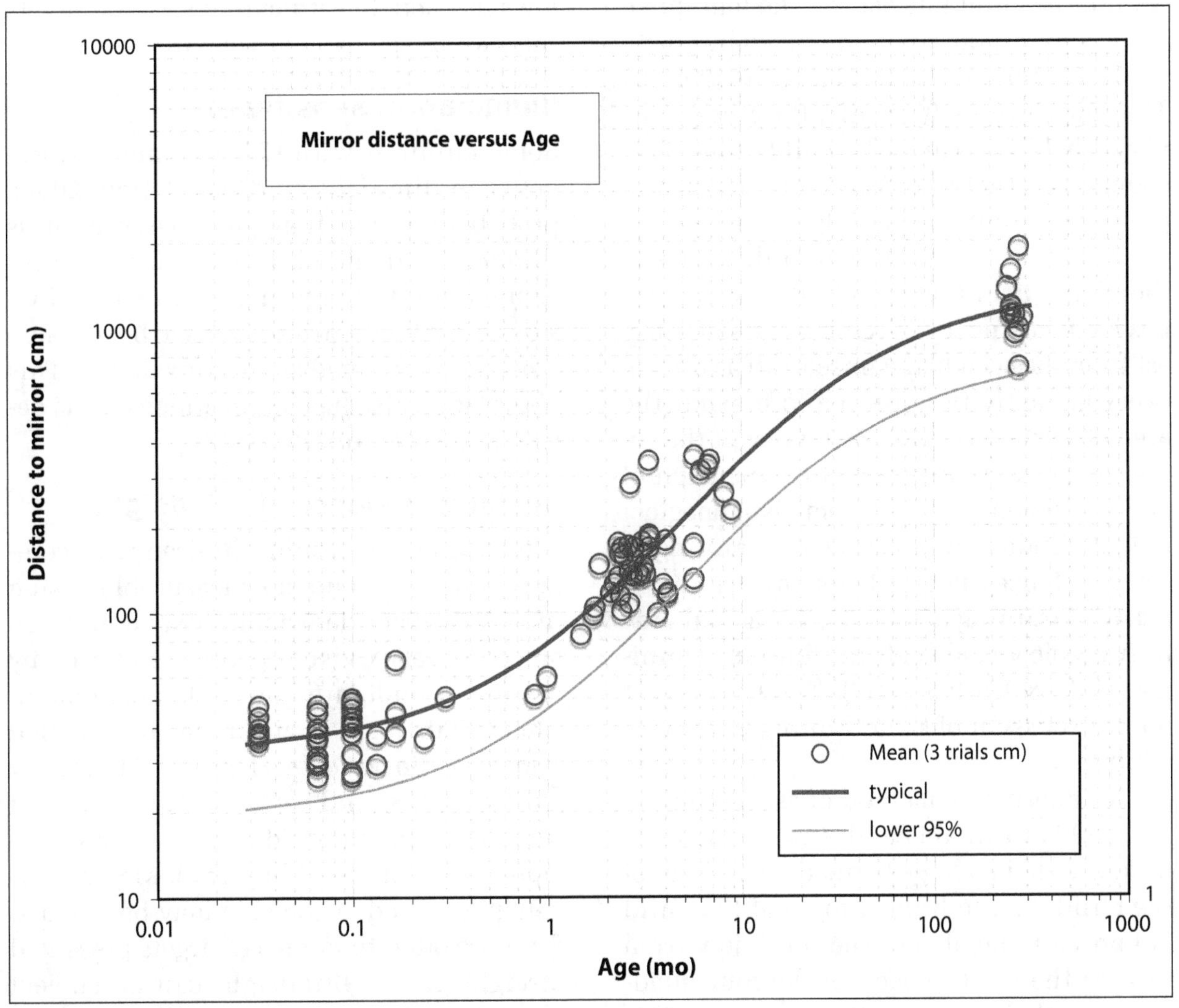


Estimation of visual acuity by measurement of the distance at which normal infants under one year of age lose attention in their own mirror image, when compared with measurement of visual acuity using Teller preferential looking cards. The following figures can be used as a practical "rule of thumb":

| | | | | |
|---|---|---|---|---|
| Snellen acuity (ft): | 20/2000 | 20/600 | 20/200 | 20/60 |
| Snellen acuity (m): | 6/600 | 6/180 | 6/60 | 6/18 |
| Mirror distance: | 28cm | 75cm | 150cm | 280cm |
| Actual distance: | 56cm | 150cm | 300cm | 560cm |

Mirror distance = the distance from the mirror at which the child loses interest.
Actual distance = double the mirror distance.

*Source*: Reproduced with permission from Bowman, R., McCulloch, D. L., Law, E., Mostyn, K., & Dutton, G. N. (2010). The "mirror test" for estimating visual acuity in infants. *British Journal of Ophthalmology, 94*(7), 882–885.

best. A large, bright, slowly moving target is brought into the child's visual field from behind the child into each of the four quadrants, and responses are evaluated by an observer in front of the child (see Chapter 12). The aim is to grossly identify the areas of the visual field for which the child is most responsive so that these areas can be used in everyday activities or in interventions.

Attention can be drawn to the areas of the visual field that the child does not appear to be using, by moving targets of interest from the seen to the unseen areas during everyday activities, aiming to expand the area of visual attention. A review of the research shows that systematic expansion of areas of vision resulting from visual neglect or inattention may be assisted by training in some instances, but studies show that the efficacy of training to increase the actual area of available visual fields in children is minimal (Zihl & Dutton, 2015). (See Chapter 24 for a discussion of such training used with adults.)

An alternative method of estimating visual fields in infants and very young children is to hold a large blank card in front of the child, and to bring a toy that the child is known to be able to see into view from behind the card in each of the four quadrants, while looking for the responses. This allows the single practitioner to screen for lack of visual function in each quadrant. One product designed for this purpose is called Puppet Face (www.beesneez.co.uk), a set of large black-on-white line drawn faces with black on the reverse side, each attached to a holder, and varying in size from large to small. A face large enough to elicit a response is suddenly revealed in each of the visual field quadrants from behind a black screen, and the positions in which the child consistently responds to the target are observed and recorded. This approach also allows teachers to estimate the size of targets that can be seen and at what distances.

## Illumination Sensitivity

Some children with CVI see and perform better in dim lighting (Good & Hou, 2006), probably because they perceive brightness differently. If the child becomes more responsive in dim lighting, the functional vision assessment process needs to be repeated with lights dimmed or curtains drawn. This observation also has implications for the design of interventions.

## Seeking Evidence of Blindsight

Infants and very young children with cerebral blindness and no measurable vision may still have detectable visual function since the reflex visual pathways (served by the upper midbrain and thalamus) remain intact. This form of vision has been called *blindsight* (Boyle, Jones, Hamilton, Spowart, & Dutton, 2005) and tends to function best for movement in the side areas of vision (peripheral vision; see Chapter 3). Moving targets positioned at the side may be reached for more often than visual targets presented straight ahead. Blindsight can be subject to fatigue (after several presentations at the side, the responses may stop), can be intermittent, and can vary from day to day and from moment to moment. (The mobile child with such blindsight can walk around obstacles. This has been called *travel vision* [Jan, Wong, Groenveld, Flodmark, & Hoyt, 1986].)

The aim is to identify, quantify, and make use of any intact persistent visual capability (with the child's most comfortable body and head posture). In general, any visual behavior that is identified in such infants and very young children will be most accessible when the child is comfortable, without pain, and in a noise-free environment that is uncluttered and free of distraction and is likely to allow them to maintain attention to only one element at a time.

### Additional Considerations for Assessment

Caregivers are often able to indicate their child's favorite toys, colors, and other preferences. These can be checked during the assessment. Parents are asked to bring favorite toys with them if the assessment is performed outside the home environment. Careful observation of the child's play can provide information about how the child functions, for example:

- Does the child need a good deal of time to respond to particular stimuli or are responses immediate?
- Does the child respond more consistently and more quickly to a familiar versus an unfamiliar person, or to a familiar versus unfamiliar toy?

This information also provides key data for determining intervention approaches. Roman-Lantzy (2007) has developed a system for examining the changes in this type of information over time.

## Vision Intervention for Infants and Very Young Children with CVI

Profound visual impairment resulting from damage to the visual brain, often with evolving cerebral palsy, intellectual challenges, and limited attention, impedes a child's early development. In addition, seizures, usually needing medical control, are common and can compound the condition. These can be followed by lack of vision that gradually improves, while treatment for seizures can cause lethargy and can impair attention.

Interventions for infants and very young children with multiple disabilities resulting from damage to the brain can focus on a range of developmental domains (see Ferrell, 2011; Lueck, Chen, Kekelis, & Hartmann, 2008; Pogrund & Fazzi, 2002). The combined application of evidence-based teaching practices and the sciences of vision, hearing, attention, and learning need to be brought to bear when supporting families with infants who have profound CVI. In this text the focus is on vision and visual perception for learning. For infants and very young children, the goals are to maximize the use of the child's existing vision, and when possible, to encourage further development of visual skills and behaviors (see Appendix 20A). The need for a more robust evidence base for these practices continues to be an issue (see Lueck, 2006; Lueck et al., 2008; Williams et al., 2014), and typical developmental sequences cannot be used as definitive guides to learning and growth for children with CVI. Warren (1994) has asserted, through careful analysis of the literature, that the development of children with visual impairments often cannot be compared with the development of typically developing children in either sequence or age of attainment. He instead calls for attention to individual differences across developmental domains, recognizing each child's developmental trajectory as meaningful and unique to that child. This concept and approach are particularly applicable to children who have CVI.

## Supporting and Collaborating with Caregivers

Parents and other primary caregivers are the main teachers of infants and very young children who have profound CVI. Their optimum development and learning occurs within the dynamics of a socially rich and positive caregiving environment. While interventionists can implement strategies directly with children during scheduled home visits or in center-based programs, it is the caregivers who can infuse critical intervention techniques into children's usual routines on a consistent, daily basis.

Early interventionists can work together with caregivers to identify typical routines in which visual skills can be promoted in a positive and socially meaningful way. They can also work together to design strategies that can be readily incorporated into those routines that promote the use of vision. Caregivers benefit from support and guidance since they are likely to be unfamiliar with the many needs of children who have profound CVI. It is important that such early support is frequent and regular so that caregivers do not become overwhelmed by all that they need to learn and do.

When caregivers first have their observations confirmed by the assessment team that their infant sees very little, their suspicions and fears are realized. For many, an overwhelming sense of helplessness can take hold. Not only do they learn this when they have a new baby (a daunting prospect in its own right), but they probably also have little or no knowledge about how to raise an infant with visual and other impairments. This can be enveloped by fear for the future and even a sense of self-blame, and can be compounded by finding out about other neurological problems that become evident as the child develops.

There are many challenges that new caregivers face:

- The template for parenting is primarily an individual experience, but for parents of a blind or profoundly visually impaired infant with CVI, the template starts off as a "blank sheet of paper."
- Early experiences lay the foundations for future development. Parents may need to be shown how these experiences can be enhanced so that their child's development is optimized.
- Infants normally reward their parents with smiles and other social behaviors that create emotional bonds, but these may not be forthcoming or be so easily recognized when a child has CVI.
- A quiet baby is usually considered a "good" baby, but these children may receive the least stimulation if they do not demand attention in the usual way. The quiet baby with CVI is the very infant who needs planned stimulation.
- On the other hand, some infants with disabilities may have irritable reactions and unpredictable behavior patterns that may be challenging for caregivers (Lueck et al., 2008).
- The psychological reactions of family members to the news that the infant has CVI can be temporarily debilitating or may continue over time in the absence of understanding and support.
- Relationships between parents, which need to be secure for everyone's sake, can become strained.
- The reactions of others, including professionals, friends, and strangers, can sometimes inadvertently send a negative

message to caregivers, who may be particularly sensitive to reactions or words that imply overtly or subtly that something is "not right" with their child since they are not developing as expected.

- Managing the care of an infant with CVI who has additional disabilities can be a full-time endeavor, balancing clinic appointments, therapy, as well as special dietary and medical interventions. This can be an economic as well as an emotional strain on the family, and the time commitment required can put jobs in jeopardy.

As can be seen, support for caregivers goes beyond the need to provide information about the visual, developmental, learning, and medical needs of the infant with CVI. Caregivers (as well as siblings and other family members) are coping with a range of new and unfamiliar issues that can affect their psychological well-being. Since caregivers are the principal teachers at this stage, it is imperative that they are given the range of support they need to address these various issues as they arise over time. This will benefit not only the caregivers, but also the infant and the whole family. With continued support and understanding, caregivers can provide an optimal environment for their child as they work in tandem with professionals to attain the best outcomes possible. (See Chapter 23 for additional information.)

## Working within the Limits of the Child's Intact Brain Functions

All individuals have limits to their perceptions. Sounds and language can be too fast or too quiet to be heard. What a person sees can be too small or move too quickly to have meaning. The typical infant has limited perception and attention at birth, but these limitations progressively diminish during the first few months of life. People typically communicate with new babies from a very close distance (in a way matched to their visual acuities), very slowly (in a way matched to their speed of processing), and with single words (matched to their capacity to perceive only a small amount of information at once).

Similarly, when someone learns to read or to drive, the process is slow initially. This is because the experience is novel, and there is no internal memory for recognition and anticipation. The situation changes quickly, however, and reading or driving becomes easier as the required information is learned, retained, and recognized. It is primarily novel information that is time consuming to assimilate. This is equally true for infants, who we intuitively know will learn best from clear, obvious, and slowly presented speech and imagery. We progressively talk more quickly when using the words we expect the child to know, only slowing for words we assume the child has yet to learn.

These ideas set the scene for how an infant or very young child who may possibly have limited mental processing capacity and limited vision needs to be cared for, stimulated, and taught. Learning takes place as their world progressively gains meaning and their perceptions become linked to prior experience and memory. Learning also takes place within a social context for babies, starting with interactions with their parents or other significant caregivers. These interactions, to be meaningful, must be conducted at the child's pace and within the child's perceptual and cognitive capabilities.

Understanding, interpretation, and learning become possible for most infants and very young children with profound CVI when information is singular, perceptible, accessible, motivating, as well as immediately following and salient to each event as it is experienced and repeated over and again. All material must be distinct, loud enough, and slow enough to be listened to, and big enough and clear enough to be seen. Eyeglasses and hearing aids therefore need to be worn if required.

Clear, slow, distraction-free enhancement of each experience with repeated, meaningful moment-to-moment use of language during times of optimal attention, matched to the known levels of attainment and knowledge, can bring about considerable strides in learning. On the other hand, auditory or visual information presented outside the child's thresholds for perception, and language that is too quiet, too fast, or too masked by background noise to be perceived, do not contribute to learning or development, because as far as the child is concerned nothing meaningful has been seen or heard.

It also needs to be kept in mind that for children whose vision varies from hour to hour and from day to day, the interventionist or teacher needs to be attuned to moments when their performance is optimal and take advantage of these moments for the administration of both assessments and interventions (Jan et al., 1987).

## Specially Prepared Environments

### *Promotion of Visual Attention*

As children with profound CVI become older, it commonly becomes apparent that they have very limited visual attention. Many such children may also have a form of Balint's syndrome (see Chapter 3) in addition to their visual impairment; they can only experience and be aware of a small number of stimuli at once. Not only can they attend to only one or two things at a time, but they can become visually unresponsive when clutter, sound, or discomfort compete for their attention. The discovery and estimation of the limits of visual attention (how much stimulation of any type is needed before visual attention diminishes) must fundamentally dictate how the child is taught. Stimulation with more input than the child can manage is clearly ineffective. Therefore, it is important to consider methods that make events perceptible by being visible and "singular" (keeping visual and auditory distraction to a minimum) from infancy, for children who may require this accommodation.

Infants can be assessed within environments that promote attention to singular events to determine if visual attention needs to be accommodated to promote vision and learning. A "tent" made of plain material without pattern, suspended so that the child and assessor are enclosed together to eliminate background stimuli (see Figure 20.2), can dramatically improve visual attention, with the child becoming animated and interested (Little & Dutton, 2015).

A carefully planned experience to encourage vision use can be designed, based on assessment results. Special environments can be set up in a tent-type situation as described, or other darkened rooms or spaces that provide systematic, planned, illuminated visual stimuli within them to encourage visual attention and vision use. This can include illumination of the assessor's face so that the child's attention can easily focus on it. A sensory room containing various types of sensory stimuli (Hulsegge & Verheul, 1987) can be tailored to the specific sensory needs

FIGURE 20.2
**A Tent to Eliminate Distraction and Promote Visual Attention**

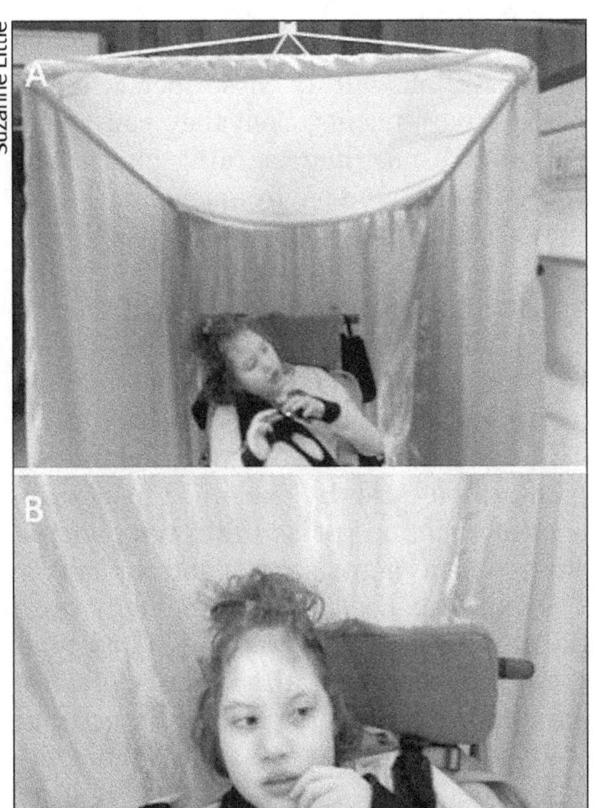


**(A)** A tent like this yellow one (shown with one wall missing) can be suspended to isolate the child and assessor, eliminating background stimuli. **(B)** The child is giving focused attention, a behavior that was not apparent prior to the use of the tent.

of children with CVI so that competing sensory stimuli are eliminated or reduced should they distract the child's attention from the visual task targeted for instruction. It is also critical that once visual attention is noted to improve under these atypical conditions, instruction is progressively and systematically transferred to more normalized situations (Lueck & Heinze, 2004). One way to begin such a transition is to move from exposure to self-illuminated objects, to objects under a spotlight in a darkened room, to objects under a spotlight in a dimly lit room, to objects against highly contrasting backgrounds under more typical lighting conditions. Research into whether sensory rooms improve functional outcomes is limited, although it is possible that this type of environment can diminish some indicators of stress in older children by managing the amount of sensory input available, related to associated relaxation effects (Hotz et al., 2006; Mount & Cavet, 1995).

Other examples of planned environments or materials that provide sensory and motor input in either typical room illumination or in specially illuminated conditions are the "little room" (Nielsen, 1991, 1992) or other specially designed play spaces (Clarke, 2013). These environments encourage children to interact with objects in their surroundings and encourage vision use for children who have some vision. They can also contribute to early conceptual and motor development for all children with visual impairments.

### *Considerations in the Use of Special Environments*

As with all learning situations, the child should be placed in the special room or environment for limited periods of time and removed from the room as soon as attention to the stimuli wanes. Activities within the sensory room, for example, are best when they require active responses from the child, particularly when the child has very basic visual skills; passive viewing experiences that do not require responses will likely not benefit children who already have these basic skills. Corresponding language experiences can help to solidify and expand concepts for children within the special environment and are to be encouraged.

Finally, it is important to remember that the most beneficial educational experiences for infants and young children occur within meaningful social interactions, and these are particularly important for children who have visual impairments, including CVI. Promoting the use of visual experiences in special environments may be needed to jump-start the use of vision, but time spent doing this needs to be monitored carefully. At the same time, it is critical to promote the use of vision in more naturally occurring environments within typical routines that encourage social exchange, especially when rudimentary vision skills are available to the child.

As noted by Lea Hyvärinen (personal communication, December, 2011):

> Visual stimulation as *passive stimulation* is appropriate when an infant/child is barely aware of vision, when the child has very little response to visual stimuli. Once the response is obtained, the goal of intervention is to develop the child's interest in *actively using vision* and a confidence in vision as a source of information about the world. This is not learned through passively watching blinking lights in a dark room or shiny objects in front of a black surface. It is learned by enabling the use of vision through the day in a variety of situations and for a variety of reasons—to better understand communication, to learn about a toy, to understand information from other senses—like looking to see what that new texture is and to understand spaces and the effect of our own actions on the world. We advocate testing and intervention that are tailored to each child in the context of all activities at home, schools, and as a part of therapies.

If the child is more attentive and interested in interactions within these specially prepared environments, then they can be incorporated into their learning plans. Any specially prepared environments must take into account that some children with CVI respond better to dim rather than overly bright, illuminated stimuli (Good & Hou, 2006), while interventions that use "black light" (ultraviolet light) to make certain objects glow may be helpful for some children. Children's visual needs and intervention plan can be carefully explained to caregivers. Intervention goals within the planned environment should be clear and observable. The final goal, however, is to gradually move the child from the specially prepared environment to more typical, socially interactive environments that promote use of vision as well as skills in other areas of development.

## Pinpointing Visual Skills and Behaviors to Support and Teach

The interventionist and caregiver must work together to identify skills that the child can perform independently. They must also identify the next logical step in a sequence of skills leading to a goal that the infant or very young child can attain with caregiver assistance. This goal is best if it is a priority for the caregivers so that it has meaning for both them and for their child, as in the following example:

**Mr. Hayashi, the early interventionist for a baby** named Peter, decided on his own that an appropriate goal for Peter would be to learn to use his vision to find and eat a particular finger food on a tray to promote visual search, inspection, and eye-hand coordination. Peter's family, however, does not typically allow their children to have finger food at this age, and the parents are reluctant to implement this activity with him. Since this goal may not be implemented on a regular basis by the caregivers, Mr. Hayashi instead works with the family to develop a more practical and meaningful goal for that particular child and family where the child is encouraged to look and reach for other objects. Peter's mother always wears several rings on different fingers that have interesting tactile properties. Mr. Hayashi and Peter's family use this information to revise the goal. Now Peter will be encouraged to locate the rings on his mother's fingers and explore them every time he is held in her arms.

This new activity allows for regular sessions of visual search, inspection, and eye-hand coordination throughout the day, and it works well within the family's usual routines and practices. Through careful selection of intervention strategies (called scaffolding techniques) such as prompts, adaptations, or environmental modifications, the child's development is promoted (Lueck et al., 2008).

The chart in Appendix 20A at the end of this chapter provides a guide for selecting interventions for young children with CVI, from birth to 24 months of age, based on the stage they have reached in their development of visual behaviors. The table shows the developmental progression of important visual skills and behaviors in three processes or types of visual behaviors: visual attending behaviors, visual examining behaviors, and visually guided motor behaviors. Teachers and interventionists can use the table to identify skills the child has mastered and then select meaningful skills within the same skills cluster (skills that usually develop around the same time) or next higher level to target for intervention. Suggested intervention approaches for working with the child to develop the targeted skills are provided.

Other suggestions for interventions to promote the attainment of visual skills can be found in the *Developmental Journal for Babies and Children with Visual Impairment*; Lueck et al. (2008); Sonksen and Stiff (1991); and Trief and Shaw (2009). See Chapters 19 and 21 for principles and instructional strategies for working with children with CVI.

## Children Who Have Blindsight

If there is evidence of blindsight, the infant or young child may need specially designed situations to promote the use of vision. The following are some suggestions:

- Enhance social interaction for children who respond to an animated smile by presenting this often and by highlighting the facial features of a caregiver or professional with high-contrast makeup or a dark mustache, matched in dimension to the measured visual acuity.
- For children who respond to a spoonful of food by opening their mouths in anticipation or by other nonverbal cues (such as subtle head, hand, or foot movements), bring in the spoon when feeding the child from each of the four quadrants of the visual field (but not straight ahead) to take advantage of any peripheral vision. Vary the direction of the spoon. If the spoon is always brought in from the same direction the infant may habituate (and not respond) to the stimulus after a short period of time. This approach can significantly shorten feeding time for some children who are fed by mouth.
- The presentation of toys that move in the child's peripheral visual fields may bring about eye or limb movements that can be encouraged, expanded upon, and sometimes used for communication.
- When darkened conditions enhance visual performance, visual activities can

be presented in dimly lit situations to promote vision use.

### Encouraging Mobility

Profound impairment of vision precludes the use of vision both to gain knowledge by watching how others move and for guidance of movement. Some infants and very young children with profound CVI are able to move but need an incentive to explore the environment safely. Those playing with the child may become visible when dressed in bright, high-contrast clothing. Encouraging the child to reach or move toward a favorite person is a great motivator for mobility. In addition, a range of toys that flash colored lights and emit noise can be consistently distributed around a room to provide another type of incentive (Fazzi et al., 2002). These provide the child with evidence of the extent and organization of the surrounding environment. One or two sounds coming from fixed locations help the child to gain and maintain orientation in surrounding space. Near elements are accessible through touch, and more distant elements become attractive for potential exploration when they are consistently and reassuringly appealing and when their position is not changed (unless the child is involved in making and remembering the change).

This process of alerting the child to the environment and then encouraging exploration can take time to develop. Caregivers need to understand that for the child with very low vision, the idea that there is a surrounding environment is a complex and time-consuming concept to learn. Care must be taken to ensure that the area around the child is not so filled with lights or noise that the stimuli are overwhelming and not motivating. Additional ideas for encouraging exploration of the environment can be found in Fazzi et al. (2002); Ferrell (2011); Lueck et al. (2008); and Pogrund and Fazzi (2002).

## Key Elements of Intervention

The following points summarize general principles and best practices in working with infants and very young children who have profound CVI. Because these children spend most of their time with family members in the home environment, it is important to share these ideas with caregivers.

### Providing a Warm and Attentive Family

Children with profound visual impairment may not interact socially in the usual ways. Finding ways to meaningfully engage and make up for the lack of engagement on the child's part is very important. Caregivers may not feel "rewarded" by the child who is not responding as expected—for example, an infant may become quiet and attentive in order to listen rather than smiling or making eye contact, or the child, when hearing a parent's voice, may make unusual and fleeting hand or foot movements that can easily go undetected. This needs to be understood and addressed. Proactive social engagement by caregivers that is both affectionate and meaningful can alter the cycle that is initiated by an infant's limited or unexpected reactions, leading to a lack of response by caregivers, and provide the social interaction that infants require for visual (as well as social and communicative) development.

### Being a 'Radio' Parent

If a person closes his or her eyes and listens to the television, the words that are spoken often do not make sense because much of the language refers to what is being seen. In contrast, when listening to the radio, closing one's eyes makes no difference, because no visual perception on the part of the listener is assumed. For the child who has minimal vision, caregivers and interventionists need to speak in "radio language," language that has descriptive phrases that the child can readily understand, with all words being meaningful since they are linked to the child's direct experiences.

### Matching Words to the Child's Experience

In addition to using radio language, all words need to become meaningful by being linked to the child's direct experiences. Clear, consistent, and repeated use of simple words, describing and immediately following each meaningful event, enhances both understanding of language and the development of speech. For example, as the child finds and picks up a spoon, the word "spoon" is spoken. When the spoon is banged on the tray, the word "bang" follows each bang. "Drop spoon" is spoken just after the spoon is dropped. For more information on early communication with very young children who have CVI, see Sidebar 20.2. (See also Chen, 2014; Chernus-Mansfield, Hayashi, & Kekelis, 1985; Kekelis & Chernus-Mansfield, 1984; Meyers & Lansky, 1991; and see Hagood, 1997 for ideas for older children that can be modified for application to infants and very young children.)

SIDEBAR 20.2

## Promoting Early Conversations with Very Young Children Who Have CVI

***Deborah Chen***

Early interactions provide the foundation for a child's social, emotional, communication, and language development. A parent's ability to identify, interpret, and respond to a child's behavioral signals initiates the child's experience with the power of communication. Young children with complex learning needs, including CVI, require particular support and repeated opportunities to participate in early conversations, to recognize the meaning of sounds and words, and thus develop language. Evidence-based strategies such as those outlined here promote language development based on research with young children with autism, developmental delays, language disorders, hearing loss, visual impairments, and multiple disabilities.

### Interpreting the Child's Behavior as Communication Output

Careful observation of the child's behavioral signals is the first step toward joint development of early conversations. The well-known Hanen Program for children with language delays advises parents and teachers to observe, watch, and listen (abbreviated as OWL) in order to recognize and interpret a child's behavioral signals and respond in a way that the child can perceive (Pepper & Weitzman, 2004). Responding to a child's vocalizations through imitation and interpretation (contingent responsiveness) is essential (Mahoney & Perales, 2005). Once a child's signals (such as movements and sounds) are identified as communicative acts, these behaviors can then be

*(continued on next page)*

gradually shaped into more conventional communication (gestures, manual signs, and speech) (Rowland & Fried-Oken, 2010). When children with disabilities have limited verbal skills, augmentative communicative devices at the child's appropriate developmental level (for example, a voice output switch or iPad; pictures or toys to manipulate) should be used to provide the child with a "voice" or expressive means of communication (Branson & Demchak, 2009).

### Ensuring the Caregiver's Comprehensible Input

*Acoustic highlighting* makes speech easier to perceive and discriminate and so supports language development. The sounds of spoken words are emphasized by eliminating background noise (turning off other sound sources such as a radio, or moving closer to the child), using short simple utterances, slowing the rate of speech, placing the target word at the end of a phrase (for example, "*Want a **ba-na-na**?*"), and adding emphasis on the key words by varying intonation (Esterbrooks & Estes, 2007). A child's vocabulary may be built and expanded though repeated exposure to different types of words in short sentences during conversations in many daily activities (Kaiser & Delaney, 2001). Vocabulary should not only include nouns or names of people and objects (mommy, baby, sponge) but also adjectives such as descriptive words (wet, sweet, bumpy), feeling words (happy, mad, tired), prepositions or location words (up, in, under), verbs or action words (squeeze, walk, drink), and words that indicate belonging (your, my, Daddy's)—all used in the context of the child's ongoing experience. A child's understanding of words and their meaning is developed by labeling the experience (for example, "Let's **squeeze** the wet sponge. **Squeeze!**") at the same time as the child experiences the referents (people, objects, actions, activities, feelings) through available vision, hearing, touch, smell, and movement.

### Early Conversations

Children with disabilities benefit from multiple planned opportunities to engage in focused interactions with responsive caregivers during the day (Mahoney & Perales, 2005). Families may be encouraged to identify specific and convenient times for these conversations. Familiar and favorite people, objects, actions, and activities are motivating conversation topics for young children. Table 20.1 lists a number of evidence-based strategies and examples to support early conversations that contribute to early language development.

**TABLE 20.1**

**Selected Strategies to Promote Early Conversations with Young Children with CVI**

| *Strategy* | *Example* |
|---|---|
| Interpret, say, and respond to what the child is attempting to say (McDuffie & Yoder, 2010) | Child leans on adult, puts arms up, and says, "*Uh.*" Adult says, "*You want up? **Up, up**, you go*" while picking the child up. |
| Interrupt favorite and familiar movement activities or action songs to promote the child's expressive language (Chen, Klein, & Haney, 2007) | Adult pushes child on swing three times then stops and waits for child to request "more" through action, gesture, or vocalization. Adult responds to child's communication "*You want **more** swing*" and pushes the swing. |
| Use the "delay procedure" to encourage the child to initiate a request for a favorite activity (Chen et al., 2007) | Adult places child on swing and waits. Child rocks body and says, "*Uh.*" Adult responds, "*Oh, you want a **push***" and pushes the swing. |

*(continued on next page)*

**TABLE 20.1** *(continued from previous page)*

| ***Strategy*** | ***Example*** |
|---|---|
| Offer choices in daily routines (Mahoney & Perales, 2005) | Adult places two bowls with food in front of child and asks, "*Want peas or carrots?*" |
| Establish joint attention with the child and a named object that is of immediate interest to the child (called triadic joint attention) (Whalen, Schreibman, & Ingersoll, 2006) | Child points to a light in the ceiling. Adult says, "*You see the **light**!*" |
| Comment on the child's focus and interest (Mahoney & Perales, 2005; McDuffie & Yoder, 2010) | Child stills when telephone rings. Adult says, "*That's the **phone**. Do you hear the **phone** ringing?*" and brings phone close to child. |
| Facilitate turn taking and two-way conversations (Mahoney & Perales, 2005) | Child holds phone to ear and says "*Ha.*" Adult responds, "*Hi! Who's this?*" Child vocalizes again. Parent says, "*Hello, Billy!*" |
| Follow the child's lead; modify interaction in response to child's cues (Mahoney & Perales, 2005) | Adult and child are rolling cars on the floor. Child crawls over to "house area" and picks up a spoon and pan. Adult says, "*Let's make something to eat.*" |
| Use "self-talk" and "parallel talk" (Girolametto, Pearce, & Weitzman, 1996; Girolametto, Weitzman, & Clements-Baartman, 1998) | Father says, "*Daddy's making **toast** for you and spreading jelly on it.*" (self-talk) Child takes a bite of toast. Parent says, "*Yum, yum, eating toast and jelly.*" (parallel talk) |
| Repeat and emphasize key words (Esterbrooks & Estes, 2007) | Reading a favorite tactile book about cats, adult says, "*Let's find the **kitty cat**. There's the **kitty cat**. Soft kitty cat!*" |
| Use various cues to increase child's understanding of words (Chen et al., 2007) | Adult says, "*Time to clean up*" and places a tub close to the child to put blocks away. Child does not respond. Adult moves tub to touch child's hand and drops block in tub and says, "***Listen**! Help me put the **blocks** in the tub.*" |
| Expand or modify one's own utterance (Thiemann & Warren, 2010) | Adult says, "***Snack** time. Time to have a **snack**. Let's **eat**.*" |
| Expand or modify the child's utterance with syntactic and semantic expansions (Thiemann & Warren, 2010) | A dog barks and child says, "*Doggie.*" Adult says, "*It's a **doggie**. Yes, **doggie** is **barking**.*" |

*Source:* Adapted from Chen, D. (2014). Promoting early communication and language development. In D. Chen (Ed.), *Essential elements in early intervention: Visual impairment and multiple disabilities* (2nd ed., pp. 447–449). New York: AFB Press.

## Sharing Vocabulary between Home and Early Intervention

As the child understands more and more words, everyone looking after the child in early intervention programs and at home needs to stay up-to-date, share, and consistently use the same progressively enlarging meaningful vocabulary in the same contexts.

## Teaching When the Child Is Attentive

It is important to ensure that teaching or intervention takes place when the child is attentive and can respond to it. Teaching can occur at any time of day during any usual daily routine or special activity to capture the moments when the child is optimally attentive (see, for example, Trief & Shaw, 2009).

## Eliminating Distraction and Minimizing Discomfort

Eliminating distraction and minimizing discomfort can be especially important during the times devoted to teaching by adapting and enhancing activities as needed and carefully shaping social interactions with the child. As already noted, the child has to be comfortable and distraction eliminated by removing background noise, pattern, and clutter. If perception is optimal in a darkened environment, make the stimuli perceptible, safe, and not overwhelming, and transition to a more typical environment whenever possible.

## Staying within the Child's Area of Visual Attention

The further away one is, the more there is to see, and the smaller the imagery. As a result there are more visual distractions and more elements in the visual scene, causing a child to lose visual interest at events occurring at greater distances. Establish the distance at which attention is easily lost and work within that distance.

## Matching the Speed of Working with the Child to the Speed at Which the Child Is Reacting

When the child has a delay in mental processing, the speed of perceiving, the speed of reacting, and the speed of bringing about a response can all be slow. This means that during interactions with the developing infant who has profound CVI, one has to recognize that the child is living in "slow time," and match one's speed of performance accordingly. Likewise, the caregivers need a complete understanding of how the child processes information so that they, too, can match their speed of presentation to the speed at which their child can perceive, understand, respond, and thereby learn.

## Gaining and Maintaining Attention to Toys

The child's attention to toys needs to be obtained and maintained to ensure that every element of every salient image is visible and every element of every sound is perceptible. This is accomplished by matching toys to measured visual capabilities. When a preferential grating acuity measure is available, details of a toy or image conveying meaning need to be larger than the line thickness of the smallest grating size that the child can see at a given distance (the child's estimated grating acuity). For example, if the minimum visible line thickness for a child is half an inch at 10 inches (24cm) away, then this must be the minimum thickness of high-contrast facial features (eye, nose, and mouth) on a doll for when the child positions it 10 inches away. This includes the lines making up the facial features and the width of gaps between these lines (see Appendix 12B). If the lines are any thinner, the features will probably not be seen. If the interventionist or caregivers are dressing up as clowns, for example, the lips need to be rendered a half-inch thick to make them visible at 10 inches, and the gap between the lips when talking has to become that wide as well. Matching these features and details to the child's visual perception allows the child's attention to be obtained and maintained, and play can start, motivating and entertaining the child with fun and laughter.

## Giving Meaning and Accessibility to the Surrounding Environment

The surrounding visual environment needs to be meaningful by being perceptible for the child with measurable vision. The surrounding soundscape and tactile environment need to be consistent and also made meaningful by providing orientation cues.

## Turn Taking and Social Interaction

For turn taking and social interaction to develop, the child must first recognize and understand that there is a surrounding external world with people in it who provide interest and reward. Children must be given opportunities to respond to incoming communications from others in any form and to learn that others respond to their attempts to communicate through such means as words, vocalizations, gestures, expressions, other body language, or touch.

## Enhancing Experiences to Make Them Perceptible, Attractive, Meaningful, and Engaging

The greatest developments take place when the child participates in stimulating, meaningful, enjoyable, and motivating experiences. Therefore, make sure that activities are perceptible to the child, attractive, meaningful, and engaging.

## Progressing from What the Child Already Knows and Can Do

Up-to-date knowledge, obtained through ongoing assessment, of what the child has learned to know and to do needs to inform each new step in the evolving intervention process so that teaching of new skills and knowledge is based on the child's existing capabilities and the next steps in the developmental progression leading to the targeted goal.

## Following the KISS Principle

The well-known KISS principle, or "**K**eep **I**t **S**low and **S**imple," can be used to summarize the following key principles of intervention with infants and very young children who have CVI:

- Each visible singular image needs to move slowly enough to be seen, and be present long enough to react to.
- Each word spoken needs to be clearly articulated at the speed that leads the child to maintain attention.
- Words that are spoken need to be consistently matched to and immediately follow the experience of the child, as the child is having that experience.
- The same vocabulary needs to be shared and used in similar ways by everyone coming into contact with the child.
- Caregivers and interventionists need to be alert to unexpected or unusual behavioral responses the child may have.
- Caregivers and interventionists need to be patient and wait for responses from the child in order to establish the beginnings of communication through turn taking.

Additional suggestions for interventions with young children with CVI can be found in Chapters 19 and 21.

# Conclusion

Infants with profound CVI need to be identified early (Dutton & Jacobson, 2001; Good, Jan, Burden, Skoczenski, & Candy, 2001) so that appropriate intervention and support can be provided as soon as possible. While there is not an extensive evidence base delineating the effects of early intervention for these children (Lueck, 2006), it is known that early intervention has a positive impact on learning and development for infants with other disabilities (Guralnick, 1998, 2011). Infants and very young children who have profound CVI require specialized assessment techniques that point toward ways to maximize the effectiveness of interventions for learning and development. For this population of children, it is the primary caregivers who need to implement intervention activities in the course of everyday routines with supportive guidance from trained professionals who can help caregivers gain insight into the world as seen through their children's eyes.

## References

Anderson, S., Boignon, S., & Davis, K. (1991). *The Oregon project for visually impaired and blind preschool children* (5th ed.). Medford, OR: Jackson Education Service District.

Atkinson, J. (2000). *The developing visual brain* (Oxford Psychology Series No. 32). New York: Oxford University Press.

Bayley, N. (1969). *Bayley scales of infant development.* New York: Psychological Corporation.

Bayley, N. (1993). *Bayley scales of infant development* (2nd ed.). San Antonio, TX: Psychological Corporation.

Bowman, R., McCulloch, D. L., Law, E., Mostyn, K., & Dutton, G. N. (2010). The "mirror test" for estimating visual acuity in infants. *British Journal of Ophthalmology, 94*(7), 882–885.

Boyle, N. J., Jones, D. H., Hamilton, R., Spowart, K. M., & Dutton, G. N. (2005). Blindsight in children: Does it exist and can it be used to help the child? Observations on a case series. *Developmental Medicine & Child Neurology, 47*(10), 699–702.

Branson, D., & Demchak, M. (2009). The use of augmentative and alternative communication methods with infants and toddlers with disabilities. A research review. *Augmentative & Alternative Communication, 25*(4), 274–286.

Calvello, G. (1990). Identifying vision impairments in infants. In D. Chen, C. T. Freidman, & G. Calvello (Eds.), *Parents and visually impaired infants.* Louisville, KY: American Printing House for the Blind.

Chen, D. (2014). Promoting early communication and language development. In D. Chen (Ed.), *Essential elements in early intervention: Visual impairment and multiple disabilities* (2nd ed., pp. 447–449). New York: AFB Press.

Chen, D., Klein, M. D., & Haney, M. (2007). Promoting interactions with infants who have complex multiple disabilities: Development and field-testing of the PLAI curriculum. *Infants & Young Children, 20*(2), 149–162.

Chernus-Mansfield, N., Hayashi, D., & Kekelis, L. (1985). *Talk to me, Part II: Common concerns* [Brochure]. Los Angeles: Blind Childrens Center.

Clarke, K. L. (2013). *Hold everything! Twenty stay-put play spaces for infants, preschoolers, and developmentally young children with sensory impairments and other special needs.* Dublin: The Ohio Center for Deafblind Education. Retrieved August 7, 2013, from http://ohiodeafblind.org/resources/products.cfm

Dutton, G. N., & Jacobson, L. K. (2001). Cerebral visual impairment in children. *Seminars in Neonatology, 6*(6), 477–485.

Esterbrooks, S. R., & Estes, E. L. (2007). *Helping deaf and hard of hearing students to use spoken language: A guide for educators and families.* Thousand Oaks, CA: Corwin Press.

Fazzi, E., Lanners, J., Ferrari-Ginevra, O., Achille, C., Luparia, A., Signorini, S., et al. (2002). Gross motor development and reach on sound as critical tools for the development of the blind child. *Brain & Development, 24*(5), 269–275.

Ferrell, K. A. (2010). Visual development. In A. L. Corn & J. N. Erin (Eds.), *Foundations of low vision: Clinical and functional perspectives* (2nd ed., pp. 299–338). New York: AFB Press.

Ferrell, K. A. (2011). *Reach out and teach: Helping your child who is visually impaired learn and grow* (2nd ed.). New York: AFB Press.

Ferrell, K. A., Trief, E., Dietz, S. J., Bonner, M. A., Cruz, D., Ford, E., et al. (1990). Visually impaired infants research consortium (VIIRC): First-year results. *Journal of Visual Impairment & Blindness, 84*, 404–410.

Girolametto, L., Pearce, P., & Weitzman, E. (1996). Interactive focused stimulation for toddlers with expressive vocabulary delays. *Journal of Speech, Language, and Hearing Research, 39*(6), 1274–1283.

Girolametto, L., Weitzman, E., & Clements-Baartman, J. (1998). Vocabulary intervention for children with Down syndrome: Parent training using focused stimulation. *Infant-Toddler Intervention: A Transdisciplinary Journal, 8*(2), 109–125.

Glass, P. (1993). Development of vision function in preterm infants: Implications for early intervention. *Infants & Young Children, 6*(1), 11–20.

Good, W. V., & Hou, C. (2006). Sweep visual evoked potential grating acuity thresholds paradoxically improve in low-luminance conditions in children with cortical visual impairment. *Investigative Ophthalmology & Visual Science, 47*(7), 3220–3224.

Good, W. V., Hou, C., & Norcia, A. M. (2012). Spatial contrast sensitivity vision loss in children with cortical visual impairment. *Investigative Ophthalmology & Visual Science, 53*(12), 7730–7734.

Good, W. V., Jan, J. E., Burden, S. K., Skoczenski, A., & Candy, R. (2001). Recent advances in cortical visual impairment. *Developmental Medicine & Child Neurology, 43*(1), 56–60.

Guralnick, M. J. (1998). Effectiveness of early intervention for vulnerable children: A developmental perspective. *American Journal on Mental Retardation, 102*(4), 319–345.

Guralnick, M. J. (2011). Why early intervention works: A systems perspective. *Infants & Young Children, 24*(1), 6–28.

Hagood, L. (1997). *Communication - A guide for teaching students with visual and multiple impairments.* Austin: Texas School for the Blind and Visually Impaired.

Hotz, G. A., Castelblanco, A., Lara, I. M., Weiss, A. D., Duncan, R., & Kuluz, J. W. (2006). Snoezelen: A controlled multi-sensory stimulation therapy for children recovering from severe brain injury. *Brain Injury, 20*(8), 879–888.

Hou, C., Good, W. V., & Norcia, A. M. (2007). Validation study of VEP vernier acuity in normal-vision and amblyopic adults. *Investigative Ophthalmology & Visual Science, 48*(9), 4070–4078.

Hulsegge, J., & Verheul, A. (1987). *Snoezelen: Another world: A practical book of sensory experience environments for the mentally handicapped.* Chesterfield, UK: Rompa.

Hyvärinen, L. (1988). *Vision in children: Normal and abnormal.* Meaford, ON: Canadian Deaf-Blind & Rubella Association.

Jan, J. E., Groenveld, M., Sykanda, A. M., & Hoyt, C. S. (1987). Behavioral characteristics of children with permanent cortical visual impairment. *Developmental Medicine & Child Neurology, 29*(5), 571–576.

Jan, J. E., Wong, P. K., Groenveld, M., Flodmark, O., & Hoyt, C. S. (1986). Travel vision: "Collicular visual system"? *Pediatric Neurology, 2*(6), 359–362.

Kaiser, A. P., & Delaney, E. M. (2001). Responsive conversations: Creating opportunities for naturalistic language teaching. In M. Ostrosky & S. Sandall (Eds.), *Teaching strategies: What to do to support young children's development: Young exceptional children monograph series No. 3* (pp. 13–23). Longmont, CO: Sopris West.

Kekelis, L., & Chernus-Mansfield, N. (1984). *Talk to me: A language guide for parents of blind children* [Brochure]. Los Angeles: Blind Childrens Center.

Little, S., & Dutton, G. N. (2015). Some children with multiple disabilities and cerebral visual impairment can engage when enclosed by a "tent": Is this due to Balint syndrome? *British Journal of Visual Impairment, 33*(1), 66–73.

Lueck, A. H. (2006). Issues in intervention for children with visual impairment or visual dysfunction due to brain injury. In E. Dennison & A. H. Lueck (Eds.), *Proceedings of the summit on cerebral/cortical visual impairment: Educational, family, and medical perspectives, April 30, 2005* (pp. 121–130). New York: AFB Press.

Lueck, A. H., Chen, D., Kekelis, L. S., & Hartmann, E. S. (2008). *Developmental guidelines for infants with visual impairments: A guidebook for early intervention* (2nd ed.). Louisville, KY: American Printing House for the Blind.

Lueck, A. H., & Heinze, T. (2004). Interventions for young children with visual impairments and students with visual and multiple disabilities. In A. H. Lueck (Ed.), *Functional vision: A practitioner's guide to evaluation and intervention* (pp. 277–351). New York: AFB Press.

Mackay, A. M., Bradnam, M. S., Hamilton, R., Elliot, A. T., & Dutton, G. N. (2008). Real-time rapid acuity assessment using VEPs: Development and validation of the step VEP technique. *Investigative Ophthalmology & Visual Science, 49*(1), 438–441.

Mahoney, G., & Perales, F. (2005). Relationship-focused early intervention with children with pervasive developmental disorders and other disabilities: A comparative study. *Journal of Developmental & Behavioral Pediatrics, 26*(2), 77–85.

McCulloch, D. L., Mackie, R. T., Dutton, G. N., Bradnam, M. S., Day, R. E., McDaid, G. J., . . . Shepherd, A. J. (2007). A visual skills inventory for children with neurological impairments. *Developmental Medicine & Child Neurology, 49*(10), 757–763.

McDuffie, A., & Yoder, P. (2010). Types of parent verbal responsiveness that predict language in young children with autism spectrum disorder. *Journal of Speech, Language, and Hearing Research, 53*(4), 1026–1039.

Meyers, L., & Lansky, P. (1991). *Dancing cheek to cheek* [Brochure]. Los Angeles: Blind Childrens Center.

Moseley, M. J., Fielder, A. R., Thompson, J. R., Minshull, C., & Price, D. (1988). Grating and recognition acuities of young amblyopes. *British Journal of Ophthalmology, 72*(1), 50–54.

Mount, H., & Cavet, J. (1995). Multi-sensory environments: An exploration of their potential for young people with profound and multiple learning difficulties. *British Journal of Special* Education, *22*(2), 52–55.

Nielsen, L. (1991). Spatial relations in congenitally blind infants: A study. *Journal of Visual Impairment & Blindness, 85,* 11–16.

Nielsen, L. (1992). *Space and self.* Copenhagen, Denmark: Sikon Press.

Pegna, A. J., Khateb, A., Lazeyras, F., & Seghier, M. L. (2005). Discriminating emotional faces without primary visual cortices involves the right amygdala. *Nature Neuroscience, 8,* 24–25.

Pepper, J., & Weitzman, E. (2004). *It takes two to talk: A practical guide for parents of children with language delays.* Toronto, ON: The Hanen Centre.

Pogrund, R. L., & Fazzi, D. L. (Eds.). (2002). *Early focus: Working with young children who are blind or visually impaired and their families* (2nd ed.). New York: AFB Press.

Roman-Lantzy, C. (2007). *Cortical visual impairment: An approach to assessment and intervention.* New York: AFB Press.

Rowland, C., & Fried-Oken, M. (2010). Communication matrix: A clinical and research assessment tool targeting children with severe communication disorders. *Journal of Pediatric Rehabilitation Medicine, 3*(4), 319–329.

Sonksen, P. M., & Stiff, B. (1991). *Show me what my friends can see: A development guide for parents of babies with severely impaired sight and their professional advisors.* London: University of London Press.

Teller, D. Y., Dobson, V., & Mayer, D. L. (2005). *Teller acuity cards II.* Chicago: Stereo Optical.

Thiemann, K., & Warren, S. F. (2010). Programs supporting young children's language development. In R. E. Tremblay, R. G. Barr, R. D. Peters, & M. Boivin (Eds.), *Encyclopedia on early childhood development.* Quebec, QC: Centre of Excellence for Early Childhood Development. Retrieved July 29, 2012, from http://www.child-encyclopedia.com/sites/default/files/textes-experts/en/622/programs-supporting-young-childrens-language-development.pdf

Tinelli, F., Cicchini, G. M., Arrighi, R., Tosetti, M., Cioni, G., & Morrone, M. C. (2013). Blindsight in children with congenital and acquired cerebral lesions. *Cortex, 49*(6), 1636–1647.

Trief, E., & Shaw, R. (2009). *Everyday activities to promote visual efficiency: A handbook for working with young children with visual impairments.* New York: AFB Press.

Warren, D. H. (1994). *Blindness and children: An individual differences approach.* New York: Cambridge University Press.

Whalen, C., Schreibman, L., & Ingersoll, B. (2006). The collateral effects of joint attention training on social initiations, positive affect, imitation, and spontaneous speech for young children with autism. *Journal of Autism & Developmental Disorders, 36*(5), 655–664.

Williams, C., Northstone, K., Borwick, C., Gainsborough, M., Roe, J., Howard, S., . . . Woodhouse, J. M. (2014). How to help children with neurodevelopmental and visual problems: A scoping review. *British Journal of Ophthalmology, 98,* 6–12.

Zihl, J., & Dutton, G. N. (2015). *Cerebral visual impairment in children: Visuoperceptive and visuocognitive disorders.* Vienna: Springer-Verlag Wien.

# APPENDIX 20A
# Functional Vision Development Charts for Selecting Interventions

The development of skills and behaviors related to visual functioning in visually impaired infants has been examined in terms of three processes: visual attending behaviors, visual examining behaviors, and visually guided motor behaviors. Indicators for these processes are listed in the corresponding charts that follow. The charts can be used to help determine critical skills and behaviors to consider for intervention with individual infants.

**Directions:**
For each process or type of behavior, determine the developmental cluster for an infant by identifying the skills and behaviors that the infant has attained. Then use the skills and behaviors within that developmental cluster, or at the next developmental cluster, as guides when devising an intervention program for the child. (Note: Some infants may have skills and behaviors in more than one cluster in a developmental process.)

**Process:**
Visual attending behaviors: The infant visually attends to environmental stimuli.
Visual examining behaviors: The infant makes cognitive judgments based on visual input.
Visually guided motor behaviors: The infant makes fine or gross motor adjustments based on visual input.

Note: Infants must have vision sufficient to participate in the activities on these charts as well as sufficient motor capabilities.

## Process: Visual Attending Behaviors

| *Cluster* | *Indicator* | *Source* | *Clarification* | *Suggestions for Intervention* |
|---|---|---|---|---|
| Cluster 1 Visual Attending Behaviors | Regards person momentarily (Infants with CVI may not look at a face but may look at a moving object) | Bayley 1 & 2 | While holding infant about 1 foot from face, infant looks at adult. Adult talks to attract infant's attention. | Encourage infant to look at the faces of caregivers. Bring the caregiver's face closer if necessary. Place the infant's hand on caregiver's face. Women can wear lipstick to heighten contrast. Caregiver can wear a shirt of contrasting color to highlight the face. |
| | Inspects surroundings | Bayley 1 & 2; Glass | Infant turns eyes or head in visual exploration of surroundings. | Provide simple, bold objects for visually impaired infant to watch. A uniform background of contrasting color is recommended for ease of viewing. Some infants will not require visual enhancement to encourage viewing. Some may require bolder, bigger stimuli at a closer distance. Others may |

*(continued on next page)*

(continued from previous page)

| Cluster | Indicator | Source | Clarification | Suggestions for Intervention |
|---|---|---|---|---|
| | | | | require presentation of softly illuminated objects in dimly lit rooms or objects spotlighted under soft illumination in dimly lit rooms. This will depend on the infant's vision capabilities and the training objective. |
| | Looks at image in mirror at progressively greater distances with increasing age. (While this behavior is seen in early ages in typical infants, this indicator may need to be first presented at later ages for infants born more than 3 weeks prematurely or with obvious ophthalmological abnormalities or uncorrected refractive errors.) NOTE: This indicator can be rechecked at different developmental ages to monitor change. | Bowman | When infant is in sitting position and wearing a brightly colored garment, hold mirror until infant attends to the reflection in it.<br>Begin at 8 inches (20 cm) from infant and engage infant to attend. If infant does not attend at 8 inches, move closer until attention is established. If infant does attend at 8 inches, move further away until infant loses interest. | The distance to use for presentation of bright and motivating toys (and when appropriate, simple, bold pictures) is two times the furthest distance at which the infant attends to his or her image in the mirror. As the infant matures, the furthest distance can be redetermined. |
| | Eyes follow moving person | Bayley 1 & 2 | While lying on floor on back, infant's eyes follow a person moving within visual field. | Encourage the infant with gentle vocalizations and tactile stimulation. |
| | Regards object very briefly | Bayley 1 & 2 | Stand behind infant and outside field of vision. Suspend toy or ring so that the lower edge is at midline and 8 inches above infant's eyes. Move toy, then hold it stationary. Infant gazes at toy at least 3 seconds in one of three trials. (May need closer distance for infants with visual impairment.) | Present objects during interactive play. For severely visually impaired infants, visual cues may need to be made larger, of higher contrast, and with good illumination. |

(continued on next page)

(continued from previous page)

| Cluster | Indicator | Source | Clarification | Suggestions for Intervention |
|---|---|---|---|---|
| | Watches lip movements | Calvello | Infant responds to normal and exaggerated lip movements by quieting, staring, or any other noticeable reaction. | Encourage interactive play with caregivers and infants. Enhance lips of women with bright or dark (high contrasting) lipstick for severely visually impaired infants. A dark mustache on a pale face can also engage the infant. Infants can be encouraged to touch the face, mustache, and/or lips as the caregiver speaks.<br>Match the speed of speech/lip movement to a speed that allows time for the infant to take in the input and respond. (Match the width of the lipstick, contrasting maximally to the color of the face, to the thickness of the lines that has been measured the infant can see, like the face of a clown. At later ages, apply the same measures and speeds to all facial features on felt and other dolls and puppets designed to be visible for the child.) |
| | Eyes follow object horizontally | Bayley 1 & 2 | Stand behind infant with object at midline and 8 inches above eyes. Attract infant's attention and slowly move object to infant's right, left, and back to midline. Infant follows one complete excursion in up to three trials even if gaze breaks away once or twice. (May need closer distance for infants with visual impairment. Some infants may need to be on their backs for this activity.) | Infant requires practice following objects that can be seen during daily routines (e.g., while eating). Infants with severe visual impairment may require enhanced objects against a high-contrast, uncluttered background. Sound may be added to encourage the infant to look and follow. Sound coming from the object (with no interference from background sound) can be added to encourage the infant to look, give attention, and follow. Illuminated objects that are not overwhelming can also be used. Some infants may need extra assistance at first by having a hand placed on an object as it moves in order to feel where it is going. Some infants may need very slow-moving objects at first. |

(continued on next page)

(continued from previous page)

| Cluster | Indicator | Source | Clarification | Suggestions for Intervention |
| --- | --- | --- | --- | --- |
| | Eyes follow object vertically | Bayley 1 & 2 | Stand behind infant with object at midline and 8 inches above eyes. Attract infant's attention and slowly move object from infant's eyes to the forehead, to the chest, then lying on back for this activity. Infant follows one complete excursion in up to three trials, even if gaze breaks away once or twice. (May need closer distance for infants with visual impairment.) | Infant requires practice following objects that can be seen during daily routines (e.g., while eating). Infants with severe visual impairment may require enhanced objects against a high-contrast, uncluttered background. Sound may be added to encourage the infant to look and follow. Sound coming from the object (with no interference from background sound) can be added to encourage the infant to look, give attention, and follow. Illuminated objects that are not overwhelming can also be used. Some infants may need extra assistance at first by having a hand placed on an object as it moves in order to feel where it is going. Some infants may need very slow-moving objects at first. |
| | Eyes follow object in circular path | Bayley 1 & 2 | Stand behind infant with object at midline and 8 inches above eyes. Attract infant's attention and slowly move toy or ring in a circle about 12 inches in diameter and in a horizontal plane. Infant should be lying on back for this activity. Infant follows circular motion in upper and lower halves of circle even if in different trials. Allow three trials. (May need closer distance for infants with visual impairment.) | Infant requires practice following objects that can be seen during daily routines (e.g., while eating). Infants with severe visual impairment may require enhanced objects against a high-contrast, uncluttered background. Sound may be added to encourage the infant to look and follow. Sound coming from the object (with no interference from background sound) can be added to encourage the infant to look, give attention, and follow. Illuminated objects that are not overwhelming can also be used. Some infants may need extra assistance at first by having a hand placed on an object as it moves in order to feel where it is going. Some infants may need very slow-moving objects at first. |

(continued on next page)

(continued from previous page)

| Cluster | Indicator | Source | Clarification | Suggestions for Intervention |
|---|---|---|---|---|
| | Reacts to objects in the periphery | Glass | When infant is looking at something straight ahead and a brightly colored toy is moved in from the side to the infant's midline at a moderate rate, in an arc about 8 inches away, the infant responds by looking at or attempting to reach for toy. (May need closer distance for infants with marked visual impairment.) | Bring toys that are visible to infant in from the sides to encourage viewing. Use visually enhanced or sound-making toys as necessary. Gently guide infant's hands to objects that are at a distance to encourage reaching when appropriate. (See comments under Inspects Surroundings on this chart.) |
| | Glances from one object to another | Bayley 1 & 2; Glass | While infant is lying on back with head propped to midline, hold bell in one hand and bell in other about 8 inches apart and 10–12 inches above infant's head with both objects in visual field. Gently shake one toy, then the other to make a soft sound. Alternate shaking three times, allowing several seconds between shakes for the infant's eyes to move from one toy to the other. Infant's eyes move from one toy to the other at least two times, even if gaze breaks away. (May need closer distance for infants with visual impairment.) | Provide these experiences with familiar sound-making objects during interactive play. Gently guide infant's hands to object rather than bringing the object to the infant's hands. For older infants, allow the infant to use a tactile bridge (e.g., a hand, arm, toy) to explore along to reach the object. |
| | Head follows object | Bayley 1 & 2 | Have infant seated. Hold object level with infant's eyes and 12 to 15 inches away. Move it in a semicircular path to child's right, left, and midline. Infant turns head to follow object through one of three trials, even if gaze breaks away. (May need closer distance for infants with visual impairment.) | Infant requires practice following objects that can be seen. Infants with severe visual impairment may require enhanced objects (related to size, color, contrast) against a high-contrast back-ground. Sound may be added to encourage the infants to look. |

(continued on next page)

(continued from previous page)

| Cluster | Indicator | Source | Clarification | Suggestions for Intervention |
|---|---|---|---|---|
| | Regards small object briefly | Bayley 1 & 2 | When seated at table, infant regards small object the size of a cube for at least 3 seconds. Tap near object to attract infant's attention. (Object size will depend on degree of visual impairment.) | Infants require practice with small objects. Use touch as well as vision for infants with severe visual impairment. Place objects visible to the infant (related to size, color, contrast) on background of high contrast in initial training phase. |
| | Eyes follow ball | Bayley 1 & 2 | When seated at table, infant turns eyes or head to watch as ball moves across midline. Ball is 12 inches away. Attract infant's attention to ball if necessary. (May need closer distance and large ball for infant with visual impairment.) | Encourage child to watch moving objects during interactive play. Objects may require visual enhancement. Sound-making objects or wind-up toys may attract infant's visual attention. (See comments under Inspects Surroundings on this chart.) |
| | Inspects own hands | Bayley 1; Glass | Observe infant's behavior during periods of unstructured activity. Infant looks attentively at one or both hands. | Place textured half-mittens over hands, with or without toys attached, use colored cloth bracelets with bells sewn between two layers of fabric to encourage viewing. Encourage this skill in different body positions. |
| Cluster 2 Visual Attending Behaviors | Attends to scribbling | Bayley 1 & 2 | Place a piece of paper in front of infant on table. Take crayon and scribble plainly with obvious writing gestures. Let child hold crayon. Child attends to demonstrated scribbling or scribbles. | Provide experiences with markers and crayons that create lines visible to the child. Place light paper with dark markers on light box for older infants with severe visual impairment. Use scented markers to add olfactory cues. |
| | Reacts to toys at distance | Hyvärinen | Infant reacts to presentation of favorite silent toys, foods, etc., when presented from 5 feet away or more. Reaction can be change in expression, excitement level, activity level, etc. | Encourage infant to expand region of visual attention if vision is available for tasks outside arm's reach. Use visually enhanced and sound-making materials for training as necessary. Be sure that the background behind presented items does not distract the infant because of competing visual clutter. |

(continued on next page)

(continued from previous page)

## Process: Visual Examining Behaviors

| Cluster | Indicator | Source | Clarification | Suggestions for Intervention |
|---|---|---|---|---|
| Cluster 1 Visual Examining Behaviors | Searches with eyes for sound | Bayley 1 & 2 | With infant lying on back, prop infant's head up in midline position, being careful not to block ears. Stand away from infant's head out of direct line of sight. Ring bell to one side, then the other side, out of the infant's visual field and 18–24 inches away. If no response, repeat using a rattle. Infant's eyes or head move in apparent search for sound, although not necessarily in the correct direction. | Bring infant's hands to sound-making objects rather than objects to the infant to reinforce the concept of their position in space. Begin by sounding object while in infant's hands or while infant's hands are in contact with toy that is touching body. Encourage movement to the object by touching the infant's shoulder (not the hand) to assist the infant in a reaching motion whenever possible. |
| | Visually recognizes caregiver | Bayley 1 & 2 | Infant visually differentiates caregiver from stranger when stranger moves from field of view and caregiver then enters it. Infant has animated expression or pays particular attention to caregiver. | Caregiver uses a consistent greeting, to begin interaction with the infant. The greeting should be at a speed that allows the infant to take in the input and allows sufficient time for the infant to respond. |
| | Reacts to disappearance of face | Bayley 1 & 2 | When infant's attention is attracted to caregiver's face, infant changes facial expression or reacts in any other way when caregiver quickly moves out of infant's range of vision. | Encourage infant to look at caregiver's face. Bring face closer to infant with severe visual impairment. Women can wear lipstick that contrasts well with the face to enhance visibility of the lips. Bring infant's hand to caregiver's face to reinforce and to encourage exploration. |
| | Displays visual preference | Bayley 2 | Present a card on which there is a simple pattern versus a card with a complex pattern (e.g., bold, black cross on white background versus thin black-and-white striped pattern). Infant looks longer at complex pattern. | Infant begins to show preferences. Continue exposure to functional stimuli the infant finds interesting. |

(continued on next page)

(continued from previous page)

| Cluster | Indicator | Source | Clarification | Suggestions for Intervention |
|---|---|---|---|---|
| | Turns head to sound | Bayley 1 & 2 | Standing behind seated infant, ring bell or shake rattle 12–14 inches from one ear, then the other ear. Repeat if necessary. Infant purposely turns head to sound at least once in three trials. | Based on earlier experiences with sound-making objects. When child turns, gently guide the infant to touch object directly. It can be helpful to allow the infant to follow along an arm or hand to the object. |
| Cluster 2 Visual Examining Behaviors | Looks for fallen objects | Bayley 1 & 2; VIIRC | Hold toy near table edge and let it drop while infant is attending. Repeat if response is not clear. Infant turns head to look for fallen toy. | Based on earlier experiences involving vision and cognition. Provide experiences for infant following visible objects moving in different directions. Objects may require visual enhancement (size, color, contrast). |
| Cluster 3 Visual Examining Behaviors | Looks at pictures (looking at two-dimensional objects may come very slowly for some infants with visual impairment) | Bayley 1 & 2 | When presented with large, clear pictures in bright colors with simple lines matched to dimension known to be seen by the infant, infant looks at specific pictures rather than quickly leafing through book. Encourage infant to look. Help hold the book for infant if necessary. | Provide experiences with pictures with key elements visible to the child. Enhance elements as needed with markers. Discuss the pictures during interactive play. Provide picture books with visible pictures (or ones that have been enhanced) for solitary play as appropriate. Use books with textures, sound effects, and peek-a-boo windows. For older infants with severe visual impairment, large outlined pictures on a light box may be the initial step. |
| | Looks for contents in container | Bayley 1 & 2 | Place small object in container and rattle container. Take objects out of container and place in front of infant. Replace objects in container and rattle again. Remove objects from container out of the infant's field of vision. Hand the container to the infant. Infant looks into the container for objects before reaching inside. | Provide opportunities for the infant to play with containers such as pots, pans, and plastic tubs along with safe objects that can be placed into and dumped out of them. |

(continued on next page)

(continued from previous page)

| Cluster | Indicator | Source | Clarification | Suggestions for Intervention |
|---|---|---|---|---|
| Cluster 6 Visual Examining Behaviors | Identifies family members at a distance | Hyvärinen | Infant can name a family member using vision from 7 feet away or more. | Encourage infant to locate and examine objects at a distance within infant's visual capabilities. Add visual enhancement as needed and present against an uncluttered background. Add sound as necessary during training. Develop a "Who's that?" game or ask the infant, "Where's Mommy?," etc. |

## Process: Visually Guided Motor Behaviors

| Cluster | Indicator | Source | Clarification | Suggestions for Intervention |
|---|---|---|---|---|
| Cluster 1 Visually Guided Motor Behaviors | Bats at dangling toy | Glass | When lying on back with a toy hanging overhead 8 inches away, infant swings at toy with hand when both hand and toy are in visual field. May need closer distance for infant to see the toy. | Provide an environment in which toys are in the infant's field of view, are readily detectable given the infant's visual impairment, and are within arm's reach. Toys should contrast well with the background (e.g., ceiling, wall, or furniture) and be positioned so that they are not directly in front of the eyes (slightly under eyes and to the right or left if the infant is lying down). In this way, the infant can choose to look at or disregard the toys. |
| | Reaches for dangling toy | Bayley 1 & 2 | While lying down, infant reaches for toy hanging about 8 inches above infant's eyes. Need not grasp toy. (May need closer distance for infants with visual impairment.) | Encourage reaching to sound-making objects. Bring infant's hands to sound source. Provide graspable hanging toys during supervised play **only,** to ensure safety. Position toys so that child can choose to look at them or look away (not directly in front of eyes). Graspable hanging toys can include canning rings, textured thick ribbon, and ponytail ribbons. (See comments under Inspects Surroundings in Visual Attending Behaviors chart.) |
| Cluster 2 Visually Guided Motor Behaviors | Reaches for caregiver's face | Calvello | Infant reaches toward caregiver's mouth, nose, eyeglasses, etc. | Based on interaction with caregiver and earlier experiences of viewing and touching caregiver's face. Name each element clearly and slowly as it is touched. |

(continued on next page)

(continued from previous page)

| Cluster | Indicator | Source | Clarification | Suggestions for Intervention |
|---|---|---|---|---|
| | Manipulates object with visual interest in object details | Bayley 1 & 2 | Hold sound-making object in front of seated infant. Sound the object and set it in front of infant. Repeat if infant does not pick up object and hand object to infant. Infant manipulates object while visually examining details. | Encourage infant to play with objects that provide sufficient visual feedback to promote prolonged visual attention. This will vary with each infant's visual needs. Consider use of size, color, and contrast. |
| Cluster 3 Visually Guided Motor Behaviors | Imitates movements | Bayley 1 & 2 | Caregiver pats unfamiliar toy on table in front of infant to elicit sound several times. Infant imitates motion. | Encourage infant to imitate movements with readily visible objects that result in a rewarding experience (e.g., sound, vibration, light, etc.). |
| Cluster 5 Visually Guided Motor Behaviors | Scribbles spontaneously | Bayley 2 | Place paper on table in front of infant with crayon on paper and the crayon tip pointing away. Infant spontaneously scribbles without demonstration or encouragement. | Encourage infant to draw with crayons, markers, scented markers, as well as paint with brushes or finger paint with pudding or paint mixed with sand. |
| Cluster 6 Visually Guided Motor Behaviors | Points to two large pictures in book | Bayley 2 | When presented with large, clear pictures in bright colors with simple lines with dimensions the infant is known to see, infant names, points, or touches two pictures as they are named. The infant can identify unfamiliar pictures as well as familiar ones. | Provide infant with a variety of picture books, books with textures, books with auditory feedback, peek-a-boo books, and books that have accompanying audiotapes. |
| | Imitates crayon stroke | Bayley 2 | Place paper on table in front of infant with crayon on paper and the crayon tip pointing away. Adult can assist in holding paper. Draw a vertical line and ask infant to copy it (e.g., Can you do it?). Then draw a horizontal line and ask infant to copy it. Infant produces stroke in any direction. | Based on earlier experiences with crayons and markers that make lines visible to the infant. Encourage scribbling, imitation of strokes in interactive play. |

(continued on next page)

(continued from previous page)

| Cluster | Indicator | Source | Clarification | Suggestions for Intervention |
|---|---|---|---|---|
| | Matches objects with pictures of those objects | Oregon | When handed objects, one at a time, infant matches three objects with corresponding pictures that are large and clear, with simple lines. Task should be demonstrated once to the infant using a different picture/object pair. Infant can point, name, or physically position objects to match pairs. | Engage in interactions in which infant matches objects to objects and objects to pictures. Objects should be readily visible to the infant. |

*Source:* Adapted from Lueck, A. H., Chen, D., Kekelis, L. S., & Hartmann, E. S. (2008). *Developmental guidelines for infants with visual impairments: A guidebook for early intervention* (2nd ed.). Louisville, KY: American Printing House for the Blind.

## Key to Sources for Developmental Behaviors

| Source | Population | Type | Reference |
|---|---|---|---|
| Bayley 1 | normally sighted infants | standardized infant development scale | Bayley, N. (1969). *Bayley scales of infant development.* New York: Psychological Corporation. |
| Bayley 2 | normally sighted infants | standardized infant development scale | Bayley, N. (1993). *Bayley scales of infant development* (2nd ed.). San Antonio, TX: Psychological Corporation. |
| Bowman | normally sighted infants | comparative study | Bowman, R., McCulloch, D. L., Law, E., Mostyn, K., & Dutton, G. N. (2010). The "mirror test" for estimating visual acuity in infants. *British Journal of Ophthalmology, 94*(7), 882–885. |
| Calvello | normally sighted infants and infants with visual impairment | literature review | Calvello, G. (1990). Identifying vision impairments in infants. In D. Chen, C. T. Freidman, & G. Calvello (Eds.), *Parents and visually impaired infants.* Louisville, KY: American Printing House for the Blind. |
| Glass | normally sighted infants who are full term and premature | literature review | Glass, P. (1993). Development of vision function in preterm infants: Implications for early intervention. *Infants & Young Children, 6*(1), 11–20. |
| Hyvärinen | infants with visual impairment | literature review and observational report | Hyvärinen, L. (1988). *Vision in children: Normal and abnormal.* Meaford, ON: Canadian Deaf-Blind & Rubella Association. |
| Oregon | infants who are visually impaired or totally blind | literature review; field test for content validity | Anderson, S., Boignon, S., & Davis, K. (1991). *The Oregon project for visually impaired and blind preschool children* (5th ed.). Medford, OR: Jackson Education Service District. |
| VIIRC | infants who are totally blind, visually impaired; includes premature infants; multiple disabilities data available but not included here | research study | Ferrell, K. A., Trief, E., Dietz, S. J., Bonner, M. A., Cruz, D., Ford, E., et al. (1990). Visually impaired infants research consortium (VIIRC): First-year results. *Journal of Visual Impairment & Blindness, 84*, 404–410. |

# 21

# Improving Functional Use of Vision for Children with CVI and Multiple Disabilities

*Marieke Steendam*

Vision is the most unifying of all the senses, detecting and coordinating near and distant perceptions of stimuli in the environment to assist with thought and action. Vision gives a more comprehensive and detailed overview than hearing. While a large percentage of children who have cerebral visual impairment (CVI) and multiple disabilities, including cognitive challenges, have profound visual impairment, even minimal visual capabilities may prove helpful to these children as they learn to understand and interact with their surroundings. Moreover, as a large proportion of children with CVI and multiple disabilities are not able to move about independently, their use of vision broadens their world. The types of intervention programs described in this chapter can often improve the ability of children with CVI to make use of their vision. If their visual skills are improved and their visual environment optimized, their quality of life and learning can be greatly enhanced, as in the following example:

**Michael, a 12-year-old boy with CVI who is severely** multiply disabled, did not receive vision intervention until he was 8 years of age. During his first assessment session at age 8, he was only seen to react to the difference between lights "on" or "off" in a dark room. A tailor-made intervention program was begun, and he gradually started to become increasingly aware of visual stimuli; he started to look at people and objects. Now Michael uses his vision in daily life to look at his cup before drinking, to look at a teacher passing by 6 to 10 feet (2 to 3 meters) away, and to play visual games. His world has become more predictable as he can now see what is about to happen.

## Intervention Programs for Children with CVI and Multiple Disabilities

This chapter describes intervention programs for children with CVI and multiple disabilities that can improve visual functioning—for example, increasing awareness of visual stimuli, improving visual attention, and teaching basic visual skills, such as fixating on objects, as well implementing compensatory strategies, all integrated into activities of daily life. When considering children with multiple disabilities in this chapter, the developmental age under discussion is between 3 months and 5 years of age. Of course there can be a big difference in levels attained by a single child in different developmental domains (visual, motor, sensory, social, and emotional). It is important to address the child at the right level within each of these areas. It should be noted that a period of vision intervention is advisable at any age, especially when there is no ocular basis for low visual functioning. Often a child starts using vision more when specifically challenged with visually interesting activities.

## Compensatory Strategies vs. Direct Teaching

In contrast to the sole use of compensatory strategies, the additional implementation of direct teaching to improve specific visual skills or behaviors has, for many years, been an issue for children who have CVI (Lueck, 2006). The use of compensatory strategies alone may not lead to optimum development of visual skills for these children. While research in this area is sparse, due to the research difficulties encountered with this group, holding back on instruction owing to lack of evidence that direct intervention improves visual skills is not the answer. As recent research shows that brain plasticity is evident through adulthood, every child should receive the benefit of intervention so that the brain is able to form new neural pathways (see Chapter 5). In the author's practice, many children have been seen to improve visual functioning significantly by direct teaching, but it is not yet known how much change can be effected by direct teaching of children at various ages and with a variety of underlying conditions, although new work is emerging (Zihl & Dutton, 2015). It is also not known which specific visual skills and behaviors are most amenable to this type of instruction. Notwithstanding, diagnostic teaching is the most viable overarching method currently available.

In diagnostic teaching with regular direct teaching sessions, the instructor reacts to the child's responses by adapting the educational program and its activities to the child's developmental and visual needs. However, direct teaching of skills and the use of compensatory strategies are intertwined. A visual skill that is developed may replace a compensatory strategy that was fine while necessary, but this compensatory strategy must be phased out when the visual skill has improved and can be used instead, as shown in the experience of Ranj:

**Ranj is a boy of 4 years with CVI and severe multiple** impairments. For drinking, both at home and at his special school, he uses an identical blue cup. He fixates on it when it is shown to him and prepares to drink by opening his mouth. After improvement of visual skills and attention, it is noted that he reacts similarly to any cup being shown to him. He does not need the identical blue cup anymore; he can recognize a cup by its shape, not only by the color. Therefore, a wider array of cups is now presented for Ranj to drink from.

## Visual Stimulation and Vision Intervention

The term *visual stimulation* is often mentioned in early intervention literature. It usually refers to placing the child in an extremely visually stimulating environment in which he or she is only expected to look at the sights presented as a passive observer.

FIGURE 21.1
**Vision Intervention**

Leo Markesteijn

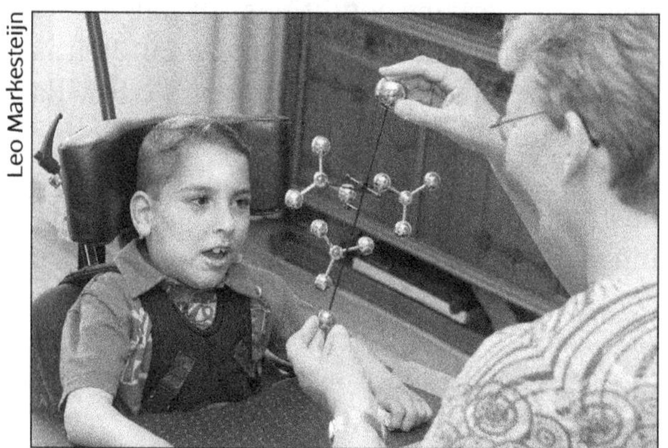

This student looking at a shiny object being twirled by the instructor is practicing visual attention, visual fixation, and following skills.

The environment might be a playpen covered with a lot of visually stimulating pictures and hanging mobiles. Or children are placed in darkened rooms with many brightly lit toys or points of light. However, for some children with CVI, this form of visual stimulation may actually prevent the child from reacting appropriately (Vervloed, Janssen, & Knoors, 2006).

Instead, an environment that consists of one or two strong visual stimuli against a plain background provides a child with profound CVI the opportunity to observe the object or objects and react through such actions as prolonged gaze, smiling, or reaching. (See the discussion of planned environments in Chapter 20.) Implementing short periods of passive visual stimulation like this can be used as an independent play activity, but improvement in visual skills from this type of limited input should not be expected.

*Vision intervention,* by contrast, is a diagnostic approach to teaching that involves continually monitoring the reactions of the child to visual stimuli by the instructor. The instructor chooses to offer a certain visual stimulus in a certain way (as discussed in the following section), the child reacts to it spontaneously, and the instructor makes adjustments that continue to engage the child and promote vision use in such a way that vision use becomes more refined and applied (Hall & Bailey, 1989; Lundervold, Lewin, & Irvin, 1987) (see Figure 21.1).

## Assessment: Developing Initial Intervention Goals

The comprehensive assessment and multidisciplinary report, as discussed in Chapters 10 and 14, identifies the child's strengths and weaknesses in a range of functional areas and relates these to skills and behaviors in daily life. Observational assessments of critical tasks in the home, school, and community along with environmental analyses of the visual demands of these tasks are presented during a meeting of the assessment/intervention team. The team members, including caregivers, then use this information to establish priority areas to address for vision intervention and formulate a specific intervention plan that will set identified goals in motion.

Chapter 14 on observational assessment introduced an assessment form that can be used to review the visual capabilities, skills, and behaviors that a child has developed (see Figure 14.5). This framework is used to devise specific intervention goals. Figure 21.2 shows this table completed for Josh, a 6-year-old child with CVI and severe cerebral palsy and developmental delay, primarily based on observational assessments.

After this assessment was completed, an educational meeting was held and the following goals for intervention were set:

FIGURE 21.2

# Areas of Functional Vision Important for Daily Activities, Completed for Josh

<table>
<tr><th colspan="4">Assessment of Visual Capabilities, Skills, and Behaviors for Daily Activities</th></tr>
<tr><td colspan="4">Name: Josh     Date of birth: April 4, 2009 (age 6 years)<br>Assessment period: September through November</td></tr>
<tr><td colspan="4">Some information from multidisciplinary report:<br>Josh has severe cerebral palsy and developmental delay, referral for assessment on visual functioning.</td></tr>
<tr><td colspan="3">Results from clinical eye examination or low vision clinical examination<br>Spectacles:<br>Yes ____ No ____<br>Full-time wear ____<br>Wear for near activities ____<br>Devices to support use of vision (optical devices, electronic enlargement, computer programs, tablet applications, other):<br>N/A</td><td>Prescription<br>OD:<br>OS:</td></tr>
<tr><th colspan="4">Formal Visual Assessment</th></tr>
<tr><th>Visual capabilities (from clinical eye examination, low vision clinical examination, and/or functional vision examination)</th><th>Assessment results for threshold measures</th><th>Required size/ contrast for optimum visibility</th><th>Comments</th></tr>
<tr><td>Object size at a specific distance</td><td>6.5 cycles/cm at 3 ft (84 cm) (VA = 0.32)*<br>3–4 mm at 1 ft (30 cm)</td><td>Line width of at least 0.1 in (2.5 mm)<br>Single dots at least 0.4 in (10 mm)</td><td>Test: Teller Acuity Cards (TAC)<br>Candy beads of different sizes</td></tr>
<tr><td>Level of contrast between adjacent stimuli required (contrast sensitivity)</td><td>25% at 2.5 ft (75 cm)</td><td>High contrast up to 100%</td><td>Test: Hiding Heidi</td></tr>
<tr><th></th><th colspan="2">Assessment results</th><th>Comments</th></tr>
<tr><td>Preferred viewing distance for near tasks</td><td colspan="2">1 ft (30 cm)</td><td></td></tr>
<tr><td>Preferred viewing distance for far tasks</td><td colspan="2">Within 2.5–3.5 ft (75–100 cm)</td><td></td></tr>
</table>

*VA = Visual acuity, 1.0 is equivalent to 20/20 or 6/6. A person with VA = 0.32 sees approximately the same details at 10.5 ft (3.2 meters) distance that a normally sighted person would see at 33 ft (10 meters). It is equivalent to 20/63 or 6/19.

*(continued on next page)*

**FIGURE 21.2** *(continued from previous page)*

| | Assessment results | Comments |
|---|---|---|
| Area of vision | Visual fields: no dysfunctions identified all around in the periphery | Confrontation method |
| Color vision | Cannot be assessed due to limited communication | |

| Visual Skills | Adequate | Varying, may need intervention | Needs intervention | Comments |
|---|---|---|---|---|
| Fixating on visual stimuli | | | Fixations of less than 5 seconds | Difficult to start and to maintain; eye contact is easier than fixation on materials |
| Following, pursuit of visual stimuli | | | X | Very difficult for Josh |
| Shifting gaze | | | X | Occasionally seen for large, strong stimuli with movement |
| Scanning | | | | Not relevant due to rest of visual skills precluding this |

| Visual Attention | Adequate | Varying, may need intervention | Needs intervention | Comments |
|---|---|---|---|---|
| Awareness of visual stimuli | | X | | Needs time to start looking |
| Sustained visual attention | | | X | Due to motor impairments and poor visual skills very hard to maintain |
| Selective visual attention<br>• Global attention: seeing a Gestalt/ zooming out | | | | Cannot be judged as yet |
| • Local attention: seeing details/ zooming in | | | | |

*(continued on next page)*

**FIGURE 21.2** *(continued from previous page)*

| ***Dorsal Stream Functions*** | ***Adequate*** | ***Varying, may need intervention*** | ***Needs intervention*** | ***Comments*** |
|---|---|---|---|---|
| Perception of movement, judgment of speed | | | | May be impaired as Josh easily startles when he is approached without sound |
| Visual guidance of movement<br>• Hands | | X | | Inability mostly due to motor impairments including spastic head tilt; intention to combine vision with the use of his hands is seen |
| • Upper limbs | | | | Same as for hands |
| • Lower limbs | | | | Insufficient function to evaluate visual guidance |
| Moving through space (judging position of body [parts] in space) | | | | Cannot be judged |

| ***Ventral Stream Functions*** (Most items deleted as they cannot be assessed as yet) | ***Adequate*** | ***Varying, may need intervention*** | ***Needs intervention*** | ***Comments*** |
|---|---|---|---|---|
| Recognition of<br>• Faces | X | | | Seems adequate, reacts to familiar people without sound |

- Josh will be able to fixate for 5–10 seconds on his favorite visual stimuli, size at least A4 (8.3 × 11 inches or ± 20 × 30 cm)
- Josh will be able to follow a favorite visual stimulus (as above) at least 45 degrees
- Josh will be able to fixate 1–5 seconds on cause-and-effect toys
- Josh will be able to independently operate five different cause-and-effect toys, adapted to his fine motor skills
- Caregivers at home and school staff will be aware of Josh's visual impairments and will know how to stimulate his vision during activities of daily life, in his school program, and in playtime

A vision instructor (most often a teacher of students with visual impairments or occupational therapist) will see Josh once every two weeks at school and once every six weeks at home to monitor, model, and modify interventions. An evaluation will be conducted after five months of intervention.

Chapter 14 also included an assessment form used to review the levels of visual attention that a child can sustain in a range of situations (see Figure 14.4). Figure 21.3 shows this form completed for Josh. Equipped with information from all available sources, the instructor and caregivers can intervene at an appropriate level, with relevant materials in an optimally matched environment. Using direct teaching, the vision instructor will use the materials mentioned previously to improve Josh's vision skills. Caregivers and other teachers will incorporate practice of visual skills in daily life at home and in class, by using visually striking objects, better contrast, and shiny materials to enhance visual attraction. They will give Josh the opportunity of visual play using a mobile and, in moments of one-to-one interaction, will repeat the direct teaching activities shown by the vision instructor as well.

These two assessments provide a framework of essential information and a starting point for the instructor. They are not forms to fill in each week to report skills attained; they are designed to guide intervention, to set updated goals, and to heighten awareness of the child's level of visual attention and how this is changing. Long-term attainment of intervention goals and the impact of visual dysfunction on all developmental areas are described in comprehensive follow-up reports.

## Establishing an Intervention Program

The design and implementation of intervention to achieve the goals set for the child with CVI and multiple disabilities is a complex process comprising three tightly interwoven aspects:

1. ***Education of all caregivers and usual school staff*** about the child's visual functioning, its theoretical basis, and its practical implications.
2. ***Application of compensatory strategies,*** including adaptations to the environment.
3. ***Regular sessions of direct teaching by the caregivers and school staff*** (preferably daily), supported by the instructor specializing in CVI.

### Education of Caregivers and School Staff

Interventions will show best outcomes when there is consistency between what happens at home and at school for children with CVI and multiple disabilities. While occasional feedback is given to caregivers when assessment sessions are under way, it is necessary to paint a complete picture of the child with CVI in a follow-up meeting of the multidisciplinary assessment team with all the child's caregivers and significant school staff. An explanation of what CVI is, as well as its effects, is needed along with discussion of the specific visual profile of the child. This provides the baseline information that caregivers and school personnel need to recognize aspects of CVI in the child and better understand the apparently illogical features of CVI and to understand the rationale of the planned intervention program.

FIGURE 21.3

## Level of Visual Attention in Activities, Completed for Josh

### Level of Visual Attention in Activities

**Name:** Josh **Date of birth:** April 4, 2009 (age 6 years)

**Assessment period:** September through November

| | Level of Visual Attention | | | | |
|---|---|---|---|---|---|
| **Activity** | ***The child primarily uses other senses in a given activity, and visual attention is minimal or nonexistent*** | ***The child fixates briefly and may follow objects momentarily in a given activity*** | ***The child looks attentively for brief periods independently or with instructor prompts in a given activity, but not for all situations or activities*** | ***The child looks attentively independently in many activities but occasionally uses other senses for exploration and accessing information*** | ***The child looks attentively and independently in most activities, although visual tasks may still present challenges*** |
| Reacting to basic visual stimuli | | | X | | |
| Eating/drinking | | | | | |
| Other skills of daily living | X | | | | |
| Communication | | | X<br>Eye contact helps in nonverbal communication | | |
| Moving around; mobility | X<br>(not independent) | | | | |
| Playing alone | X | | | | |
| Playing in one-to-one situations | | X | | | |
| Doing tasks alone | Not applicable | | | | |
| Doing tasks in one-to-one situations | Not applicable | | | | |
| **Description of signs of fatigue, including average duration of occurrence:** | Needs 5–10 minutes to warm up when vision intervention starts After 25–30 minutes of visual activities, he is very tired and closes his eyes most of the time | | | | |

*Source:* Adapted from Steendam, M. (2007). *Weet jij wat ik zie? Cerebrale visuele stoornissen bij kinderen, een handleiding voor professionals* [Do you know what I see? Cerebral visual disorders in children, a manual for professionals]. Huizen, The Netherlands: Royal Dutch Visio (Koninklijke Visio).

This approach helps to motivate people to commit to the intervention program. The following suggestions can be used at a meeting to convey this type of information:

- Video segments of the child's assessment sessions can be used as examples of visual behaviors, as well as provide a way to share experiences.
- Wearing simulation glasses matched to the child's visual impairment while doing short activities in which the child often engages helps people to understand the child's ability to see details, both near and distance, and the child's field of vision.
- Other simulations of the child's experiences can be used to demonstrate features of CVI. For example, the book *Where's Waldo?* (Handford, 1987; known in the UK and Europe as *Where's Wally?*), in which readers search for the Waldo character embedded in various complex full-page scenes, shows how difficult it is to find a single detail in a very busy picture, and helps explain the problem that the child with CVI has when searching for and identifying one out of a small number of items on a page.
- Books, pamphlets, Internet sites, and social media groups with information about CVI can also be provided to interested parties.

This education meeting provides a basis for subsequent communication between caregivers and teachers later during the intervention. Whenever the child's situation or staff change, it may be necessary to organize a new educational meeting.

## Application of Compensatory Strategies

Compensatory strategies are adaptations to support improvement of the general level of visual functioning of the child or help the child to execute a specific task successfully. It is important to recognize and encourage appropriate compensatory strategies that the child develops spontaneously and not hinder them because the teacher may not immediately understand their adaptive value.

Compensatory strategies for children with CVI have to be matched to the specific impairments of each child, to the different activities a child engages in, and to the different environments each child encounters. Ongoing observation of the child can determine whether the child has started to use new, spontaneous compensatory strategies or whether the child has assimilated compensatory strategies taught in earlier instruction sessions.

Following is an overview of compensatory strategies; more explanations about the application of these strategies follow later in the chapter.

### *Adaptations to the Environment*

- Adapt the level of room lighting to facilitate successful completion of the intended activities; be aware of the influence of natural light.
- Use a plain, contrasting background, both on and around the tabletop.
- Simplify the environment to be within the child's optimal functional capacity to handle clutter and crowding.
- When the environment cannot be adjusted optimally, be aware of the impact that various environmental stimuli (such as sound, smell, touch) can have on the visual behavior of the child.

### *Compensatory Strategies Based on the Child's Assessed Sensory Capabilities*

- Make sure that details on all materials are above threshold for visual acuity. As a guideline, use materials with details or lines that are three times bigger or wider than the corresponding measured visual acuity at a specific distance.

- Use the best area of the child's functioning visual field.
- Use movement to attract attention.
- Use optimal color and contrast to enhance materials.
- Use all other senses: auditory, tactile, proprioceptive, vestibular, and olfactory (smell) to support use of vision or be used instead of vision.
- Adapt speed of visual presentation and speech to child's speed of processing.

### *Compensatory Strategies Based on the Child's Cognitive Capabilities*

- Use memory and habituation.
- Use reasoning skills.
- Use social skills.

The following case study shows how a student created his own compensatory strategies and how the teaching staff worked with him to fine-tune and extend them:

> **MARK, 11 YEARS OLD, CANNOT RECOGNIZE PEOPLE BY THEIR** faces. Whenever he is walking in the corridors of his school to the playground, he keeps greeting everyone because he wants to know who they are. His teacher tells him it is not necessary to know all the people he passes and that doing so reduces his playtime outside. Mark is happy to discontinue his greeting ritual in the corridor after that.
>
> However, school staff members give Mark many opportunities to use his own compensatory strategies in his classroom. He is encouraged to greet people who enter the room in order to recognize them by their voice. He also remembers salient elements of the class schedule: the occupational therapist comes on Wednesday morning; the vision instructor always carries a big yellow bag. So Mark is using memory, habituation, and reasoning skills as well as his social skills as compensatory strategies.

Similar strategies are described by Borch (2002).

In essence, compensatory strategies for children with CVI who have multiple impairments can be summarized into three categories:

1. Simplify visual stimuli
2. Simplify the environment
3. Adapt the tempo to that of the child

## Regular Sessions of Direct Teaching

Direct teaching sessions consist of the systematic presentation of specific materials to the child in order to elicit visual responses or the systematic promotion of potentially productive visual skills and behaviors that the child has developed but hardly uses in the absence of special sessions of vision intervention.

The core of the intervention program is integration of visual activities into daily life. For very young children, this means that the program is implemented primarily by the daily caregivers. For children in school programs for all or part of the day, general education staff and teachers or paraprofessionals in special education classrooms also implement the program. A specialized vision instructor designs the program in collaboration with caregivers or school staff to ensure daily implementation of the program and also works with the child in regular one-to-one sessions. The one-to-one sessions with the vision instructor will vary in frequency depending on the needs of the child and educational resource allocations in a country or region.

Ideally, one of the child's caregivers or a school staff member is present during one-to-one sessions so that a person familiar to the child is available. This also allows the caregiver or staff member and the special vision instructor to learn from each other. The special vision instructor can use his or her time to try out new activities, answer any questions, and adjust the regular program in consultation with the caregiver or school staff member, so as to maximize the learning experiences for the child. It needs to be made clear to everyone that infrequent, short teaching sessions by the special vision instructor will not result in significant improvement in visual skills unless these are taken forward and implemented regularly by others who see the child on a daily basis. More frequent sessions are needed. This also provides a way to take advantage of the many other unplanned opportunities that come up during the day when visual skills can be taught within typical routines, as shown in the following example (adapted from Lueck, Dornbusch, & Hart, 1999):

A STRICT INTERVENTION PROGRAM WAS SET UP FOR 1-year-old Bruce who had CVI. His mother indicated that her son did not follow objects at first, but later, after about 31/2 months, he started to follow toys and people and showed a greater degree of visual attention to objects in his environment. The planned intervention motivated his mother, and she encouraged her son to be visually attentive at other times of the day with other objects and with people. This extra training in everyday life was incorporated in a very natural way, and likely added to Bruce's improved visual skills.

It is not easy to introduce an intervention program that must be executed on a regular basis by the caregivers or school staff. People directly involved with the child need to be committed to start an intervention program that includes regular, preferably daily, intervention sessions that are incorporated into activities of daily life as well as during special visual game time. Most important, they must have the time and opportunity to do it. The special vision instructor has to plan an intervention program that meshes with each child's school and home situation and has to be very realistic about what can be achieved. In this plan, it is preferable to have shorter or fewer sessions that can be maintained over a prolonged period than to set the standard too high. No one is happy with a sense of failure if planned goals are not achieved; this may even lead to people stopping intervention altogether.

As the child with CVI is often unable to transfer new skills from home to school or vice versa, it is important that all those interacting with the child are aware of what the child has learned and how the child has learned these skills. In this way, skills can be taught using the same methods, apart from some additional small adaptations required as necessary for each situation. The special vision instructor can play an important role in the transfer. In early intervention programs, for example, the special vision instructor can often visit both home and school, and can exchange experiences that have taken place in each situation.

### *Methodology for Direct Teaching during Regular Sessions*

Systematically developing intervention activities for a child with CVI is not simple. The child may react quite differently from one day to another. Even though the child may have looked carefully at colorful toys during one session, on the next day the child may only look at large shiny sheets of paper. A lot of flexibility is required on the part of the instructor to determine the child's capacity for visual attention. Even within one session, the instructor or caregiver must be able to adapt to the child's changing levels of attention, interest, and skill at each moment. Sometimes a child needs 5 to 15 minutes of warmup time to regain the level of performance he or she attained during the previous session. The instructor or caregiver must gauge the child's level at each moment and adjust the lesson accordingly.

Opportunities that arise spontaneously to promote visual skills, however, should not be overlooked. Caregivers or instructors must gain confidence in their observational skills and the ability to make quick adjustments to their lessons in order to capture every unplanned opportunity to promote learning. Understanding that ongoing observation of the teaching and learning process forms the basis for optimal intervention, caregivers and instructors must be encouraged to develop and trust their observational skills and judgment. With this acquired confidence, not only will they be implementing the activities as planned, they will simultaneously be observing the child and the child's reactions to directions, materials, and the environment, ready to adjust lessons and to respond to the immediate needs of the child.

For example, a cat walking by may be more interesting to a child than a toy on the tabletop. Actively following the cat with the child may be a perfect way to train visual skills. Or, when outside, walking past colorful gardens and then stopping to admire the color, shape, and scent of the flowers is another perfect, spontaneous moment of intervention. The goal is better visual functioning, and the tool is a program with systematic, regularly scheduled activities, but taking advantage of the many spontaneous moments for practice provides an added dimension to instruction.

## Building Blocks of the Intervention Program

The individualized program for regular intervention sessions relies on three interrelated but separate practices that, joined together, encourage the development of visual skills and behaviors. This "three-dimensional" process consists of *development, diversity,* and *duration*—the "3 D's." There is no specific order of presentation for these aspects within a session; however, it is important to ensure that all three approaches are used.

### *Development* of Increasingly Complex Visual Skills and Behaviors

Providing stimuli and activities of increasing complexity develops and expands students' visual skill levels. The progression of increasing complexity is as follows:

1. Encouraging basic visual skills (see Figure 21.4)
   - Learning to fixate, follow, and shift gaze
   - Moving from visual attention activities to visually guided movement and visual examining activities (Lueck, 2004)
2. Encouraging attention to stimuli of increasing complexity
   - From big stimuli to smaller stimuli
   - From objects to pictures of objects
   - From simple pictures to complex pictures
   - From one picture to more pictures
   - From simple to more complex practical tasks
3. Increasing the complexity of the environment
   - From semi-dark to normal illumination

FIGURE 21.4
**Visual Attention**

Marieke Steendam and Bart Makkinga

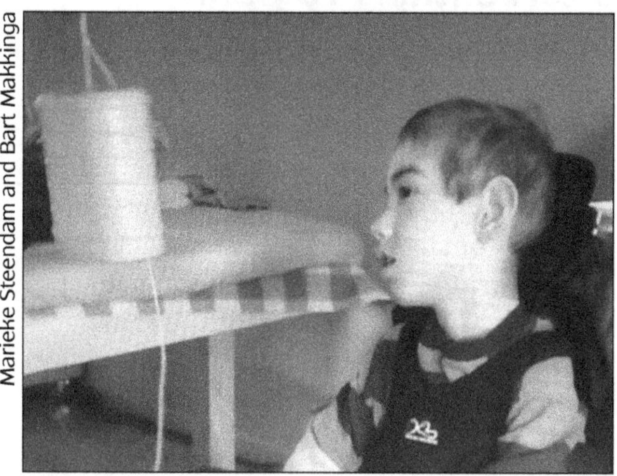

This student is looking at a moving, bright yellow container that is being slightly shaken and slowly moved around to help improve visual attention, visual fixation, and following skills.

- From looking at stimuli nearby to expanding the viewing distance to cover a whole room
- From a stimulus-free room to an environment with multisensory distractions

## *Diversity* of Visual Stimuli

Many children with CVI prefer to look at certain visual stimuli more than others. These highly motivating stimuli help in practicing visual skills, much more than less favorite ones. While less riveting stimuli may not initially motivate a child to interact, once a visual skill is developed, it is important to promote its use across a broader and more diverse range of visual stimuli, particularly those in typical environments. In daily life, the quantity of visual stimuli is immense, and expanding the scope of stimuli that the child will react to spontaneously is important, as in the following example:

*JOE'S FAVORITE SUBJECT IS TRAFFIC; ANYTHING TO DO WITH cars, buses, or trains captures his attention. He is able to spot these even in very busy situations, like around a train set in his classroom's play area. He shows quite good skill with visual search, fixation, following, and recognition when anything relating to traffic is concerned. He finds it difficult, however, to use these skills for other objects and pictures such as fruit, animals, or puppets. Acceptance of diversity is a big challenge, and the standard of skills expected to develop has to be set at a much simpler level for Joe in conjunction with material other than traffic-related objects and pictures. By using both types of teaching situations but expecting different levels of performance, Joe can enjoy games and practice in both situations. He practices many skills by himself with his traffic toys, and by offering him other materials, he improves his visual skills in these other situations, with the hope that he will eventually achieve equal skills in both areas.*

## Increasing the *Duration* of Visual Activities

The third key focus is on prolonging the duration of fixation and pursuit behaviors, as well as all tasks involving the use of vision, specifically:

- Fixating for longer periods, as well as following for longer periods and less haphazardly
- Shifting gaze more often and more quickly
- Prolonging the duration of activities involving vision and engaging in a higher frequency of visual activities each day

It is not possible to prearrange how these three aspects will be managed from one lesson to another, since each learning session can vary. In one session, for example, the child can be (a) learning how to shift gaze when viewing two big sheets of shiny cardboard (a difficult skill with easy material); (b) learning to fixate and follow a black-and-

FIGURE 21.5
**Play Activities**

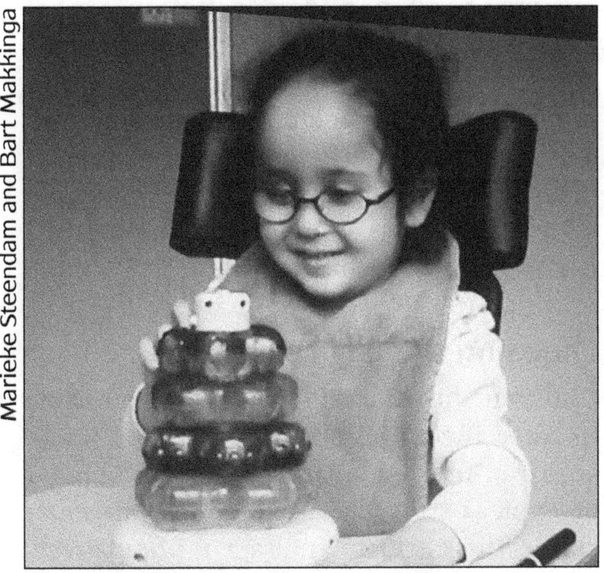

Marieke Steendam and Bart Makkinga

Some children enjoy games with sound and light stimuli. This one allows this girl to practice visual and visually guided motor skills.

white 3-inch (8-cm) ball (an easy skill with difficult new material); (c) reading a book that has stylized bold pictures (introduction to books and pictures and to fixating and shifting gaze); and (d) taking rings off a light and music tower (visually guided motor action with strong visual and auditory feedback) (see Figure 21.5). As children's skills progress in these activities, the length of time they can maintain visual attention and the number of visual activities they can pursue during the day also increase.

## Variables Influencing Interventions

Motivating and enticing the child to look is a primary goal when setting up direct teaching intervention sessions. The variables described here must be taken into consideration in the lesson's design. It may seem daunting to have to integrate all these elements into one session, but with experience, a skilled vision instructor will automatically coordinate many of these components when implementing lessons and when suggesting specific activities to the caregivers or instructors.

### Developing a Positive Relationship

The development of a mutually rewarding relationship with the child forms the basis for any effective intervention. Very little productive learning can take place without positive interactions, however subtle, between the instructor or caregiver and the child. Time must be invested to achieve this interpersonal chemistry. Children with multiple disabilities are usually very intuitive and respond directly to a person's positive energy; materials and activities often come in second place to the relationship between the instructor and child.

### Playful Activities

The importance of play and having fun during the interaction with the instructor or caregiver cannot be stressed enough, as it leads the child to strive to achieve an objective. Human beings learn so much better while having fun! As vision is so hard to use for children with profound CVI, activities must be sought that use toys and other objects that appeal to the child. Moreover, the child's enjoyment of an activity is infectious and will spur the instructor on, as is the case with Jonathan:

JONATHAN, A 3-YEAR-OLD BOY BORN WITH HYDROCEPHALUS, does not use his vision a lot; usually hearing is his primary sense. He can fixate and follow for short periods in a semi-dark room when viewing shiny materials, bright colors, and lights, but there is one object he favors over all others. Even though the color is not bright, he will look for his beige comforter if he is told it is there, searching for it visually and following it when it is moved in his field of vision before it is given to him. Although the instructor feels it looks very uninteresting visually, because Jonathan is so eager to find the comforter, she quickly warms to working with it as a visual target for the intervention. She recognizes that it is the child's drive and motivation to achieve that is pivotal to gaining skills.

## Alertness

A child who is not alert will not be able to learn. The instructor should estimate the child's level of general alertness at the start of every session. Only offer visual activities if the child is alert (allow for a warmup time of up to 5 to 15 minutes). It may be necessary to use sensory integration techniques, such as vestibular stimulation (being moved) and proprioceptive stimulation (deep pressure) to heighten alertness. These approaches should only be applied after consultation with appropriate staff.

## Tempo of the Child

Keeping to the child's tempo during each moment is the only practicable speed for visual activities for a child with CVI. This requires the instructor or caregiver to be observant and aware of the child's needs at different times and to match physical movements and verbal input to those needs. Waiting for a reaction requires patience. Three to 15 seconds' delay for a response is common for children with CVI and multiple disabilities; some need up to 60 seconds to react.

## Method of Instruction

The method of instruction chosen may be different for each child and for each activity, and it may even be different on different days for the same child. In general, a familiar activity needs little prompting, but a new one may need more demonstration, verbal instruction, or both. Complex activities need more instruction than simple ones. If listening demands too much attention, the child may not be able to focus on the visual elements of a task. The challenge is to determine which method to apply to promote optimal learning in different situations.

## Choosing the Environment

Children with brain damage are often unable to filter incoming stimuli properly. Some children may easily become overwhelmed by typical stimuli. The environment must entice the child to interact without overstimulation, because when overstimulated, the child will not be able to process anything and may withdraw or become hyperactive. A learning situation that contains the right balance of stimuli promotes a degree of alertness that allows stimuli to be processed, organized internally, and integrated to foster learning.

The optimum environment for learning is elicited during the assessment. Initially, it often needs to be decluttered without background pattern or sound. Elements can gradually be added to the situation to eventually resemble, as closely as possible, the natural environment. Although the ultimate goal of intervention is to have the child use his or her vision in typical environments, when learning, modifications that make environmental input manageable are often necessary.

## Posture

Maintaining good body posture with sufficient support for the child is critical. This allows the child to use precious energy and attention for learning rather than maintaining position. At the same time, the child should be as active as possible to promote optimal alertness and visual attention. Standing frames or side-lying mattresses should be considered in addition to sitting positions, and the comfort of sitting in a familiar person's lap should not be underestimated for young children.

### Structure and Predictability

Using structure and predictability helps the child to perform better. Start and stop each activity in a clear way, build in certain rituals to lessons that the child enjoys. Make sure the child understands what is expected, and use a set sequence when presenting activities. Children at all levels of development appreciate this, but this is especially important for children with CVI and multiple disabilities.

### Fatigue

Visual tasks are tiring for children with CVI. It is important to adjust existing activities or to change them entirely when the child becomes fatigued. Furthermore, elements of the intervention program can be modified to reduce the potential to tire. These include length of session, frequency of sessions, and level of difficulty of visual activities. Children with CVI and multiple disabilities should be allowed to have nonvisual time to recharge their batteries, interspersed with quiet times where they have hardly any sensory input at all.

## Materials and Activities

The choice of materials and activities used in instruction depends on the child, the situation, and the goals set. The ultimate starting point is to provide what the child enjoys, so that the child will look more readily, for longer periods, and with an interest in understanding what is seen. The instructor must find key stimuli that pique the child's visual interest in order to "kick-start" internal motivation. To help with this, the instructor can explore the characteristics of visual stimuli using the assessment presented in Figure 14.5 (Chapter 14) to determine parameters for choosing and varying the visual stimuli.

### Materials

There is no set rule when it comes to familiarity or novelty of material and activities as these can vary for each child. The goal is to promote active participation. As with other variables in instruction, it is best to follow the child's lead; one child will need familiar lesson content, while another will prefer novel experiences, as Isabel did:

ISABEL IS A 15-YEAR-OLD GIRL WITH CVI AND MULTIPLE disabilities. She often looks away from a task or activity that she is involved in doing. One day a child psychologist came to observe Isabel to determine her level of development. She brought along her own kit of materials for Isabel for observation. This time Isabel did not look away when playing. To find out why, two favorite toys were brought in from the classroom. Isabel constantly looked away again while playing with them. It turned out that Isabel did not need to look at these toys as she was very familiar with them. She seemed to choose the least demanding way to interact with the toys. With novel toys, however, she had to use her vision in order to learn about them and could apply this. Giving new and more varied materials to Isabel allowed her to practice her eye-hand coordination more. Also, slightly altering the way familiar toys were presented—for example, balls to take out of a bucket, rather than cubes, or spreading materials across her table to pick up—challenged her to look more, as well.

Many materials can be used to engage a child's attention for vision intervention. Key concepts for children who require support in this area are strong visual attraction, sufficient size, and absence of small details. Eight- by 12-inch cardboard sheets (size A4, or 20 × 30 cm) of shiny, black-and-white patterns, fluorescent and bright colors are indispensable in the vision instructor's materials library. Christmas decorations (tinsel), shop decorations, household materials, and anything with a strong visual impact and a fair size can be used. Shopping trips for the instructor become a different experience as one notices items that attract the eye to add to the vision materials kit. It is important, however, once basic visual attention skills have been established, to gradually introduce materials and toys that are commonly found in a child's natural environment so that the child has repeated practice in visual skills with these items throughout the day.

Children may surprise their instructor by showing a visual reaction to something that was not intended to be a visual stimulus. The observant instructor will then repeat this motivating stimulus, and integrate it into the regular intervention program, as in the following example (adapted from Steendam, 2007):

> **It was difficult to find a stimulus that would** encourage Kelly, a 3-year-old girl with CVI and multiple disabilities, to reach out for an object or to move about. The first time she reached out, it was to a banana; she loves food. And to get her moving about, a beige-colored pillow from the couch turned out to be her motivator; she spontaneously started to crawl after it in a playful situation.

## Categories of Activities

In addition to the materials mentioned in the paragraph above, activities can be chosen from three main categories:

1. Play activities
2. Activities of daily living and other skills or activities during the day
3. Developmental activities related to early learning

In typical practice, these categories of activities are not so clearly defined. The learning outcome depends on the way the activity is implemented and how the child interacts with its components. The caregiver or instructor needs to have a wide range of materials on hand, as previously discussed, in order to make immediate adaptations to the child's level of visual functioning during each moment. (See Appendix 21A for additional intervention ideas that can be tailored to individual needs to enable and stimulate vision in children with multiple disabilities.)

### *Play Activities*

Activities to promote learning of new visual skills must be appealing and not stressful because some vision skills and behaviors can be hard to use for many children with CVI. Many commercially available toys are full of sound, music, lights, and buttons, but some may be so busy that children with CVI cannot benefit from them. Fewer details and distractions in a toy are often better. Baby toys and baby books with black-and-white patterns and strong contrast seem to be best for children who have multiple disabilities and are learning to use their vision.

For older children, however, it is important to shift to activities that are meaningful and age-appropriate. For example, playing a matching card game with peers is more appropriate than matching pictures from a set of preschool game cards, or sorting colored crayons in preparation for an art project, or working with appropriate games on a computerized tablet.

### Activities of Daily Living

There are many activities in daily life that provide opportunities to start the use of vision intervention activities in regular sessions in the classroom and during family life. Moments in everyday routines, such as those involving eating and drinking and diaper changing, are often ideal situations for one-to-one instruction for younger children. Food preparation, laundry, and classroom "jobs" offer excellent opportunities to use vision for older children. Some examples include the following:

- Use a drinking cup to work on fixation and following. Using the same cup with a color that is attractive to the child in all drinking situations in school and home helps train the child with CVI to recognize it. Showing the cup in the child's area of best vision and waiting for the child to fixate on it before giving that child a sip provides a way to encourage vision use. If the child is able to hold the cup, it is important to encourage the child to look at the cup first before handing it to the child. Hold the cup in a different position every time and pull back slightly if the child does not look. Be supportive verbally, encouraging the child to look, moving the cup to and fro to make it stand out and giving a lot of praise when the child looks while reaching.
- When changing diapers, remove the diaper from a specially decorated box that is within the child's field of vision. Then slowly move the diaper toward the child so the child can follow it. As a reward, rub the soft, clean diaper on the child's bare legs or tummy for a tactile game before putting it on. (Of course there are moments of high stress with very dirty diapers when this ritual cannot be used.)
- The route from the main entrance of the school to the classroom can be complicated for a child with CVI. As a daily exercise, walk the route together with the child; encourage him or her to look at points of orientation (landmarks) along the way. As the child looks at objects as they are named, talk about their visual and other characteristics, such as the color of the floor and the color of the different doors and objects on the walls. This takes little extra time, but does demand focused attention from both the adult and child. Don't forget to check what landmarks the child readily sees, as they may be very different from what the caregiver sees. For example, the child may focus on the red circle of the fire hose reel on the lower part of the wall, rather than the blue classroom door next to it.
- Encourage children to set the table at home or school during meal times. A child can learn to locate each place at the table and set up a plate, glass, and fork for each place setting. If the child cannot remember where to position the implements, a placemat with a picture of place setting can be created as a guide so that the child can match each dish, glass, and utensil to the picture of it on the placemat. This activity involves identifying each utensil or dish visually, locating each place setting and moving around to it, matching objects to pictures if a placemat guide is used, and visually setting down each item with or without the special placement as a guide, and it practices

eye-hand coordination. It may help to initially have the items placed on a highly contrasting tabletop, tablecloth, or placemat. The effect of rotating the chair by about 10 degrees, so that the better functioning side of the body is closer to the table, can make a difference if there is better attention on that side as well (see Figure 3.5 in Chapter 3).

### *Early Learning and the Use of Developmental Activities*

It is easy to use activities like games, worksheets, and construction materials that are common in preschool or kindergarten. They must be relevant to the child and suited to the child's developmental range. A lot of these activities are very visually oriented, especially games and worksheets. Often, with some adaptations, these materials can be used by children with visual impairments. The visual input can be simplified, with visual details matched to functional acuity, enhanced contrast, or certain aspects made accessible by touch. The rules can be adapted as well. A game of memory or lotto, for example, can be used for matching pictures and can be a rewarding and pleasant exercise for the child. Sorting the colored parts of construction blocks may be much more interesting than sorting colors on a worksheet. Using these types of developmental materials can enhance the execution of visual learning tasks and stimulate the child to use vision in other activities as well.

For older children, similar games or worksheets can be used, but if necessary with subjects that are more age-appropriate: for example, using a store's logo to create a matching game, or choosing model cars or items in a sorting game. Involving older children in creating the games can be a rewarding activity in itself.

The following case study (adapted from Goetz & Gee, 1987) illustrates how such activities can be used to stimulate vision use:

**A 3-YEAR-OLD GIRL WITH PROFOUND CVI WAS GIVEN THE** following six developmental activities to practice to encourage visual attention skills:

1. Insert puzzle piece
2. Stack rings over pole
3. Put lid on pot
4. Stack glasses
5. Insert coin in piggy bank
6. Hang cup on hook

All the activities had specific segments in which the use of vision could contribute to successful task performance.

At first the activities were offered a few times without any special focus on vision use. If the girl was able to finish the task with or without the use of vision, she was complimented and could play with the material. As the sessions progressed, the instructor began to encourage the girl to use her vision to complete each task. If the girl did not use her vision to look at a specified portion of the task before completing it, the task was interrupted by the instructor. The instructor then encouraged the girl to attend to the task visually, using verbal cues or by tapping on a critical element of the task at a key moment (such as tapping the handle of a cup that was to be placed on a cup hook). With this method, the girl eventually performed the tasks, using her vision more frequently and completing the tasks with greater success.

The materials used in these activities need to be selected so that the features to be viewed on any toy, game, or book can be readily seen by the child. For example, if they are to be seen, the width of the lips and the size of the eyes on the face of a doll must be about three times larger than the child's visual threshold (that is, about three times larger than the smallest size the child can see at the distance at which the doll is held) or these features will not always be seen (see Chapter 12).

Developmental games and tasks for children with CVI are often full of a multitude of elements, many of which cannot be seen by children with simultanagnosia. Before offering such tasks, it is important to determine the goal of the activity. If the goal is to finish the task as quickly as possible, then it is essential to reduce visual clutter in order to render all salient elements visible. If the purpose is to practice selective attention, the instructor can leave some visual clutter in the game to encourage sequential visual search (using strategies that have already been taught to the child), while assuring the child that speed of completion is not important.

## Specific Interventions for Visual Capabilities, Skills, and Behaviors

Visual capabilities, skills, and behaviors, as described in Figure 14.5 and applied in Figure 21.2, are used here as a framework to describe aspects of intervention. While this information provides a guide to point instructors in the right direction, it has to be applied individually to each child and learning situation.

### Visual Skills

Vision intervention at early stages of visual development consists of two main areas, depending on the level of visual attention of the child: (1) teaching visual attention, including awareness of visual stimuli, and then, as the child progresses, sustained and selective visual attention, and (2) teaching basic visual skills (fixation, following, shifting gaze, and scanning). (Additional suggestions for interventions to promote specific visual skills and behaviors are provided in Appendix 21A.)

### Visual Attention

#### *Awareness of Visual Stimuli*

Attracting awareness to a visual stimulus is needed primarily for children who, for most of the time, have a very low level of visual attention (the first two levels of visual attention described in Figures 14.4 and 21.3). For other children, this approach may be needed at the start of a session, to get the visual system "warmed up."

Visual preferences of newborn babies tend to be for black-and-white patterns (wide stripes or checkerboard patterns), while facial features are favored stimuli for children up to 2 months of age. After this, the child starts to be interested in bright colors, as well as more complicated patterns. After about 3 months, children become progressively more interested in simple and clear pictures (Steendam, 1989).

Research related to children aged 18 to 72 months with CVI and cerebral palsy for preferences for color and movement found the following results (Cohen-Maitre & Haerich, 2005):

- A colored stimulus (red, yellow, blue, or green) will attract more attention than a gray stimulus with the same luminance.
- Movement attracts more attention than a stationary colored stimulus, even if the moving stimulus is gray.
- Of all these variables, color and movement together best attract and maintain focused attention in children with CVI.

This information can be incorporated into the selection of stimuli to promote emerging visual skills. Some examples include:

- Sources of light such as a light box (a backlit surface onto which translucent

toys, colored designs on translucent paper, paper cutouts, or translucent, colored pictures can be placed), penlights, toys that light up, Christmas light ropes, and spotlights onto toys
- Moving stimuli
- Black-and-white patterns
  - Starting with wide stripes, moving on to finer stripes
  - Checkerboard patterns and dot patterns
- Shiny card surfaces and shiny objects
- Fluorescent and bright colors
- Facial contours, both schematic pictures as well as real faces, such as the caregiver's face enhanced by makeup

The strategy of instruction makes a difference too:

- Support the child in maintaining attention on an object, by moving it, tapping on it, or touching the child's hand if the child is holding the object.
- Adding sound to attract initial visual awareness may work for some children. Other children may not look at all when stimulated by sound.

In practice, gaining a child's awareness of stimuli and practicing specific visual skills are intertwined. When a child has become aware of a certain stimulus, the instructor can immediately encourage fixation and following. As the child becomes more aware of visual stimuli, these can be used to learn a range of visual skills and behaviors, from basic to more complex.

While a child may be able to perform tasks at a certain attentional and cognitive level, visual skills may need to be taught as part of tasks that have less demanding cognitive requirements, as in the following example:

**Anishia is a 2-year-old girl with CVI and slight** developmental delay who has a variable level of visual functioning. She can pick up small pegs to put in a pegboard or complete a simple puzzle. She looks for only a fraction of a second to pick up the right piece. She is able to do a pegboard game or puzzle, but otherwise shows minimal use of her vision. Wanting to improve her visual skills, especially the duration of fixation, her instructor starts to offer her large, vivid visual stimuli such as tinsel, a rotating box with shiny surfaces, and a black-and-white patterned ball. The developmental level of these materials is much less demanding than the level of puzzles and pegboards, but with these less-demanding activities, Anishia can more easily start to expand her visual skills. She fixates for much longer, follows better, and starts to shift gaze. The ultimate goal is to get her to use her newly developed visual skills in the more demanding tasks that she is able to do, so that her cognitive skills are challenged at the same time.

### Sustained Visual Attention

Visual attention in children with profound CVI starts with basic awareness of visual stimuli but gradually extends to the more advanced skills of sustained attention and selective visual attention. The ability to sustain attention on an object or action is necessary to reach levels of visual processing in complex situations. Vision intervention techniques to promote sustained attention focus on expanding the duration of attention while varying the complexity of the visual stimuli, as discussed earlier in this chapter.

### Selective Visual Attention

There are hardly any tests currently available to pinpoint problems with selective visual attention (see Chapter 6) in children with CVI and multiple disabilities. Information from the observational assessment can provide some clues about selective visual attention. In neuropsychology, selective attention is divided into local attention and global attention. Individuals have to switch continually between local and global attention (see Chapter 6) to understand what is seen. When this ability is impaired, the person (assuming he or she has the requisite acuity) may only see details but not the whole Gestalt of an object or picture, like the P's in the example in Figure 6.2 (using local attention) or, conversely, may see only the P (using global attention) and not see the small letters. To see both, flexibility between these systems is necessary.

In children with CVI and multiple disabilities, this neuropsychological division may not always be distinct as a result of simultanagnosia (Drummond & Dutton, 2007; see Chapters 3 and 6), one of the most common problems in children with CVI, but one that may go unrecognized. These children can only see a small number of items at once and cannot simultaneously see all the details, so, for example, cannot find a favorite toy in a toy box. An affected child may recognize the curly tail of a pig in a picture, but have no idea that the whole scene actually depicts a pig in a farmyard because he or she cannot perceive a sufficient number of elements of the picture to attribute overall meaning.

There has been no definitive research on the intervention methods to improve the performance of children who have problems with selective visual attention, but in the experience of the author, the following strategies have been found useful:

- Start intervention at a basic level, with one simple object or picture that is readily seen (at least three times the threshold of the child's level of visual acuity).
- This is followed by gradually adding more details that can be seen, such as introducing more pictures or objects, and allowing progressively less space in between them, while adding more "visual clutter" to the visual activities.
- With new tasks, this requires a process of reduction, starting again with single elements and gradually adding more new elements.
- The use of pictures depends on the cognitive level of the child. Children must first understand that pictures are representations of real objects before they can be used in intervention plans. Instructors may need to begin with objects.
- Next, have children match simple objects to photos of the objects (that are within the child's visual capacities to see readily) against a plain background of high contrast. If photographs are used, they need to be in color, since black-and-white photos are more difficult to decipher visually.
- Using very similar, simple pictures of the objects is the next step, but some children are more able to discern simplified pictures than photos, so both should be tried.

The ability to identify pictures and photos can be very helpful to children who need to use them for their communication systems, as seen in the example that follows:

**Jake is an 8-year-old boy who can only speak a few** words. The speech pathologist tried to start a communication system for him with pictures, but discovered that he does not recognize the pictures all the time. The instructor made a matching game with 15 everyday objects, toy animals, and other familiar items in duplicate, along with photos of the objects against a plain, contrasting background, also in duplicate. After a few trials with the matching game using the objects, Jake showed that he understood the concept of matching. Every time the game was started, Jake needed time to investigate the toys again, as a result of his developmental level. He also learned how to pick one object out of five in front of him on the table, using the same name for each object every time.

The game was then expanded to matching a photo to the object, and eventually Jake was able to match all 15 photos with objects. However, Jake needed time to become familiar with new objects and their photos. Once Jake was able to match photos, the speech pathologist was able to set up a communication system for Jake with objects and photos that would slowly phase out the use of objects altogether.

### *Compensatory Strategies to Promote Visual Attention*

The following are some compensatory strategies that can be used in addition to direct instruction:

- Reducing the number of images or objects helps a child to see a variety of images on a page or objects in an array. This is a subtle process that requires a lot of observational skill and judgment by the instructor or caregiver to add or subtract the right elements at the right time.
- It is often thought that the size of the objects or pictures should be larger when crowding is an issue. However, it is often not the size of the objects that counts, but the space between the objects and their number. Therefore, spreading out the items can help the child focus better on the pictures or objects.
- Superfluous visual information can be covered by
  - rearranging the pictures digitally
  - cutting and pasting with scissors and glue
  - photocopying a picture onto a plain sheet of paper
  - using two L-shaped black or white cards to make a frame around a part of a picture, to easily adjust the opening around a designated area.

### Perception of Movement

The ability to see movement is processed in various parts of the brain. It is very rarely completely damaged in children with CVI (Ahmed & Dutton, 1996). Processing movement, as in seeing a moving target, may be impaired as well. This can cause the child to startle frequently, since a person (or animal) may appear to emerge suddenly when stopping right in front of the child. A small number of children with profound CVI only see static or slow-moving targets, and recognition of this phenomenon can guide diagnostic teaching to ensure that the speed of movement of targets is within the child's visual capabilities. For children who do perceive movement, however, movement may be a very useful tool, as it attracts visual attention (Cohen-Maitre & Haerich, 2005) (see Figure 21.6).

FIGURE 21.6
**Perception of Movement**

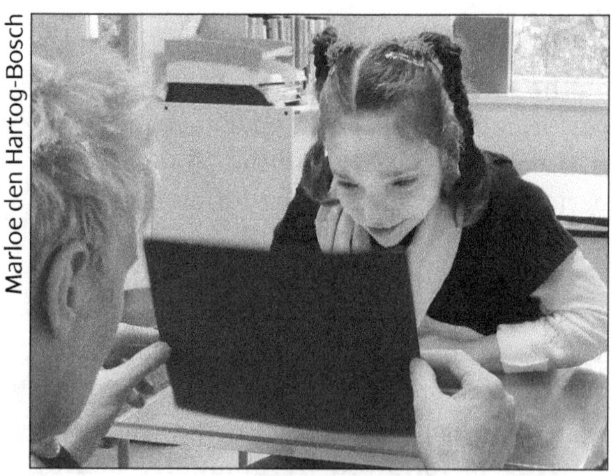

Marloe den Hartog-Bosch

Slightly moving the picture that this girl is looking at helps to prolong the duration of looking.

### *Interventions Related to Movement Perception*

Seeing movement is not a goal in itself. From the very limited literature about children and adults who do not see movement, this is usually caused by permanent damage of the brain and cannot be improved by training. It is more important to be aware of this condition and to teach the child and caregivers how to handle it by means of compensatory strategies.

### *Compensatory Strategies for Lack of Movement Perception*

The following are some compensatory strategies that can be used when a child does not see movement:

- Adapt the speed of visual stimuli in tasks and training to the speed the child can process.
- Moving about in the corridors or playground at school can pose challenges to the ability to process movement and speed. Work with an orientation and mobility (O&M) specialist to teach children how to use other senses. A play push toy or a long cane may be recommended to move around safely, without demanding too much of the visual processing system.
- Instruction to caregivers and peers is important too because they need to understand how they may startle the child by moving quickly, then stopping, which makes them appear suddenly. Talking while approaching from the front, and allowing more time to be detected are simple strategies for them to adopt.
- Learn the speed at which moving balls and toys can be seen, since some children may have difficulty perceiving such fast-moving objects.
- Recognize the implications for traffic and moving around in busy places if a child's perception of movement is impaired.

## Visually Guided Motor Tasks

Visually guided motor tasks involve eye-hand coordination, eye-foot coordination, and guiding the body through the environment. Apart from any motor impairments they might have, children with CVI may lack efficiency in using their motor skills based on visual information. They may grasp a cup as if they are blind, or they may look or turn away when reaching for or grasping something. If formal assessment has shown that the child views material using peripheral (side) vision, causing a head tilt, then this behavior maximizes vision use and should not be discouraged. If the child turns away with no opportunity to use central or peripheral vision, then one explanation is that the child cannot use vision at the same time as using other senses such as proprioception, or the sense of movement of the body.

### *Intervention to Enhance Visually Guided Motor Skills*

A child who hardly uses vision at all needs to have the combined use of vision and motor skills built up carefully in an intervention program, starting primarily with visual activities alone.

When a child is beginning to be aware of his or her body, touch may elicit a visual reaction, but may also deter the child from looking, since the child may focus attention on the sense of touch, rather than his or her vision. This has to be observed carefully. Before starting to combine vision with touch, be sure the child has no tactile hypersensitivity.

Some ideas to make the child's body a more motivating visual target include these:

- Putting on shiny or fluorescent gloves
- Painting with shaving cream or finger paint
- Joint play with the hands; four hands may be even more attractive than two
- Putting a brightly colored and "trembling" toy in the child's hand
- Putting a "space blanket" (emergency blanket) between the child's hands or feet
- Touching parts of the body with a toy, inviting the child to look at the toy while sensing the touch

Children who use their vision spontaneously are usually ready to combine vision with reaching or grasping if their motor development allows it. A lot of practice and repetition is the best intervention for weak visually guided motor skills.

At this stage of a child's visual development, there may be a gap in the degree to which visual skills are used in the performance of visual-motor tasks done independently by the child versus those done with assistance in a one-to-one session with an instructor. Playing alone, the child with CVI is often not able to combine vision and motor performance. This can result in a lower performance level.

Some ways to encourage children to combine vision and motor performance include the following:

- Handing objects to the child in games or daily life activities, such as eating and drinking, is a good strategy for encouraging the child to look and touch. As with all objects, the caregiver needs to vary the position of each object as it is handed to the child, so that the child learns to search in all directions. Be sure to wait until the child views the object before handing it over or starting the action (for example, bringing a cup to the mouth). If the child has visual field limitations, do not hold the objects in the affected visual field.
- Using a light box may encourage visual guidance of movement by attracting the visual attention of the child to specific objects or pictures. But beware of the bright light taking the child's attention away from the task (Lueck et al., 1999).
- Using bigger material may encourage visually guided movements. Building a tower of blocks that are about 1 × 1 inch (3 × 3 cm) is easier in terms of motor skills than blocks of about ½ × ½ inch (1 × 1 cm), and is less demanding on visual guidance.
- Adapting activities to a level the child can perform with success diminishes frustration and resistance.
- Supplementing visual guidance of movement with tactile guidance is a good compensatory strategy; for example:
  - Gently allow the child to explore along your hand to get to the desired target if visual guidance alone is not enough to grasp the object.
  - Allow the child to slide his or her hand along a table to reach the desired target.
  - Let the child's body touch the table; this subconsciously informs the child through touch of the height and location of the table in three-dimensional space.

## Moving through Space (Position in Space)

Most children with CVI and multiple disabilities often have severe motor problems and have difficulty moving through space as a result. When a child with CVI can move about independently by crawling, walking, or using an electric wheelchair, the accuracy of the child's movement through space is important to consider. Many children with CVI who are mobile are able to use their vision fairly well while moving around, especially compared to their level of visual accomplishments in the performance of developmental games at the table. Suggestions for encouraging movement through space include these:

- Using a physical "buffer" to act as a tactile guide and to supplement visual guidance while moving about can help the child detect obstacles and supports independence.
- A young child can use a little cart or push toy, and an older child can learn to use a long cane. O&M specialists can provide instruction for these travel devices.

### *Interventions and Compensatory Strategies Related to Movement in Space*

When a child starts to use more visual skills, determining position in space for visually guided movements becomes progressively more important. The following are suggestions for interventions and compensatory strategies related to movement in space:

- Most children with CVI will spontaneously use touch and proprioception when picking up an object. Picking up items from the tabletop is easier than taking something that is held in the air.
- Putting something in exactly the same spot makes repetition and successful task completion easier through the use of proprioception and memory.
- Using a placemat with silhouettes of cup, plate, and cutlery as guides for placement during meals can help a child set up for meals.

Environmental adaptations can be made to landmarks and obstacles so that they are

- large enough for the child to see,
- of clear contrast, and
- at eye level.

Negotiating passageways easily can be a difficult task for some children with CVI as seen in the following example (adapted from Steendam, 2007):

**Erik is 21 years of age, with multiple impairments** including cerebral palsy with quadriplegia, an ocular condition, CVI, and problems in communication. He rides an electric wheelchair by using his head to push steering buttons on both sides of the headrest and his foot to accelerate and brake. Erik has problems judging distances and he seems "scared" of walls, parked wheelchairs, and other obstacles. He stares at them as he is afraid of bumping into them as he travels in his wheelchair. While doing so, he pushes the steering button with his head and steers the wheelchair directly into what he fears. By putting a black stripe about 2 inches (5 cm) wide along the middle of the corridor at school, Eric has a visual "anchor" to look at and steer along, rather than having to judge distances, and has gained the ability to follow the black stripe for safe travel.

### *Some Remarks about Traffic*

Children with developmental delays may vary in their ability to negotiate in traffic without assistance, and complications resulting from CVI may be an additional reason for this. The ability to detect rapid movement may be damaged, but it can also be a concern in terms of children's understanding of the relationship between themselves and moving objects (such as cars, bicycles, or a child running). Even more, orientation skills may be impaired as well. An O&M specialist must be involved if there are questions about these issues (see Chapter 17 for more information about O&M with children who have CVI).

## Seeing Color

Color vision is not often functionally impaired in children with CVI (Jan & Groenveld, 1993). However, in children with late-onset acquired brain damage, an isolated color blindness (achromatopsia) may be seen, although it is extremely rare (Steendam, 1989). Therefore, color can be used in compensatory strategies for children with CVI and can support many visual tasks.

## Recognition of Objects and People

In children with CVI and multiple disabilities, it is not always initially clear whether aspects of recognition are functioning or impaired. Visual recognition requires the necessary development level in addition to a number of visual skills, including visual acuity, contrast sensitivity, visual attention, visual search ability, and the capacity to retain and recall visual information (see Chapters 2 and 3). As the child develops, the capacity to recognize needs to be evaluated with each of these aspects in mind. In the clinical experience of the author, intervention to treat specific recognition disorders (ventral stream dysfunctions) appears not to be effective, and therefore compensatory strategies need to be used to handle these deficits in specific situations.

Some children may not recognize biological forms such as people's faces and facial expressions as well as pictures of animals, but may easily identify store logos (see Chapter 3). It is important to properly assess all aspects of a child's visual functioning before assuming that a particular aspect is disturbed.

Caregivers can provide useful information about the child's ability to recognize. If an older child can communicate verbally, asking the child how he or she recognizes something can be very helpful. Testing out a range of variables, such as those presented in Sidebar 21.1, helps to establish features that the child can use to recognize what he or she is looking at. This information can be communicated to all caregivers and instructors.

SIDEBAR 21.1

### Features That Contribute to Visual Recognition

Making children aware of features such as the following, whether isolated or combined with other features, can help them recognize objects, people, and animals both in real life and in pictures:

#### Real Life

***People:***

- size
- color of hair, skin, etc.
- hairdo
- style of makeup
- stature
- way of walking or moving
- details of appearance such as earrings or bracelets
- style of clothing or shoes
- smell (for example, perfume or shampoo)
- connection to certain situations

***Animals:***

- size
- color

*(continued on next page)*

SIDEBAR 21.1 *(continued from previous page)*

- stature (number of legs, type of figure, or type of snout)
- details such as ears or tail
- familiarity
- situation

***Objects:***

- size
- color
- details standing out
- familiarity
- situation

**Pictures and Photos**

- contrast
- size of picture
- size of figure in picture
- width of lines
- contour
- color
- familiarity
- situation
- complexity of drawing or composition
- complexity of scene (for example, one item by itself versus an item within a complex picture)
- detailed features, such as a pig has a curly tail, cows have black spots
- specific Gestalt (for example, a pictogram of a group session in class may become a certain symbol rather than a drawing of children sitting in a circle)
- relationship to something of high interest (for example, recognizing toy cars but not other toys)

Flexible thinking is important so that specific aspects of games or tasks are replaced to accommodate the child's current recognition abilities; for example, using objects or logos in matching tasks instead of pictures, use of color coding, and use of voice recognition. Training in seeking and recognizing identifiers for people is encouraged. All the general tips in intervention and compensatory strategies mentioned earlier in this chapter also apply.

## Evaluating and Adjusting Intervention

Intervention needs to be evaluated after a period of time. In the author's experience, for children with CVI and multiple disabilities, a period of at least 4–6 months of regular intervention is necessary to allow appropriate time and opportunity for changes to occur. Even for older children who have not had access to vision intervention or whose vision intervention was discontinued some time in the past, the period of 4–6 months may be useful to stimulate the child to use vision more. As already noted, at any age, a period of vision intervention is advisable, especially when there is no ocular basis for low visual functioning. Usually, the caregivers and staff at school will incorporate intervention activities more into the child's daily life once they see that the child is using vision in activities over this period of time.

For children with a very low level of visual functioning, formal assessments to record changes in vision need to be no less than one year apart. Repeated assessment may show longer periods of visual fixation, improved visual attention, and more eye contact in addition to more enjoyment of visual activities. The latter quality of visual functioning is difficult to describe but can be easily seen on video recordings.

Evaluation needs to be done together with the caregivers and instructors to determine the influence of vision in daily life activities. The intervention goals are the first issue to evaluate, but with children with CVI and multiple disabilities, looking beyond the set goals is just as important. In the author's experience, wonderful side effects of vision intervention may occur. For example, Yarah, who had goals aimed at improving visual attention and skills within arm's reach, also started to follow her caregivers, walking around the room 6.5 to 10 feet (2 to 3 meters) across.

As children with CVI and multiple disabilities develop, learn, and change, their intervention programs must change with them. These changes must be noted regularly through careful, sensitive observations throughout the instructional process. Behavioral changes that are significant can be very small and subtle. Often developmental steps cannot be easily predicted for children with brain damage, as they may be different or may occur over different time intervals. In addition, not all aspects of visual functioning may be revealed during the assessment but become evident during the intervention phase. For example, recognition of faces is not always easy to ascertain when a child lacks sufficient communication skills. Changes and new developments in a child's behavior, however small, require immediate adjustments to curricular presentation methods to optimize further learning. This *diagnostic teaching* (see Chapters 10, 16, and 19) is an instructional method that recognizes that assessment and instruction are inseparable.

When definitive development in visual functioning is noted, new goals and instructional strategies can be established. Ideally, the visual goals are eventually integrated into the overall educational goals established for the child.

## Ending Intervention and Continuing Use of Vision

If no change has been noted at any level of visual functioning for 4 to 6 months of intensive intervention, and the child's visual levels remain static, specific vision intervention is generally brought to an end. However, all caregivers must maintain an emphasis on the use of available visual skills in daily life and activities at home and in school. When specific attention is given to the use of vision in activities for children with CVI and multiple disabilities, qualitative analysis has shown their visual skills continue to improve, but without the emphasis on vision use in activities the level of visual functioning may even diminish (den Hartog-Bosch, 2006, 2011).

## Conclusion

Children with CVI and multiple disabilities can benefit from even small improvements in their use of vision to increase learning opportunities and promote quality of life. Based on assessment results, a multifaceted intervention program can be implemented that includes (1) education for the caregivers and instructors, (2) regular intervention sessions—ideally, daily—implemented by caregivers and instructors along with a specialized vision instructor, and (3) use of specific compensatory strategies. Diagnostic teaching methods provide a way to monitor and update vision instruction methods to ensure that intervention programs continually match the changing capabilities of each child in a variety of environments. The design of intervention programs requires a great deal of skill on the part of instructors who must coordinate the complex interplay of vision with motor, cognitive, social-emotional, and communication skills.

## References


Ahmed, M., & Dutton, G. N. (1996). Cognitive visual dysfunction in a child with cerebral damage. *Developmental Medicine & Child Neurology, 38*(8), 736–739.

Atkinson, J., & Braddick, O. (1982). Sensory and perceptual capacities of the neonate. In P. Stratton (Ed.), *Psychobiology of the human newborn* (pp. 191–220). New York: Wiley.

Banks, M. S., & Salapatek, P. (1983). Infant visual perception. In P. Mussen (Ed.), *Handbook of child psychology: Vol II* (pp. 435–571). New York: Wiley.

Borch, T. G. (2002, July/August). *The use of different strategies to compensate for difficulties in recognition of people for a child with CP and CVI.* Paper presented at 11th ICEVI World Conference, Noordwijkerhout, The Netherlands. Retrieved from http://icevi.org/publications/ICEVI-WC2002/intro.html

Boyle, N. J., Jones, D. H., Hamilton, R., Spowart, K. M., & Dutton, G. N. (2005). Blindsight in children: Does it exist and can it be used to help the child? Observations on a case series. *Developmental Medicine & Child Neurology, 47*(10), 699–702.

Cohen–Maitre, S. A., & Haerich, P. (2005). Visual attention to movement and color in children with cortical visual impairment. *Journal of Visual Impairment & Blindness, 99*(7), 389–402.

den Hartog–Bosch, M. (2006). *Visuele stimulatie binnen het project Activiteitenbegeleiding* [Visual stimulation within the project supervised activities]. Huizen, The Netherlands: Royal Dutch Visio.

den Hartog–Bosch, M. (2011, June). *Enhancement of visual abilities of multiply disabled children with CVI.* Paper presented at 13th Biennial Meeting of the Child Vision Research Society, Huizen, The Netherlands.

Drummond, S. R., & Dutton, G. N. (2007). Simultanagnosia following perinatal hypoxia: A possible pediatric variant of Balint syndrome. *Journal of American Association for Pediatric Ophthalmology and Strabismus, 11*(5), 497–498.

Goetz, L., & Gee, K. (1987). Teaching visual attention in functional contexts: Acquisition and generalization of complex visual motor skills. *Journal of Visual Impairment & Blindness, 81,* 115–117.

Good, W. V., & Hou, C. (2006). Sweep visual evoked potential grating acuity thresholds paradoxically improve in low-luminance conditions in children with cortical visual impairment. *Investigative Ophthalmology & Visual Science, 47*(7), 3220–3224.

Hall, A., & Bailey, I. L. (1989). A model for training vision functioning. *Journal of Visual Impairment & Blindness, 83,* 390–396.

Handford, M. (1987). *Where's Waldo?* Boston: Little, Brown and Company.

Hyvärinen, L., & Jacob, N. (2011). *WHAT and HOW does this child see?* Helsinki, Finland: VISTEST Ltd.

Jan, J. E., & Groenveld, M. (1993). Visual behaviors and adaptations associated with cortical visual and ocular impairment in children. *Journal of Visual Impairment & Blindness, 87,* 101–105.

Kern, H. (2003). Eine entwicklungs—und förderdiagnostik des sehens für menschen mit mehrfacher behinderung—konzept und inhalte. In T. Klauss & W. Lamers (Eds.), *Alle kinder alles lehren . . . Grundlagen der paedagogik für menschen mit schwerer und mehrfacher behinderung* (pp. 295–307). Heidelberg, Germany: Universitätsverlag Winter.

Lueck, A. H. (2004). Overview of intervention methods. In A. H. Lueck (Ed.), *Functional vision: A practitioner's guide to evaluation and intervention* (pp. 257–275). New York: AFB Press.

Lueck, A. H. (2006). Issues in intervention for children with visual impairment or visual dysfunction due to brain injury. In E. Dennison & A. H. Lueck (Eds.), *Proceedings of the summit on cerebral/cortical visual impairment: Educational, family, and medical perspectives, April 30, 2005* (pp. 297–300). New York: AFB Press.

Lueck, A. H., Dornbusch, H., & Hart, J. (1999). The effects of training on a young child with cortical visual impairment: An exploratory study. *Journal of Visual Impairment & Blindness, 93*(12), 778–793.

Lundervold, D., Lewin, L. M., & Irvin, L. K. (1987). Rehabilitation of visual impairments: A critical review. *Clinical Psychology Review, 7*(2), 169–185.

Luria, A. R. (1970). *Die höheren kortikalen funktionen des menschen und ihre störungen bei örtlichen hirnschädigungen* [The higher cortical functions of man and their disturbances in local brain damage]. Berlin, Germany: Deutscher Verlag der Wissenschaften.

Malkowicz, D. E., Myers, G., & Leisman, G. (2006). Rehabilitation of cortical visual impairment in children. *International Journal of Neuroscience, 116*(9), 1015–1033.

Münssinger, U., & Kerkhoff, G. (1995). *Therapiematerial zur behandlung visueller explorationsstörungen bei homonymen gesichtsfeldausfällen und visuellem neglect* [Therapy materials for the treatment of visual disorders in exploration homonymous visual field defects and visual neglect]. Dortmund, Germany: Verlag Modernes Lernen.

Solzbacher, H. (2010). *Von der dose bis zur arbeitsmappe—Ideen und anregungen für strukturierte beschäftigungen in anlehnung an den TEACCH-Ansatz* [From the box to the workbook—Ideas and suggestions for structured activities based on the TEACCH approach]. Dortmund, Germany: Borgmann Media.

Steendam, M. (1989). *Cortical visual impairments: A handbook for parents and professionals.* Sydney, Australia: Royal Blind Society of New South Wales.

Steendam, M. (2007). *Weet jij wat ik zie? Cerebrale visuele stoornissen bij kinderen, een handleiding voor professionals* [Do you know what I see? Cerebral visual disorders in children, a manual for professionals]. Huizen, The Netherlands: Royal Dutch Visio.

Vervloed, M. P., Janssen, N., & Knoors, H. (2006). Visual rehabilitation of children with visual impairments. *Journal of Developmental & Behavioral Pediatrics, 27*(6), 493–506.

Zihl, J., & Dutton, G. N. (2015). *Cerebral visual impairment in children: Visuoperceptive and visuocognitive disorders.* Vienna: Springer-Verlag Wien.

Zihl, J., & Priglinger, S. (2002). *Sehstörungen bei kindern—Diagnostik und frühförderung* [Visual impairment in children—Diagnosis and early intervention]. Vienna: Springer-Verlag Wien.

# APPENDIX 21A
# Menu of Intervention Ideas

*Anne Henriksen*

The aim of the suggestions for intervention presented here, as a supplement to the strategies discussed in the chapter, is to motivate and enable children with CVI and multiple disabilities to use their vision. Complete blindness is rare; most children have some vision, and in most cases it is possible to enhance their use of vision. Some children can use their vision without much or any adaptation of the environment, while others need a special environment because they are not able to look under "typical" conditions. For many, it is important to provide materials that promote development of different basic visual skills (attention, fixation, following, shifting gaze, and scanning), visual guidance of motor activities, and visual perceptual functions (recognition). Adjustments to the learning environment are described first, followed by concrete intervention ideas for promoting specific visual functions.

## The 'Dark Room'

The dark room provides a way to eliminate visual clutter, enhance contrast (Kern, 2003), render visual information accessible as single presentations, and enhance vision for those whose vision is optimal in darkened conditions (Good & Hou, 2006). The dark room is a quiet room with the walls painted black; a darkened room without clutter on the walls may be adequate as well. It has a dark floor and dark furniture. All sorts of shining objects and lights appear brighter in a darkened environment and are seen singly. For many children who appear blind under other lighting conditions, these adapted conditions might be the first time in their lives when they realize they are able to see. This enables them to start to develop visual skills that they have not shown before. It should be noted that working in the "dark room" is not the same as working with "black light" (ultraviolet light shining on materials that glow under it or give off reflected fluorescent light).

Structured activities presented one at a time in the dark room can promote a wide range of visual skills, especially the promotion of visual attention: eye movements to follow, locate, and scan for objects; and visually directed limb and body movement. It is possible to use a range of different materials such as shiny toys, flashlights (torches), or presentations prepared for computers or touch-screen tablets (see Figure 21.7), employed one at a time initially, then perhaps two at a time. The use of such specially designed environments needs to be progressively diminished to help children slowly adapt to more natural situations and materials. This can be done initially by gradually increasing background illumination to more realistic everyday lighting conditions.

## The 'Portable Office'

The "portable office" helps eliminate competing visual input. It is a wooden wall with three sides that can be put up on the table to exclude visual distractions (see Figure 21.8). It should be big enough to make it possible to install additional light, and to work with

FIGURE 21.7
**Dark Room**

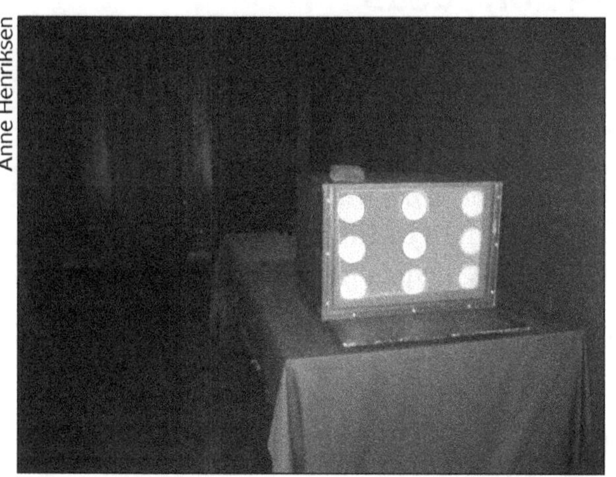

Anne Henriksen

The walls, floor, and furniture of the room are dark in order to reduce visual complexity and improve contrast. An image is projected on a screen from behind, so that no shadow occurs when a child is sitting close to it, and the screen is installed in a box so that it is stable (Kern, 2003). Here, the image on the screen shows dots against a contrasting background to foster visual attention.

FIGURE 21.8
**Portable Office**

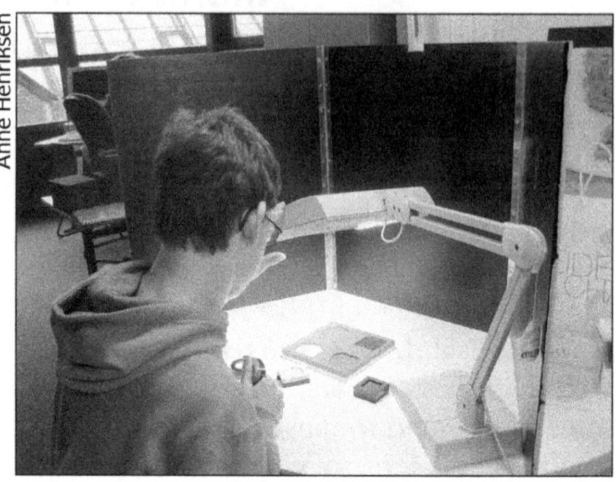

Anne Henriksen

A portable office screens out competing visual stimuli for a student working on a visual task.

different materials. Some study cubicles that are similar to the portable office may be available commercially, or a quiet corner in the classroom may be made into a defined area using the side of a cupboard.

## Use of Computers

The use of computers has many advantages for children with multiple disabilities and low vision. The computer screen is internally illuminated so the student does not sit in his or her own shadow. Images can also be projected onto a large area. A computer monitor on an arm can be presented quite close to the child, affording magnification and minimizing clutter and distraction. The screen can also be positioned optimally for the child in a wheelchair.

A switch that the child can operate, such as those used to promote augmentative communication, can enable the child to change the images on the screen. Working with a switch provides a good opportunity for the child to independently activate changes on the screen. This has an immediate and consistent effect, since the child receives reliable feedback and can take as much time as needed to look at each slide. It may take a while for children to develop an understanding of how the switch functions. It is important to give enough time for the child to gain experience with the switch to explore how to interact with it and learn what happens when activated. A touch screen also provides a direct link between action and effect and affords a good means of enhancing eye-hand coordination and encouraging directed attention. Many instructors are now using special applications for children on tablet computers (see Appendix 18A in Chapter 18 for more information).

### Designing Materials for Working with the Computer

Many different kinds of software are available for young children and for children with multiple disabilities, but not many follow the principles required for children with low vision: high magnification, high contrast, and lack of visual distractions from the key visual task. In addition, these programs may not consider the needs and interests of each child. Therefore, in many cases, it is often better to develop individualized material for each child. This is easy when using computer presentation software such as PowerPoint, Open Document, or Keynote. When creating presentations on the computer to enhance visual development, it is possible to consider the child's interests (for example, by using familiar and motivating material) and the child's special needs (such as the required size and contrast of an object, its position in the visual field, and the background and complexity of the material). It is possible to create presentations with pictures or picture books with slow- or fast-moving objects and to add sounds, music, or spoken language. Special apps for tablet computers can be used with children with CVI as well (see Appendix 18A).

## Intervention Ideas to Promote Visual Capabilities, Skills, and Behaviors

The following intervention ideas are grouped together under the headings of the different visual goals to be promoted. In reality, intervention for an individual child would probably not include interventions for only one visual skill area, but it is helpful to categorize them in this way. In addition, the images associated with each intervention idea are intended as examples that will enable readers to create their own colorful materials.

### Visual Attention

Very young children and children with multiple disabilities are attracted by moving and high-contrast visual stimuli, as well as stimuli that have sharp edges and that change quickly—for example, that blink or spin. Various flashlights and lights can be used in a dark room, or bright pictures can be presented by means of computer.

### Stimulus Localization

This task encourages the child to locate a stimulus in different areas of vision. Make sure the child is in the best position to become aware of the stimulus. Offer a bright visual stimulus on the monitor or shine a light in front of the child's face (being sure not to overwhelm the child with the light). Do the same from different directions in the child's peripheral visual field (above, below, left, and right). If a response can be seen, vary the stimulus as well as the position of the stimulus by choosing smaller lights, objects, or pictures, depending on the child's capabilities. If no response is demonstrated, let the light blink or move it closer to the child or choose larger objects or pictures.

### Fixation

Fixation is the ability to direct gaze toward an object of interest and keep it in view. The ability to fixate continues to develop in early infancy (Atkinson & Braddick, 1982) and is closely related to other visual functions, such as following, scanning, and especially eye-hand coordination. There are many ways to promote fixation on the computer or on different materials.

FIGURE 21.9
**Promoting Fixation**

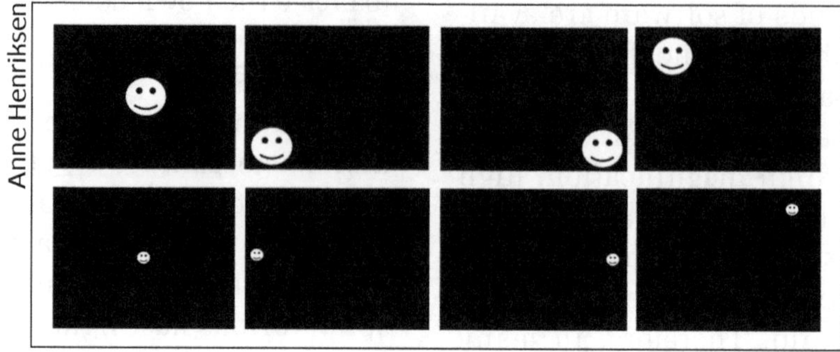


In the center of the screen is a big smiling face in high contrast (faces are extremely motivating to look at). When the child activates a switch, the face disappears and then reappears in another area of the visual field. The sequence is repeated, with the faces slowly becoming smaller. This activity helps children learn to take up and maintain fixation in different areas of the visual field with stimuli of varying sizes.

At the initial stages, large images of different colors on the computer or large, bright stimuli presented centrally and at close range can be offered (see Figure 21.9). Switching penlights or flashlights on and off against a dark background, or the use of objects, such as balls, with rich colors on a black table can also stimulate fixation. Be sure not to overload the child with bright light. A colored toy cap on the penlight or flashlight tip can be added to reduce the brightness of the light and add interest to the task.

If a child is able to hold fixation for a longer time with these initial materials, photos or smaller, familiar objects (such as a small flashlight, small toys, or food items) can be used in varying light conditions and at a greater distance. Once fixation is connected with grasping, be sure that the light stimulus is fixated on before the child grasps the toy, so that vision is used prior to the motor action. Once the child is able to hold fixation on these visual stimuli presented centrally, the fixation task can be made more challenging by presenting the materials more toward the peripheral area of a child's area of vision. It is important to have a good understanding of a child's available visual fields for these tasks.

### Visual Following Movements

Many children with motor disabilities have difficulty controlling their eye movements and executing smooth visual following. Inability or serious delay in bringing about following movements may be an outward sign of simultanagnosia, inability to pay attention due to medication or fatigue, lack of initiative, low visual acuity, or disordered gaze control. Missing, delayed, or jerky following movements to one side can indicate a visual field defect or neglect, while losing fixation may indicate bilateral central lack of vision (scotomas) (Zihl & Priglinger, 2002, p. 108). Lack of following movements can also result from Balint's syndrome (see Chapters 3 and 8). If a child does not react to

FIGURE 21.10
**Visual Following**

Anne Henriksen

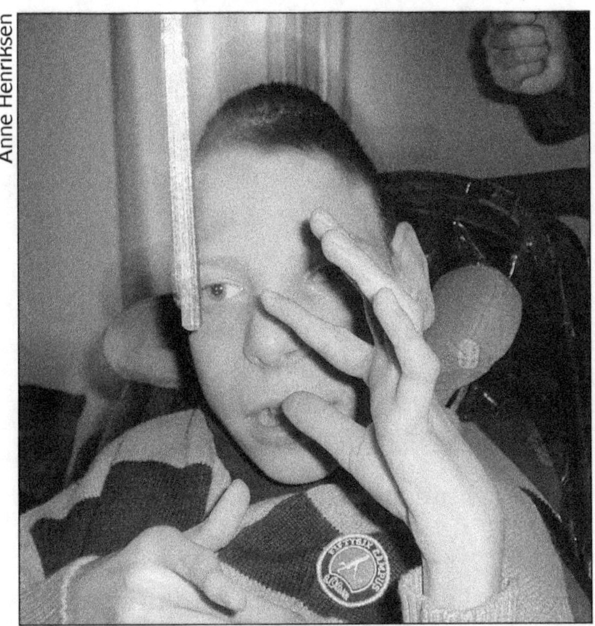

Bright objects moved in front of the eyes enhance visual following movements.

small stimuli, large stimuli should be used. In the case of profound Balint's syndrome, children rarely show saccades or following movements in horizontal directions side-to-side, and it is also not possible to "guide" them to either side, unless the target they are looking at is eliminated, when attention can be drawn to a new single target in a new location.

Some children with CVI and hemianopia have movement perception in the peripheral visual field (which may be intermittently evident) even if this is their "blind" visual field. These children are not able to fixate or respond to a centrally placed target, but can respond to a moving target in the peripheral visual field (Boyle, Jones, Hamilton, Spowart, & Dutton, 2005). To determine this, present a moving light source, or an object on the monitor, moving horizontally, vertically, and diagonally (see Figure 21.10). Watch carefully to see if the child is able to carry out continuous following movements, with or without additional head movements. Make sure that the child is in an appropriate position that facilitates an upright head posture without additional effort. Then encourage the child to expand visual attention and following in and slightly beyond these areas of vision.

### Shifting Gaze and Attention from One Object to Another

Shifting attention from one object to another can be stimulated by presenting two objects alternately. Inability to shift gaze might result from lack of interest or attention, a defect in the visual field, dorsal stream dysfunction, an eye movement disorder, or coordination problems. Once it is determined that children can make the necessary eye movements to shift gaze, the instructor can proceed to devise ways to develop this skill.

Shift of gaze requires the ability to be aware of several stimuli. At first only single elements can be perceived by a child with profound simultanagnosia. By simplifying visual tasks and encouraging the child to direct attention, first from one object or picture to another, then to shift gaze among three objects or pictures, this skill can be promoted. A child should be able to shift gaze easily between two objects or between two pictures several times. Two objects (toys) or pictures, identical in size and interest if possible, are held in front of the child or pictures of two objects are shown (see Figure 21.11). If the child does not shift gaze automatically from one object to the other it is necessary to attract the child's attention to one of them by quickly turning a lighted object off and on or shaking the object, giving

FIGURE 21.11
**Promoting Shift of Gaze**

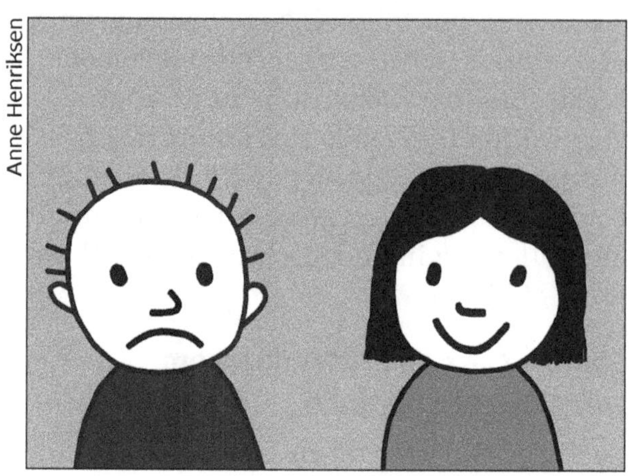


The two figures in the picture promote a shift of gaze from one to the other. It is not necessary to understand the content of the image (girl versus boy and happy versus sad); it only serves as a medium to promote looking from one object to the other.

FIGURE 21.12
**Scanning**

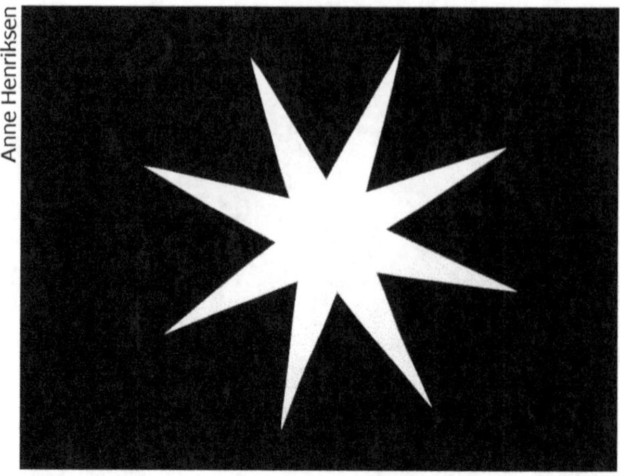


Scanning is necessary to find the points of this star.

sufficient time to gain attention, and before attracting attention to the other object. If possible, choose objects that are familiar to the child.

### Scanning the Features of an Object or Picture

Visual scanning—making a series of fixations to inspect a visual target or area—is one of the most important basic visual activities. Children begin visual scanning movements of faces at 9 days of age. The eyes, mouth, and hairline are the most preferred points (Luria, 1970). By the age of 4 weeks, perception of the outline of figures is possible (Banks & Salapatek, 1983). From the age of 8 weeks on, children investigate the inner portions of figures, and at 12 weeks of age they notice unusual visual details such as the unexpected interruption of a shape or a line (see Kern, 2003).

Materials for enhancing scanning should include simple facial features as well as large black-and-white stimuli to encourage detection of edges and lines. Later, simple shapes can be added, such as circles, triangles, or stars, and black-and-white or colorful outlined images, as well as simple facial expressions (see Figure 21.12). When scanning improves, increasing detail within the images can be included (see Malkowicz, Myers, & Leisman, 2006).

### Motion Perception

Motion perception, or the detection and discrimination of movements, is central for communication and mobility (Hyvärinen & Jacob, 2011). Several different kinds of problems exist with motion perception. Some children do not see objects that are standing still, while others have difficulties in seeing moving objects. If children are able to recognize moving objects, they often move their head or body in order to see well. This ability can be useful when teaching other visual

FIGURE 21.13
**Eye-Hand Coordination**

Anne Henriksen

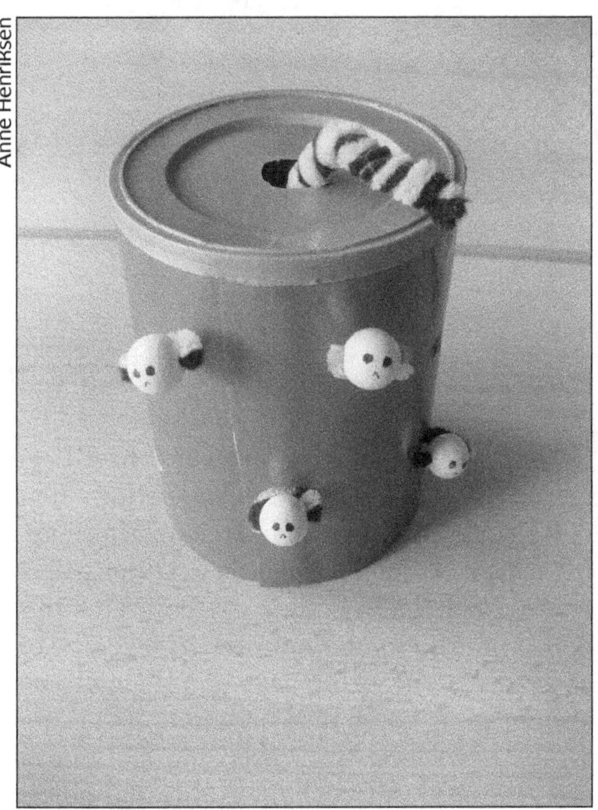

Coordination of precise looking and precise grasping is required to insert the objects—worms, balls, magnets—into the openings of the tin.

abilities, such as form perception or color recognition, as they will more likely respond to forms or colors in motion. If a child prefers moving objects, there are many ways to offer moving objects on the computer screen. For example, a moving light source or a moving object can be presented on the monitor horizontally, vertically, and diagonally.

### Visually Guided Movement

The ability to use the eyes in connection with hands (or feet) in order to reach objects or move toward objects is an important ability. In many children with multiple disabilities, eye-hand coordination might be delayed, impaired, or inaccurate. Some children have difficulties in viewing and reaching simultaneously; these children seem to look first, then turn their heads away and grasp without looking. When children have very limited motor abilities, a monitor with a touch screen is a good aid to enhance eye-hand coordination. Each time the child touches the screen, a new visual experience is presented.

Children who have developed motor coordination will be able to play with different kinds of high-contrast boxes, tins, spoons, dishes, and other visually interesting materials. Many ideas can be adapted from the TEACCH approach (Treatment and Education of Autistic and related Communication Handicapped Children), developed at the University of North Carolina (see http://teacch.com). This approach offers many practical ideas for working with children with cognitive disabilities, such as designing schedules and sorting and matching tasks (see Figure 21.13 and Solzbacher, 2010). As these ideas are not originally designed for children with visual impairments, some examples are in low contrast, and some are visually overloaded. If these suggested methods are to be implemented for children with CVI, the materials need to be large enough, of sufficiently high contrast, and reduced in complexity so that the child can see them readily.

### Visual Clutter

Children who have difficulties with visual clutter often have problems finding objects, unless they are presented in front of a clear background. These difficulties increase the more the background colors or forms blend

FIGURE 21.14
**Figure-Ground Perception**

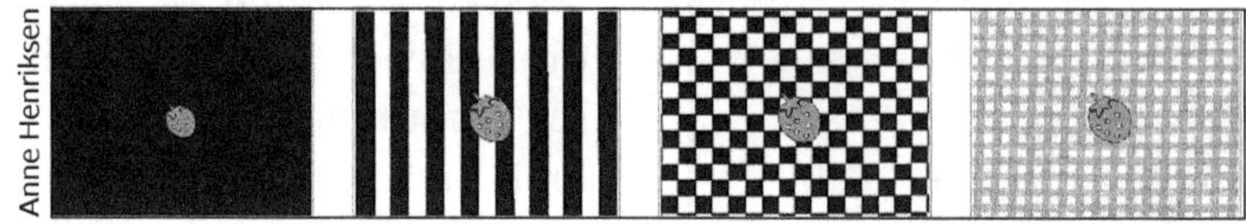


The strawberry in these pictures is "hidden" against a background that becomes progressively more complex as it changes color from black, to black and white, to red and white.

in with the figure in the foreground. To start, single-color objects with clear background are necessary for children with difficulties in figure-ground perception; later, the background can become more and more complex. Children with the cognitive capability to understand a hide-and-seek game can play with a figure that is "hidden" within the background. Initially the child is asked to find figures that stand out clearly in front of a well-structured background. The target figure is progressively hidden in a more complex background so that it becomes more and more difficult to find (see Figure 21.14). Movement of the target, which in this program can be made to twinkle, blink, or turn, makes detection easier.

### Recognition of Shapes, Objects, Pictures, and Photos

Recognition of photos, pictures, shapes, and objects requires the ability to differentiate between same and different, and known and novel. When working on shape or object recognition it is good to start with tactile material and only two shapes or objects. Adding other forms is possible when the concept of the first two forms is clear. The pieces of the LEA Puzzle (see Figure 21.15) are very useful for tactile discrimination because they look quite similar from different perspectives, and they can be presented with and without color coding of the shapes. The circle and the square are the easiest to differentiate. If a child is able to see better when objects are moving, the next step, after having learned from these tactile experiences, is to work with moving clearly colored symbols on the computer monitor. The degree of abstraction and difficulty should slowly be enhanced by using more symbols, by taking away the colors, by presenting stationary objects with and without additional color, and finally by presenting pictures of the symbols.

### Color Preference

Some children with CVI have a strong attraction to specific colors. It is useful to find out about preferred colors, since attention can be attracted to objects when using these special colors. Sometimes it is difficult to determine color preferences in children with severe multiple disabilities. One option is to offer two shapes or objects of similar interest, but in different colors (as in preferential looking tests), and to observe the reaction of the child. If the child is consistently attracted to a certain color, even when positioned on the left or right side of the monitor, or if the child shows any other kind of response, it could be a sign of color prefer-

Anne Henriksen

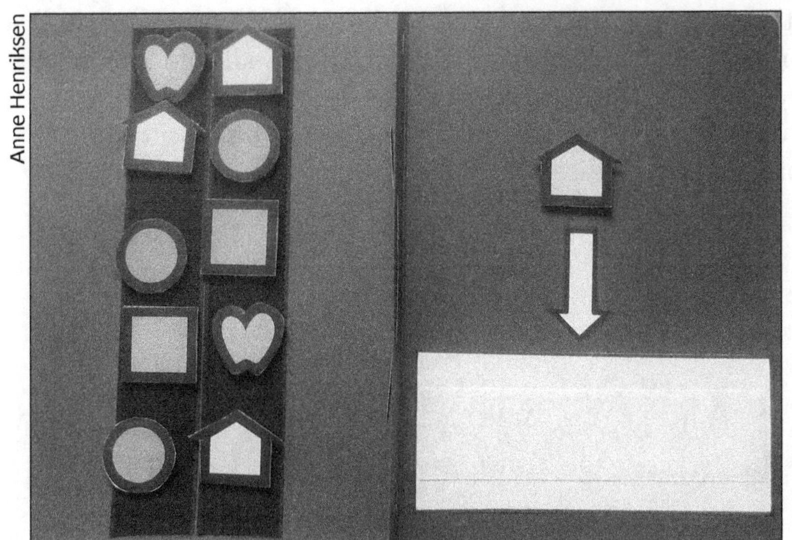

FIGURE 21.15
**Form Perception**

Shapes from the LEA Puzzle are used to teach form perception. One shape is placed on the right side of the Velcro background. The child is asked to find a matching shape from the various forms on the left side and to place it on the white Velcro strip under the arrow.

ence. The same type of investigation can be done on the monitor with a smiling face in different colors.

### Area of Vision

It is difficult to assess the location and extent of visual field defects in very young children and children with multiple disabilities. The Table Test is an adaptation from visual field training for adults with hemianopia (Münssinger & Kerkhoff, 1995) that can be used with children who can follow a complex set of directions. It may not be suitable for children with considerable cognitive delay. It uses 20 play animals: 10 animals that each have a "partner" that looks exactly the same to be used in pairs (5 pairs total) and 10 single animals that function as "distractors." Fifteen of the animals (excluding 5 of the animals that have a partner) are spread out on a table to encourage children to use their vision in all areas of their visual field. The children are supposed to find the partner of an animal. They can be told the following story: "A farmer is driving a tractor. He has an animal in the back of his tractor and is looking for the partner of this animal so that he can take them both home." The child has to find the second animal and put it into the toy tractor that is part of the test (see Figure 21.16). If children have difficulties finding the "partner" animal, they should be encouraged to drive the toy tractor to each

FIGURE 21.16
**Table Test for Visual Fields**

Anne Henriksen

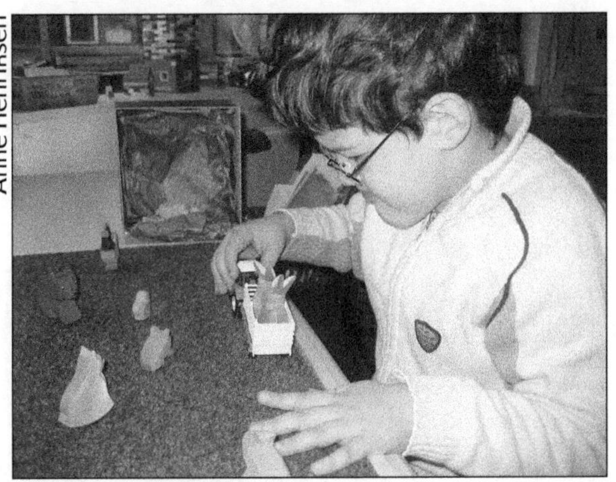

The Table Test for visual fields involves matching like objects—pairs of similar animals—that are spread out on a contrasting background.

corner and to search in all areas of the visual field. Rotation of the child's chair may be needed by those with evidence of lack of visual attention on one side of the body (see Figure 3.5 in Chapter 3). The number of animals and the size of the animals presented will depend on the child's visual and cognitive capabilities. Some teachers may wish to try the game with children who have cognitive disabilities but with fewer pieces to match.

# 22

# Parent-Recommended Strategies to Assist Children with CVI

*Debbie Cockburn and Gordon N. Dutton*

The behaviors of children with cortical visual impairment (CVI) whose visual acuities are between 20/80 and 20/100 or better who have disorders of visual field and visual processing are often attributed to clumsiness, lack of attention, or bad behavior, when the observed behaviors actually relate to their disorders of visual guidance of movement (optic ataxia) or perceptual visual dysfunction (see Chapter 3). See Tables 3.2–3.9 in Chapter 3 for a list of behaviors that can be misinterpreted when due in part, or in full, to CVI and when other potential causes have been examined through careful assessment. (A detailed discussion of the consequences of this kind of misinterpretation appears in Chapter 23.)

Parents with long-term experience of looking after children with CVI can serve as a rich resource of strategies, many of which have been learned by trial and error, for coping with the difficulties that result from these disorders. The information presented in this chapter highlights common difficulties and a range of adaptations, approaches, and strategies that parents have found effective for their own children (Dutton, McKillop, & Saidkasimova, 2006; McKillop & Dutton, 2008). This parent-sourced information has been built up over a period of over 20 years of seeing and helping these children.

Just as each child with CVI is different, the appropriate approaches will also be different and will match each child's unique set of needs. The list of parent-recommended strategies in this chapter can be considered by the educational assessment and planning team, including the caregivers, when determining appropriate adaptations to recommend and integrate into the child's overall management and care plan. They can reduce stressful demands placed on the child and can help to enhance the child's overall performance at home, at school, and in the community. Some of the approaches suggested here may well prove helpful for children with visual acuities lower than 20/100 as well.

## Difficulty Recognizing Known People and Facial Expressions

### Difficulty Recognizing People

- Have the teacher wear a colored identifier, such as a colored neck scarf, that is visible from all angles.
- Teach the child to look at color of shoes, hairstyle, or hair color as alternative identifiers if this is feasible.
- Help the child to develop skills of voice recognition.
- Notify the child of an intention to change hairstyle, and explain the change after, if required.

### Difficulty Interpreting Facial Expressions

- Ensure that all staff members know the child has difficulty interpreting facial expressions and provide training.
- Train the child in the meanings of facial expressions once it has been established that they can be seen.
- Prolong facial expressions when required, and reinforce them with spoken cues and possibly with exaggeration.
- Encourage the child to focus on the tone of voice and the words being used.
- Supplement facial expressions with matching language; for example, while smiling say, "Well done! I'm pleased you have finished so quickly." The language informs the child of the meaning of the smile.

## Persistent Difficulty Assigning Names to Colors

- Test color vision to be sure that color discrimination is normal.
- Use conceptual linkage to assign conceptual meaning to the abstract concept of color (for example, "grass-green," "sky-blue," "lemon-yellow").
- Diminish use of conceptual linkage when a color is learned.

## Difficulty Recognizing Shapes and Objects

### Recognizing Shapes

- Match three-dimensional shapes to two-dimensional images.
- Reinforce visual recognition with tactile recognition.

### Recognizing Objects

- Spread out objects that need to be found and identified so there is no overlap of items.
- Do not criticize when the child does this.
- Ensure possessions are stored in known locations to aid locating and identifying them.
- Train the child in tactile recognition.
- Hang clothes rather than fold them to maximize visibility and recognition of the whole items.

## Impaired Visual Function in the Lower Visual Field

### Tripping Over Obstacles

- Ensure floor space is kept clear by having good storage facilities.
- Consider changing the floor surface to one that is plain and without a pattern.

### Difficulty Negotiating Steps and Stairs

- Ensure that there are secure handrails at the correct height on both sides of the stairs.

- Arrange for the child to be first or last in a group when using the stairs.
- Let the child be first or last when leaving class to avoid crowding on the stairs.

### Colliding with Low Furniture

- Avoid moving the furniture, and involve the child when it has to be moved.
- Keep the amount of furniture in the room to a minimum.
- Keep the amount of visual distraction in the room to a minimum.
- Consider using "trails" or "footprints" on the floor as a guide for children with more severe disabilities.

## Inability to See and Gain Meaning from Fast-Moving Images

- Use alternative teaching media if a television presentation is too fast to learn from.

## Inaccuracy of Guidance of Reach Using Vision Alone

### Incorrect Reach and Grasp, Sometimes Missing or Knocking Items Over

- Minimize the number of items to be seen at once.
- Use items that contrast well in color with the unit surface.
- Show the child how to use the nondominant hand to first locate and touch the item being reached for with the dominant hand. (This supplements visual guidance of reach with tactile guidance.)
- Show the child how to run the reaching hand over the unit surface to help locate the item.
- Teach the older child how to extend the little finger of the moving hand to contact the unit surface both when reaching and when putting items down.
- Show the child how touching the unit the item is on (such as the countertop a toy is on) with part of the body can make reach more accurate.
- Practice with games and toys that require targeting and controlled dexterity.

## Difficulty Finding Elements in Scenes with a Lot of Visual Information or Finding Items against Similar Backgrounds

### Difficulties with Crowding of Text

- Match the amount of information on each page to the child's ability to see and interpret.
- Mask adjacent text (for example, by using a typoscope); some children can use the fingers on two hands to do this.
- Keep surrounding clutter and pattern to a minimum, particularly in the direction the child is looking from his or her workstation.

### Difficulty Seeing an Item Pointed Out in the Distance

Note that often, the further away one looks, the more there is to see.

- Use clear verbal prompts for large visual targets in order to cue the child. For example, "If you look at the big church, then look past it, you will see your friend."
- Give the child sufficient time to process information, and do not rush the child.

- Share the screen of a digital camera and zoom function to locate and point out what is being shown.
- Go with the child to view the item at closer range.

### Difficulty Finding People in the Playground or Classroom

- If the child stands at the side of the playground unable to engage, train the class to understand the nature of the child's vision and how to best support the child.
- Give additional verbal information. (For example, "Your friend Jenny is at the gate in a pink jacket.")
- Train the child in voice recognition to help identify and find friends.
- Make sure teachers and friends introduce themselves in busy locations.
- Use prearranged meeting points.
- If a child is unable to find a parent who is collecting the child from school, the parent should wear bright-colored clothing that stands out.
- Give the older child permission to use a mobile phone and show him or her how to use it to find friends.

### Difficulty with Team Sports, Difficulty Finding and Identifying Team Members

- Inform physical education staff so they can select optimal activities. (Failure in school sports can diminish confidence and self-esteem.)

### Difficulty Finding a Wanted Item if There Is Too Much Visual Information

- Keep number of items—for example, in a locker—to a minimum.
- Choose items to be of different bright colors, to aid in finding them.
- Store items horizontally or vertically in specific places so that search is in one direction.
- Design a storage system and train the child in keeping items in specific locations.
- Train the child in putting everything back in correct locations.
- Teach salient methods of visual searching, supplemented by touch when needed.
- Give verbal directions when necessary.

### Difficulty Locating Items of Clothing in Changing Room

- Teach the child to hang clothes on peg in the order that they are removed, and to reverse the order for getting dressed again.

### Difficulty Filling Cups and Pouring Liquids

- Use a clear plastic cup with the level marked, for example, with nail varnish.
- Use a thumb over edge of cup as a tactile indicator for cold liquids (when appropriate).
- Teach the child to listen for the progressively higher pitch of the sound of the liquid as the vessel is filled, and to learn when to stop filling at the optimum pitch level.
- Consider using a fluid level indicator.

## Difficulty Knowing Where Sound Is Coming From

- Calling out to locate another person tends not to work; use mobile phones or walkie-talkies to find one another and communicate.

## Behavioral Difficulties in Crowded Locations

- When there is too much visual or auditory stimulation, such as in school classrooms, corridors, or dining areas, schedule activities and classroom changes to avoid crowds.
- Use a quiet, undecorated "chill-out room" as appropriate.
- Minimize noise and visual clutter in the area where the child is looking in class.
- Train staff to recognize and understand behavior and take appropriate action.

## Difficulty at Mealtimes

### Leaving Food on Plate

- Position favorite foods where they are usually missed to stimulate exploration.
- Develop a routine of rotating the plate to look for the food.
- Use plain plates with no pattern and colors that contrast well with the food.
- Displace the place setting to the side that is best seen.

### Distress with Multiple Food Items on the Plate

- To avoid visual crowding of food items on a plate, serve items of food on separate plates or one item after another.
- Sauces and gravy over food can prevent separate items being seen and can be unpopular, so try pouring them over single items only, or not at all.

The many adaptations described in this chapter not only render everyday living easier for affected children, but have also been found by the authors to have enhanced emotional well-being. The accommodations relieved many of the minor stresses that the children had hitherto experienced on a day-to-day basis prior to the adaptations being implemented.

## References

Dutton, G. N., McKillop, E. C., & Saidkasimova, S. (2006). Visual problems as a result of brain damage in children. *British Journal of Ophthalmology, 90*(8), 932–933.

McKillop, E., & Dutton, G. N. (2008). Impairment of vision in children due to damage to the brain: A practical approach. *British and Irish Orthoptic Journal, 5,* 8–14.

# 23

# Supports for Children and Families

*Mary T. Morse and John L. Morse*

In many countries, special education is now considered a partnership between parents and professionals sharing their specialized knowledge and collaborating to observe children, solve problems, and implement services. Accomplishing this task for students who have difficult-to-understand conditions requires communication, understanding of the conditions, coordination, and, most of all, trust. This is particularly true for students who have cerebral visual impairment (CVI), a difficult-to-understand, brain-based visual condition. This chapter discusses a variety of social and adjustment challenges that children with CVI and their families may face, and offers some supportive strategies to address these challenges that can be implemented by early intervention and school personnel.

CVI is not a label that describes a singular visual diagnosis. Rather, CVI is a label that indicates that visual concerns are brain-based and, as such, may manifest with other challenging conditions, as well as a wide variety of associated visual behaviors in children, ranging from those with no useful vision to those who have normal to near-normal visual acuity. This latter group can be the most difficult to understand for parents, educators, the general public, and the children themselves (Dutton, 2003). The children appear visually normal and, in the authors' experience, most use vision as their primary learning modality, with auditory and/or olfactory (smell) information as backup systems. However, many of these students are unaware, at least most of the time, that they do not operate with a fully intact visual system or a fully intact auditory system (G. N. Dutton, personal communication, February 19, 2012), as will be discussed in this chapter.

Many infants, school-age children, and adults, but not all, have significant disabilities in addition to their diagnosed CVI. These may include seizures, cerebral palsy, severe feeding problems (with many requiring feeding by a gastrostomy, or G-tube, inserted near the navel), and high health risks. Such high health risks may include frequent respiratory illnesses, cardiac issues, deafness, and more. CVI, in addition to these other disabilities, tends to place heavy physical, emotional, and financial burdens on families.

In many countries, including the United States, families no longer have the strong, accessible family support systems they did a century ago. Thus, friends and local, state, and federal services frequently have to assume the functions of these missing support services. As a result, services for young children, school-age children, and adults with disabilities have become a political issue because of the need for public assistance to provide support in areas that were once considered to be exclusively within the family domain. Based on personal conversations with various families over the past four decades, the lack of availability of the extended family can further contribute to a family's sense of loss and isolation since they may feel they do not have access to the support they need.

Appendix 23A provides three personal stories about growing up with CVI and describes experiences with the diagnostic process, subsequent development, intervention services, and the interventions themselves. Two stories are told by parents, and one is an interview with an adult who has CVI. This chapter discusses the same journey from the point of view of the professionals who work with these children and their families and provides suggestions about how professionals can provide support to them.

## The Road to Diagnosis

> . . . Misunderstanding of CVI and how the child sees or doesn't see are the biggest issues we parents face when seeking an appropriate education for our children with CVI (personal discussion with a parent, October 10, 2011).

CVI is a difficult visual condition to diagnose and to understand. Many children with multiple problems from birth or early infancy have a range of urgent problems that need to be addressed. Issues surrounding vision may not be at the forefront since other, more pressing conditions, some of them life-threatening, may require immediate medical attention. In addition, more obvious ocular conditions may overshadow the identification of coexistent CVI. Moreover, the medical profession might not suspect CVI in light of what appears to be a normal infant or young child. Questionable observable visual behaviors might be interpreted to be the result of another condition. Or, as Hyvärinen (1992) points out, "The present visual acuity values and visual field recordings, which are used for classification, do not always correctly depict visual function even in older children." For many infants and children, the label frequently appears incongruent with behaviors observed by individuals unfamiliar with CVI.

When CVI is diagnosed, the professionals involved may not be aware of potential coexisting *hidden disabilities,* such as auditory processing issues, that may be manifested in early childhood or in later years. For example, one of the authors (Mary Morse) has seen over 1,000 infants, toddlers, and school-age children eventually diagnosed with CVI. Some had no vision, most had variable visual responses, but many had near-normal visual acuity and visual fields—some of the time. However, all had one behavior in common: an intense interest in music and the melodic intonation of voices. In addition, all had a range (varying from a small to a large amount) of difficulty in processing language and displayed difficulties with pragmatics, the social nuances of language (Aitken, 2010). This dual difficulty may be because auditory and visual processing are closely interconnected (G. N. Dutton, personal communication, February 19, 2012; Guzzetta, Conti, & Mercuri, 2011). Thus, many individuals with CVI may also have varying degrees of difficulty with processing auditory information (Aitken, 2010), and this possibility should be considered within the framework of a comprehensive evaluation. When the interpretation and processing of information from these two sensory systems is not functioning optimally, a child or adult with CVI may frequently be viewed as distractible, not attending, or noncompliant.

In addition, many people with CVI who appear fully sighted may have other "invisible challenges" that are behavioral consequences of CVI. These are not readily apparent but may manifest as learning differences, personal safety issues, self-concept issues, communication difficulties, atypical behavior, movement disorders, and hindered social relationships, all of which can affect social and emotional development from birth through the school years.

## Support Needs for Children with CVI and Their Families at Different Developmental Stages

In the authors' experience, four stages in children's general development mark four major vulnerable periods for families who have a child with CVI:

- the early intervention years,
- the early school years,
- the middle and high school years, and
- the period of transition to adult services.

During each of these periods, families face certain common needs:

- emotional support,
- information about the visual condition and possible health issues,
- information regarding available resources,
- a simple overview of future educational models,
- training on how to advocate with doctors, therapists, educators, and others on their child's behalf, and
- how to enlist help from family and friends.

Concurrent with this bombardment of information is the need for the family and caregivers to learn how to work with the wide range of professionals who offer necessary services for their child. Aside from the services provided by eye care professionals and educators, this may also include counseling services for the child if he or she experiences isolation from family members and friends.

### The Journey Begins: The Early Intervention Years

Some infants may have obvious disabilities at birth, and many of these conditions can overshadow the possibility or immediate importance of a visual impairment. Other infants may not have any obvious disabilities at birth and CVI may not reveal itself during the course of early development. In either case, once a disability is identified, life for the family becomes a waiting game for the acquisition of information, diagnoses, and prognoses, and the focus on medical issues can distract from parenting and habilitation. Infancy is an essential period of adjustment during which critical bonds of attachment and early communication typically occur. For families who have babies in the process of having their condition diagnosed, this is a period of great vulnerability. Problems that may result during this period are not isolated events but may impact the newborn child, the immediate family, and the extended family for life (Tuttle & Tuttle, 2004).

For many of these families, this journey involves allowing a range of professionals into their home on a regular basis to provide and demonstrate suggested visual activities; tactile, gross, and fine motor skills; early concept building; communication skills; and techniques to promote continued development as well as train other senses. These professionals also promote play skills (which may require adaptive intervention methods), early literacy, social skills, spatial skills, and more. During these extensive interventions, a large number of people encroach on the family's time and home space to provide these services. During this most vulnerable period, parents may be encouraged to seek out other parents for support, to review, research, and learn more about CVI and other issues pertaining to their child's specific needs. Simultaneously, parents are asked to implement various techniques to develop and utilize their child's visual capacity as fully as possible. All of this is a lot for most parents who fully expected to bring home an infant who would just need physical care, soothing touches, and continuous love.

As the infant grows older, families will need information and support for the transition from early intervention in the home to preschool situations or entry into elementary school. They will need to learn new ways to work with school staff. They will also need information regarding the various types of educational placement options and other available community supports.

The first three years are a fragile time for parents who have a child born with disabilities. Parents are at the beginning of a long journey. It is an overwhelming and frequently traumatic period of waiting for medical information, traveling long distances for medical appointments, hearing new and unfamiliar medical terms, and learning how to care for medical needs they never knew existed. For most families this is a physically, emotionally, and financially draining experience. The first person to deliver the news about the child having a disability will have the greatest impact on how the parents understand future information. This is a time when parents need to hear not just information regarding vision, but also information about other developmental areas such as communication methods, what their child's behaviors might mean, what to do to help their child live and progress, available services, and much more. To paraphrase a conversation with Lea Hyvärinen, parents need to become experts in the problems of their child; they can be taught to observe and support the development of their child (L. Hyvärinen, personal communication, Summer, 2007).

Upon learning of their child's CVI, grieving is most difficult when parents are faced with a disability that may not be readily apparent, has an uncertain prognosis, includes the presence of an undetermined amount of available vision, and may involve additional disabilities. Many difficulties may not manifest themselves for years, whether they are academic, social, communicative, or other. Such is the case for Larry and his parents in the following case study. Some suggested ways to support families during early intervention years can be found in Sidebar 23.1.

**LARRY IS A HANDSOME 3-YEAR-OLD BORN AT 28 WEEKS** gestation, who remained in the neonatal intensive care unit for several months. During this period, Larry's parents were told he had suffered a stroke in utero and most likely would have some disabilities. At 4 months, his parents were told he had a seizure condition; at 4½ months they received news that he had a mild form of cerebral palsy; and at

SIDEBAR 23.1

## Supports for Families in Early Intervention Years

### The Challenge

Parents need to manage both medical and unique developmental needs.

### Some Solutions

The following supports may assist families of young children with CVI. These suggestions have been written into Individual Service Plans for Families and Individualized Education Programs over the years by Mary Morse, one of the chapter authors.

- Well-coordinated care and respect from the medical profession with reports that are easily understandable to the family.
- Early intervention specialists, including a teacher of students with visual impairments, who are experienced in working with infants and toddlers with CVI and in working in homes, rather than just working in schools or hospitals.
- Support from family members, including grandparents, siblings, and extended family.
- Support groups or one-to-one support from another person with similar experiences, depending on the individual's needs and preferences.
- Active case management systems involving a range of community services.
- Early intervention specialists attending doctor appointments with the family—in person or by video conferencing or teleconferencing.
- User-friendly medical and early intervention reports and the inclusion of parents in every phase of the coordination (Morse, 1990).
- Respect for the family's knowledge of their child, concerns about their child, and their opinions.
- Information about and access to resources about parent and consumer organizations related to children who have visual impairments.
- Support for siblings
  - The school psychologist can be a very good resource for older siblings of children who have CVI. It is likely that there is a group of students within the school, or within the school district, who have siblings with disabilities, not necessarily CVI but a range of other disabilities. Developing group discussion sessions and sharing feelings might alleviate feelings of guilt the siblings may have regarding their ambivalence and come to understand that their feelings are legitimate (Morse & Whelley, 2007).
  - In the authors' experience, it is important to help parents understand that mundane chores like grocery shopping can become a special time for siblings who do not have disabilities. Revealing conversations are frequently spontaneous and come about during unplanned times. Such conversations, short though they may be, allow parents the opportunity to recognize their child's feelings by listening, acknowledging, providing a sympathetic touch, or showing understanding in other ways that are special to that family. Such open talks usually result in feelings of relief for both parents and siblings. Even when grocery shopping, doing dishes, or attending a special event, there is time to talk openly, with each offering support and expressing understanding in their own way.
  - Identifying resources to assist parents in supporting their children who do not have disabilities.

*Source:* Except as otherwise noted, the above statements were adapted from Edwards, C., & Da Fonte, A. (2012). The 5-point plan: Fostering successful partnerships with families of students with disabilities. *TEACHING Exceptional Children*, *44*(3), 6–13.

9 months, the pediatric ophthalmologist said that brain imaging revealed that with the exception of an eye turn, Larry's ocular structures looked good. However, he went on to say, it was too early to know if Larry would be able to use his vision as well as other children, and he explained the brain's role in processing visual information. Like many other parents who had similar experiences, Larry's parents waited and waited for "the next shoe to drop"—for the next piece of bad news.

Around this same time, Larry was rushed to the hospital on two separate occasions; once when his grandmother was caring for him and again when he was under the care of a certified nurse assistant. As a result, his parents are desperately afraid to let him out of their sight, and do not use any respite services. Their level of trust of service providers and others caring for their child—even close family members—is low.

Although they intellectually understand Larry's visual condition, they find it hard to believe that this very visually oriented child has a visual impairment. Even though he had a second small stroke in the occipital area when he was 2 years old, he walks, talks, and seems to see even the smallest item of interest. Larry's parents want to know if their child will be able to read, but the pediatric ophthalmologist and the teacher of students with visual impairments say it is too early to tell. Thus, the parents continue to remain uncertain. Their life appears to be on hold, and they remain focused on this one child while they make every possible attempt to give what little attention they have remaining to their two other children. They appear to be physically and emotionally exhausted.

How is it possible for parents to grieve when they are unsure of what they are grieving for, or to accept, when they are unsure about what they need to accept? Their seemingly impossible task is to struggle with their emotions and feelings and to simultaneously be expected to give to others 24 hours per day, seven days a week.

It is difficult for parents to be expected to deal with their reactions and simultaneously make adjustments in their daily routines that will affect the whole family. Concomitantly, siblings frequently are affected when another child in the family has CVI. They may be affected even more if CVI is accompanied by other disabilities, both hidden and obvious. At times, siblings may feel overlooked, while at other times they may feel protective. Usually, this ambivalence is normal, but sometimes it may be helpful for siblings to receive professional counseling to maintain optimum mental health. (See Sidebar 23.1 for more suggestions about supporting siblings.)

## The Early School Years

Parents also "graduate" when their child leaves home-based early intervention services to go into the big world of school-based services. For many parents, this transition is traumatic because the home is their turf; but school belongs to the community, is less personal, is less accessible, and is governed by rules and standards different from home. Many parents report that they experience a sense of having less control, an uncertain "letting go," and a personal loss when their very young child has so many experiences away from home and with people they barely know. This is a critical time for building trust between the school and the home, and requires continued efforts by everyone involved (home, school staff, service providers, and other agency personnel) to ensure a positive result.

For some children with CVI, this may be when they begin to realize that they are different from other children. These children may not understand all they see and hear. And their orientation and movement through the environment may be difficult and appear awkward to others. The nature of their CVI and hidden disabilities may provide them with a different visual and

SIDEBAR 23.2

## Supporting the Child and Family in the Early School Years

### The Challenge

CVI, in addition to other disabilities, tends to place heavy physical, emotional, and financial burdens on families and school staff.

### Some Solutions

The following methods may assist families with young children who have CVI. These suggestions can be utilized by parents, medical professionals, therapists, and others, as determined in meetings with the child and family. These suggestions have been written into Individual Service Plans for Families and Individualized Education Programs over the years by Mary Morse, one of the chapter authors.

- Ask the parents to explain any additional disabilities and what physical care and adaptations are needed.
- Have the school nurse obtain permission to communicate directly with physicians for additional explanations and with school-related questions.
- If the child has a physical disability and uses a wheelchair, have the physical therapist teach all classroom staff appropriate and safe techniques for positioning the student and transferring the student from one position to another (for example, from wheelchair to toilet).
- If the child has feeding problems or has a gastrostomy, or G-tube (also know as a PEG tube), ask parents to demonstrate the feeding process. Many students with this disability have feeding specialists involved. Ideally, the specialist would also be available for questions and to demonstrate techniques.
- If the child has seizures, request that the nurse demonstrate what to do at the start, during, and after a seizure, and how to chart them.
- Post important individualized safety rules in accessible locations so all school staff will know what to do in an emergency. Many school programs post one copy on the back of a wheelchair, with another on the stander or in other locations used by the child.
- Ideally, all school personnel should have CPR (cardiopulmonary resuscitation) training.
- Attend in-service training sessions related to multiple disabilities.
- Never lose sight of normal growth and development. The student is not an accumulation of his or her disability diagnoses. Each is an individual.

intuitive perspective compared to their peers' and teachers' perspectives and make it difficult to communicate and share common interests. An example follows, and Sidebar 23.2 offers some suggestions for support in this area.

**Antonio is in second grade. He has a rare syndrome** that includes cerebral palsy affecting the lower extremities, great difficulty when attempting visually guided gross and fine motor activities, ptosis, myopia, articulation problems, and bilateral inability to move his eyes horizontally. In addition, he has been medically diagnosed with CVI. He fatigues quickly when using his vision, as evidenced by turning his head away from activities, although he usually remains attentive to sounds.

Antonio is charming, and, during his preschool years, used his charm to divert adult attention from activities he felt he could not perform. Beginning in first grade, the teacher of students with visual impairments provided in-service training to all staff regarding the impact of CVI in combination with Antonio's other challenges. In addition, the teacher of students with visual impairments provided consultation on ways to adapt activities and materials, such as modifying Antonio's schedule to allow for extra time to complete activities, introduction of a video magnifier, provision of an adapted computer with appropriate software for his visual needs, as well as an iPad for Antonio to use. The school supplied the classroom with a smart board, and the classroom teacher became interested in learning to use all these devices. Antonio's classmates were fascinated with the equipment, and Antonio, in turn, happily found himself the center of a lot of peer attention. More important, Antonio found that with these technology devices—combined with his teacher's expectations for performance—he began to read, albeit much more slowly than his classmates. However, he still fatigued faster than his classmates when using his vision, as demonstrated by his looking away from visual tasks, talking to himself, closing his eyes, and so forth.

Nevertheless, Antonio was making progress. Even though he required extra time, he was learning to read. Even though he walked slowly, he had friends. Even though his handwriting was hard to decipher, he was cognitively learning how to make facsimiles of letters and numbers. This was a win-win situation for all. His teacher was thrilled with the technology and the challenge of having Antonio in her class. His parents began to perceive Antonio as a child who could learn, and not as a baby. And Antonio began developing a positive self-image of himself as a learner.

## The Middle and High School Years

Middle school and high school is a turbulent period for any teenager and their parents and even more so for students who have CVI and hidden disabilities. These students become much more aware of their differences from same-age peers and, as a result, there is a very high risk for social isolation, anger, and depression. Providing educational services for those students who have additional disabilities or medical conditions may become an extremely difficult challenge (Kef, 2002). To paraphrase many of the students with CVI whom both authors have talked with, making true friendships seems impossible because of the lack of mutual interests and abilities. Below is an example of some of these issues, as experienced by one child, along with some suggested solutions.

**Nate, an only child, is a 15-year-old high school** student who has been diagnosed with CVI as well as having seizures, asthma, and motor disabilities for which he uses a motorized wheelchair. He wears eyeglasses for myopia and has esotropia. The past year has been difficult for Nate, as evidenced by his tremendous mood swings and at times uncontrollable and destructive behavior.

On observation, Nate appears visually disengaged during academic activities even though he is obviously listening. He tries to answer questions when asked, and many times comes up with the correct response. It is difficult for him to answer questions, as it takes him time to process the question, plan the necessary oral-motor breathing patterns, and implement them. Often, by the time he has completed this arduous task, someone else has answered for him or the subject matter has already changed. Nate has almost no reading or math skills in spite of an IQ in the low average range. He fatigues easily when using his vision, even when playing games on the computer, an activity he dearly loves. He seems to prefer talking books or personal readers to reading print.

When provided with academic work, Nate does not use his vision and hearing simultaneously. Depending on his comfort level in answering academic questions, he is able to look and speak at the same time, but he has great difficulty in sustaining eye contact. He uses a power chair and is very adept at weaving his way around chairs, desks, and people. Perhaps the saddest aspects of his disabilities are first, that traditional teaching methods have not been successful with Nate, and second, that he has no friends. Nate clearly wants to socialize with his same-age peers, as seen by a dramatic change in his demeanor when occasionally invited to join a few classmates during after-lunch social time. During these few times, his face gleams with joy as he tries to bat a balloon or engage in some other activity. In reality, Nate has little in common with other teenagers because he cannot engage in the same athletic pursuits, he is not an equal academically, and his unusual visual behaviors distance him even further.

### *Some Possible Solutions for Nate*

Knowledge of Nate's preferences can suggest some solutions to his challenges with schoolwork and socializing. Nate enjoys "The Three Stooges" and other old TV shows. A project could be developed around this interest that would embed vocabulary, number concepts, categorizing and subcategorizing, using the library, and planning and giving a demonstration to the class. Working with a peer who receives help from the special education teacher in understanding both Nate's difficulties and his talents, this thematic unit might involve researching how many TV shows the "Stooges" made, what the real names of the men were, and something about their personal lives. Nate and the peer might prepare a short paper (which could be tape recorded if he wished) on what the two find so entertaining about these shows. The theme could be carried further by having them write their own show (or tape recording it if it is easier).

Nate also has a wonderful imagination and likes gardening in window boxes. He might work with a peer in creating a recreational area on the school's flat rooftop. This type of creativity could turn into a math lesson by obtaining the measurements of the rooftop, planning the varying types of recreational opportunities, designing where they should be located (keeping in mind accessibility issues), and drafting a plan to scale. This unit might require Nate and the peer to do some research in the library and to obtain costs for various aspects. Such a project could involve math, reading, cooperative planning, social interaction, and creativity. The plan could then be presented to the class.

Finally, in a variation of a peer-collaboration approach (Tinzmann, Jones, Fennimore, Bakker, Fine, & Pierce, 1990), all the students in Nate's class (Nate included) could collaborate to form a lunchtime club, with the special education teacher as the facilitator. The teacher might call a class meeting and raise the question of having a "club" in the resource room during the lunch period. Nate and the peers are invited to suggest as many ideas as they want, no matter how unrealistic. All ideas are listed on the board. Subsequently, the students look over the list and decide, as a group, which ideas are unrealistic or have the least chance of success at this time. Those ideas are crossed off the board. The remaining ideas are prioritized in order of importance or anticipated degree of success. The top two or three ideas are selected as a start and are analyzed as to what, when, where, who, and so forth. This systematic method teaches all the involved students analytical thinking, a process for reaching group consensus and analysis.

Methods that involve same-age peers and help groups analyze options are also extremely helpful when there are activities that might potentially exclude those with disabilities. Same-age peers can be very creative. Some have developed the means for giving a book report when the student with disabilities cannot speak, or going on a field trip up a mountain when the student with disabilities uses a wheelchair. Since the same-age peers helped develop the plans, they tend to take more ownership in becoming actively involved in working with classmates like Nate who have disabilities.

### *Promoting Inclusion in the Classroom*

As already noted, the population of students with CVI is heterogeneous with regard to age, gender, type of visual impairment, degree of vision present, onset of the condition, additional disabilities, educational status, receptivity to special services, and level of adjustment. The fact that many students appear to have normal vision, but demonstrate a short attention span or "distractibility" as well as other atypical behaviors is particularly problematic. Moreover, many students with CVI typically demonstrate inconsistent and inefficient use of the visual system (Dutton & Bax, 2010). As a result, students with CVI may present a range of unique behaviors that can affect social interactions. A student's ability to participate in inclusive school programs can, therefore, be varied and inconsistent depending on the nature of the task, the visual-motor demands of the activity, the complexities of what is to be viewed, and the history of what was tried, what worked, and what was successful or not successful from the student's perspective. All these factors play a major role in the life of students with CVI, especially students who are considered academic learners and are expected to graduate from school with a high school diploma. (Some ways to support children with CVI in regular education programs can be found in Chapter 19.)

## Making the Transition to Adult Services

Transition services are a coordinated set of activities that promote movement from school to postschool activities, such as employment, postsecondary education, vocational training, independent living, and community participation. Such services must be based on the cultural mores of the country or region as well as the individual student's preferences, interests, and needs. "Futures planning" is one process that can be used to promote transition to adult activities. This process provides students with disabilities, including those with CVI, with support from significant others and empowers them to focus on their goals, abilities, dreams, and needs in order to chart plans for the future (HMS School, n.d.; Moss & Wiley, 2003). The school psychologist, guidance counselor, or social worker might have training in implementing this helpful process that will act as a guide for curricular choices during a student's final high school years. In working through this process, the following content might be considered in the plans to achieve a student's chosen goals:

- Specific instruction in core educational courses
- Community experiences
- Development of employment and other postschool adult living objectives
- Acquisition of daily living skills
- A functional vocational evaluation when appropriate

As they make the transition from high school to whatever situation comes next, students with CVI and their families require access to support services to ensure that each student's chosen lifestyle, based on personal preferences and capabilities, is of high quality, promotes desired levels of independence, and provides the student with a sense of purpose and meaningful social stimulation. In the United States, many students with CVI who previously received services to address their visual needs (such as services from a teacher of students with visual impairments and an orientation and mobility [O&M] specialist, specialized equipment, and adapted reading materials) may find they are no longer eligible for disability assistance under adult service systems once they complete high school. This may be because they do not meet the criteria for entitlement to adult services based on the typical criteria for visual impairment–a specific degree of reduced visual acuity and visual field restrictions (see Chapter 1). Some may not be able to find adult services that can accommodate their multiple needs if they have a complex array of disabilities that includes a visual impairment. Other students with CVI and their families will be able to access opportunities through special government or private programs or services. Available services will depend on the country or specific regions of a country in which they are located. Specific opportunities may include placement in specialized settings with daily enrichment activities, supervised apartment living, and worksite supervision. However, postsecondary opportunities involve more than a job and a place to live. For individuals with CVI who are able to live independently or semi-independently, social issues and pressures may need to be addressed through postsecondary placements and services, as discussed in some of the following sections.

## Managing Adjustment Concerns for Students with CVI

### Understanding the Student's World

The most typical hallmark of children with CVI is variation. The way they experience their world can change from day to day or minute to minute. A real part of this variation is caused by changes in brain functions resulting from the condition itself. This can affect vision, other sensory systems, cognition, and motor functions. Variation also may be caused by medications, fatigue, and composition of the environment. In addition, tasks that are routine for typical children may not be readily accomplished by a child with CVI. It can happen that a child who can perform an apparently more demanding task may fail to complete what seems to be an easier one. Others need to realize that a task that appears to be easier may actually be more difficult for the child with CVI if functions needed by the child to complete the "easier" task are among the functions that are impaired (Hyvärinen, 2004; Hyvärinen & Jacob, 2011).

Making the effort to understand how the student experiences his or her world can also provide abundant insights into issues associated with social interaction skills. From the students' perspective, they may have heard the following comments:

- "Pay attention."
- "You read the first paragraph beautifully but you are not trying as hard on the second paragraph."
- "Go play with your friends instead of walking aimlessly."
- "Be more careful and you won't trip on the stairs so much."
- "Stop and look before crossing the street or moving about the school hallway."
- "Sit up straight when you are reading instead of continuing to slide down into your chair."
- "Look at me when I am talking to you."

These and other such comments have been heard by both authors from numerous parents and teachers during many classroom observations and educational team meetings. Moreover, these comments are frequently rephrased and written into students' Individualized Education Programs. For many students, hearing such comments from teachers and parents so many times diminishes their self-concept, self-confidence, and feelings of competence. Statements like these tend to interfere with a student's level of independent functioning, ability to relate spontaneously with peers, and their behavior both at home and during school hours. As G. N. Dutton (personal communication, February 19, 2012) explains, "Children with damage to the brain are often not aware of the nature of their problems. When they cannot do something, they are unaware that they are unaware (anosognosia), and this compounds the sense of isolation brought about by such criticism, as they do not, and cannot, know why they are being criticized." Unfortunately, these students are not immune from bullying or, at a minimum, being ignored or isolated by their peers. Sadly, some students can give up by the time they reach middle school.

## Understanding and Accepting Vision and Learning Needs

Students with CVI may experience difficulty when attempting to learn how to master their environment. This is especially the case for those with variable visual functioning who walk, talk, and appear ready for the identical academic experiences as same-age peers. Given the difficulties with building an accurate and reliable concept of the world around them, some students with CVI may have more questions and less understanding of their visual limitations than those with more severe and obvious handicaps (Morse & Whelley, 2007). These students may understand less about what they can and cannot do than students who are totally blind. Much of this lack of understanding is a result of the variability of CVI and coexisting, but not understood, invisible disabilities. As just mentioned, these students are usually unaware that they are unaware (anosognosia), and this compounds the sense of isolation. Furthermore, some students may not know that what they see and hear and how they react is atypical. Sometimes, these students find that it is easier to "cover up"—to themselves and to others—their true need for adapted methods and materials as they attempt to comply with requests and assignments and simultaneously "fit in" with their peers (Morse, 1983).

While some students with CVI may appear to the general public to be totally blind, in the authors' experience, a large proportion of students with CVI give the appearance of being sighted. The attitudes and demands made by people around them often make it difficult for this latter group of students with CVI to perceive themselves as either "sighted" or "blind." These conflicting attitudes about visual capabilities and supportive needs may have a great impact on the struggle for independence versus dependence—a process that is normal during the teenage years but one that can be exacerbated for students who have disabilities. As a result, many students with CVI may experience tension and frustration as they struggle to understand their condition and when and how to adapt to it (Hatlen, 2004).

Behaviorally, adjustment issues can manifest in different ways. For example, when asked to do a difficult task, and expecting to fail, some of these students may make only a half-hearted attempt. Others may make no attempt to comply, or try to convince themselves it is not worth the effort. These ignored or half-hearted attempts to comply may further increase already present feelings of tension and frustration. This further impacts the internal struggle for independence versus the need for dependency. Students with CVI may respond to verbal reactions, gestures, and remarks made to them in typical interactions by either avoiding certain situations or by blocking out or not attending to the negative feedback heard from other students and adults. This process may be reinforced by overprotective behaviors offered by meaningful others who have full sight (Griffin-Shirley & Nes, 2005). Avoiding tasks or situations may be helpful in some instances, but it limits opportunities that might provide students with reassurances that when they tried something, their attempt worked, and positive feelings about themselves were generated (Sacks, Kekelis, & Gaylord-Ross, 1992).

Creating a strong informational base and support network for the child and the family early on in the child's life may help to ease any potential adjustment issues, as well as aid with the transition from early intervention services to school and eventually to adult life. Some possible solutions that address the invisible challenges faced by students with CVI, their families, and school staff may include the following:

- *Support from providers of early intervention services.* These professionals can work closely with families who have received an early diagnosis of CVI to promote their understanding of their children with CVI from diagnosis to intervention needs. They also may provide an overview of the supports that will be available over the years. Although this information may be overwhelming for families, it also may provide a source of comfort to know that services will be available to their child and to them for many years to come. Although such support is highly dependent on the country or regions of a country, a knowledgeable and supportive family is crucial to the optimal growth and development of children who have CVI, no matter where the family lives.
- *Support groups for caregivers.* Caregivers can provide support to one another to promote communication and learning among families.
- *In-service training for school personnel by a vision specialist trained and experienced with CVI.* Follow-up services to this training are recommended especially when there is a change to a new school or there is staff turnover.
- *Educational resources.* Webinars, conferences, and online courses on CVI for parents and school personnel may also be very helpful.
- *Support from parent-school partnerships.* Over the years and in partnership with school staff, parents can teach their child techniques for self-advocacy.

Sidebar 23.3 presents some methods to support families through parent-school partnerships.

## Vocal Communication and Body Language

It is important to remember that we send and receive messages not only from *what* we say but *how* we say it. The subtleties and nuances of facial expressions, postures, and gestures are important and serve as clarifiers and interpreters as we listen to what others say to us. As difficult as it can be to interpret these expressions accurately for those with full sight and hearing, it is even more difficult for individuals with CVI who have compromised visual systems combined with possible auditory processing difficulties. Vi-

SIDEBAR 23.3

## Promoting Parent-School Partnerships

### The Challenge

Partnerships between parents and school need to be promoted as a key method of supporting students and helping them adjust to their life with CVI.

### Some Solutions

Teachers of students with visual impairments, special education teachers, psychologists, guidance counselors, and therapists may find these suggestions helpful in promoting partnerships between school and parents of children with CVI:

- Meet with parents before the beginning of the school year or as soon after as possible to ask them about their perceptions of their child: areas of strength, areas of concern, interests, and health. Also ask them about any disability-related questions and sources of information and accommodations they make at home for their child that may be helpful at school.
- Encourage parents to ask questions about you, your qualifications, and how you teach. Give families a schedule that indicates when you are available for phone conferences or emails. Ask parents if they would like to set up a communication schedule.
- Use home-school communication notebooks to share information and ideas between families and school staff. Discuss with parents the format they would find most helpful.
- Respect the family's roles, cultural background, and knowledge of their child.
- Listen to the family's concerns and keep them informed with regard to their child's performance in school. Do not make assumptions about what a family needs.
- Contact parents as concerns arise in school and encourage parents to contact you concerning events at home that may impact the student's functioning in school.
- As appropriate, ask parents if they need support at home. Become knowledgeable in non-school community resources that may support parents such as respite services, funding sources, and others. Many disability agencies have compiled information you can obtain ahead of time and keep on hand so that it is available when needed. Many university training programs for teachers and social workers are willing to make this an assignment in undergraduate and graduate classes.
- Do not compare the student with CVI to other students or to your own children.
- Encourage the guidance counselor, school psychologist, or school social worker to offer "parent trainings and education nights to address specific concerns shared by many families as, for example, managing behavior at home, providing summer activities, working on academics over breaks" (Edwards & Da Fonte, 2012, p. 12).

*Source:* Adapted in part from Edwards, C., & Da Fonte, A. (2012). The 5-point plan: Fostering successful partnerships with families of students with disabilities. *TEACHING Exceptional Children*, *44*(3), 6–13.

sual information may be perceived differently or in a distorted fashion and, when combined with frequent unreliable auditory information, the resulting message may be interpreted by the student with CVI in a very different manner than the way in which it was intended. Thoughts may not be fully expressed, as the speaker may assume that the listener understands or is able to "catch the gist" before it is even fully verbalized (Feldman & Rimé, 1991). Such assumptions cannot be made with students who have CVI.

Given the limited, unreliable, or fluctuating visual messages individuals receive as a result of CVI, it may not be possible for a student to acquire accurate indicators of conversations and catch the nuances of body language. Shrugs, raised eyebrows, looks of puzzlement, and so forth may be missed, particularly if they are brief, considering the insufficient time often available for their detection and recognition. This renders the difficulties intermittent and more difficult to understand. Some students with CVI may not be able to discriminate facial expressions. (Methods to assess the optimal communication distance and the ability to see facial expressions in young children can be found in Chapters 13 and 20.)

Furthermore, students with CVI potentially face another obstacle that might arise if they have associated auditory processing difficulties. Missed vocal cues that can verify, explain, and elaborate on what is being said may affect a student's understanding, social relationships, learning, and behavior. Another person's change in tone of voice, variable pitch, increased pauses, or incomplete utterances may provide important information within conversations but may be missed by the student with auditory processing difficulties. Furthermore, the words spoken in an interaction, which some say impart only a small percentage of a conversation's message, are often the least reliable source for understanding the emotional content of what is being said (Feldman & Rimé, 1991). Words alone may not be sufficient to convey a message accurately, especially when there is a high degree of emotional content present. The derivation of emotional meaning from vocal communication has been found, for example, in typical infants who are able to interpret voice sounds emotionally, before they understand language. In addition, visitors to most foreign countries can sense the emotional state of speakers even though they may not understand the words spoken (Feldman & Rimé, 1991). Students with CVI who cannot discriminate and correlate nuances between words that are said and how the verbal information is expressed through vocalization changes and body language may be at a disadvantage. As a further complication, there may be limited opportunity or encouragement for the student to ask for clarification to clear up what was said and any possible misunderstandings. Some of these issues are seen in the example of Carole:

**Carole tested in the intellectually gifted range** when she was in late preschool. However, many of her behaviors were perplexing to her parents and to school staff. Her visual acuity and fields of vision initially measured in the near-normal range but appeared to be less so when she was tired, in unfamiliar environments, in open space, or when requested to perform visual-motor tasks that required fine and prolonged fixation, tracking, and scanning (for example, reading). In addition, she rarely made eye contact, rarely called people by their names, and demonstrated awkwardness in moving around the classroom, even in planning how to seat herself in her desk chair.

It was not until Carole was assessed by a pediatric ophthalmologist and a teacher of students with visual impairments, both of whom specialized in evaluation of children with CVI, that it was discovered that she had numerous challenges associated with CVI. She read beautifully but could only sustain the effort for about 5 minutes without a break, unless she was seated on a couch and surrounded by pillows to stabilize her position. Despite her near-normal visual acuity, she could not identify familiar relatives and close friends without the benefit of voice, but she could see a small bug on her mother's blouse. She tried to compensate by identifying people by their shoes (an unreliable source of information); she had great difficulty with pragmatics (social nuances of language), but tried hard to make friends. She identified students in her class by their proper names by associating which car they got out of upon arrival at school.

Once contact was made with a peer, Carole had great difficulty in maintaining a conversation. She was considered very clumsy and disorganized. There were numerous times when Carole would walk into peers, never noticing they were in her path. True friends were hard for Carole to maintain. She became even more disorganized in crowded environments, talked in a louder voice, and required the use of a cane to safely navigate store aisles.

Unfortunately, in spite of her parents' outstanding efforts on her behalf, Carole suffered from extreme anxiety that had an impact on her behavior, health, and emotional state. She appeared fully sighted to others, but her variable vision and the associated invisible disabilities were not identified and took their toll. In Carole's situation, the least inclusive option of home schooling became necessary because of her stress with so many people in one building, teachers not being able to understand the subtleties of her disability, and a school environment and routine that were overly arousing and distressing for her. Such an extreme outcome could perhaps have been avoided if Carole's CVI and associated hidden disabilities had been better understood and managed.

## Social Participation

Students with CVI may want to participate fully in social environments and have friends, but they may not know how to accomplish this feat. Families and professionals need to recognize these desires and teach students specific ways to accomplish these social goals. A summary of possible social issues for students with CVI can be found in Sidebar 23.4.

SIDEBAR 23.4

### Possible Social Issues for Students with CVI

- Misinterpreting verbal messages. Verbal messages may be interpreted by the student with CVI in a very different manner than intended as a result of the inability to see or interpret gestures or body language, or the inability to access information due to associated auditory processing difficulties.
- Difficulty or inability to discriminate one face from another and associate it with that person's name. This difficulty can result from an ocular problem (such as reduced visual acuity or contrast sensitivity) or from the brain's inability to make such interpretations (prosopagnosia).
- Difficulty or inability to interpret facial expressions and body language.
- Difficulty or inability to follow group conversations. For children who have auditory issues, this may result from too many people talking at one time, not understanding the subtle nature of what is being discussed, or the discrepancies between the tone of voice and the actual words spoken.
- Difficulty or inability to negotiate in crowded areas perhaps as a result of difficulties with spatial orientation or not being able to visually perceive individual people or objects crowded together.
- Difficulty or inability to locate items or people in a group. It can be quite scary for individuals with CVI if they cannot find their best friend or parent in a group, and it may have a strong impact on social interaction.
- Lack of awareness that their reactions in social situations are atypical.

*(continued on next page)*

SIDEBAR 23.4 *(continued from previous page)*

- Lack of awareness of the reactions of others to what they say or do.
- Lack of awareness of how others perceive them.
- Lack of awareness that they may perceive the world differently from others.
- Difficulties in understanding the meaning behind words and phrases (pragmatics).
- Giving the appearance of indifference and lack of interest.
- Engaging in unconstructive behaviors when faced with difficult situations.
- Possible overreliance on others for support and direction.
- Difficulty with trust.
- Bullying. Bullying has become an issue of great concern for many students, including those with or without obvious disabilities. In the United States, many states have adopted anti-bullying regulations. Bullying students with disabilities occurs more often than bullying students without disabilities (Elias, 2012). Among other factors, teachers should understand that students with disabilities often have different appearances and behaviors. Many students with CVI have problems with visual search and recognition, which makes social engagement difficult. Thus, they may become socially isolated or lack relationships that help protect them from bullying. They may also be less likely or able to defend themselves.

Suggestions to address these issues can be found in Sidebar 23.5 and are made with the hope that parents and teachers will call on a range of professionals from other disciplines (such as speech-language pathologists, counselors, psychologists, occupational therapists, physical therapists, and physical education teachers) who may be able to work with a particular child to help implement the suggestions. The acquisition of competent social skills is an ongoing process. These skills are not easily learned and must be continuously fine-tuned throughout a child's life. Teachers can be most helpful by offering encouragement and indicating their availability to assist the child. The teacher and the student may "talk through" the pros, cons, and alternatives before the student makes a decision. Teachers may be supported in these efforts by parents, school psychologists, and other allied service providers.

Some students with CVI, at different times in their lives, may need to be referred for counseling services. Once appropriate supports are put into place, children, families, and staff will come to understand the nature of behavioral expressions of CVI and the best ways to support the well-being of students with this condition. Unfortunately, it is understood that the availability of counseling services will vary depending on the country, geographic region, and adequacy of funds. In many countries there is a shortage of school psychologists, guidance counselors, and social workers experienced in working with students who have visual impairments in general, and even fewer experienced in working with students who have CVI (Morse & Whelley, 2007).

## Personal Safety Issues

### Safe Mobility

In the authors' experience, it has been noted that some students do not seem aware of

SIDEBAR 23.5

## Possible Solutions to Social Issues for Students with CVI

Many of the following suggested solutions are adapted from those developed for students who have nonverbal learning disorders (Thompson, 1997).

- Collaborate throughout the school so that all staff are aware of students with CVI and their needs. This includes classroom staff, school counselors, guidance counselors, psychologists, secretaries, maintenance workers, bus drivers, etc.
- Implement home-school collaboration so that the school and family work in ways that are consistent to address the social and learning needs of students who have CVI.
- Have the school psychologist, guidance counselor, or social worker develop school counseling programs that meet the needs of students with CVI.
- Form clubs where special education personnel, students without disabilities, and special needs students work together on projects of community importance. Many communities have been able to raise and use funds, including federal stimulus money, to support such programs. In some communities where such collaboration has occurred, there has "been a culture shift at the school . . . as teenagers who otherwise might be tempted to poke fun at students with disabilities instead enjoy spending time with them" (Philips, 2012).
- Some students with CVI will need specific strategies for social skill acquisition, opportunities for experiential learning, and assurances that learned social skills will be retained through practice and reverification.
- Many students with CVI need models on how to act and respond in various social situations (such as not shouting out statements in public places, caution in regard to talking to strangers, and types of topics to avoid discussing in public). Teach the student with CVI how to request verbal feedback from their peers and from adults when they are unsure of what is happening around them.
- Ask the school psychologist to begin a social skills club where a small group of students with varying social difficulties can learn to interact in a socially acceptable manner. In such a group, the students will be able to observe and practice acceptable behavior. Moreover, these exchanges, offered within a safe and supportive environment, will allow the students to think about potential courses of action and try them out in a safe environment before using them in a more general setting.
- In many situations, the student with CVI will require instruction for behaviors normally dependent on vision (such as waiting in line versus cutting in line or appropriate behaviors in the restroom).
- Provide practice sessions before taking a field trip. Discuss where the trip will be, the most likely social interactions that may occur on the trip, and varying responses the student might consider. At times, it may be helpful for adults to "put into words" what they think the child with CVI may be feeling. This is especially important for young children.
- Teach the student to review what they plan to do or what they have already done. Simultaneously, provide realistic and truthful reinforcement. This will serve as a reminder that it is permissible for the student to ask questions when he or she is unsure of what has been heard and that adults care and are available for assistance.
- Consider "reverse role-playing," in which a student and an adult assume the role of the other to increase awareness of how others may feel.

*(continued on next page)*

**SIDEBAR 23.5** *(continued from previous page)*

- Encourage students with CVI to document their strengths, areas of concern, and possible courses of action. Their thoughts may be contained in a journal or notebook for them to routinely peruse and share with an adult. Strengths and successes should be reviewed as well as planned courses of action.
- It may be beneficial for the student with CVI to have either a "big brother" or "big sister" or to be a "big brother" or "big sister" to a younger child (under adult supervision). This type of opportunity would do much to increase a student's feeling of self-confidence and level of accomplishment.

moving objects, while other students become aware of objects more when either they or the object are moving (see Chapter 3). Both situations have an impact on safe mobility, be it in school hallways or in the community. These students may bump into furniture and people. They may not notice stationary automobiles. However, when a car or bicycle is moving toward them, these students must be able to judge the distance and speed in order to be safe. The services of an O&M specialist are of great importance for these students.

For those students who do not see moving objects, the situation is even more serious. These students also benefit from the services of an O&M specialist to help them use their other senses. Without such services, the students are at high risk for serious injury. It is suggested that students with CVI who are independent travelers receive an evaluation of motion perception by both a trained teacher of students with visual impairments and an O&M specialist (Hyvärinen & Jacob, 2011). (See Chapter 17 for additional information about O&M and CVI.)

## Discriminating Familiar and Unfamiliar People

There are individuals who are unable to discriminate one person from another based solely on vision (prosopagnosia) (see Chapter 3). In most situations, these individuals are not identified as having prosopagnosia, even by their families. Many times, these individuals, whether children or adults, are thought to have some other problem. They themselves know no other life and, once again, are unaware of what they are unaware of (G. N. Dutton, personal communication, February 19, 2012).

Although this condition may sound rare, it is thought to be relatively common in the general public (1 in 50 people), as discussed during a television interview by the neurologist and writer Oliver Sacks, who himself has prosopagnosia (Finkelstein, 2012). The students with CVI who have this condition and are known to the authors seem to live a stressful life, trying to rely on the association of the memory of voices and specific visual characteristics of different people. Such characteristics might be hair color and style, body shape, unique manner of walking, specific items that some people wear (such as jewelry or eyeglasses)—all characteristics that may vary and appear different depending on lighting, contrast, and the person's position such as frontal view versus partial profile versus full profile (Hyvärinen & Jacob, 2011). Children who have prosopagnosia may show no fear of strangers. Thus, they require an assessment of the extent of their facial recognition problem, strategies to help them identify people, and instruction regarding personal safety when unaccompanied by a familiar person.

## Teachers Supporting Teachers through Communities of Practice

Very few general education teachers in today's schools have had training to teach students with special needs, let alone in teaching students with CVI, although this is changing. Teachers who have students with CVI in their classrooms might find it helpful to read the many articles found on the Internet, attend workshops and conferences, and join appropriate e-mail lists, where they can connect with other teachers who are working with this population. Teachers might also find it helpful to contact national and regional agencies for the blind as well as universities to identify resources, courses, workshops, and conferences that may enhance understanding of this very complex visual condition.

## Conclusion

Children with CVI, along with their parents, other caregivers, and service providers, face numerous challenges during the journey from infancy through the school years. Each phase of this journey has its unique hurdles and challenges, which the approaches and solutions outlined in this chapter have attempted to address. The examples provided present some real situations that others have encountered. Each reader of this chapter will have unique challenges of their own with this difficult-to-understand, brain-based visual condition. Hopefully, this chapter provides a starting point for thinking about ways to provide a range of supports on behalf of children and students diagnosed with CVI and those who travel the path with them.

## References

Aitken, S. (2010). Strategies to help children who have both visual and hearing impairments. In G. N. Dutton & M. Bax (Eds.), *Visual impairment in children due to damage to the brain* (pp. 245–256). London: Mac Keith Press.

Dutton, G. N. (2003). Cognitive vision, its disorders and differential diagnosis in adults and children: Knowing where and what things are. *Eye, 17,* 289–304.

Dutton, G. N., & Bax, M. (Eds.). (2010). *Visual impairment in children due to damage to the brain.* London: Mac Keith Press.

Edwards, C., & Da Fonte, A. (2012). The 5-point plan: Fostering successful partnerships with families of students with disabilities. *TEACHING Exceptional Children, 44*(3), 6–13.

Elias, M. (2012, January 12). Addressing bullying of students with disabilities. *Edutopia.* Retrieved December 22, 2014, from http://www.edutopia.org/blog/anti-bullying-students-disabilities-maurice-elias

Feldman, R. S., & Rimé, B. (Eds.). (1991). *Fundamentals of nonverbal behavior: Studies in emotion & social interaction.* New York: Cambridge University Press.

Finkelstein, S. (Producer). (2012, March 18). *60 Minutes: Face blindness, part 1* [Television broadcast]. New York: CBS News. Retrieved from http://www.cbsnews.com/videos/face-blindness-part-1/

Griffin-Shirley, N., & Nes, S. (2005). Self-esteem and empathy in sighted and visually impaired preadolescents. *Journal of Visual Impairment & Blindness, 99*(5), 276–285.

Guzzetta, F., Conti, G., & Mercuri, E. (2011). Auditory processing in infancy: Do early abnormalities predict disorders of language and cognitive development? *Developmental Medicine & Child Neurology, 53*(12), 1085–1090.

Hatlen, P. (2004). Is social isolation a predictable outcome of inclusive education? [Speaker's Corner]. *Journal of Visual Impairment & Blindness, 98*(11), 676–678.

HMS School. (n.d.). Transition planning/futures planning. Retrieved from http://hmsschool.com/resources/transition-planningfutures-planning/

Hyvärinen, L. (1992, July/August). *How to classify paediatric low vision*? Presentation at the International Council for Education of the Visually Handicapped Conference, Bangkok, Thailand.

Hyvärinen, L. (2004). Cerebral visual impairment lecture series [CD-ROM]. Logan, UT: Utah State University, SKI-HI Institute.

Hyvärinen, L., & Jacob, N. (2011). *WHAT and HOW does this child see?* Helsinki, Finland: VISTEST Ltd.

Kef, S. (2002). Psychosocial adjustment and the meaning of social support for visually impaired adolescents. *Journal of Visual Impairment & Blindness, 96*(1), 22–37.

Morse, J. L. (1983). Psychosocial aspects of low vision. In R. T. Jose (Ed.), *Understanding low vision* (pp. 43–54). New York: American Foundation for the Blind.

Morse, J. L., & Whelley, P. (2007, July). *Adjustment issues facing children with a visual impairment, their parents, and involved service providers.* Presentation at the 29th International School Psychology Association Colloquium, Tampere, Finland.

Morse, M. T. (1990). *A qualitative study of the use of health and medical information in planning and providing educational services to young children with disabilities.* (Doctoral dissertation, Florida State University.) Retrieved from Dissertations and Theses database (UMI No. 9112108).

Moss, K., & Wiley, D. (2003). *A brief guide to personal futures planning: Organizing your community to envision and build a desirable future with you.* Austin: Texas School for the Blind and Visually Impaired, Texas Deafblind Outreach.

Philips, R. H. (2012, January 15). Autistic students excelling at Spanish Fort High [Blog]. Retrieved December 22, 2015, from http://blog.al.com/live/2012/01/autistic_students_excelling_at.html

Sacks, S. Z., Kekelis, L. S., & Gaylord-Ross, R. J. (Eds.). (1992). *The development of social skills by blind and visually impaired students.* New York: AFB Press.

*Student v. Fairfield Board of Education.* (2007). Retrieved from www.sde.ct.gov/sde/lib/sde/PDF/DEPS/Special/Hearing_Decisions/06_134.pdf

Thompson, S. (1997). *The source for nonverbal learning disorders.* East Moline, IL: LinguiSystems.

Tinzmann, M. B., Jones, B. F., Fennimore, T. F., Bakker, J., Fine, C., & Pierce, J. (1990). *What is the collaborative classroom?* Oak Brook, IL: North Central Region Educational Laboratory. Retrieved December 24, 2014, from http://methodenpool.uni-koeln.de/koopunterricht/The%20Collaborative%20Classroom.htm

Tuttle, D. W., & Tuttle, N. R. (2004). *Self-esteem and adjusting with blindness: The process of responding to life's demands* (3rd ed.). Springfield, IL: Charles C. Thomas.

# APPENDIX 23A
# In Their Own Words: Personal Stories of Children with CVI

*Frances Dibble, Bernadette Jackel, and Fiona Lovett*

Each child with CVI is different. Three of their stories are presented here. Each child and family has faced different challenges in order to obtain appropriate services and address issues related to their multiple medical and physical conditions. Harrison's story focuses on his early years, Michael's on his transition to young adulthood, and Jacob tells about his experiences and insights as an adult.

## Harrison

### *Fiona Lovett*

Harrison was born on October 20, 1998, after a textbook pregnancy and delivery. Yet, as ideal as the pregnancy was, there was something different about Harrison from the start. I began to record concerns about his development and visual behavior when I noticed that he did not make eye contact while feeding. I could not ignore the voice inside me telling me that something was not quite right.

Follow-up home health professionals and doctors agreed that something was amiss when, at the eight-month medical check-up, he had not achieved several developmental milestones. Thus began our family's long journey with therapists and many health professionals to address Harrison's diagnosis of global developmental delay.

Visually, Harrison did not make eye contact, nor did he get excited when family members walked into a room. Therapists and doctors assessed him and made recommendations, but none could give a complete diagnosis or root cause for his condition until we were referred to a pediatric ophthalmologist knowledgeable about the symptoms Harrison exhibited.

Our notes and observations helped the ophthalmologist make the diagnosis of cerebral visual impairment (CVI). We could explain how we gained Harrison's attention by touching him and saying his name, that he favored slow-moving, well-articulated cartoons on television, that he disliked busy places, and fast movements did not capture his attention. Results of an MRI corroborated the diagnosis of CVI and revealed that Harrison had suffered a stroke-like injury to his brain about 24 weeks into the pregnancy. Though this news was not what any parent wants to hear, we felt relief with a definitive diagnosis and validated that our observations were real.

The medical file we keep on Harrison has thickened. Diagnoses include *periventricular leukomalacia, cerebral palsy, osteochondritis dissecans,* and *joint hyper-mobility of the hands.* Harrison walks with an awkward gait. Tight leg muscles and inflamed cartilage in his knees cause pain and reduced mobility. He has difficulty with his handgrip and fine motor function, making it extremely tedious to handwrite; we expect that he will learn to use the keyboard as his best form of writing. Multiple conditions associated with Harrison's profound CVI include *lower visual field impairment, simultanagnosia, impaired visual guidance of movement (optic ataxia), prosopagnosia (or face blindness), dyskinetopsia, lack of stereopsis,* and *visual fatigue.* (Definitions of these terms can be found in Chapter 3.)

Objects such as curbs, stairs, walkways, uneven surfaces, food on a plate, pencils on a table, fasteners on clothes, and print at the bottom of a page can be out of Harrison's view due to a lower field vision loss. He cannot view a lot of visual information at one time, and it is nearly impossible for him to visually identify a friend or family member in a group setting. Harrison always needed a bold callout and arm wave in order to locate me waiting outside the primary school yard at the end of the school day.

Harrison's inability to recognize faces and facial expressions often causes misinterpretation of the emotions that smiles, frowns, angry, or sad looks are intended to convey. A person's clothing style, hairstyle, and voice quality give him more information in identifying a friend than the typical quick glance. He cannot see fast-moving objects such as balls flying through the air, traffic, or recognize classmates running on the playground. We have found it helpful for him to focus on a toy or some other closely viewed object while riding in a vehicle.

Harrison attended a mainstream nursery school and was supported by specialists working with him in the classroom, including the support of a teacher of students with visual impairments. When it was time to transition to primary school, a full team consisting of an educational psychologist, learning support coordinator, physical therapist, occupational therapist, teacher of students with visual impairments, speech teacher, along with specialized equipment, including an FM system, video magnifier, sloping desk chair, and a computer with a screen reader and software, supported Harrison in the mainstream setting. But it was not easy for him there.

Despite introductory meetings with Harrison's specialists and a warm reception by the school's principal, the classroom teacher gave us daily reports of his lack of concentration and told us that he was unteachable. The assistant hired to support him was redirected to help with general duties in the classroom, leaving Harrison on his own and by himself. Fortunately, we had built a supportive medical and educational team prior to his start in primary school and were able to gather the team together to problem solve and correct this situation.

Though Harrison experienced many challenges, he remained a fun-loving and well-liked classmate. He received an award for his determination and good character and became a class officer during his last year in primary school. Classmates accepted him and learned how to speak and listen to him, but he did not have friends.

In living with Harrison, we have learned to prepare, prepare, and prepare when planning family outings. We learned to shop during quiet times, and to locate in advance, toilets, calm areas, and escape routes, and to arrive early before the crowds. We learned to sit at eye level rather than higher in the bleachers when going to ball games so that Harrison's lack of lower visual field would not interfere with his seeing the players. We learned how to organize his bedroom and play area to maximize his ability to find his belongings and to dress himself as independently as possible. Clothes laid out on the floor each night with labels facing down still make a big difference in how independently he can dress himself in the morning when everyone in the family is busy preparing to go out the door. While we learned to adapt to Harrison's needs at home, the thought of the challenges facing him at a large public high school became daunting.

For this transition, the educational team, which now included a family advocate, met before Harrison matriculated from the upper primary level in order to map out the next educational plan in preparation for his high school years. Considerations included Harrison's need for a small class size in a calm and quiet environment. He needed specialists who could handle his increasing technology needs and staff who could understand the nuances of a cerebral visual impairment. He needed to be pushed to his potential with a sensitive staff that could accommodate and adapt the curriculum and aspects of the environment to his learning needs.

After much negotiation, we all agreed that Harrison might benefit most from attending a specialized school for students with visual impairments. While his start at the school was not all clear sailing, his teachers understood his needs, he was learning every day, and, most joyously, he made true friends.

Our hope is that Harrison's story will help parents and professionals alike to listen, observe, and learn, and if something seems amiss, trust that instinct to find the source of the question. Finally, students benefit when parents, teachers, and specialists work and plan together to solve problems that arise due to a visual brain difference. If I could go back and give myself one piece of advice it would be to believe in myself and trust my instincts more deeply.

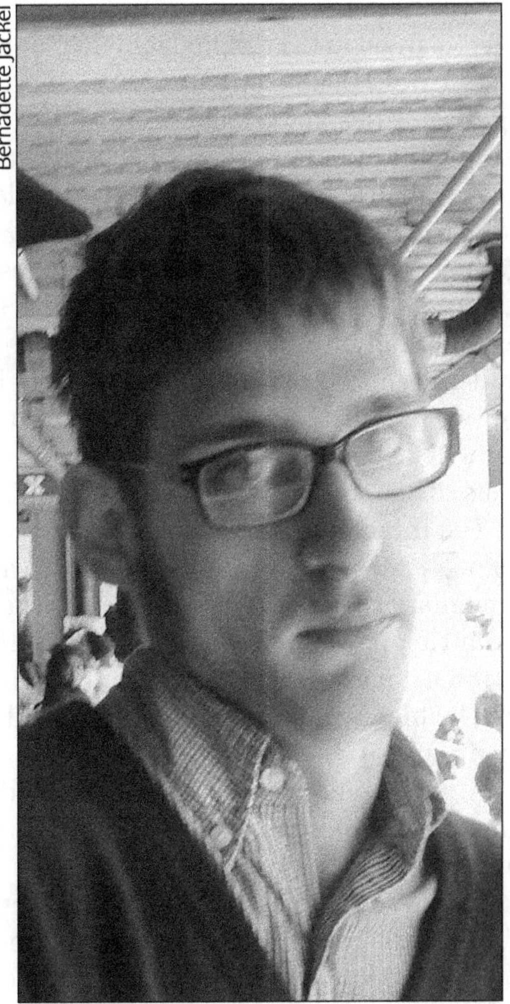
Bernadette Jackel

Michael

## Michael

### *Bernadette Jackel*

Michael, now 23 years old, lives in a semi-independent living setting. The path to this achievement was not without its challenges. After two decades of parenting, we realize issues of one kind or another will continue to come up for Mike.

From the start, from Mike's earliest years, we learned that when school teams understood his needs as a student with a cerebral visual impairment (CVI), he made gains and learned, but when they did not, he was more isolated than included and could not achieve his potential.

Mike was born three months premature and remained in the hospital for two months. We were told that he might have some learning disabilities but all else seemed fine, including his eyes. But when he was admitted to the pediatric intensive care unit a few days after discharge with an apnea attack, and again six months later following episodes of infantile spasms, we learned then that the early prediction of mild learning problems suddenly shifted to the likelihood of his being severely disabled with a chance that he might not walk. This was a life-changing day for us.

The infantile spasms and the damage to the occipital lobe were due to hypoxia and ischemia, or lack of oxygen to the brain. A pediatric ophthalmologist diagnosed Mike with what was described as "cortical blindness," which was supported by an MRI during his stay in the hospital.

A developmental evaluation concluded that, except for communication, Mike was showing delays in all areas and that he would respond best to auditory and tactile stimulations because his visual impairment had an impact on his overall development. A few years later the same psychologist evaluated him again. One recommendation stood out for us, and while the need is not quite as rigorous today as it was then, this recommendation continues to be a major consideration in the way Mike learns new skills:

> With regard to Michael's learning style, it is suggested that he best understands what is required when a uni-sensory channel is provided. In other words, it is important that the learning operations of alerting, looking, listening, and doing function as separate entities and not simultaneously. Once Michael is ready to perform, it is most appropriate to encourage a multisensory channel approach to learning. He needs to view what he is doing, talk about his work, and explore with his hands. Michael frequently appears confused when given directions to motor activities. Comprehension is ensured provided demonstrations are offered with no simultaneously offered verbal directions. He will best understand verbal directions provided he is not trying to perform a visual-motor activity simultaneously. He needs to ensure his availability for instruction by eye gazing at the adult.

Mike's visual difficulties were not well understood in the elementary-school years. Specialists reported that ". . . he doesn't have a true visual impairment because there is nothing wrong with his eyes; his learning difficulties are due to brain damage, not a visual impairment." Some considered Mike's problems to be volitional.

Mike made educational gains, but there were many contentious team meetings during these years. Our district agreed to a trial year at a residential school for visually impaired and blind students, a change that benefitted Mike academically, socially, and emotionally. After much negotiation and attempts to come to agreement, a due process hearing officer ruled in Mike's favor for his return to this school. (See *Student v. Fairfield Board of Education,* 2007 for this decision.)

Mike graduated with a high school diploma as a functional reader. He keeps up with the world by watching television, listening to the radio, and utilizing the computer. We think that he is most likely capable of holding a job that will give him the opportunity to be a contributing member of society, but not one that will afford him a living.

Mike has since transitioned into a semi-independent living situation that will afford him happiness, self-worth, and as much independence as his disability will allow. He will need supports throughout his life but far fewer than he would have needed had he not received some good early childhood interventions.

Unfortunately, the lack of understanding about CVI has most recently surfaced again when we learned that his visual acuity and visual field impairment do not meet the federal definition of blindness, resulting in his discharge from our state vision services at the age of 21. He is eligible for general adult services, but staff members from these agencies do not have experience with clients with visual impairments, especially not with cerebral visual impairment.

For example, an agency representative conducted a job assessment that required Mike to stock shelves, scan items, place labels on shelves, and remove expired items from shelves. The agency's job coach concluded that Mike would never be competitively employable and wrote, "Michael would not look at the shelf before placing an item on it . . . Michael had a difficult time reading the expiration dates even with his handheld reader." Reports about his visual functioning were available before the assessment, but they had not been read. Sadly, Mike's visual impairment was disregarded, again.

Two years have passed since Mike transitioned to his new home. In that time, there has been turnover among residents and staff that required ongoing teaching, and raised the question of the most appropriate and compatible roommate for him. Staff show their appreciation for the presentations that I give to them about CVI, telling me that their questions about Mike's capabilities get cleared up and that they can support his independence more appropriately.

Mike is very happy in his living situation. He met a girl through his association with the adult agency and wants to ask her to marry him. This new development is a fabulous one for Mike; admittedly we dared not think about it too much when he was young. Mike would like to have children, but we feel that neither of them could rear a child on their own. As his legal guardian, this raises issues concerning his self-autonomy and self-determination. We've had several serious conversations with him about marriage and parenthood. Presently Mike volunteers for a variety of nonprofit organizations including a police and fire department, a food/clothing bank, and by grocery shopping for four homebound senior citizens. He has a paid position at a McDonald's franchise near his home and travels independently to and from work.

Mike also has a full social life nights and weekends, with activities including workouts at the gym, happy hour at the local sports bar, visiting his girlfriend, going for dinner and a movie with friends, attending music, theater, and sporting events.

There have been many, many moments in Mike's life when we wondered how we could survive the next medical or educational crisis. The stress of getting a complete medical diagnosis, working with multiple medical and educational professionals, learning about CVI, and attempting to support the school teams in their understanding of it took its toll. At times we felt lost.

Upon reflection, though, Mike has gained an education and we have gained a perspective about life that few ever get. We don't dwell on what might have been and love Mike for who he is. We see him as a young man with a disability, not a disabled young man. He loves sports, music, video games, and anything to do with law enforcement and traveling. We've been fortunate to have a large support system of family and friends, and we've kept our humor. Our hope is that our story, told briefly in these few pages, underscores how difficult it is for a child with CVI to get an appropriate education due to the misunderstanding of this visual impairment. We hope that the next generation of parents, teachers, and health professionals will work together with more information and acceptance of this disorder.

## Interview with Jacob

### *Frances Dibble*

Jacob, now 31 years old, with a master's degree in social work, told me some of his life experiences over lunch one afternoon, experiences of how the ambiguity and the uncertainty of visual fluctuations play havoc in his everyday life. Jacob lived at home with his parents during his years of attending graduate school and later when seeking employment, all the while developing interests in disability advocacy, political systems, radio, dance, and the arts, and setting his goal to live with friends and to build a meaningful career in social work. In 2013, he moved to Santa Barbara, California, to accept a paid position as a community organizer with the Independent Living Resource Center, stating, "I have my dream job and hope to continue advocating for social justice in the world."

Jacob was diagnosed with cerebral palsy at birth, and later with "cortical visual impairment." His speech, gross and fine motor skills, mobility, and visual functioning have been affected. When Jacob was a preschool student, he was often the focus of teacher discussions because of the perplexities of his visual functioning; he could see, but not when we thought he might, nor when we least expected he could. Now Jacob is able to articulate what we had observed then. He hopes to provide some insight for parents with a child diagnosed with CVI, and what it takes for students with CVI to come to school every day ready to learn. He explained, "It can be difficult. My eyesight changes every minute. I can be studying and my eyes get very tired quickly. My eyesight changes all the time, every minute, sometimes making it too difficult to continue using my eyes."

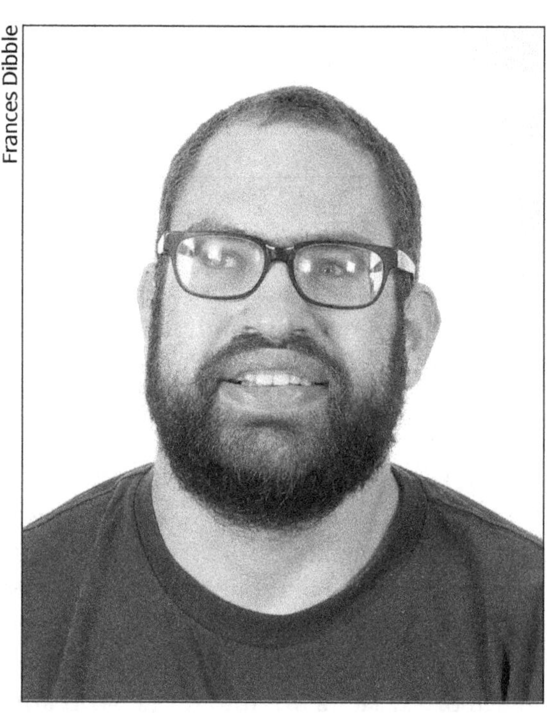
Frances Dibble

Jacob

Jacob told of the time when he did not recognize a friend in a familiar setting where he had anticipated seeing her. He and the friend from a graduate studies class commuted together to their internship program a few mornings a week. One afternoon Jacob expected to meet her in their graduate studies class but didn't see her there, so he sent her a text message to see what had happened. To his surprise, she returned a message telling him she was seated a few chairs away, adding that she wondered why he had not greeted her when he walked by. After class he had a chance to explain that he had not recognized her because this time her hair was loosely styled rather than tied back in her signature ponytail, the way he had learned to easily recognize her. "She had her hair down, and I thought she was a different person. I felt so strange."

Jacob explained that this was far from the first time he missed seeing or mistook someone he knew. He has learned to ask questions that will help him identify people because he cannot recognize them by looking at their faces. He might ask, "Have we been introduced before?" which stimulates conversation and gives him time to place the person in context, and to study style of hair, dress, and mannerisms to ensure that he correctly identifies the speaker.

Jacob hopes that those who read this book gain knowledge and understanding of visual disorders of the brain and of the specific effects this particular impairment has on a person's everyday life. He hopes teachers develop specific and engaging curricula for students with visual brain disorders that would include lessons on how to initiate, maintain, and repair conversations as related to the challenges of living with visual fluctuations. He hopes that those students with additional disabilities, who cannot easily advocate for themselves, will benefit from the new understanding of those who read this book.

Jacob is not alone. Bernadette and Fiona hope that their experiences will lead other parents to trust in themselves, to trust their observations and intuition in pursuing medical and educational assessments when things seem "not quite right," and to partner with school teams to address the challenges that arise.

# 24

# Insights from Adult Neuro-Vision Rehabilitation and Rehabilitative Considerations for Children

*John Kingston*

Each child with cerebral visual impairment (CVI) has a unique set of visual difficulties and behavioral issues, with the greatest variation to be found among those who have lesser degrees of visual dysfunction. This means that it is not possible to create a didactic model of teaching that is suitable for all. Rather, each child requires a unique plan that melds with his or her everyday life. This chapter presents a detailed account of the intervention strategies developed for adults with brain injuries and provides a model of approach that includes many elements potentially transferable to the care of children.

Recent developments in the care of members of the armed forces with visual impairment as a result of brain injury have led to the search for novel strategies to improve skills that can affect overall quality of life. In 2007, the Comprehensive Neurological Vision Rehabilitation (CNVR) program was established within the U.S. Department of Veterans Affairs Palo Alto Health Care System to address the needs of active duty service members returning from Iraq and Afghanistan with brain-based vision loss, such as from blast or traumatic injuries. The inpatient program, based within the Western Blind Rehabilitation Center, also saw a need for services for veterans with vision loss resulting from a variety of other brain injuries such as cerebrovascular accident or stroke. The program has since addressed a wide spectrum of visual impairments resulting from brain injury.

The program uses innovative technology and multisensory training methods to treat the unique and individual needs of the patients. In an effort to suggest the types of approaches for possible future studies with children, this chapter describes insights from experiences of that interdisciplinary team. The rehabilitation of vision in adults is a developing subject, and this chapter outlines some strategies that have been utilized, with a description of their methods, rationale, and outcomes.

While a substantial evidence base for vision training for children with CVI has yet to be developed, the remarkable potential for neuroplasticity in the young (see Chapter 5) means that it is likely that, with carefully designed training approaches matched to the needs of these children, such methods will prove effective in the long term. Zihl and Dutton (2015) suggest a variety of methods that may form the basis for successful interventions based on work with adults and initial work with children.

This chapter presents two case studies within the context of the Comprehensive Neurological Vision Rehabilitation program. One case presents rehabilitation strategies in the event of an open head injury affecting the visual brain, and the other discusses rehabilitation for a brain injury resulting from a cerebrovascular accident.

## History and Treatment

In adults, successful rehabilitative training of eye movements to help compensate for lack of reading skill resulting from visual field loss was first reported in 1917 (Poppelreuter, 1917/1990). It was not until the 1980s that this work was systematically taken forward. Zihl (2011) showed that training of eye movements to search in the area of missing vision to compensate for visual field impairment could prove effective in expanding the area of perception in both those with visual field loss and those with loss of visual attention and visual neglect (see Chapter 3).

Treatment of visual field loss and visual neglect in adults has been categorized into three approaches: restitution, substitution, and compensation.

- ***Restitution*** refers to direct training of basic visual abilities (such as fixation, pursuit, and saccade training), and pharmacological treatment, among others.
- ***Substitution*** pertains to the use of optic or prosthetic devices, such as prisms, adapted lighting, and magnification, or environmental changes.
- ***Compensation*** refers to the training in compensatory skills such as visual search strategies, saccadic training for visual field defects, training eye movements for reading, teaching head movements for field loss, attention training, visual scanning therapy, optokinetic stimulation, training with cueing, and eye patches, among others.

A combination of these approaches is often more practical, such as combining scanning training (compensation) with use of prisms (substitution) (Ting et al., 2011).

## Visual Field Loss and Loss of Visual Attention

Vision is a personal, internal, and subjective experience. It is most effective with intact normal visual acuities, contrast sensitivity, visual fields, and movement perception, as well as with typical visual perceptual and cognitive functioning. Also critical to typical visual functioning are normal eye movement systems that optimally align the eyes, lock them onto the target of interest (fixation), allow the eyes to follow moving targets (pursuit), and help them look elsewhere with fast eye movements (saccades). These eye movement systems contribute to visual abilities such as reading or determining traffic movement and distance when crossing a street. Since vision is processed in multiple areas of the brain, even mild brain damage can lead to a variety of visual deficits and disorders of eye movement that significantly alter the experience of vision.

Homonymous hemianopia affects either the right or left visual field of both eyes and is common with damage to the occipital lobe. While stroke is the leading cause in adults, hemianopia occurs in children with traumatic brain injury, cerebral palsy, cerebral hemorrhage, or those who have tumors affecting the visual pathways in the brain (Donahue & Haun, 2007; Kedar, Zhang, Lynn, Newman, & Biousse, 2006; Mezey et al., 1998; see Chapter 3). The prevalence of hemianopia in children is unknown, as children (like adults) do not tend to complain of a visual field defect.

Adults with hemianopia experience a perceptual loss, and affected individuals are often not aware of the missing visual information. They lack the peripheral field to be alert to stimuli on the side of the hemifield loss as a result of occipital lobe damage. The person experiencing this does not see the missing visual space as being blurred or dark; it simply does not exist within their visual space.

While normal visual acuities may be present in cases of hemianopia, the danger with hemifield loss is that the visual field does not extend across the entire body's space. This can result in collisions with undetectable objects or an inability to notice moving hazards entering a person's body space from the affected side. For someone with left hemianopia, a far gaze to the right would shift the area of blindness across the entire body space, resulting in complete absence of vision directly in front of the body, which is necessary to guide movement and prevent contact with obstacles.

In addition, the ability to decode visual information such as depth perception or orientation cues may be impaired. Functional implications also include difficulties with activities of daily living, such as locating household items or not noticing all the food on a plate. Social interactions may be affected, especially in a group, as an individual with visual neglect will be unaware of those seated on the affected side. A total absence of the left peripheral visual field combined with a fully functioning right peripheral field often results in a heightened alertness to stimuli in the right visual field due to intact right peripheral vision which is alert to movement.

Children with this condition may have never experienced full visual fields and compensate for hemianopia through head and eye movements, combined with the use of blindsight, which may develop to a remarkable degree (see Chapter 2). In children, however, it is commonly visual neglect that is more problematic, with neglect affecting the left field of vision tending to be more evident and severe. Neglect is not automatically compensated for by head and eye movements, but children may adapt by turning the body (see Chapter 3). Lower visual field impairment or neglect can be found in some children, often accompanied by dorsal stream dysfunction (see Chapter 3 for a discussion of lower field impairment and visual neglect in children).

Difficulties with visual attention may exist with or without the presence of visual field loss. Attention plays a necessary role in learning, memory, and reasoning (Bate, Mathias, & Crawford, 2001). Impaired visual attention is common in children with CVI (Smith & Chatterjee, 2008). Difficulties may exist with shifting attention among various stimuli, or children may experience an overload of sensory information and may have difficulty with visual clutter.

In 1990, Posner and Petersen brought forward the concept that the orienting of visual attention occurs in three distinct stages: disengagement, movement, and engagement. The first step is taking attention away, or disengaging, from whatever is currently being visually examined; next is the physical shifting of attention from one spot to another (movement); and this is followed by engaging, or focusing of attention, on the new object or space.

Rehabilitative techniques, such as those to train visual scanning, can incorporate these stages of visual attention by providing visual activities in which the individual must first disengage attention from a visual target, then shift attention to another location in visual space, and finally focus attention onto a new visual target. The shift of attention often encourages head and eye movements. The head and eye movements help to compensate for a reduction in the visual field, but additional body rotation helps compensate for the lack of visual attention on one side.

Table 24.1 presents training procedures used for training in a variety of basic skills, including targets and tools used. Their uses are explored in the case studies below. The techniques represented in the case studies demonstrate instruction in visual attending behaviors (fixating, shifting gaze, scanning, localizing, tracking, tracing), visual examining behaviors (inspecting, identifying, matching), and visually guided motor behaviors (reaching, turning toward/moving toward targets or objects).

It is not known at this point which of these techniques can be applied to children with CVI, but these examples are intended to provide ideas for strategies that may be considered and evaluated for application to a pediatric population. However, it is important to note that some of the tools used (see Table 24.1), such as alphabet pencils and letter charts, have already been used with children.

The following sections present two detailed cases that demonstrate various

TABLE 24.1

## Training Tools, Purpose, and Procedures

| ***Training Tool*** | ***Description*** | ***Purpose*** | ***Procedures*** |
|---|---|---|---|
| Alphabet Pencils<br>**Figure 24.1** | Two pencils with the alphabet printed vertically A-Z on one side and Z-A on the reverse side. Print is small and requires good visual acuity. | 1. To develop smooth and accurate eye movements (saccades). | 1. Hold pencils at a distance and practice looking from the left to the right pencil reading each letter, alternating between the two.<br>2. Distance between pencils can be increased for larger saccades or moved closer for smaller saccades.<br>3. Increase the speed of shifting from letter to letter. Include a metronome and focus on controlling the saccade to the metronome beat.<br>4. Time sessions to monitor progress and outcomes. |

*(continued on next page)*

**TABLE 24.1** *(continued from previous page)*

| *Training Tool* | *Description* | *Purpose* | *Procedures* |
|---|---|---|---|
| Parquetry Blocks 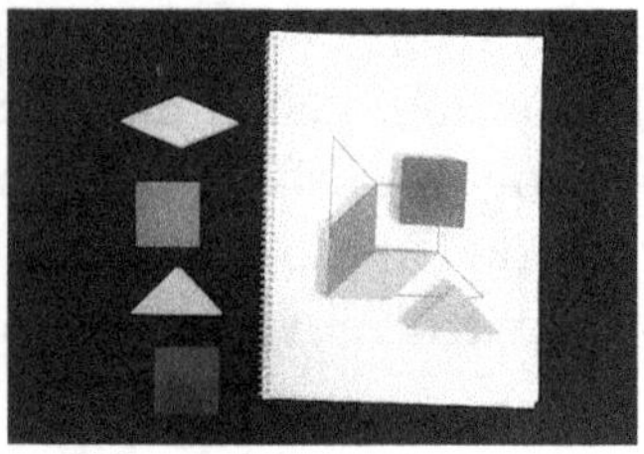<br>**Figure 24.2** | Multicolor wooden blocks in the shapes of a triangle, diamond, and square. | 1. To provide meaningful visual and tactile discrimination and examination opportunities.<br>2. To develop hand-eye coordination, fine motor control, and visualization abilities.<br>3. To explore spatial concepts and practice spatial problem-solving abilities. | 1. Examine and name shapes.<br>2. Combine into puzzles.<br>3. Provide matching and sequencing copy tasks.<br>4. Use workbooks that outline puzzle combinations and have student place the blocks directly onto the workbook (see Figure 24.2) or onto plexiglass. |
| Letter Charts 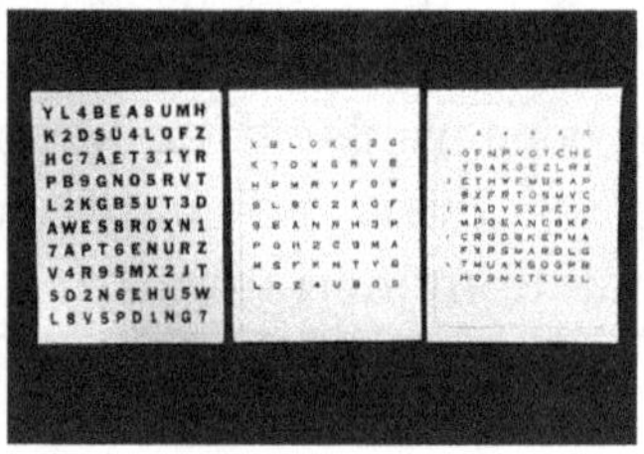<br>**Figure 24.3** | Paper wall charts with letters and numbers, 10 rows of 10 letters and numbers, or more. Charts can be purcased or created. | 1. To develop smooth and accurate eye movements (saccades).<br>2. To develop accommodative convergence. | 1. Read first and last letter for each row.<br>2. Read top and bottom letter of each column.<br>3. Read first and next to last letter for each row.<br>4. Read whole chart left to right and top to bottom.<br>5. Use for near and far.<br>6. Perform sitting, standing, or balancing.<br>7. Read to metronome.<br>8. Combine numbers, symbols, or words.<br>9. A smaller handheld version of the chart can be used for accommodation training—practicing reading while alternating between the near and far charts. |
| Targets 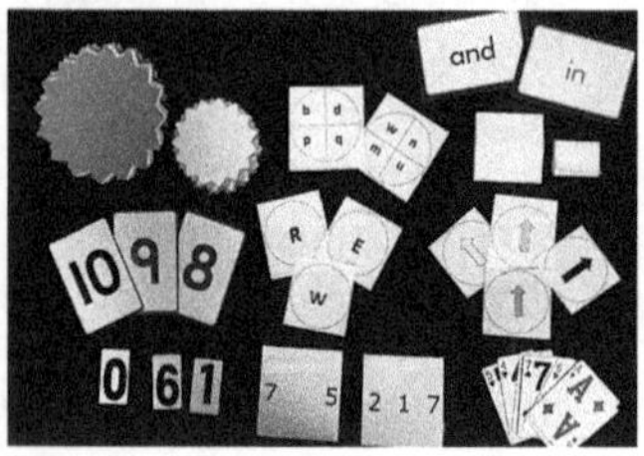<br>**Figure 24.4** | Targets can include single letters, numbers, symbols, or arrows, as well as multiple letters, numbers, or symbols. They can be purchased (e.g., flashcards, sticky notes, playing cards) or made. | 1. To encourage compensatory scanning techniques.<br>2. To provide a target to encourage movement of visual attention and engagement of vision onto the target. | 1. Encourage scanning for field loss by presenting a target (target training) in desired field during dynamic training.<br>2. Develop scanning for doorways, intersecting hallways, and elevation changes. |

*(continued on next page)*

**TABLE 24.1** *(continued from previous page)*

| *Training Tool* | *Description* | *Purpose* | *Procedures* |
|---|---|---|---|
| | | 3. To provide additional processing and perceptual tasks during dynamic training. | 3. Increase complexity of environment as habitual scanning is achieved.<br>4. Develop awareness for orientation signs and landmarks.<br>5. Include spatial concepts with arrows. |
| Tactile Scan Board<br>**Figure 24.5** | A 20″ × 30″ foam core board, easily purchased at craft or office supply stores. Larger sizes are also available. Alternatively, a large piece of wood or tray could also be used. | 1. To develop systematic scanning.<br>2. To provide a tactile anchor for left awareness.<br>3. To enhance contrast for targets. | 1. Numerical sequencing.<br>2. Alphabetical sequencing.<br>3. Card games.<br>4. Matching and problem-solving puzzles.<br>5. Increase size of board. |
| Tracking Worksheets<br>**Figure 24.6**<br>**Figure 24.7** | Paper worksheets contain single letters, symbols, and words in regular and large print. | 1. To develop systematic scanning.<br>2. To develop awareness of need for scanning and systematic approach.<br>3. To develop smooth and accurate eye movements.<br>4. To scan effectively not to miss information.<br>5. To increase ability to attend to information with visual clutter.<br>6. To develop anchoring techniques.<br>7. To practice saccades.<br>8. To develop more efficient use of vision. | 1. Use a pen/marker/highlighter to circle or cross out letters, symbols, or words.<br>2. Increase page size.<br>3. Utilize tactile anchor.<br>4. Encourage systematic scanning into missing visual field.<br>5. Errorless learning, student guided in the activity.<br>6. Progress to more difficult worksheets (e.g., words ending in a similar right sequence of letters—pen, ten, then, hen). |

assessment and intervention methods used successfully with adults in the Comprehensive Neurological Vision Rehabilitation program at the Western Blind Rehabilitation Center, Veterans Administration Hospital, in Palo Alto.

## Denny: Demonstrating Visual Field Loss

Denny, a 28-year-old male, was admitted two months postinjury with a right frontal, parietal, and occipital lobe injury resulting from a motor vehicle accident. He sustained left homonymous hemianopia, double vision, left hemiparesis (weakness on left side of his body), and visual inattention to the left as a result of his significant head injury.

### Assessment

Optometric examination reported jerky saccades and pursuits, with delayed initiation of voluntary saccades. He displayed rapid-onset fatigue with his eye movements, and was unable to completely read more than 10 lines of print. His visual acuities with correction were 20/20 (6/6) right, 20/25 (6/7.5) left. Denny demonstrated a strong and defensive resistance to recognizing his visual field loss, insisting he could see "the same as before the accident."

Also included in the initial set of evaluations were a full battery of neuropsychological testing, as well as assessments and training with physical therapists, occupational therapists, and speech-language therapists.

Denny was admitted from an acute ward within the hospital to the Comprehensive Neurological Vision Rehabilitation program and participated in additional assessments performed by rehabilitation therapists, certified low vision therapists, and orientation and mobility (O&M) specialists, all of whom had extensive training in and experience with brain injury and some with additional training in ocular motor therapy techniques and tools.

An intake with questions and answers was performed in all areas to determine goals and issues. Low vision therapists administered the Rivermead Conventional Subtest's pen and paper scanning sheets (Wilson, Cockburn, & Halligan, 1987). O&M specialists administered the Neuro Vision Technology (NVT) Panel assessment, and the Mobility Assessment Course (MAC) (see Table 24.2). These tests confirmed Denny's poor awareness of his left visual field and confirmed unsystematic scanning patterns, with greater attention to the right. Also, Denny was observed bumping into doorframes and obstacles on his left side when walking in the ward.

In addition to visual field loss and inattention, Denny had difficulty orienting to the world around him, and attending to things in his immediate vicinity; his vision problems were compounded by damage to the frontal lobe so that Denny tended to be very literal and demonstrated extremely concrete thinking.

The Mobility Assessment Course determined how much visual information Denny observed while walking indoors. Denny was asked to walk along a route consisting of four connecting hallways (see Table 24.2 and Figure 24.11) with 4″ × 4″ yellow targets placed on the right and left walls (see Figures 24.9 and 24.10). Four of the targets included orientation signs with arrows and the words "turn right" or "turn left."

The Mobility Assessment Course score included how many targets were visually located on the left and right sides of the hall-

TABLE 24.2

## Assessment Tools, Purpose, and Procedures

| *Assessment Tool* | *Description* | *Purpose* | *Procedures* |
|---|---|---|---|
| Rivermead Behavioral Inattention Test (BIT)—Conventional Subtests<br> 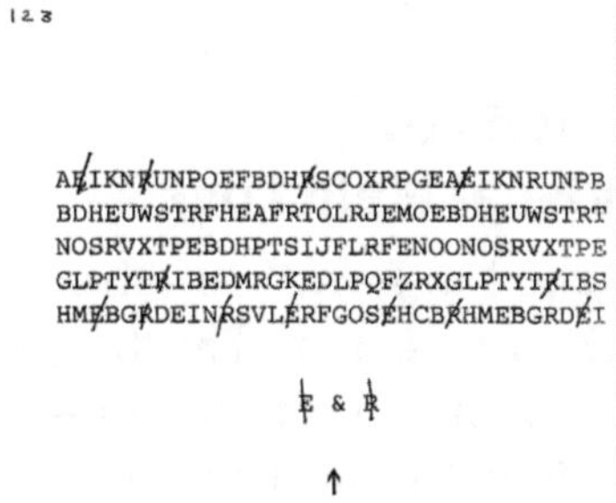<br>**Figure 24.8** | An objective behavioral test of everyday tasks, which can assist in identifying neglect. The BIT contains six conventional subtests and nine behavioral subtests. The conventional subtest with the worksheets for line bisection, line crossing, letter cancellation, star cancellation, figure and shape copying were implemented. Pearson Educational Limited sells copies of this assessment. | 1. To assess for left neglect.<br>2. To evaluate scanning strategy.<br>3. To evaluate saccades and ability to move between letters and lines of text. | 1. Pen-and-paper assessments are presented at midline to evaluate scanning patterns and attention to left and right.<br>2. Worksheets are used with a pen to bisect lines, cancel letters and symbols, and copy shapes. |
| Mobility Assessment Course (MAC) 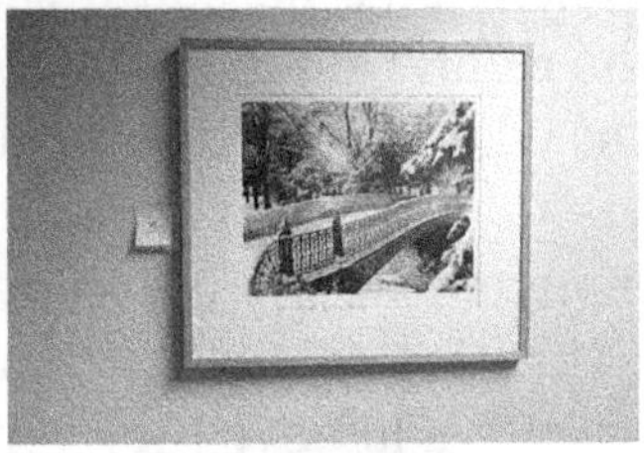<br><br>**Figure 24.9** 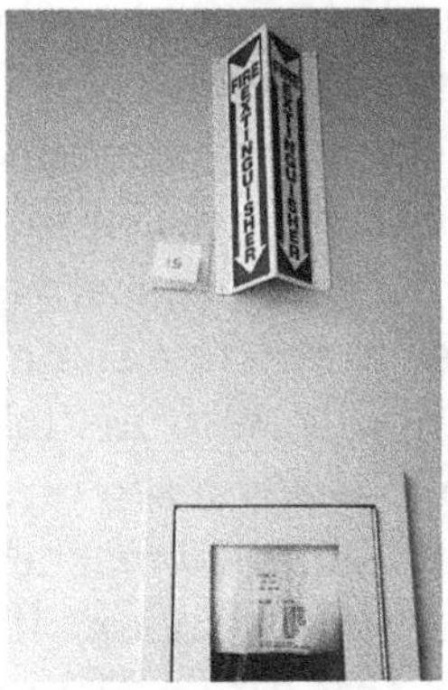<br><br>**Figure 24.10** 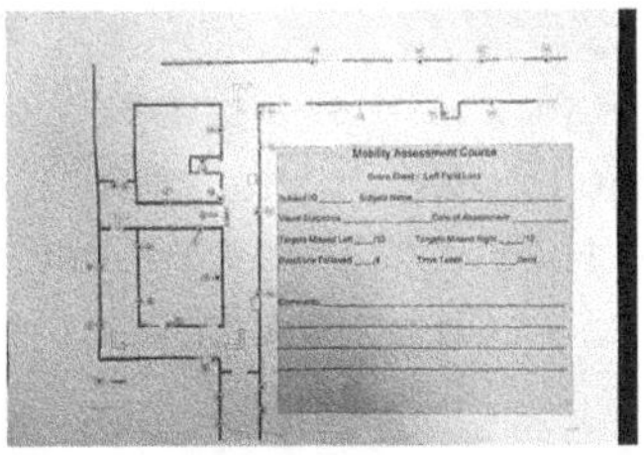<br><br>**Figure 24.11** | A timed, dynamic assessment to measure how many targets and orientation signs a person can locate while walking.<br>Articles regarding the MAC include those by George, Hayes, Chen, and Crotty (2011); Kingston, Katsaros, Vu, and Goodrich (2010); and Verlander et al. (2000) (see References). | 1. To establish a dynamic mobility measure baseline prior to scanning training.<br>2. To establish an outcome measure post O&M training. | 1. Used with patients with field loss to establish a baseline pretraining and to provide a posttraining measure.<br>2. Targets are placed out of normal view and require scanning with head movements to locate information.<br>3. Results are recorded for target location, time to complete, and number of orientation signs located and followed.<br>4. Consists of standardized route, targets, orientation signs, and directions. Includes a practice route with four targets. No training takes place on a MAC route. |

way, how many directional signs were followed, and the time taken to complete the route. Targets were placed so that Denny had to turn his head to best see them. For example, targets were placed on doors next to the nearest door jam so that they could not easily be seen without a head turn.

Denny completed the course in 4 minutes and 17 seconds while locating 41 percent of the targets on the left, and 54 percent of the targets on the right. When feedback was given about his performance on the task, Denny was not satisfied with his low scores and verbalized, "Maybe I really have a vision problem."

Further demonstration of Denny's field loss was provided using the Neuro Vision Technology Panel, which consists of a light panel containing two rows of ten LED multicolored lights controlled by a training software program (see Table 24.3 and Figure 24.12), and which allowed Denny to experience his field loss in relation to the lights on the board. While seated a foot away from the panel, with the lights at eye level, he touched and turned his head to see lights presented in his left visual field. Fields were first tested with central fixation. Denny's field of vision while centrally fixating allowed him to see the lights only on the right side of the panel.

During an exercise demonstrating the width of his visual field, Denny was shown that, by turning his head to view the far left end of the light panel, he could see most of the lights on the panel since they were now positioned in his intact right visual field. But when looking at the far right perimeter, he could only see four lights, since most of the panel was now positioned in his left visual field, the area of Denny's field loss.

After completing these assessments, Denny's motivation to learn to compensate for his visual field impairment increased. As he learned to use his vision in a new way, he occasionally required functional demonstrations of the width of his visual field to enhance his motivation to apply scanning strategies.

### Additional Methods to Demonstrate Visual Field Loss

Targets were attached to a wall in a line at eye level, with Denny seated. The targets were sticky notes with the numbers 0–10, with the number 5 at the midline. Denny was instructed to look at the number 5 and to describe how many other notes he could see. Denny could only see the numbers to the right of the 5. Denny was then asked to look toward the zero on the left and compare how many sticky notes he could see versus looking to the right. He reported seeing more sticky notes when turning his head to the left.

Denny was instructed to sit in a chair facing forward. His instructor had him compare his visual field with a left eye turn versus a left head turn. First, Denny was told to turn only his eyes, as far as he could to the left, and to let his instructor know as soon as he could see him. The instructor approached from Denny's left and walked past Denny's chair (and beyond Denny's body space) before Denny was able to see him. Then Denny was instructed to turn his head to his left shoulder "and to tell me when you see me." Denny saw the instructor before he reached Denny's left shoulder, as his instructor did not walk past the chair this time. Denny said, "I can see you sooner if I turn my chin to my shoulder."

During leisure activities Denny was asked to describe the details of the room. On a trip to the movie theater, Denny reported only being able to see half of the screen. He

TABLE 24.3

## Innovative Technology Used for Assessment and Training with Adults in Neuro-Vision Rehabilitation

| *Device* | *Description* | *Purpose* | *Procedures* |
|---|---|---|---|
| Neuro Vision Technology (NVT) Panel 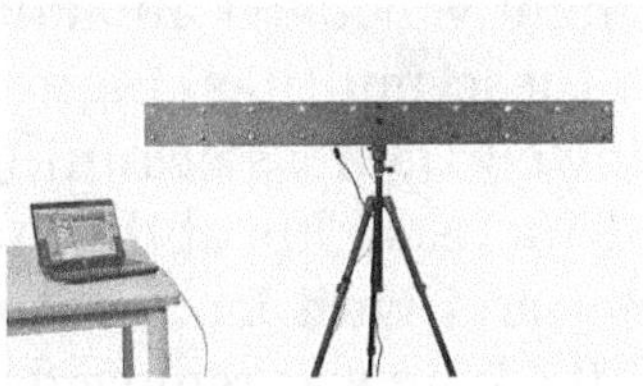<br>**Figure 24.12** | A neuro-vision rehabilitation tool, the light panel contains two rows of ten LED multicolored lights controlled by a training software program. | 1. Increase ability to attend to stimuli and increase speed of scanning while seated and standing.<br>2. Develop muscle memory/kinesthetic feedback for head turn needed to compensate for missing field.<br>3. Increase visual spatial problem solving and visual memory.<br>4. Increase ability to attend to stimuli in the presence of changing stimuli of LED lights.<br>5. Increase multitasking skills and parallel processing.<br>6. Develop scanning strategies before dynamic scanning with targets. | 1. Client sits 1 foot from the panel for visual field assessment and scanning training. LED lights provide stimuli in left and right visual fields.<br>2. Assessment captures measures for speed of scanning; visual field analysis and demonstration; response to stimuli in both visual fields; visual spatial, visual memory, and other perceptual concepts. |
| Interactive Metronome (IM) 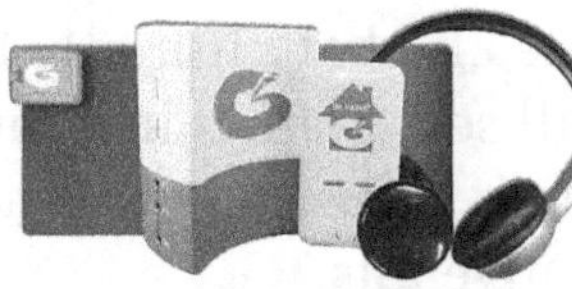<br>**Figure 24.13**<br>IM hand and foot triggers 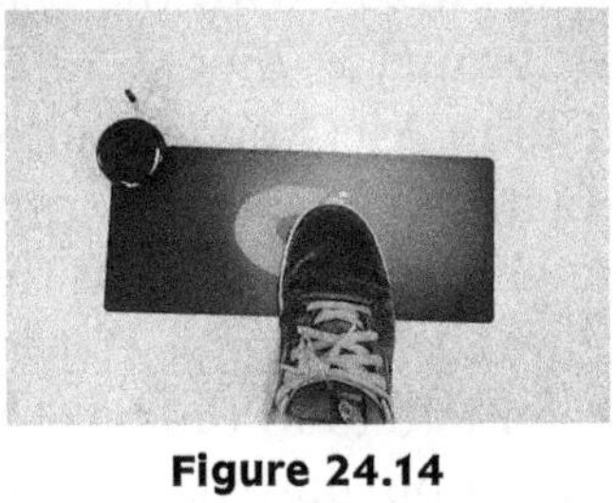<br>**Figure 24.14** | A neuro-rehabilitation tool used to address attention, coordination, motor planning, gait, balance, and multitasking abilities. | 1. Improve ability to attend.<br>2. Improve parallel processing.<br>3. Improve coordination.<br>4. Integrate left and right sides of the body.<br>5. Increase demand for ocular motor training exercises with letter charts or other tools. | 1. Triggers are used, attached either to the hands for clapping to the beat of the metronome or to foot trigger pads to be stepped on, to the beat of the metronome.<br>2. Assessment captures measures for hands and feet, including balancing and alternating between left and right sides of the body.<br>3. Training incorporates auditory and visual feedback for improving performance. |

was encouraged to scan to the left and describe the details on that side of the theater as well.

## Vision Training

To educate about brain injury along the visual pathways, Denny was provided with colored markers in an exercise to color in a diagram of the visual pathways from the eyes to the brain. Tactile brain models and tennis balls with different tactile cords (for nasal and temporal pathways) were used to represent the visual pathways as they travel through the brain. These methods encouraged Denny to try to explain his field loss in his own words and provided him with concrete and functional examples of the need for visual scanning to compensate for his field loss for safer mobility.

Denny participated in daily Neuro Vision Technology Panel training sessions to start to develop a systematic scanning pattern by looking toward the left perimeter light followed by scanning to the right without missing lights. Initial sessions took place while he was seated in a quiet environment. Instructors focused on training methods that highlighted proprioceptive feedback from Denny's neck muscles in order to encourage Denny to move his head as well as his eyes to achieve better visual outcomes.

As prompts to scan toward the left decreased, other visual perceptual tasks were added, such as matching light patterns on the left and right, and counting or calling out colors of lights. Activities to encourage the use of Denny's left hand and foot were implemented as recommended by occupational therapy. Using his hands to explore and touch the lights during problem-solving tasks, such as determining which lights to switch on to create a matching pattern of lights, were included.

Task performance focused on accuracy rather than speed. With practice, Denny's speed increased for all exercises, and additional tasks were added; for instance, Denny clapped when he saw a white light, or stomped his right foot when there was a green light. Crossing midline tasks were added for other lights, until every light generated an additional task. While these multitasking exercises initially slowed Denny's scanning speed, they helped increase his ability to scan for lights faster and with more accuracy when the multitasking was removed.

Concurrently, Denny participated in daily vision therapy sessions with a focus on methods for improving fixation, saccades, and pursuits. Training included the use of letter charts (Hart Charts) and alphabet pencils, among other tools (see Table 24.1). Various types of pen-and-paper worksheets were used, including word-tracking worksheets, maze puzzles, letter and symbol cancellation worksheets, and search-and-find puzzles. Ball-tossing games for pursuit training and hand-eye coordination were also implemented into training sessions. One of Denny's personal goals was to reach 100 consecutive direct hits of a paddle and ball. Initially he could only hit the ball seven times in a row, but by the end of his training he had advanced to 94 consecutive hits.

Studies have linked improvements in attention, motor control, timing, rhythm, and reading with metronome training, in which movements are synchronized with the beat of the metronome (Buhusi & Meck, 2005; Shaffer et al., 2001; Taub, McGrew, & Keith, 2007). The use of a metronome was incorporated into ocular motor exercises such as the letter charts and alphabet pencils. Denny was instructed to read letters to the beat of the metronome with the purpose of moving his eyes to the beat as he read. These skills improved with performance. (Metronome apps are now available for free online and on smartphone and tablet apps.)

Video feedback has been used successfully with adults (Tham & Tegner, 1997) as it provides them with a chance to review their own performance and identify strengths and weaknesses. Activities were videotaped throughout training so that Denny could review his own progress. Videos were reviewed by Denny and his instructors. Denny could pick out instances where he could have scanned to his left, for example, before getting off the elevator and where hallways intersected.

## Dynamic Training

To assist in the transfer of skills from static to dynamic situations, all the above visual training tasks were practiced while standing, marching in place, or during balancing exercises in conjunction with Denny's physical therapy sessions. Standing increases the complexity of tasks and enhances the progression into navigating in a world in motion.

O&M sessions included practice with locating targets on the left. Denny was told to look for targets along hallways that his O&M specialist had placed on the left, and eventually the right side of the hallway, to encourage complete scanning. Simple, large, brightly colored targets such as sticky notes were used at first. Gradually more complex targets were introduced, including those with letters, numbers, arrows, and symbols. (See Table 24.1 for other examples of targets.)

Various dynamic perceptual tasks (perceptual tasks while moving) were added while practicing scanning. An example of this was having Denny call out when he had a "match" while he was scanning for a variety of arrow targets with patterns placed in the hallways. Denny was asked to locate all the targets, call out the directions of each arrow (left, right, up, or down), and then indicate when he found a matching pattern. Denny was allowed to carry a sample of the "match" target with him, but was encouraged to use visual memory as best he could.

By keeping track of daily target sessions, Denny and staff could monitor his progress. For instance, finding 10 out of 12 targets gradually increased to locating all the targets. While walking, if Denny missed a target, he was immediately stopped and prompted to scan for its location. As Denny improved at this task, targets were placed in more demanding environments, such as busier hallways and at intersections to encourage left to right scanning for approaching traffic.

Target training advanced to the outdoors for Denny, where the fabricated targets were replaced by naturally occurring "targets" in the environment. For instance, when Denny walked with his O&M specialist along a sidewalk near parked cars on his left, he was asked to read the first and last figure of each license plate. During store training, Denny's instructor had him scan each aisle on the left, looking for aisle signs and other shoppers, or systematically scanning items on shelves. Training graduated into negotiating residential neighborhoods, scanning driveways for the presence or absence of vehicles, and other avoidable obstacles. With mastery of these skills, Denny progressed into the instruction of visual scanning techniques for safe street crossings.

When traveling further into the community, Denny received instruction about the use of his smartphone with GPS, camera phone, and digital recorder as tools to assist with memory. He took pictures of important visual landmarks along his route and was taught to plot routes using Google Maps for directions and preroute planning.

The Mobility Assessment Course posttest verified Denny's improvement for dynamic tasks. After training, Denny increased his scores on the course to 75 percent of right and left targets equally (up from 54 percent right and 41 percent left). This demonstrated an improvement on the left side, and now he was seeing an equal amount on both sides. He also improved his performance on the time to complete the course, a minute (1 minute and 14 seconds total time) faster than pretraining measures.

Denny completed four weeks of daily inpatient therapies including ocular motor training (fixation, pursuits, and saccades) and scanning training, among other therapies. He completed a total of 18 sessions (six static Neuro Vision Technology light panel sessions and 12 dynamic mobility sessions). O&M sessions lasted between 60 and 90 minutes, while ocular motor training sessions were typically 45 minutes each day. At discharge, Denny demonstrated improved ocular motor function and control, smooth pursuits, improved saccades, and an increased ability to maintain steady fixation. Although treatment resulted in improved visual performance, the more remarkable gain was Denny's insight into his own vision impairment.

### At One-Year Follow-Up

Denny returned for follow-up one year later. While he lacked any spontaneous recovery of his visual field, he demonstrated more flexible thinking and was more patient with tasks. He identified difficulties with crowds and more complex environments such as airports. He was also thinking about going back to school and needed strategies for reading for long periods of time.

Follow-up scores using the Mobility Assessment Course were obtained. He showed a slight decline in scanning for targets (67 percent of the left and right targets), while still locating an equal number of targets on either side. His identification of orientation signs showed a reduction by 50 percent, and he took additional time to complete the course (2 minutes and 28 seconds total).

The focus of follow-up training was to include mobility and scanning training in more complex environments such as airports, nearby universities, and busy business environments. In addition, Fresnel prisms were added to his eyeglasses. These prisms are attached to the lenses and assist by shifting the image from his missing visual field into his intact visual field. Denny learned how to use the prisms for quick visual checks as an individual does with the rearview mirror of a car. He practiced using the prisms to detect stimuli and then turn his head to view them more carefully. Long cane training was provided for selective use in crowded and complex areas to give Denny coverage of his body space should he become distracted or not scan quickly enough for the demands of the changing environment. It also served to signal to the public that he had a visual impairment.

Another innovative technology used was a neurorehabilitation tool called Interactive Metronome (IM) (see Table 24.3). This device was incorporated into Denny's training to encourage use of his right hand, arm, and leg, as well as to further enhance his ocular motor skills. To accomplish this, Denny was asked to perform visual tasks while engaged in activities with the metronome. For example, while reading a Hart Chart to the beat of the metronome while standing, Denny was asked to alternate between clapping his hands to the beat of the metronome and stepping on a foot pedal in time with the metronome beat. He enjoyed the challenge and the new approach to familiar activities.

Denny was also trained in the use of text-to-speech technology to assist with the prolonged reading assignments required for school. He also answered questions about reading passages to evaluate his comprehension.

At completion of his follow-up training, Denny's Mobility Assessment Course scores were 2 minutes and 8 seconds to complete the course, 100 percent accuracy for sign identification, and 92 percent accuracy locating left and right targets. This demonstrated improved performance for both left and right target identification (from 67 percent to 92 percent), and he completed the course 20 seconds faster than his initial time at the beginning of follow-up training. He also improved on the location of all orientation signs during the course and continued to see equal amounts on both sides.

## Casey: Multisensory Approaches

Casey, a 61-year-old male, was admitted to the rehabilitation program three years post-injury and went through eight weeks of daily training. He had developed left homonymous hemianopia (loss of the left half of the field of vision in both eyes) and right superior quadrantanopia (loss of the right upper quarter of the field of vision in both eyes) as a result of multiple strokes. Casey also had left hemiparesis, or weakness on the left side of his body.

### Assessment

An optometric examination noted fast eye movements that were short of the target, were slow in searching, and tended to undershoot when seeking the target. Reflexive saccades were also hypometric, undershooting to the right and left. Visual acuities were 20/60 (6/18) in both eyes with correction.

In addition, Casey was found to have difficulty finding things in cluttered visual scenes and reduced visual memory. He saw the world in black and white due to impaired color vision processing. Casey was also diagnosed with constructional dyspraxia (difficulty with spatial relationships) and had left/right confusion.

Rivermead Conventional Subtests (see Table 24.2) were administered. Errors were made in association with poor scanning and a random approach to visual search patterns. On the letter cancellation task, Casey made errors related to poor scanning and found 13 letters out of 40. On the star cancellation task he missed 17 stars out of 54. He demonstrated a random approach to all tasks and neglected to complete the left half of the line-by-line bisection task, as well as missing two rows on the right on that task.

Casey was assessed with the Neuro Vision Technology Panel, which demonstrated a slow speed of visual processing and random scanning patterns without spontaneous initiation of looking movements toward the left end of the light panel. It took him a considerable amount of time and energy to locate the lights and respond. He had a difficult time visually locating lights when turning his head. The team, therefore, decided to focus on training with other tools, as discussed below. However, showing Casey his visual field limitations in relation to the lights assisted in his understanding of the need for training in scanning.

Pen-and-paper training (see Table 24.1) included letter, number, and symbol tracking worksheets. Casey was asked to point to each number as he read. Covering all but the first line with a white piece of paper helped reduce visual clutter. Once the task was understood he was able to proceed with minimal prompting, and was asked to circle or cross out letters with a pen.

The Rivermead was performed post-training and Casey improved on the letter tracking task; he found 24 out of 40, improving his score to 60 percent, up from 33 percent on the pretest. Casey's ability to recognize numbers and read two- to three-letter words assisted functionally when applied to reading room numbers, orientation signs, and money management.

## Spatial Skills

Improvements with perceptual problems have been described as a sequel to combining block design training with training scanning and search (Young, Collins, & Hren, 1983). Parquetry blocks were used for visuospatial assessment and training. Casey was presented with three blocks and asked to visually examine the shapes. He was unable to visually identify and name the square, diamond, or triangle. But when using both visual and tactile exploration, the block shapes could be identified.

Casey's instructors placed blocks on his left side to encourage him to scan to the left. Casey was asked to sort the blocks. Some prompting for visual examination was initially required for these tasks, especially when Casey had to identify, compare, and process which two shapes were a match.

As identification and matching of shapes became less challenging, instructors created puzzles by combining blocks together. Prompting was required to examine each block by touch and vision and to determine at what points they were touching. For example, two triangles joined together with each long side of the triangle touching one other created a square. Casey was guided in visual examining behaviors, as well as tactile exploration of each shape, to determine which shape was on each side. The shapes were then examined to identify which was above and which below. Gradually, prompting was reduced for these tasks and Casey was able to independently copy three- and four-block combinations.

## Anchoring Techniques

Anchoring provides a means of maintaining a position of reference. It was shown in the 1960s that individuals with left neglect could be taught to place a finger of the left hand on the left margin of a book and then look toward the finger before reading each new line (Lawson, 1962) if they were able to use and attend to their left hand. The idea was to present a "visual guide" (Pigott & Brickett, 1966) in the affected field as a reference or starting point for scanning. (Analogous techniques are utilized with the Neuro Vision Technology Panel described in the previous case study, where the far left light becomes the anchor point.)

Examples of other types of anchoring techniques include the use of hemianopia reading guides, which are commercially available. These are shaped like the letter *L* and provide a guide for where to start (for left visual field loss) or stop (for right visual field loss). Using a ribbon, string, or a sticky note placed on the left or right side of a book can also provide such a reminder. While items can be bought or made, using a finger to monitor the margin can be effective because it is simple, does not require a tool, and encourages the use of touch as an additional frame of reference in the development of the skill.

## Tactile Scan Board

Other techniques for tactile-visual examination include the use of a black foam core board to add a tactile anchor to the left (see Table 24.1). Much of Casey's near training tasks were used on the foam core board called a Tactile Scan Board. The board was 20 × 30 inches (51 × 79 cm) in size and provided a defined background for visual scanning skills instruction so that Casey knew where scans began and ended. Casey was instructed to touch the left edge of the board to help develop a kinesthetic memory for visual scanning.

Activities on the Tactile Scan Board included sorting flashcards in sequential order. Bold-print flashcards with the numbers 1–10 were placed in two rows of five on the board, starting from the top left perimeter.

Casey was instructed to begin scanning at the top of the board from left to right. It was suggested that he use his finger to point to each number and move his finger in unison with his eyes. The low vision therapist asked him to read each number out loud and provided correction when errors were made. He was asked to begin by scanning with the goal of rearranging the number cards into sequential order. When Casey reached the end of the row, he was instructed to look toward his left hand, which was used to monitor the left edge of the Scan Board and served as a tactile reference point prior to the initiation of scanning each time. Casey also practiced exercises in which he systematically scanned single-letter flashcards and placed them in alphabetical order, or scanned the cards to spell names and short words. Large-print playing cards were used for games such as solitaire, concentration, or memory, as well as sorting suits. Casey had enjoyed card games prior to the stroke, and they were something he could also do for recreation and with family members and friends.

## Software Training

Casey also participated in basic computer training on a laptop computer so that he could continue to play computerized visual perceptual training games when he returned home. The chosen software was used to establish baseline scores for training games mentioned below and to monitor scores throughout training.

For visual memory training, the Arrow Game was used, in which Casey watched arrows flash on a computer screen for an adjustable number of seconds; he then had to respond by entering the same number and sequence of arrows using the arrow keys on the keyboard. A row of three arrows each pointing in different horizontal and vertical directions appeared and flashed on the screen for a period of 5 seconds. After the arrows disappeared, Casey had to enter the same sequence using the arrow keys. Each session lasted three minutes. Initial scores on this game were averaged, with 44 percent accuracy. Since this task requires some initial training in where to look and respond, his first attempts were averaged to establish a baseline score. At the completion of training, his accuracy scores on the Arrow Game improved to 81 percent. As the amount of time the arrows flashed was reduced from 5 to 4 seconds, the duration of each session was increased from 3 to 5 minutes.

In another computer game, the Flipper Game, Casey was presented with an image and then four choices to select either the matching or the inverted image. This game required Casey to mentally reverse images and to incorporate left and right and up and down (top and bottom) spatial concepts. The scores for the first three games were averaged for a baseline score of 65 percent correct. The average amount of time spent on this task was 27 minutes, and the average number of images attempted in that time was 18. His average response time per image was 75 seconds.

Casey completed a total of 11 sessions using this game. At discharge Casey had improved on this game to 91 percent correct. He spent 30 minutes on the game and gave answers for 23 images. His average response time decreased to 60 seconds.

### Metronome Training for O&M

The Interactive Metronome was used to train Casey to coordinate long cane movements with the movement of his feet in order to keep his steps synchronized, or "in step," with his long cane. Being in step provides advance warning for detection of obstacles and elevation changes. When traveling with a long cane, in order to be in step, the cane user must use a coordinated rhythm. Initial attempts to train in-step methodology using traditional O&M methods did not allow Casey to experience the continuous feedback of what it feels like to be in step since he lacked coordinated rhythm. Casey performed this by alternating tapping his feet on the Interactive Metronome foot trigger to a controlled beat. His O&M specialist provided hand-over-hand guidance for his wrist movements. As Casey progressively matched the rhythm, the instructor released the hand-over-hand guidance. Concurrently, the appropriate width of the arc made by moving his cane from side to side was reinforced during these sessions.

Each session ended with a dynamic application, using a long cane in the hallway. After three lessons of about 800 repetitions each day on the Interactive Metronome, Casey was noted to begin self-correcting and synchronizing his in-step moves independently. After about a week of daily training, he demonstrated appropriate arc width and in-step techniques when walking independently on the ward. Further O&M training was added, as this basic long cane skill progressively needed less conscious effort on Casey's part, and attention could be applied to environmental information such as the use of landmarks to assist with orientation.

Casey demonstrated many gains over his 8-week period of daily training, as the pre- and posttraining scores presented earlier demonstrated. While complete independent mobility in unfamiliar areas had yet to be achieved, he was able to incorporate these techniques on familiar travel routes. The plan for Casey was to return home to transfer skills into his daily routine, continue with computer training with assistance from his family, and to return for further training in the near future.

## Considerations for Children with CVI

The training approaches for adults discussed in this chapter operate under the assumption that vision is an integrated brain function. These approaches link visual guidance of movement, visual attention, recognition, understanding, memory, and imagination (mental imagery). The acquisition of new or lost strategies requires some degree of cortical reorganization or plasticity (Kerkhoff, 2000). Visual training to learn such skills, however, cannot be done *to* people. It has to be done *by* them. The promotion of optimum neuroplastic development needs participants who are self-driven and motivated. Compensatory scanning, for example, requires motivation to learn a new skill, a new way of seeing. For children, these approaches work best if embedded in play, games, and meaningful tasks that are motivating and fun. Yet there still needs to be constructive feedback; the role of feedback in the reinforcement of neural pathway enhancement plays a significant role.

While all strategies discussed in this chapter relate to adults, it must be stressed that children are not little adults. Children are still growing and developing. All of their incoming senses contribute to learning through the accumulation of holistic, interconnected experiences. Since vision does not operate in isolation from other senses and impacts all domains of development, all facets of a child's skills and development must be understood and evaluated in the context of home, school, and community environments. Educational approaches for children need to address specific skills and their application in tasks that are functional, meaningful, and motivating, with methods matched to developmental levels. Strategies offered to children need to be flexible and change as the children change. Future approaches in the development of training protocols for children with CVI need to take into account the cumulative, complex, and multifaceted nature of this process.

## References


Bate, A. J., Mathias, J. L., & Crawford, J. R. (2001). The covert orienting of visual attention following severe traumatic brain injury. *Journal of Clinical and Experimental Neuropsychology, 23*(3), 386–398.

Buhusi, C. V., & Meck, W. H. (2005). What makes us tick? Functional and neural mechanisms of interval timing. *Nature Reviews Neuroscience, 6*(10), 755–765.

Donahue, S. P., & Haun, A. K. (2007). Exotropia and face turn in children with homonymous hemianopia. *Journal of Neuro-Ophthalmology, 27*(4), 304–307.

George, S., Hayes, A., Chen, C., & Crotty, M. (2011). The effect of static scanning and mobility training on mobility in people with hemianopia after stroke: A randomized controlled trial comparing standardized versus non-standardized treatment protocols. *BMC Neurology, 11*, 87.

Kedar, S., Zhang, X., Lynn, M. J., Newman, N. J., & Biousse, V. (2006). Pediatric homonymous hemianopia. *Journal of the American Association for Pediatric Ophthalmology and Strabismus, 10*(3), 249–252.

Kerkhoff, G. (2000). Neurovisual rehabilitation: Recent developments and future directions. *Journal of Neurology, Neurosurgery, & Psychiatry, 68*, 691–706.

Kingston, J., Katsaros, J., Vu, Y., & Goodrich, G. L. (2010). Neurological vision rehabilitation: Description and case study. *Journal of Visual Impairment & Blindness, 104*(10), 603–612.

Lawson, I. R. (1962). Visual-spatial neglect in lesions of the right cerebral hemisphere. A study in recovery. *Neurology, 12*, 23–33.

Mezey, L., Harris, C. M., Shawkat, F., Timms, C., Kriss, A., West, P., et al. (1998). Saccadic strategies in children with hemianopia. *Developmental Medicine & Child Neurology, 40*(9), 626–630.

Pigott, R., & Brickett, F. (1966). Visual neglect. *The American Journal of Nursing, 66*(1), 101–105.

Poppelreuter, W. (1990). *Disturbances of lower and higher visual capacities caused by occipital damage.* (J. Zihl & L. Weiskrantz, Trans.). Oxford: Oxford University Press. (Original work published in 1917.)

Posner, M. I., & Petersen, S. E. (1990). The attention system of the human brain. *Annual Review of Neuroscience, 13*, 25–42.

Shaffer, R. J., Jacokes, L. E., Cassily, J. F., Greenspan, S. I., Tuchman, R. F., & Stemmer P. J., Jr. (2001). Effect of interactive metronome training on children with ADHD. *American Journal of Occupational Therapy, 55*(2), 155–162.

Smith, E., & Chatterjee, A. (2008). Visuospatial attention in children. *Archives of Neurology, 65*(10), 1284–1288.

Taub, G. E., McGrew, K. S., & Keith, T. Z. (2007). Improvements in interval time tracking and effects on reading achievement. *Psychology in the Schools, 44*(8), 849–863.

Tham, K., & Tegner, R. (1997). Video feedback in the rehabilitation of patients with unilateral neglect. *Archives of Physical Medicine and Rehabilitation, 78*(4), 410–413.

Ting, D. S. J., Pollock, A., Dutton, G. N., Doubal, F. N., Ting, D. S. W., Thompson, M., et al. (2011). Visual neglect following stroke: Current concepts and future focus. *Survey of Ophthalmology, 56*(2), 114–134.

Verlander, D., Hayes, A., Mcinnes, J., Liddle, R., Liddle, G., Clarke, G., . . . Walsh, P. (2000). Assessment of clients with visual spatial disorders: A pilot study. *Visual Impairment Research, 2*(3), 129–142.

Wilson, B., Cockburn, J., & Halligan, P. (1987). Development of a behavioral test of visuospatial neglect. *Archives of Physical Medicine and Rehabilitation, 68*(2), 98–102.

Young, G. C., Collins, D., & Hren, M. (1983). Effect of pairing scanning training with block design training in the remediation of perceptual problems in left hemiplegics. *Journal of Clinical and Experimental Neuropsychology, 5*(3), 201–212.

Zihl, J. (2011). *Rehabilitation of visual disorders after brain injury* (2nd ed.). East Sussex, UK: Psychology Press.

Zihl, J., & Dutton, G. N. (2015). *Cerebral visual impairment in children: Visuoperceptive and visuocognitive disorders.* Vienna: Springer-Verlag Wien.

# GLOSSARY

**Absolute orientation perception** The ability to understand one's own orientation with respect to the surrounding space.

**Accommodation** Automatic adjustment to the shape of the lens of the eye in order to bring objects into focus as the viewing distance varies.

**Agnosia (visual)** Decreased or absent ability to visually recognize or identify shapes, objects, or people.

**Akinetopsia** A condition in which an individual can only see things when they are not moving.

**Alexia** Difficulty in the naming of letters or words.

**Alternative communication** Nonverbal means of expression, such as smiling, head turn, gestures, vocalizations, pointing with the hand or foot, changes in posture, or communication through tactile means.

**Amblyopia** Impaired vision in one or both eyes, with no anatomical cause, due to impaired development of vision as a sequel to untreated optical (refractive) error, impaired image formation due to an eye disorder such as cataract, or impaired eye alignment (strabismus). Also known as *lazy eye.*

**Anisometropia** Difference in refractive error between the two eyes.

**Anomia** Inability to name objects or to recognize the written or spoken names of objects.

**Anopia** A defect in the visual field.

**Anosognosia** State of being unaware of one's own agnosia.

**Apraxia of gaze** Disorder of attention due to bilateral damage to the posterior parietal (dorsal stream) territory of the brain, leading to lack of visually driven eye movements.

**Assistive technology** Equipment used to help individuals compensate for visual and other impairments. Legally defined in the U.S. as "Any item, piece of equipment, or product system, whether acquired commercially, modified, or customized, that is used to increase, maintain, or improve functional capabilities of individuals with disabilities." (Assistive Technology Act of 2004, 29 U.S.C. Sec 2202[2]).

**Astigmatism** A type of refractive error that focuses light at different points in front of or behind the retina rather than a single point, and results in blurred vision at all distances, due to the subtle asymmetric, non-spherical shape of the cornea.

**Atrophy** Loss of tissue due to wasting.

**Auditory processing** How the brain recognizes and interprets auditory information.

**Autism spectrum disorder (ASD)** A neurodevelopmental disorder that can include disturbances in the areas of social interaction and communication along with restricted, repetitive, and stereotyped patterns of behavior (including motor mannerisms), interests, and activities, as well as rigid adherence to nonfunctional routines. Autism spectrum disorders are characterized on the basis of clusters of behaviors.

**Backward chaining** The process of learning the stages of a task one by one, starting from the last stage of the task and working toward the beginning of the task.

**Balint's syndrome** A condition due to bilateral posterior parietal lobe damage resulting in optic ataxia, simultanagnosia, and oculomotor apraxia.

**Bifocal lens** A spectacle lens with two separate and distinct areas, each with a different strength or power of lens. The top portion of the lens is used for distance viewing, and the lower portion for near viewing.

**Bilateral** Affecting both sides.

**Blindness** Absence of vision. *Total blindness* is complete absence of vision and is rare.

**Blindsight** Slight awareness of, or reflex reaction to, moving targets, lights, and colors in an area of apparently absent visual field.

**Braillewriter** A mechanical device that, with a combination of six keys, can produce any letter in embossed braille.

**Brain stem** The area at the base of the brain that, along with the midbrain above it, carries the nerve fibers running in both directions between the brain and the body and receives and processes input from the cranial nerves, including those that serve hearing and eye movements.

**Central acuity** The capacity of the visual system to see in the central visual field.

**Central fixation target** A target placed in the center of a visual field test.

**Cerebellum** A timekeeping brain structure that ensures that control of emotion by the frontal lobes, movement of the body processed by the parietal lobes, and vision processed by the occipital lobes are synchronized and coordinated.

**Cerebral blindness** Profound impairment or absence of vision due to bilateral damage to the visual pathways posterior to the lateral geniculate bodies that may be accompanied by damage to other regions of the brain that serve vision. Also known as *cortical blindness.*

**Cerebral visual impairment (CVI)** Visual impairment due to damage or disorder of the visual pathways and visual centers in the brain, including the pathways serving visual perception, cognition, and visual guidance of movement. Sometimes also referred to as *cortical visual impairment.*

**Chorioretinal (or retino-choroidal)** Affecting the retina and underlying choroid.

**Ciliary muscles** Internal eye muscles that focus the lens.

**Closed-circuit television (CCTV)** *See* Video magnifier.

**Cloud storage** Networked and virtual storage of data files on the Internet, usually hosted by third parties.

**Cognitive visual dysfunction** Disordered function of the brain related to damage to the visual-associative areas and/or their incoming pathways leading to misinterpretation of the visual world either with respect to where things are, or what they are.

**Color anomia** Inability to name colors due to neuro-logical dysfunction.

**Comprehension (of text)** Engaging in the complex process of making sense from text; reading with the purpose of learning, understanding, or enjoyment.

**Confrontation visual field testing** A way of estimating visual fields by employing a target in the child's peripheral visual field and observing orienting eye-head movements, or asking the child to point at or locate the moving target in each location tested.

**Congenital** Existing at or before birth.

**Constant deviation** Condition in which both eyes, and often the head, are constantly turned to the left, right, up, or down. Also *tonic deviation.*

**Contralateral** The opposite side of the body.

**Contrast sensitivity** The ability of the visual system to distinguish the difference in brightness between two adjacent surfaces.

**Convergence** The ability to turn the eyes inward as an object approaches them.

**Concave** Curved inward.

**Convex** Curved outward.

**Cortical** Pertaining to the cerebral cortex.

**Cortical visual impairment** *See* Cerebral visual impairment.

**Crystalline lens** The lens within the eye whose shape is altered by the ciliary muscles to bring objects into focus.

**Decoding** The ability to use phonics skills to translate a word from print to speech in an alphabetic writing system, usually by using knowledge of sound-symbol correspondence.

**Developmental age** A mea-sure of a child's level of

development according to social, emotional, intellectual, and physical growth.

**Developmental disability** Mental or physical disability arising as a consequence of a disorder of development.

**Diagnostic teaching** Individualized method of teaching that uses assessment data in the teaching and learning process to determine the next steps in intervention.

**Diffusion tensor imaging (DTI)** An imaging technique that facilitates the study of anatomical connections in the brain by mapping the movement of water molecules.

**Diplegia** Paralysis or weakness of the lower limbs.

**Discrepancy analysis** A method that first determines typical subtasks needed to perform a specific activity or routine and then identifies those subtasks that require the implementation of alternate approaches for a particular student with disabilities to complete them successfully.

**Dorsal stream** The pathway between the occipital and posterior parietal lobes that maps the surroundings and brings about visual guidance of movement. Sometimes known as the "where" pathway, it functions at a subconscious level.

**Dorsal stream dysfunction** Condition in which the function of the dorsal stream is disrupted, causing impaired visual guidance of movement and limiting the number of entities that can be seen in crowded scenes.

**Dyskinetopsia** A condition in which impaired perception of movement is relative and not absolute. (*See also* akinetopsia.)

**Dyslexia** A language-based learning disability that can be associated with difficulties in reading, spelling, writing, and sound-symbol association.

**Eccentric viewing** Looking slightly above, below, or to one side of an object in order to place a visual image onto an optimum area of the visual field for viewing.

**Echolalia** Repetition of phrases, words, parts of words, or vocal sounds. It can be immediate (occurring immediately or shortly after hearing a stimulus) or delayed.

**Echolocation** The use of sound echoes to perceive the structure of the surroundings and to guide a person's movement through space.

**Electroencephalography (EEG)** Along with its magnetic counterpart, magnetoencephalography (MEG), this procedure noninvasively records brain activity from the surface of the scalp to provide an indirect evaluation of brain function.

**Emmetropia** Condition in which the light coming from a distant object to the eye is focused accurately on the retina to make a crisp, focused image without the need for refractive correction.

**Encephalopathy** Disorder of the brain due to disease, causing damage and malfunction.

**Esotropia** A condition in which one eye is horizontally turned inward; also known as *convergent strabismus* (US), or *convergent squint* (UK). Results in a lack of stereopsis.

**Executive functions** Higher-order mental skills that are used to control and coordinate cognitive abilities and behaviors to achieve a particular goal.

**Exotropia** A condition in which one eye is horizontally turned outward; also known as *divergent strabismus* (US) or *divergent squint* (UK). Results in lack of stereopsis.

**Expanded core curriculum (ECC)** Curricular areas unique to students with visual impairments that facilitate access to educational curricula and independent living and that may require direct instruction throughout developmental and school years.

**External hard drive** Digital data storage space in a physical device such as a memory card or USB flash drive.

**Farsightedness** *See* Hyperopia.

**Fine motor** Small, accurate movements that involve the small muscles in the body such as those in the hands and fingers.

**Fixation** The ability to maintain the eyes on a target.

**Fluency** The ability to read accurately, quickly, and with proper expression and rhythm.

**Forward chaining** Moving through the successive stages of a task from beginning to end.

**Fresnel prisms** Prisms attached to spectacle lenses that are used to assist in the treatment of double vision and various eye movement disorders.

**Frontal lobes** Area at the front of the brain, part of which (the prefrontal cortex on both sides, or the front portion of the frontal lobes) serves the executive functions of thinking, planning, and controlling behavior.

**Functional MRI (fMRI)** A neuroimaging procedure that permits observation of the brain in action when performing a particular task by tracking changes in brain metabolism. Foci of enhanced activity in the brain scan seen while the task is being carried out show the principal parts of the brain involved.

**Functional skills** Skills that students with multiple disabilities learn that provide them with the opportunity to work, play, socialize, and take care of personal needs to the highest attainable level.

**Functional vision** The ways in which a person uses available visual skills and abilities in typical tasks of daily life.

**Functional visual impairment** Damage to the visual system that impedes the ability to learn or perform usual tasks of daily life, given a child's level of maturity and cultural environment.

**Generalization of skills and behaviors** The ability to perform skills and behaviors learned within the context of one activity and location and with specific people in another context, in a different location, and with different people.

**Gestalt** Immediate mental construct of an overall (global) scenario formed from a collection of separate elements.

**Gross motor** Movement that involves the large muscles of the body such as those in the arms and legs (e.g., crawling, running, or jumping).

**Habilitation** Services that enable a person to learn, keep, or improve skills and functional abilities that have never developed or have not developed in a typical manner.

**Habituation** A process by which an individual becomes so accustomed to a repetitive stimulus or activity that they lose interest in it.

**Haptic** Relating to the sense of touch.

**Hemianopia** Lack of perception of one half of the visual field. Also called *hemianopsia.*

**Hemifield** One half of a sensory field.

**Hemiparesis** Weakness on one side of the body.

**Hemiplegic** Paralysis on one side of the body.

**Higher visual functions** The combination of visual perception, visual cognition, guidance of movement, and the capacity to choose to give visual attention.

**Homonymous** Affecting the same part of the visual field of each eye.

**Homonymous hemianopia** A visual field defect in which the same half of the field of view is not seen by each eye.

**Hydrocephalus** A condition due to impaired circulation of cerebral spinal fluid (CSF), causing increased intracranial pressure, commonly with increased CSF volume expanding the water spaces in the brain (the ventricles).

**Hyperopia (or hypermetropia)** A type of refractive error that results in blurred images when the length of the eye from front to back is too short, or the optical power of the eye is insufficient to bring an object into focus. Also known as *long-sightedness* or *farsightedness.*

**Hypertropia** An upward eye turn.

**Hypometric** Voluntary muscle movements that fall short of their intended goal.

**Hypoplasia** Underdevelopment of a body part.

**Hypotropia** A downward eye turn.

**Hypoxia** Lack of oxygen.

**Impaired pursuit** Disordered ability to pursue a moving target with the eyes.

**Independent living skills** A broad label encompassing every skill an individual needs to have at some time in life to be as independent as possible. Typically divided into five categories: personal management, home management, communication, leisure and recreation, and orientation and mobility.

**Intermittent deviations** Turning of both eyes together in one direction for a variable duration, often with an accompanying head turn. Also *paroxysmal deviation.*

**Invisible disabilities** Disabilities that are not immediately apparent; may include physical, visual, or mental impairments. Also known as *hidden disabilities.*

**Ischemia** Insufficient supply of blood.

**Joint attention** An exchange that involves a child's and a partner's awareness of the other's mutual focus of attention on a third object or event, shared through mutual gaze, gesture, or language.

**Kinesthesia** Perception and knowledge of the movement of one's limbs.

**Kinetic perimetry** A method to measure visual field function that projects stimuli (e.g., spots of light) that move from a peripheral to a more central location until they are seen.

**Labyrinthine system** The subconscious automatic system in the inner ear and brain stem that is responsible for controlling and maintaining balance.

**Lateral geniculate bodies** Small knee-shaped structures deep inside the brain that act as relay stations to convey visual information from the eyes through the brain.

**Learning media assessment (LMA)** Assessment that identifies a student's primary and secondary media for learning.

**Literal alexia** Inability to recognize certain individual letters due to damage to the brain.

**Location perception** Knowing where an object is located.

**Long-sightedness** *See* Hyperopia.

**Low vision** Visual impairment that is severe enough to impede a person's ability to learn or perform usual tasks of daily life but still allows some functionally useful visual discrimination. It covers a range from mild to severe visual impairment, but excludes total blindness.

**Magnetic resonance imaging (MRI)** A neuroimaging procedure that shows the anatomical features of the brain in great detail and can be used to study brain structure following injury.

**Magnocellular pathway** A major pathway of the visual system that primarily transmits visual information in the peripheral visual field to the brain and serves movement perception, as well as facilitating visual guidance of movement.

**Michelson contrast** A method of reporting contrast values for the difference between the darkest and lightest parts of a pattern and commonly used when gratings (stripes) are the test target.

**Midline** The median plane of the body.

**Mirror neuron system (MNS)** A system in the brain that facilitates understanding and imitation of the actions of others.

**Motion perception** The capacity to see movement.

**Myopia** A type of refractive error that results in blurred images on the retina when viewing objects in the distance. Also known as *nearsightedness* or *short-sightedness.*

**Nearsightedness** *See* Myopia.

**Norm-referenced test** An assessment tool that has been standardized in a way that enables comparison of the results of test takers in relation to a group that has already taken the test.

**Null point** The position of the eyes in which the oscillations of a person's nystagmus are least. Often accompanied by a compensatory head posture.

**Nystagmus** Unintentional or involuntary to-and-fro movement of the eyes.

**Object permanence** The understanding that objects still exist when they cannot be seen, heard, touched, smelled, or sensed.

**Occipital lobes** Posterior (back) portions of the cerebral cortex in each hemisphere responsible for processing vision and sending visual information to other parts of the brain.

**Occipitoparietal dysfunction** A disorder involving the occipital and parietal lobes of the brain, resulting in impairment of the functions of both structures.

**Occupational therapy (OT)** A treatment methodology that develops and maintains activities of daily living and work skills.

**Ocular** Of or relating to the eye.

**Ocular alignment** A description of the position of the eyes. If the eyes are out of alignment, strabismus is present.

**Ocular visual impairment** Visual impairment caused by a disorder of the eye or optic nerve (but not the brain).

**Oculomotor apraxia** Limited ability to move the eyes fast (saccadic movement) from one target to another.

**Oculomotor dysfunction** Impaired control of eye movements leading to visual difficulties such as visual fixation or visual tracking problems, ocular misalignment, and impairment of accommodation.

**Olfaction** Sense of smell.

**Ophthalmologist** A physician or surgeon who specializes in refractive, medical, and surgical care of the eyes and visual system.

**Optic ataxia** Impaired accuracy of movement of the limbs and body through visual space because visual guidance of movement is impaired.

**Optic chiasm** The X-shaped structure formed by the joining up of the optic nerves, which cross and then become the optic tracts just below and leading into the brain.

**Optic nerves** Nerves that transmit visual information from the retina of each eye to the brain.

**Optic radiations** A collection of nerve axons that carry information from the lateral geniculate bodies to the visual cortex in the occipital lobes.

**Optic tract** Bundles of nerve fibers that emerge from the back of the optic chiasm on each side that carry visual information to the lateral geniculate bodies.

**Optical character recognition (OCR)** A process that converts scanned or photographed images of text into a format that is readable by the computer. This process digitizes printed text for electronic editing, storage, and access by text-to-speech technology.

**Optokinetic** Related to eye movements.

**Optometrist** A health care provider who specializes in the measurement of refractive errors and other visual functions, prescribes eyeglasses or contact lenses, and (in some countries) diagnoses and manages conditions of the eye.

**Optotypes** Letters and symbols used to test visual acuity.

**Oral-motor apraxia** Difficulty coordinating muscle movements of the mouth (particularly the lips, jaw, and tongue) needed for speech.

**Orientation and mobility (O&M)** Training that enables an individual with visual impairments to travel as safely and independently as possible when navigating through various environments.

**Orientation perception** The capacity to know where one is, has been, and will be going, as well as the position and location of possessions.

**Orthoptist** A specialist in the measurement and management of disorders of eye movements and binocular vision.

**Parallax** The perception of the relative alignment of objects in relation to the position of viewing. A phenomenon that helps compensate for lack of stereopsis.

**Parietal lobes** The parts of the brain that integrate incoming sensory information with the execution of body movements and process language (usually on the left side).

**Paroxysmal deviation** *See* Intermittent deviation.

**Partial participation** When a student can participate in a portion of a task but cannot complete all of its component parts independently.

**Parvocellular pathway** A pathway in the brain served by small retinal and brain cells that transmits fine, detailed visual information primarily in the central visual field.

**Perception** The ability to see, hear, or become aware of something through the senses.

**Perceptual visual dysfunction** A condition in which the brain is unable to process visual information correctly. Sometimes used synonymously with *perceptual visual impairment.*

**Perinatal** Around the time of birth.

**Peripheral target** A target placed at the outer edge of a person's visual field.

**Peripheral visual field** The area of vision outside the center of an individual's gaze.

**Periventricular leukomalacia** Damage to white matter adjacent to the lateral ventricles in the brain.

**Periventricular white matter** The white matter near the ventricles of the brain.

**Phasic** Occurring in stages or phases; functioning intermittently.

**Phonemic awareness** The ability to hear, recognize, and manipulate the smallest units of sounds that differentiate meaning in language.

**Phonics** The process of linking sounds to letter symbols and combining them to make words.

**Pixelation** Appearance of a digital image whose individual elements, or pixels, are clearly discernible, as when an image is enlarged without increasing the number of pixels, which results in an image that is not sharp or clear.

**Prefrontal cerebral cortex** The anterior part of the frontal lobes of the brain that contributes to initiation and coordination of thoughts and actions.

**Progressive lens** A spectacle lens that provides correction for distance and near vision in a single lens with a continuous, invisible change in lens power and no abrupt separation between distance and near focus portions.

**Proprioception** Knowledge of one's own position of the body and limbs through feedback from ligaments, skin, and muscles.

**Prosopagnosia** Inability to recognize faces.

**Pupil (of an eye)** The hole in the center of the iris that allows light to enter the eye and, by its change in size, controls the amount of light passing through.

**Pursuit eye movements** Smooth eye movements made while following an object. Also known as *smooth pursuit movements.*

**Quadrantanopia** A defect in the visual field that affects a quarter of the visual field, demarcated by vertical and horizontal lines passing through the center of the visual field.

**QWERTY keyboard** A standard, traditional keyboard for the Latin alphabet.

**RAM (random access memory)** A computer's temporary memory required to operate software.

**Recognition acuity** Ability to recognize and distinguish a specific visual target from other similar stimuli; often measured using letter charts.

**Refractive error** A focusing inaccuracy within the eye such that light rays do not come into clear focus on the retina, resulting in a blurred image. (In children and young adults the refractive error of hyperopia may be corrected by accommodation, and therefore may not lead to a blurred image.)

**Rehabilitation** Training to improve skills or behaviors that have been lost or decreased due to disease or injury.

**Relative orientation perception** Ability to see subtle differences between orientations.

**Response to intervention (RTI)** A multitiered approach in which struggling learners are provided with interventions that increase in intensity based on the individual student's response to instruction.

**Retina** The inner sensory nerve layer next to the choroid that lines the posterior two-thirds of the eyeball. The retina reacts to light and transmits visual information by means of nerve impulses to the brain.

**Retinopathy of prematurity (ROP)** A disorder of the retina related to abnormal vascular development that occurs as a sequel to premature birth. It is arrested in most cases following appropriate screening and treatment.

**Saccades** Fast eye movements from one fixation to another.

**Sans serif** A font that does not have small, projecting lines at the ends of characters.

**Scanning** Making a series of visual fixations in order to visually inspect a large area.

**Scotoma** A non-seeing area in the visual field.

**Screen magnification program** A software program that allows the user to change the level of magnification and contrast of a computer monitor.

**Self-determination** Belief in one's ability to control one's own life and reach goals based on an understanding of one's own abilities, strengths, and weaknesses.

**Serif** A small line at the ends of letters and numbers.

**Shift of gaze** Changing visual fixation to a new object of interest.

**Short-sightedness** *See* Myopia.

**Simultanagnosia** Inability to see more than one or two items within the visual scene at the same time due to damage to the posterior parietal region of the brain.

**Spastic diplegia** A form of cerebral palsy resulting in weakness and stiffness of the lower limbs.

**Spectacles** Eyeglasses that hold corrective lenses.

**Spina bifida** A congenital disability that results when the spinal column does not close completely during development in the womb.

**Static perimetry** A method to measure visual field function that presents stimuli (e.g., spots of light) in fixed locations that are progressively brightened until visible.

**Stereopsis** Fine depth perception that results from the brain's interpretation of the slight difference between the disparate pictures of the same visual scene provided by the two eyes.

**Strabismus** Misalignment of the eyes; eyes do not look in the same direction.

**Structured play** Circumstances that are engineered to elicit specific target play behaviors that may shed light on a child's functional needs. Also known as *structured learning situations.*

**Tactile defensiveness** An aversion to touch due to oversensitivity.

**Task analysis** A process in which the sequence of components needed to complete a specific task efficiently by a typical student is identified.

**Temporal lobes** The areas of brain under the temples that analyze the input from the senses. They provide the memory banks that underpin knowledge and recognition.

**Thalamus** A structure situated between the cerebral cortex and the midbrain involved in processing and relaying sensory and motor signals to the cerebral cortex. The thalamus plays an important part in bringing about reflex visual attention.

**Threshold acuity** The lower limit of visual acuity measured with each eye separately for the purposes of diagnosis and follow-up of visual disorders.

**Tonic** In a state of continuous unremitting action; denoting especially a prolonged muscular contraction. Vision is a tonic sense.

**Tonic deviation** *See* Constant deviation.

**Topographic agnosia** Disorientation in one's surroundings. Impairment results from ventral stream damage and problems forming a mental map of the environment. Also known as *topographic disorientation.*

**Tracking** Maintaining fixation on a moving object of interest using pursuit eye movements.

**Transcranial magnetic stimulation (TMS)** A process that emits electronic pulses to trigger brain activity. Seeks to determine a causal relationship between a specific brain area and a specific task by selectively inhibiting or enhancing brain activity in specific parts of the brain.

**Typoscope** Reading window that facilitates reading efficiency by blocking out surrounding words and only showing a small number of words to be read. Usually black in color to absorb light and reduce glare.

**Unilateral** Affecting one side of the body.

**Universal design** Design with sufficient flexibility to meet the needs of all users, whether able-bodied or disabled.

**Ventral stream** Visual pathway between the occipital and temporal lobes, sometimes known as the "what" pathway, which supports the process of visual recognition. Dysfunction can cause impaired recognition of objects and persons and impaired orientation in surrounding and extended space.

**Ventricles** Fluid-filled cavities in the brain.

**Vestibular** Related to movement and balance.

**Video magnifier** A low vision device that uses a camera to project and magnify text or other content onto a video screen, often used for reading by people who have low vision and to zoom in on distant objects and make near objects appear larger. Also known as *closed-circuit television (CCTV)*.

**Vision loss** Lack of vision due to acquired damage to a previously intact visual system.

**Visual acuity** A measure of the ability of the visual system to see, or resolve, the component parts of an image as being separate from one another, when tested at maximum contrast.

**Visual attending behaviors** Behaviors that have a major visual component, including fixating, following, shift of gaze, scanning, localizing, and tracing.

**Visual attention** The ability to focus on specific elements in a visual scene by selecting or being drawn to salient information and filtering out less salient information.

**Visual brain** The totality of brain elements serving or supporting vision that serve to map, search, give attention to, recognize, and interpret visual input.

**Visual cognition** The capacity to process what is seen, to think about its significance, and to manipulate and use both incoming image data and remembered imagery in the context of creative thought.

**Visual dysfunction** Disorder of visual perception, visual guidance of movement, and/or visual attention.

**Visual evoked potential (VEP)** Computerized recording of electrical activity at the back of the brain used to assist in diagnosis and in the estimation of visual acuity and contrast sensitivity.

**Visual examining behaviors** Behaviors that have a major visual-cognitive component and include inspection, identification, and matching of visual material.

**Visual field** Area of space visible to the eyes when looking straight ahead.

**Visual functions** Measurable components of vision, including visual acuity, contrast sensitivity, color perception, visual fields, and the perception of movement.

**Visual guidance of movement** Mapping of incoming visual information in the mind that is used to guide movement of the limbs and body.

**Visual impairment** Damage to the visual system that impedes the ability to learn or perform usual tasks of daily life, given a child's level of maturity and cultural environment. Includes both low vision and blindness.

**Visual latency** The time taken to receive and process incoming visual information in the brain.

**Visually guided motor behaviors** Behaviors with a major visual-motor component, including reaching for, turning toward, and moving among obstacles toward visual targets.

**Visual memory** The ability to remember a visual image or form after viewing.

**Visual-motor processing** Coordination of goal-directed motor actions in relation to a visual target.

**Visual neglect** Inattention to one side of visual space and/or to one side of the body.

**Visual pathways** Bundles of nerve fibers that carry visual information to different locations in the brain.

**Visual perception** Ability to interpret the immediate environment by processing incoming information that is sent from the eyes to the brain.

**Visual processing** The brain's recognition and interpretation of information taken in through the eyes.

**Visual recognition** The ability to recognize and identify objects, faces, geometric shapes, and colors, as well as their pictures and images.

**Visual stimulation** An approach that places a child, as a passive observer, in an environment in which selected visual stimuli are presented with the intention of bringing about attention and enhancement of visual development.

**Visual system** Network that produces sight, including both the eyes and the brain.

**Visuospatial perception** The capacity to appreciate, understand, and map the three-dimensional characteristics of the surroundings, both for subjective appreciation and to facilitate movement through space.

**Weber contrast** A method of reporting contrast values for the difference in brightness between an object or image and its background; commonly used with letters as the test target.

# INDEX

Note: Page numbers followed by *f* indicate figures; followed by *t* indicate tables.

## B

## C

## G



## H

## J



## K



## L

## Q



## R

## T

## U



## V

## W



## Y



## Z

www.ingramcontent.com/pod-product-compliance
Lightning Source LLC
LaVergne TN
LVHW081314201224
799558LV00003B/5
*9780891286394*